Blueprints
Q&As for Step 3

Blueprints Q&As for Step 3

Series Editor:

Michael S. Clement, MD, FAAP
Mountain Park Health Center
Clinical Lecturer in Family and Community Medicine
University of Arizona College of Medicine
Consultant, Arizona Department of Health Services
Phoenix, Arizona

Authors:

Aaron B. Caughey, MD, MPP, MPH
Assistant Professor, Division of Maternal-Fetal Medicine
Department of Obstetrics & Gynecology
University of California, San Francisco
Division of Health Services and Policy Analysis
University of California, Berkeley
Berkeley & San Francisco, California
Obstetrics & Gynecology

Jeffrey L. Foti, MD, FAAP
Attending Pediatrician, Bill Holt Pediatric Infectious Disease Clinic
Phoenix Children's Hospital
Phoenix, Arizona
Clinical Assistant Professor, University of Arizona School of Medicine
Tucson, Arizona
Pediatrics

Deirdre J. Lyell, MD
Assistant Professor, Obstetrics & Gynecology
Stanford University School of Medicine
Attending Physician
Stanford University Medical Center
Stanford, California
Obstetrics & Gynecology

James Brian McLoone, MD, DFAPA
Chairman, Department of Psychiatry and
Director, Psychiatry Residency Training Program and Medical Student Clerkship
Banner Good Samaritan Medical Center
Clinical Professor of Psychiatry
University of Arizona College of Medicine-Phoenix Campus
Phoenix, Arizona
Psychiatry

Edward W. Nelson, MD
Professor of Surgery
University of Utah School of Medicine
Attending Surgeon
University of Utah Medical Center
Salt Lake City, Utah
Surgery

Janice P. Piatt, MD
Medical Director, Bill Holt Pediatric Infectious Disease Clinic
Associate Director, Pediatric Clinic
Phoenix Children's Hospital
Phoenix, Arizona
Pediatrics

Brenda L. Shinar, MD
Assistant Program Director
Department of Internal Medicine
Banner Good Samaritan Medical Center
Phoenix, Arizona
Clinical Professor of Internal Medicine
University of Arizona College of Medicine
Tucson, Arizona
Medicine

Susan H. Tran, MD
Resident Physician, Obstetrics & Gynecology
Kaiser San Francisco Hospital
San Francisco, California
Obstetrics & Gynecology

Wolters Kluwer | Lippincott Williams & Wilkins
Health
Philadelphia • Baltimore • New York • London
Buenos Aires • Hong Kong • Sydney • Tokyo

Acquisitions Editor: Nancy Anastasi Duffy
Managing Editor: Cheryl W. Stringfellow
Marketing Manager: Jennifer Kuklinski
Creative Director: Doug Smock
Associate Production Manager: Kevin Johnson
Compositor: International Typesetting and Composition

351 West Camden Street
Baltimore, MD 21201

530 Walnut Street
Philadelphia, PA 19106

9 8 7 6 5 4 3 2 1

Library of Congress Cataloging-in-Publication Data

Blueprints Q&As for step 3. Medicine, obstetrics & gynecology,
psychiatry, pediatrics, surgery / Aaron B. Caughey . . . [et al.].—1st ed.
p. ; cm.
Includes bibliographical references and index.
ISBN-13: 978-0-7817-7821-3
ISBN-10: 0-7817-7821-2
1. Medicine—Examinations, questions, etc. 2.
Physicians—Licenses—United States—Examinations—Study guides.
I. Caughey, Aaron B. II. Title: Blueprints Q and As for step 3.
[DNLM: 1. Clinical Medicine—Examination Questions. WB 18.2 B6579
2008]
R834.5.B5822 2008
610.76—dc22

2007035025

DISCLAIMER

Care has been taken to confirm the accuracy of the information present and to describe generally accepted practices. However, the authors, editors, and publisher are not responsible for errors or omissions or for any consequences from application of the information in this book and make no warranty, expressed or implied, with respect to the currency, completeness, or accuracy of the contents of the publication. Application of this information in a particular situation remains the professional responsibility of the practitioner; the clinical treatments described and recommended may not be considered absolute and universal recommendations.

The authors, editors, and publisher have exerted every effort to ensure that drug selection and dosage set forth in this text are in accordance with the current recommendations and practice at the time of publication. However, in view of ongoing research, changes in government regulations, and the constant flow of information relating to drug therapy and drug reactions, the reader is urged to check the package insert for each drug for any change in indications and dosage and for added warnings and precautions. This is particularly important when the recommended agent is a new or infrequently employed drug.

Some drugs and medical devices presented in this publication have Food and Drug Administration (FDA) clearance for limited use in restricted research settings. It is the responsibility of the health care provider to ascertain the FDA status of each drug or device planned for use in their clinical practice.

To purchase additional copies of this book, call our customer service department at **(800) 638-3030** or fax orders to **(301) 223-2320.** International customers should call **(301) 223-2300.**

Visit Lippincott Williams & Wilkins on the Internet: http://www.lww.com. Lippincott Williams & Wilkins customer service representatives are available from 8:30 am to 6:00 pm, EST.

Contributors

Sarah Beaumont, MD
Chief Resident, Internal Medicine/Pediatrics
Banner Good Samaritan Medical Center
Phoenix Children's Hospital
Phoenix, Arizona
Medicine

Ryan Bradley
Class of 2004
University of California, San Francisco
San Francisco, California
Obstetrics & Gynecology

Brendan Cassidy, MD
Pediatric Ophthalmologist
Phoenix Children's Hospital
Phoenix, Arizona
Pediatrics

Randal Christensen, MD, MPH
Clinical Assistant Professor
University of Arizona
Tucson, Arizona
Faculty Physician
Phoenix Children's Hospital
Phoenix, Arizona
Pediatrics

Melvin L. Cohen, MD
Director of Medical Education
Phoenix Children's Hospital
Phoenix, Arizona
Clinical Professor, Pediatrics
University of Arizona School of Medicine
Tucson, Arizona
Pediatrics

Rafe C. Connors, MD
Resident, Department of General Surgery
University of Utah School of Medicine
Salt Lake City, Utah
Surgery

Tracy L. Crews, MD
Chief Resident, Psychiatry
Banner Good Samaritan Medical Center
Phoenix, Arizona
Psychiatry

Tala Dajani, MD
Fellow, Pediatric Endocrinology
Phoenix Children's Hospital
Phoenix, Arizona
Pediatrics

Darren G. Deering, DO
Chief Resident, Department of Internal Medicine
Banner Good Samaritan Medical Center
Phoenix, Arizona
Medicine

Derek Deibler, MD
PGY-3 Psychiatry Resident
Banner Good Samaritan Medical Center
Phoenix, Arizona
Psychiatry

Stephen J. Fenton, MD
Resident, Department of General Surgery
University of Utah School of Medicine
Salt Lake City, Utah
Surgery

Kimberly A. Gibson, MD, MPH
Resident, Department of Obstetrics & Gynecology
Kaiser Permanente, San Francisco
San Francisco, California
Obstetrics & Gynecology

M. Rosanna Gray-Swain, MD
Resident, Department of Obstetrics & Gynecology
Washington University
St. Louis, Missouri
Obstetrics & Gynecology

Joel A. Hahnke, MD
Pediatric Chief Resident
Phoenix Children's Hospital
Phoenix, Arizona
Pediatrics

Ronald C. Hansen, MD
Chief, Pediatric Dermatology
Phoenix Children's Hospital
Phoenix, Arizona
Pediatrics

John R. Hartley, DO, FAAP
Attending Physician, General Pediatrics
Phoenix Children's Hospital
Phoenix, Arizona
Pediatrics

Amy E. Helmer, BA
Class of 2004
University of California, San Francisco
San Francisco, California
Obstetrics & Gynecology

Michelle Huddleston, MD
Clinical Assistant Professor, Pediatrics and Internal Medicine
University of Arizona School of Medicine
Tucson, Arizona
Attending Pediatrician and
Clinical Director of Adolescent Clinic
Phoenix Children's Hospital
Phoenix, Arizona
Pediatrics

John Kashani, DO
Banner Good Samaritan Medical Center
Office of Medical Toxicology
Phoenix, Arizona
Pediatrics

Adam R. Koelsch, MD
Chief Resident, Department of Psychiatry
Banner Good Samaritan Medical Center
Phoenix, Arizona
Psychiatry

Frank LoVecchio, DO, MPH
Medical Director
Banner Good Samaritan Poison Control Center
Maricopa Medical Center, Department of Emergency Medicine
Phoenix, Arizona
Pediatrics

Margaret R. Moon, MD, MPH
Director, General Pediatrics Outpatient Clinic
Phoenix Children's Hospital
Phoenix, Arizona
Pediatrics

J. Robb Muhm, Jr., MD, MBA
Clinical Assistant Professor
University of Arizona School of Medicine
Tucson, Arizona
General Pediatrician
Phoenix Children's Hospital
Phoenix, Arizona
Pediatrics

Elizabeth Baytion Munshi, MD
PGY-3 Psychiatry Resident
Banner Good Samaritan Medical Center
Phoenix, Arizona
Psychiatry

Kay C. Pinckard-Hansen, MD, FAAP
Faculty, General Pediatrics Department;
Teaching Attending Physician; and
Pediatric Consultant, Rehabilitation Program
Phoenix Children's Hospital
Phoenix, Arizona
Pediatrics

Michael Recht, MD, PhD
Director of Hematology
Director, The Hemophilia Center
Division of Hematology/Oncology
Phoenix Children's Hospital
Phoenix, Arizona
Pediatrics

Mukesh Sahu
Class of 2004
University of California, San Francisco
San Francisco, California
Obstetrics & Gynecology

Adam Schwarz, MD
Clinical Associate Professor of Pediatrics
University of Arizona School of Medicine
Director, Education Program
Division of Pediatric Critical Care
Phoenix Children's Hospital
Phoenix, Arizona
Pediatrics

Brian L. Shaffer, MD
Resident, Department of Obstetrics & Gynecology
University of California, San Francisco
San Francisco, California
Obstetrics & Gynecology

Tressia Shaw, MD
Chief Resident, Internal Medicine/Pediatrics
Banner Good Samaritan Medical Center
Phoenix Children's Hospital
Phoenix, Arizona
Medicine

Lishiana Solano-Shaffer, MD
Resident, Department of Obstetrics & Gynecology
Kaiser Permanente, Oakland
Oakland, California
Obstetrics & Gynecology

Paul C. Stillwell, MD
Director, Pediatric Pulmonology
Physician in Chief
Phoenix Children's Hospital
Phoenix, Arizona
Pediatrics

Jeffrey Weiss, MD
Chief, Section of General Pediatrics
Phoenix Children's Hospital
Phoenix, Arizona
Professor, Clinical Pediatrics
University of Arizona School of Medicine
Pediatrics

Mark Yarema, MD, FRCPC
Fellow, Department of Medical Toxicology
Banner Good Samaritan Medical Center
Phoenix, Arizona
Pediatrics

Acknowledgments

MEDICINE

There are many people who helped to make this project a reality. Thank you to my contributors, Darren Deering, Sarah Beaumont, and Tressia Shaw. Thank you to my mentors and colleagues at "Good Sam," Dr. Alan Leibowitz, Dr. Bob Raschke, Dr. Michelle Park, and Dr. Grant Hertel. Thanks to Kate Heinle at Blackwell Publishing for her advice, and to Frank Wallace for his computer genius. Most of all, thanks to my wonderful family for their love, encouragement, and support of my endeavors, and to my husband, Ron, who completes me.

Brenda L. Shinar

There are several people I would like to thank: first of all, my family, whose love and unwavering support have made me the person I am today; my friends, who put up with me during this project; Sarah and Tressia for being there when the going gets tough; Donna, for having the first faith in me as a physician and as a friend; Barb and Kristin—for everything you have done for me through the years; and to "J. Crew" for all the happiness you have brought into my life. This project is dedicated to my parents—words can never repay the gifts that you have given me.

Darren G. Deering

First, I would like to thank Brenda Shinar for her guidance in this project. Without the help of my "sisters" Tressia and Doreen, this task would have been impossible. A special thanks goes to Donna for her support, guidance, and friendship. Last but not least, I thank my parents, Matthew, Jackson, and my husband, Doug.

Sarah Beaumont

There are many people who have been great influences in my life. I would especially like to thank my wonderful colleagues and friends Sarah, Darren, Donna, and Jodi. Thanks to Brenda Shinar for including me in this project. But most of all, I would like to acknowledge my family—thanks Mom, Dad, and Amy for always believing in me and supporting my endeavors.

Tressia Shaw

OBSTETRICS & GYNECOLOGY

We would all like to thank the staff at Blackwell Publishing, particularly Kate Heinle and Nancy Duffy, for involving us in this project. I would also like to thank my friends and family for their support and encouragement. In particular, Mom and Dad, Mommaroonie and Pops, Mike & Viv, the girls, Rob & Rosaline, Kim & Mike, Nancy, Ethan, Samara, Soyoung & Cameron, Donna & Doug, Linda, Tina, Patricia, the Bhirridge, the Kaiser SF residents and staff, and of course, my guys, Pi and The Bun, who make the journey meaningful.

Susan H. Tran

This project is dedicated to the medical students, residents, faculty, and staff at Stanford Medical Center and the Brigham and Women's Hospital, and most of all to Jacob, Isabel, and Max.

Deirdre J. Lyell

I would like to acknowledge my colleagues including the residents and faculty in the Departments of Obstetrics and Gynecology at UCSF and the Brigham and Women's Hospital, Peter Callen, Mary Norton, and Gene Washington whose support makes my work possible. I also thank my mother, father, Ethan, Samara, Big & Mugsy, my new family—Ngan, Lieu, Mike, Vivian, Rob, Kim & Nancy, and Mamy whose unflagging support during all of my projects keeps me on task and productive. This book is dedicated to The Bun and his college education.

Aaron B. Caughey

PEDIATRICS

Phoenix Children's Hospital, Pediatric Radiology Archives, for supplying a majority of the radiologic images used in this book. David Carpientieri, MD, Pathologist, Phoenix Children's Hospital, for assistance in obtaining and supplying images used in this book. This book is dedicated to Louis and Maria, for your continued love and support.

Jeffrey L. Foti

PSYCHIATRY

A heartfelt thanks to Melissa Hardy for her patience, perseverance, and humor assisting with the preparation of the text and to our Psychiatry residents and medical students at Good Samaritan for their inquisitiveness and fresh thinking.

James B. McLoone

SURGERY

The goal of this review was to provide the appropriate scope and quality of information to adequately prepare students for the surgical portions of the USMLE Step 2 exam. The extent to which that goal has been accomplished is entirely attributable to the efforts of my resident authors, Rafe and Steve, and our faculty reviewers, Michelle and Courtney. Most important, we are all indebted to Mary Mone, our collaborator, counsel, and conscience throughout.

Edward W. Nelson

Contents

Abbreviations

AAA	abdominal aortic aneurysm
ABC	airway, breathing, circulation
ABG	arterial blood gas
ABI	ankle brachial index
AC	abdominal circumference
ACAS	Asymptomatic Carotid Atherosclerosis Study
ACE	angiotensin-converting enzyme
ACOSOG	American College of Surgeons Oncology Group
ACS	abdominal compartment syndrome
ACTH	adrenocorticotropic hormone
AD	Alzheimer disease
ADD	attention deficit disorder
ADH	antidiuretic hormone
ADHD	attention deficit hyperactivity disorder
AED	automatic external defibrillator
AF/AV	anteflexed, anteverted
AFB	acid-fast bacillus
AFI	amniotic fluid index
AFP	alpha-fetoprotein
AGA	appropriate for gestational age infant
AHA	autoimmune hemolytic anemia
AI	aortic insufficiency
AIDS	acquired immunodeficiency syndrome
AIHA	autoimmune hemolytic anemia
ALL	acute lymphocytic leukemia
All	allergies
ALS	amyotrophic lateral sclerosis
ALT	alanine aminotransferase
AMA	advanced maternal age
AML	acute myelogenous leukemia
AN	acanthosis nigricans
ANA	antinuclear antibody
Anti-HBC	antibody to hepatitis B core
AOM	acute otitis media
AP	anteroposterior
APC	adenomatous polyposis coli
APOE	apolipoprotein E
aPTT	activated partial thromboplastin time
APUD	amine precursor uptake and decarboxylation
ARDS	adult/acute respiratory distress syndrome
AROM	artificial rupture of membranes
AS	aortic stenosis or ankylosing spondylitis
ASAP	as soon as possible
ASCUS	atypical squamous cells of undetermined significance
ASD	atrial septal defect
ASO	anti-streptolysin O
AST	aspartate aminotransferase
ATN	acute tubular necrosis
AV	arteriovenous, atrioventricular
AVM	arteriovenous malformation
AV node	atrioventricular node
AZT	zidovudine
β-hCG	beta human chorionic gonadotropin
BAL	bronchoalveolar lavage; dimercaprol (British antilewisite)
BE	base excess
BID	*bis in die* (twice a day)
BMI	body mass index
BMP	basic metabolic panel
BP	blood pressure
BPD	biparietal diameter, bronchopulmonary dysplasia
BPH	benign prostatic hypertrophy
BPM	beats per minute
BPP	biophysical profile
BRAT	banana, rice, applesauce, toast
BRBPR	bright red blood per rectum
BRCA-1 and 2	breast cancer gene mutations 1 and 2
BTL	bilateral tubal ligation
BUN	blood urea nitrogen

BW	body weight
C	Celsius; centigrade
Ca	calcium
CA	coronary artery
CABG	coronary artery bypass graft
c-Abl	nonreceptor tyrosine kinase protein
CAD	coronary artery disease
CAH	congenital adrenal hyperplasia
cAMP	cyclic adenosine monophosphate
CAP	community-acquired pneumonia
CBC	complete blood count
CBT	cognitive behavioral therapy
cc	cubic centimeter
CCU	coronary care unit
CDC	Centers for Disease Control
CEA	carcinoembryonic antigen
CF	cystic fibrosis
CHF	congestive heart failure
CI	cardiac index
CIN II	cervical intraepithelial neoplasia grade 2
Cl	chloride
CLL	chronic lymphocytic leukemia
cm	centimeter
CML	chronic myelogenous leukemia
CMP	complete metabolic panel
CMV	cytomegalovirus
c-myc	protooncogene
CNS	central nervous system
CO	cardiac output
CO_2	carbon dioxide
COPD	chronic obstructive pulmonary disease
CPAP	continuous positive airway pressure
CPK	creatine phosphokinase
CPK-MB	creatine phosphokinase MB isoenzyme, creatinine phosphokinase-myocardial band
CPM	central pontine myelinolysis
CPPD	calcium pyrophosphate dihydrate
CPR	cardiopulmonary resuscitation
Cr	creatinine
CRF	corticotropin-releasing factor
CRP	C-reactive protein
CSF	cerebrospinal fluid
CST	contraction stress test
CT	computed tomography (cat scan)
CTA	computed tomography angiography
CVA	cerebral vascular accident
CVP	central venous pressure
CXR	chest x-ray
d	day
DA	dopamine; duodenal atresia
D&C	dilation and curettage
DCIS	ductal carcinoma in situ
DDAVP	vasopressin
DDH	developmental dysplasia of the hip
D&E	dilation and evacuation
DEA	Drug Enforcement Agency
DES	diethylstilbestrol
DEXA	dual-energy x-ray absorptiometry
DHEA	dehydroepiandrosterone
DHEAS	dehydroepiandrosterone sulfate
DI	diabetes insipidus
DIC	disseminated intravascular coagulation
DID	dissociative identity disorder
DIP	distal interphalangeal (joint)
DKA	diabetic ketoacidosis
dL	deciliter
DLB	dementia with Lewy bodies
DM	diabetes mellitus
DMSA	2,3 dimercaptosuccinic acid
DNA	deoxyribonucleic acid
DSM	Diagnostic and Statistical Manual
DTaP	diphtheria, tetanus, acellular pertussis
DTR	deep tendon reflex
DUB	dysfunctional uterine bleeding
DVT	deep venous thrombosis
EBV	Epstein-Barr virus
ECF	extracellular fluid
ECG	electrocardiogram
ECHO	echocardiogram
ECMO	extracorporeal membrane oxygenation
ECT	electroconvulsive therapy
ED	emergency department
EDC	estimated date of confinement
EGD	esophagogastroduodenoscopy
ELISA	enzyme-linked immunosorbent assay
EMBx	endometrial biopsy
EMG	electromyogram
EMS	emergency medical service
ENT	ears, nose, and throat
EPS	extrapyramidal symptoms
ER	emergency room
ERCP	endoscopic retrograde cholangiopancreatography
ERU	endorectal ultrasound
ESR	erythrocyte sedimentation rate
EtOH	ethanol, alcohol
ETT	endotracheal tube
F	Fahrenheit
FEV_1	forced expiratory volume in 1 second
FFP	fresh frozen plasma
FHR	fetal heart rate
FIGO	International Federation of Gynecology and Obstetrics

FiO_2	fraction of inspired oxygen
5-FU	5-fluorouracil
5-HIAA	5-hydroxyindoleacetic acid
FL	femur length
FLM	fetal lung maturity
FNA	fine-needle biopsy
FOBT	fecal occult blood testing
FSGN	focal segmental glomerulonephritis
FSH	follicle-stimulating hormone
FTA-ABS	fluorescent treponemal antibody absorption
FTT	failure to thrive
G	gravida
g	gram
G6PD	glucose 6-phosphate dehydrogenase
GA	gestational age
GABA	gamma-aminobutyric acid
GAD	generalized anxiety disorder
GAS	group A streptococcus
GBS	group B streptococcus
GCS	Glasgow Coma Scale
GDM	gestational diabetes mellitus
GE	gastroesophageal
GER	gastroesophageal reflux
GERD	gastroesophageal reflux disease
GHB	gamma hydroxybutyrate
GI	gastrointestinal
GIFT	gamete intra-fallopian tube transfer
GnRH	gonadotropin-releasing hormone
GTD	gestational trophoblastic disease
GU	genitourinary
H_2	histamine 2 receptor
HA	headache
HAART	highly active anti-retroviral therapy
HAV	hepatitis A virus
HBSAb	hepatitis B surface antibody
HBSAg	hepatitis B surface antigen
HC	head circumference
HCC	hepatocellular carcinoma
hCG	human chorionic gonadotropin
HCM	hypertrophic cardiomyopathy (also called HOCM)
HCO_3	bicarbonate
Hct	hematocrit
HCV	hepatitis C virus
HDL	high-density lipoprotein
HEENT	head, eyes, ears, nose, throat
HELLP	hemolysis, elevated liver enzymes, low platelets
her-2 neu	human epidermal growth factor receptor-2
HgbA1C	hemoglobin A1C
HHV-8	human herpes virus-8
HIDA scan	hydroxy iminodiacetic acid scan
HIPAA	Health Insurance Portability and Accountability Act
HIV	human immunodeficiency virus
HMG-CoA	hydroxy-methylglutaryl-coenzyme A
HNPCC	hereditary nonpolyposis colon cancer
HOCM	hypertrophic obstructive cardiomyopathy
HPF	high-power field
HPI	history of present illness
HPP	history of present pregnancy
HPV	human papillomavirus
HR	heart rate
HRT	hormone replacement therapy
HSG	hysterosalpingography
HSV	herpes simplex virus
HT	serotonin
HTLV-1	human T-cell lymphotropic virus-1
HUS	hemolytic uremic syndrome
HVA	homovanillic acid
I^{131}	iodine 131
IAP	intraabdominal pressure
IBD	inflammatory bowel disease
ICP	intracranial pressure
ICSI	intra-cytoplasmic sperm injection
ICU	intensive care unit
Ig	immunoglobulin
IGF	insulin growth factor
IL	interleukin
IM	intramuscular
INH	isoniazid
INR	international normalized ratio
IPTH	intact parathyroid hormone
IPV	inactivated polio
IQ	intelligence quotient
ITP	immune thrombocytopenic purpura
IUD	intrauterine device
IUFD	intrauterine fetal demise
IUGR	intrauterine growth restriction
IUI	intrauterine insemination
IUP	intrauterine pregnancy
IV	intravenous
IVC	inferior vena cava
IVDA	intravenous drug abuse
IVF	in vitro fertilization
IVH	intraventricular hemorrhage
IVIG	intravenous immune globulin
IVP	intravenous pyelography
J	Joules
JNC-VII	Joint National Commission VII
JRA	juvenile rheumatoid arthritis
K	potassium
Kcal	kilocalorie

KCL	potassium chloride
Kg	kilogram
KOH	potassium hydroxide
k-ras	protooncogene
KUB	kidneys, ureters, bladder (a plain abdominal -ray)
L	liter; lumbar
LAD	left anterior descending
Lb	pound
LCIS	lobular cancer in situ
LDH	lactate dehydrogenase
LDL	low density lipoprotein
LES	lower esophageal sphincter
LFTs	liver function tests
LGA	large for gestational age infant
LH	luteinizing hormone
Li	lithium
LMP	last menstrual period
LP	lumbar puncture
LSD	D-lysergic acid
LSO	left salpingo-oophorectomy
LUQ	left upper quadrant
LV	left ventricle
LVAD	left ventricular assist device
LVH	left ventricular hypertrophy
m	meter
MAC	membrane attack complex
MALT	mucosa-associated lymphoid tissue
MAOI	monoamine oxidase inhibitor
MCH	mean corpuscular hemoglobin
MCHC	mean corpuscular hemoglobin concentration
MCP	metacarpophalangeal (joint)
MCV	mean corpuscular volume
MDMA	ecstasy
MEN	multiple endocrine neoplasia
mEq	milliequivalent
Mg	magnesium
mg	milligram
mg/dL	milligrams per deciliter
MGUS	monoclonal gammopathy of undetermined significance
MHC	major histocompatibility complex
MI	myocardial infarction
MIBG	metaiodobenzylguanidine
min	minute
mIU	milli-International Unit
mm	millimeter
mm Hg	millimeters of mercury
mmol	millimole
MMR	measles, mumps, rubella
MMSE	mini-mental state examination
MR(I)	magnetic resonance (imaging)
MRA	magnetic resonance angiography
MS	multiple sclerosis
MTC	medullary thyroid cancer
MTP	metatarsophalangeal (joint)
μU	micro International Unit
NA	sodium
$NaHCO_3$	sodium bicarbonate
NASCET	North American Symptomatic Carotid Endarterectomy Trial
NBT	nitroblue tetrazolium test
NE	norepinephrine
NEC	necrotizing enterocolitis
NG	nasogastric
ng	nanogram
NGT	nasogastric tube
NJ	nasojejeunal
NKDA	no known drug allergies
NLD	necrobiosis lipoidica diabeticorum
NMS	neuroleptic malignant syndrome
n-myc	protooncogene
NPO	nil per os (nothing by mouth)
NPV	negative predictive value
NS	normal saline
NSABP	National Surgical Adjuvant Bowel and Breast Project
NSAID	nonsteroidal anti-inflammatory drug
NST	nonstress test
NT	nontender
O_2	oxygen
OA	osteoarthritis
OCD	obsessive-compulsive disorder
OCP	oral contraceptive pill
OCT	oxytocin challenge test
OME	otitis media with effusion
1,25 OH_2D_3	1,25-dihydroxyvitamin D
OPSI	overwhelming postsplenectomy infection
OR	operating room
OSA	obstructive sleep apnea
OTC	over the counter
P	pulse; para; parity
PA	posterior-anterior; pulmonary artery
paO_2	partial pressure of O_2 in arterial blood
Pap	Papanicolaou (smear)
PCo_2	arterial carbon dioxide pressure
PCOD	polycystic ovarian disease
PCOS	polycystic ovarian syndrome
PCP	phencyclidine; Pneumocystis carinii pneumonia; primary care physician
PCR	polymerase chain reaction
PCWP	pulmonary capillary wedge pressure

PD	Parkinson disease
PDA	patent ductus arteriosus
PE	physical exam; pulmonary embolus
PEEP	positive end-expiratory pressure
PET	positron emission tomography
PFT	pulmonary function tests
PGE1M	prostaglandin E1M—Cytotec/misoprostol
PGE2	prostaglandin E2
PGF2α	prostaglandin F2-alpha
PGynHx	past gynecologic history
pH	hydrogen ion concentration
PICU	pediatric intensive care unit
PID	pelvic inflammatory disease
PIP	peak inspiratory pressure; proximal interphalangeal (joint)
PLTS	platelets
PMDD	premenstrual dysphoric disorder
PMHx	past medical history
PMN	polymorphonuclear (white blood cell)
PNS	parasympathetic nervous system
PO	per os (by mouth)
PO_2	arterial oxygen pressure
pO_2	oxygen partial pressure
PO_4	phosphate
POBHx	past obstetric history
POC	products of conception
POMC	pro-opiate melanocorticotropin
PPD	purified protein derivative
PPROM	preterm premature rupture of membranes
PPV	positive predictive value
PR	per rectum
PRN	*pro re nata* (as needed)
PROM	premature rupture of membranes
PSA	prostate-specific antigen
PSC	primary sclerosing cholangitis
PSGN	poststreptococcal glomerulonephritis
PSHx	past surgical history
PT	prothrombin time
PTC	percutaneous transhepatic cholangiography
PTH	parathyroid hormone
PTHC	percutaneous transhepatic cholangiography
PTH-rp	parathyroid hormone-related peptide
PTL	preterm labor
PTSD	posttraumatic stress disorder
PTT	partial thromboplastin time (same as aPTT)
PTU	propylthiouracil
PVC	polyvinyl chloride
PVD	peripheral vascular disease
QD	*quaque die* (every day)
QID	*quarter in die* (four times a day)
R	respirations
RA	rheumatoid arthritis; room air
Rb	retinoblastoma
RBC	red blood cells
RCC	renal cell carcinoma
RDW	red cell distribution width
REE	resting energy expenditure
REM	rapid eye movement
RET	rearranged during transfection oncogene
RF	rheumatoid factor
RL	Ringer lactate
RNA	ribonucleic acid
ROM	rupture of membranes
RPR	rapid plasma reagin
RR	respiratory rate
RSO	right salpingo-oophorectomy
RSV	respiratory syncytial virus
RUQ	right upper quadrant
RV	right ventricle
RVAD	right ventricular assist device
S	sacrum
s	seconds
SAB	spontaneous abortion
SAD	seasonal affective disorder; social anxiety disorder
SaO_2	arterial oxygen saturation
SBE	subacute bacterial endocarditis
SBO	small bowel obstruction
SCC	squamous cell carcinoma
SCD	sequential compression device
SCFE	slipped capital femoral epiphysis
17-OH	17 hydroxy
SG	Swan-Ganz
SGA	small for gestational age infant
SIADH	syndrome of inappropriate antidiuretic hormone
SICU	surgical intensive care unit
SIDS	sudden infant death syndrome
SLE	systemic lupus erythematosus
SMI	seriously mentally ill
SMR	sexual maturity rating
SNS	sympathetic nervous system
SPEP	serum protein electrophoresis
SROM	spontaneous rupture of membranes
SRU	solitary rectal ulcer
SSE	sterile speculum exam
SSI	superficial skin infection
SSRI	selective serotonin reuptake inhibitors
STD	sexually transmitted disease
SVE	sterile vaginal exam

SVR	systemic vascular resistance
SVT	supraventricular tachycardia
T	temperature; thoracic
T_3	triiodothyronine
T_4	thyroxine
TAB	therapeutic abortion
TAH-BSO	total abdominal hysterectomy and bilateral salpingo-oophorectomy
TB	tuberculosis
TBSA	total body surface area
TBW	total body water
TCA	tricyclic antidepressant
TD	tardive dyskinesia
TEE	trans-esophageal echocardiogram
TEF	tracheoesophageal fistula
TFT	thyroid function test
TIA	transischemic attack
TIBC	total iron-binding capacity
TID	*ter in die* (three times a day)
TIPSS	transjugular intrahepatic porto-systemic shunt
TM	tympanic membrane
TNF	tumor necrosis factor
TNM	tumor/node/metastasis
TOA	tubo-ovarian abscess
Tob	tobacco
TP	total protein
TPN	total parenteral nutrition
TRH	thyroid-releasing hormone; thyrotropin-releasing hormone
TSH	thyroid-stimulating hormone
TSS	toxic shock syndrome
TSST	toxic shock syndrome toxin
TTE	trans-thoracic echocardiogram
TTN	transient tachypnea of the newborn
TTP	thrombotic thrombocytopenic purpura
TURBT	transurethral resection bladder tumor
TURP	transurethral resection of the prostate
UA	urinalysis
UC	ulcerative colitis
UGI	upper gastrointestinal tract
U/L	International Units per liter
UPEP	urine protein electrophoresis
URI	upper respiratory infection
US	ultrasound
UTI	urinary tract infection
VDRL	Venereal Disease Research Laboratory
V_E	minute ventilation
VLDL	very low density lipoprotein
VMA	vanillylmandelic acid
V/Q	ventilation/perfusion
VS	vital signs
VSD	ventricular septal defect
V_T	tidal volume
VTE	venous thromboembolism
VZIG	varicella-zoster immunoglobulin
VZV	varicella-zoster virus
WBC	white blood cells
WPW	Wolff-Parkinson-White syndrome
XR	x-ray

Normal Ranges of Laboratory Values

U.S. traditional units are followed in parentheses by equivalent values expressed in SI units.

Blood, Plasma, and Serum Chemistries

Acetoacetate, plasma—<1 mg/dL (0.1 mmol/L)
Alanine aminotransferase (ALT, GPT at 30°C) (Ob/Gyn)—8–20 U/L
Alanine aminotransferase (ALT) (Pediatrics)—2–40 IU/L
Albumin—3.8–5.4 g/dL
Alkaline phosphatase—42–362 IU/L
Alpha-fetoprotein, serum—0–20 ng/mL (0–20 µg/L)
Aminotransferase, alanine (ALT, SGPT)—0–35 U/L
Aminotransferase, aspartate (AST, SGOT)—0–35 U/L
Ammonia, plasma—40–90 µg/dL (23-–47 µmol/L)
Amylase (Pediatrics)—21–86 IU/L
Amylase, serum (Medicine)—0–130 U/L
Amylase, serum (Ob/Gyn)—25–125 U/L
Antinuclear antibody—<1:40
Antistreptolysin O titer—<150 units
Antistreptolysin O titer (school-aged child)—170–330 Todd units
Arterial blood gas, child
  pCO_2—35–40 mm Hg
  pH—7.35–7.45
  pO_2—90–95 mm Hg
  HCO_3—22–26 mEq/L
Ascorbic acid (vitamin C), blood—0.4–1.5 mg/dL (23–86 µmol/L); leukocyte—<20 mg/dL (<3.5 µmol/L)
Asparatate aminotransferase
  (AST, GOT at 30°C)—8–20 U/L
  (AST)—10–41 IU/L
Bicarbonate—22–28 mEq/L
Bicarbonate, serum—23–28 mEq/L (23–28 mmol/L)
Bilirubin, serum (Medicine, Surgery)
  Total—0.3–1.2 mg/dL (5.1–20.5 µmol/L)
  Direct—0–0.3 mg/dL (0–5.1 µmol/L)
Bilirubin, serum (adult) Total // Direct (Ob/Gyn)—0.1–1.0 mg/dL // 0.0–0.3 mg/dL
Bilirubin, total (Pediatrics)—0.2–1.1 mg/dL

- Blood gases, arterial (room air)
  - Po_2—80–100 mm Hg
  - Pco_2—35–45 mm Hg
  - pH—7.38–7.44
- C-reactive protein (CRP)—0.3 mg/dL
- Calcium (Surgery, Pediatrics)—8.8–10.8 mg/dL
- Calcium, serum (Ca^{2+}) (Ob/Gyn)—8.4–10.2 mg/dL
- Calcium, serum (Medicine)—9–10.5 ng/dL (2.2–2.6 mmol/L)
- Carbon dioxide content, serum—23–28 mEq/L (23–28 mmol/L)
- Carcinoembryonic antigen—<2 ng/mL (2 µg/L)
- Carotene, serum—75–300 µg/dL (1.4–5.6 µmol/L)
- CD4 absolute count/% (12 months–6 years)
  - No suppression—1000/L/25%
  - Moderate suppression—500–999/L/15–24%
  - Severe suppression—500/L/15%
- Cerebrospinal fluid, child (CSF)
  - Glucose—40–80 mg/dL
  - Protein—5–40 mg/dL
  - RBC—0 RBCs/µL
  - WBC—0–7 WBCs/µL
- Ceruloplasmin, serum—25–43 mg/dL (250–430 mg/L)
- Chloride—95–105 mEq/L
- Chloride, serum—98–106 mEq/L (98–106 mmol/L)
- Cholesterol—<170 mg/dL
- Cholesterol, high-density lipoprotein (HDL), plasma—≥40 mg/dL (1.04 mmol/L), desirable
- Cholesterol, low-density lipoprotein (LDL), plasma—≤130 mg/dL (3.36 mmol/L) desirable
- Cholesterol, serum—Rec: <200 mg/dL
- Cholesterol, total, plasma—150–199 mg/dL (3.88–5.15 mmol/L), desirable
- Complement, serum
  - C3—55–120 mg/dL (550–1,200 mg/L)
  - Total—36–55 U/mL (37–55 kU/L)
- Copper, serum—70–155 µg/dL (11.0–24.3 µmol/L)
- Creatine kinase, serum (Medicine)—30–170 U/L
- Creatine kinase, serum (Ob/Gyn)—Female: 10–70 U/L
- Creatine kinase (CPK) (Pediatrics)—10–70 U/L
- Creatinine, serum (Medicine)—0.7–1.3 mg/dL (61.9–115.0 µmol/L)
- Creatinine, serum (Pediatrics)—0.6–1.2 mg/dL
- Delta-aminolevulinic acid, serum—15–23 µg/dL (1.14–1.75 µmol/L)
- Electrolytes, serum
  - Bicarbonate (HCO_3^-)—22–28 mEq/L
  - Chloride (Cl^-)—95–105 mEq/L
  - Magnesium (Mg^{2+})—1.5–2.0 mEq/L
  - Potassium (K^+)—3.5–5.0 mEq/L
  - Sodium (Na^+)—136–145 mEq/L
- Ethanol, blood—<50 mg/dL (11 nmol/L)
- Fibrinogen, plasma—150–350 mg/dL (1.5–3.5 g/L)
- Folate, red cell—160–855 ng/mL (362–1937 nmol/L)
- Folate, serum—2.5–20.0 ng/mL (5.7–45.3 nmol/L)
- Follicle-stimulating hormone, serum/plasma
  - Female: premenopause 4–30 mIU/mL
    - midcycle peak 10–90 mIU/mL
    - postmenopause 40–250 mIU/mL

Glucose, plasma—fasting, 70–105 mg/dL (3.9–5.8 mmol/L;
2 hours postprandial <140 mg/dL (7.8 mmol/L)
Glucose, serum—Fasting: 70–110 g/dL
2-h postprandial <120 mg/dL
HIV viral load—<50 copies/mL
Homocysteine, plasma—Male: 4–16 μmol/L; female: 3–14 μmol/L
Immunoglobulins
IgG—640–1,430 mg/dL (6.4–14.3 g/L)
IgG_1—280–1,020 mg/dL (2.8–10.2 g/L)
IgG_2—60–790 ng/dL (0.6–7.9 g/L)
IgG_3—14–240 mg/dL (0.14–2.40 g/L)
IgG_4—11–330 ng/dL (0.11–3.30 g/L)
IgA—70–300 mg/dL (0.7–3.0 g/L)
IgM—20–140 mg/dL (0.2–1.4 g/L)
IgD—<8 mg/dL (0.1–0.4 mg/L)
IgE—0.01–0.04 mg/dL (0.1–0.4 mg/L)
Iron, serum—60–160 μg/dL (11–29 μmol/L)
Iron-binding capacity, serum—250–460 μg/dL (45–82 μmol/L)
Lactate dehydrogenase, serum (Medicine)—60–100 U/L
Lactate dehydrogenase, serum (Ob/Gyn)—45–90 U/L
Lactic acid, venous blood—6–16 mg/dL (0.67–1.80 mmol/L)
Lead, blood (Medicine)—<40 μg/dL (1.9 μmol/L)
Lead, blood (Pediatrics)—<5 μg/dL
Lipase—16–63 IU/L
Lipase, serum—<95 U/L
Luteinizing hormone, serum/plasma
Female: follicular phase 5–30 mIU/mL
midcycle 75–150 mIU/mL
postmenopause 30–200 mIU/mL
Magnesium—1.5–2.0 mEq/L
Magnesium, serum—1.5–2.4 mg/dL (0.62–0.99 mmol/L)
Manganese, serum—0.3–0.9 ng/mL (300–900 ng/L)
Methylmalonic acid, serum—150–370 nmol/L
Osmolality, plasma—275–295 mOsm/kg H_2O
Osmolality, serum—275–295 mOsm/kg
Parathyroid hormone, serum, N-terminal—230–630 pg/mL
Phosphatase, acid, serum—0.5–5.5 U/L
Phosphatase, alkaline, serum—36–92 U/L
Phosphate (alkaline), serum (p-NPP at 30°C)—20–70 U/L
Phosphorus, inorganic, serum—3.0–4.5 mg/dL (0.97–1.45 mmol/L)
Potassium, serum—3.5–5.0 mEq/L (3.5–5.0 mmol/L)
Prolactin, serum (hPRL)—<20 ng/mL
Protein—5.7–8 g/dL
Protein, serum
Total—6.0–7.8 g/dL (60–78 g/L)
Albumin—3.5–5.5 g/dL (35–55 g/L)
Globulins—2.5–3.5 g/dL (25–35 g/L)
$Alpha_1$—0.2–0.4 g/dL (2–4 g/L)
$Alpha_2$—0.5–0.9 g/dL (5–9 g/L)
Beta—0.6–1.1 g/dL (6–11 g/L)
Gamma—0.7–1.7 g/dL (7–17 g/L)
Rheumatoid factor (Medicine)—<40 U/mL (<40 kU/L)

Rheumatoid factor (RF) (Pediatrics)—<1:20
Sodium, serum—136–145 mEq/L (136–145 mmol/L)
Thyroid-stimulating hormone, serum or plasma—0.5–5.0 μU/mL
Thyroidal idodine (^{123}I) uptake—8–30% of administered dose/24 h
Thyroxine (T_4), serum—5–12 μg/dL
Triglycerides—<150 mg/dL
Triglycerides—<250 mg/dL (2.82 mmol/L), desirable
Urea nitrogen, blood (BUN)—8–25 mg/dL
Urea nitrogen, serum (BUN) (Ob/Gyn)—7–18 mg/dL
Urea nitrogen, serum (Medicine)—8–20 mg/dL (2.9–7.1 mmol/L)
Uric acid, serum (Medicine)—2.5–8.0 mg/dL (0.15–0.47 mmol/L)
Uric acid, serum (Ob/Gyn)—3.0–8.2 mg/dL
Vitamin B_{12}, serum—200–800 pg/mL (148–590 pmol/L)

Cerebrospinal Fluid
Cell count—0–5 cells/μL (0–5 × 10^6 cells/L)
Glucose—40–80 mg/dL (2.5–4.4 mmol/L); <40% of simultaneous plasma concentration is abnormal
Protein—15–60 mg/dL (150–600 mg/L)
Pressure (opening)—70–200 cm H_2O

Chemistry

Alanine aminotransferase (ALT)	Male: 13–72 U/L, female: 9–52 U/L
Alkaline phosphatase	38–126 U/L
Amylase	30–110 U/L
Aspartate aminotransferase (AST)	Male: 15–59 U/L, female: 14–50 U/L
Bicarbonate (HCO_3^-)	19–25 mmol/L
Bilirubin total	0.2–1.3 mg/dL
Bilirubin direct	0.0–0.3 mg/dL
Calcium	8.4–10.2 mg/dL
Carbon dioxide	22–29 mmol/L
Chloride (Cl^-)	98–107 mmol/L
Creatinine	Male: 0.8–1.5 mg/dL, female: 0.7–1.2 mg/dL
Glucose	64–128 mg/dL
Lactate	0.7–2.1 mmol/L
Lactate dehydrogenase (LDH)	300–600 U/L
Magnesium (Mg^{2+})	1.6–2.3 mg/dL
Osmolality	280–303 mOsm/kg
Phosphorus (inorganic)	2.4–4.3 mg/dL
Potassium (K^+)	3.3–5.0 mmol/L
Sodium (Na^+)	136–144 mmol/L
Urea nitrogen (BUN)	Male: 9–22 mg/dL, female: 6–22 mg/dL

Endocrine
Adrenocorticotropin (ACTH)—9–52 pg/mL (2–11 pmol/L)
Aldosterone, serum
  Supine—2–5 ng/dL (55–138 pmol/L)
  Standing—7–20 ng/dL (194–554 pmol/L)
Aldosterone, urine—5–19 μg/24 h (13.9–52.6 nmol/24 h)
Catecholamines—epinephrine (supine): <75 ng/L (410 pmol/L); norepinephrine (supine): 50–440 ng/L (296–2600 pmol/L)
Catecholamines, 24-hour, urine—<100 μg/m^2 per 24 h (591 nmol/m^2 per 24 h)

Cortisol
  Serum—8 A.M.: 8–20 μg/dL (221–552 nmol/L); 5 P.M.: 3–13 μg/dL (83–359 nmol/L)
  1 h after cosyntropin—>18 μg/dL (498 nmol/L); usually 8 μg/dL (221 nmol/L) or more above baseline
  Overnight suppression test—<5 μg/dL (138 nmol/24 h)
Dehydroepiandrosterone sulfate, plasma—Male: 1.3–5.5 mg/mL (3.5–14.9 μmol/L); female: 0.6–3.3 mg/mL (1.6–8.9 μmol/L)
11-deoxycortisol, plasma—Basal: <5 μg/dL (145 nmol/L); after metyrapone: >7 μg/dL (203 nmol/L)
Estradiol, serum—Male: 10–30 pg/mL (37–110 pmol/L); female: day 1–10, 50–100 pmol/L; day 11–20, 50–200 pmol/L; day 21–30, 70–150 pmol/L
Estriol, urine—>12 mg/24 h (42 μmol/day)
Follicle-stimulating hormone, serum—Male (adult): 5–15 mU/mL (5–15 U/L); female: follicular or luteal phase, 5–20 mU/mL (5–20 U/L); midcycle peak, 30–50 mU/mL (30–50 U/L); postmenopausal, >35 mU/mL (35 U/L)
Growth hormone, plasma—After oral glucose, <2 ng/mL (2 μg/L); response to provocative stimuli: >7 ng/mL (7 μg/L)
17-hydroxycorticosteroids, urine (Porter-Silber)—Male: 3–10 mg/24 h (8.3–28 μmol/24 h); female: 2–8 mg/24 h (5.5–22.1 μmol/24 h)
Insulin, serum (fasting)—5–20 mU/L (35–139 pmol/L)
17-ketosteroids, urine—Male: 8–22 mg/24 h (28–77 μmol/24 h); female: up to 15 μg/24 h (52 mmol/24 h)
Luteinizing hormone, serum—Male: 3–15 mU/mL (3–15 U/L); female: follicular or luteal phase, 5–22 mU/mL (3–15 U/L); midcycle peak, 30–250 mU/mL (30–250 U/L); postmenopausal, >30 mU/mL (30 U/L)
Metanephrine, urine—<1.2 mg/24 h (6.1 mmol/24 h)
Parathyroid hormone, serum—10–65 pg/mL (10–65 ng/L)
Progesterone
  Luteal—3–30 ng/mL (0.10–0.95 nmol/L)
  Follicular—<1 ng/mL (0.03 nmol/L)
Prolactin, serum—Male: <15 ng/mL (15 mg/L); female: <20 ng/mL (20 mg/L)
Renin activity (angiotensin-I radioimmunoassay), plasma
  Normal diet: supine, 0.3–1.9 ng/mL per h (0.3–1.9 μg/L per h); upright, 0.2–3.6 ng/mL per h (0.2–3.6 μg/L per h)
Sperm concentration—20–150 million/mL (20–50 × 10^9/L)
Sweat test for sodium and chloride—<60 mEq/L (60 mmol/L)
Testosterone, serum—Adult male: 300–1200 ng/dL (10–42 nmol/L); female: 20–75 ng/dL (0.7–2.6 nmol/L)
Thyroid function tests (normal ranges vary)
  Thyroid iodine (^{131}I) uptake—10–30% of administered dose at 24 h
  Thyroid-stimulating hormone (TSH)—0.5–5.0 μU/mL (0.5–5.0 mU/mL)
  Thyroxine (T_4), serum
    Total—5–12 μg/dL (64–155 nmol/L)
    Free—0.9–2.4 ng/dL (12–31 pmol/L)
    Free T_4 index—4–11
  Triiodothyronine, resin (T_3)—25–35%
  Triiodothyronine, serum (T_3)—70–195 ng/dL (1.1–3.0 nmol/L)
Vanillylmandelic acid, urine—<8 mg/24 h (40.4 μmol/24 h)
Vitamin D
  1,25-dihydroxy, serum—25–65 pg/mL (60–156 pmol/L)
  25-hydroxy, serum—15–80 ng/mL (37–200 nmol/L)

Gastrointestinal
D-xylose absorption (after ingestion of 25 g of D-xylose)—Urine excretion: 5–8 g at 5 h (33–53 mmol); serum D-xylose: >20 mg/dL at 2 h (1.3 nmol/L)
Fecal urobilinogen—40–280 mg/24 h (68–473 μmol/24 h)

Gastric secretion—Basal secretion: male: 4.0 ± 0.2 mEq of HCl/h (4.0 ± 0.2 mmol/h); female: 2.1 ± 0.2 mEq of HCl/h (2.1 ± 0.2 mmol/h); peak acid secretion: male: 37.4 ± 0.8 mEq/h (37.4 ± 0.8 mmol/h); female: 24.9 ± 1.0 mEq/h (24.9 ± 1.0 mmol/h)
Gastrin, serum—0–180 pg/mL (0–180 ng/L)
Lactose tolerance test—Increase in plasma glucose: >15 mg/dL (0.83 mmol/L)
Lipase, ascitic fluid—<200 U/L
Secretin-cholecystokinin pancreatic function—>80 mEq/L (80 mmol/L) of HCO_3 in at least one specimen collected over 1 h
Stool fat—<5 g/day on a 100-g fat diet
Stool nitrogen—<2 g/day
Stool weight—<200 g/day

Hematology
Activated partial thromboplastin time—25–35 sec
Bleeding time—<10 min
Coagulation factors, plasma
  Factor I—150–350 mg/dL (1.5–3.5 g/L)
  Factor II—60–150% of normal
  Factor V—60–150% of normal
  Factor VII—60–150% of normal
  Factor VIII—60–150% of normal
  Factor IX—60–150% of normal
  Factor X—60–150% of normal
  Factor XI—60–150% of normal
  Factor XII—60–150% of normal
Erythrocyte count (Medicine)—4.2–5.9 million cells/μL (4.2–5.9 × 10^{12} cells/L)
Erythrocyte count (Ob/Gyn)—Female: 3.5–5.5 million/mm^3
Erythrocyte sedimentation rate (Westergren)—Female: 0–20 mm/h
Erythrocyte sedimentation rate, child (ESR)—0–10 mm/hr
Erythrocyte survival rate (^{51}Cr)—$T^1/_2$ = 28 days
Erythropoietin—<30 mU/mL (30 U/L)
D-dimer—<15–200 ng/mL (15–200 mg/L)
Ferritin, serum—15–200 ng/mL (15–200 mg/L)
Glucose-6-phosphate dehydrogenase, blood—5–15 U/g Hgb (0.32–0.97 mU/mol Hgb)
Haptoglobin, serum—50–150 mg/dL (500–1500 mg/L)
Hematocrit, child—12.5–16.1 mg/dL
Hematocrit (Surgery)—Male: 40.8–51.9%, female: 34.3–46.6%
Hematocrit (Medicine)—Male: 41–51%; female: 36–47%
Hemoglobin A_{1C}—≤ 6%
Hemoglobin—Male: 14.6–17.8 g/dL (140–170 g/L); female: 12.1–15.9 g/dL (120–160 g/L)
Hemoglobin, child—36–47%
Hemoglobin, plasma—0.5–5.0 mg/dL (0.08–0.80 μmol/L)
Leukocyte alkaline phosphatase—15–40 mg of phosphorus liberated/h per 10^{10} cells; score = 13–130/100 polymorphonuclear neutrophils and band forms
Leukocyte count—3,200–10,600/mm^3
Leukocyte count—Nonblacks: 4,000–10,000/μL (4.0–10 × 10^9/L); blacks: 3,500–10,000/μL (3.5–10 × 10^9/L)
Leukocyte count and differential

Leukocyte count	4500–11,000/mm^3
Segmented neutrophils	54–62%
Bands	3–5%
Eosinophils	1–3%

Basophils — 0–0.75%
Lymphocytes — 25–33%
Monocytes — 3–7%

Lymphocytes
CD4+ cell count—640–1175/μL (0.64–1.18 × 10^9/L)
CD4+ cell count—335–875/μL (0.34–0.88 × 10^9/L)
CD4:CD8 ratio—1.0–4.0
Mean corpuscular hemoglobin (MCH)—28–32 pg
Mean corpuscular hemoglobin concentration (MCHC)—31–37 g/dL Mean corpuscular hemoglobin concentration (MCHC)—32–36 g/dL (320–360 g/L)
Mean corpuscular volume (MCV) (Ob/Gyn, Medicine)—80–100 fL
Mean corpuscular volume (MCV) (Pediatrics)—75–95 μm^3
Osmotic fragility of erythrocytes—Increased if hemolysis occurs in >0.5% NaCl, decreased if hemolysis is incomplete in 0.3% NaCl
Partial thromboplastin time (activated) (Ob/Gyn)—25–40 seconds
Partial thromboplastin time (PTT) (Pediatrics)—25–40 sec
Partial thromboplastin time (Surgery)—26–37 s
Platelet count (Medicine)—150,000–350,000/μL (150–350 × 10^9/L)
Platelet count (Peds, Ob/Gyn)—150,000–400,000/mm^3
Platelet count (Surgery)—177,000–406,000 K/μL
Platelet lifespan (^{51}Cr)—8–12 days
Protein C activity, plasma—67–131%
Protein C resistance—2.2–2.6
Protein S activity, plasma—82–144%
Prothrombin time (PT) (Medicine)—11–13 sec
Prothrombin time (PT) (Ob/Gyn, Pediatrics)—11–15 sec
Prothrombin time (PT) (Surgery)—12–15.5 sec
Red cell distribution width (RDW)—11.5–14.5%
Reticulocyte count—0.5–1.5% of erythrocytes; absolute: 23,000–90,000 cells/μL (23–90 × 10^9/L)
Schilling test (oral administration of radioactive cobalamin-labeled vitamin B_{12})—8.5–28.0% excreted in urine per 24–48 h
Sedimentation rate, erythrocyte (Westergren)—Male: 0–15 mm/h; female: 0–20 mm/h
Volume, blood
Plasma—Male: 25–44 mL/kg (0.025–0.044 L/kg) body weight; female: 28–43 mL/kg (0.028–0.043 L/kg) body weight
Erythrocyte—Male: 25–35 mL/kg (0.025–0.044 L/kg) body weight; female: 20–30 mL/kg (0.020–0.030 L/kg) body weight

Pulmonary
Forced expiratory volume in 1 second (FEV_1)—>80% predicted
Forced vital capacity (FVC)—>80% predicted
FEV_1/FVC—>75% (0.75)

Urine
Amino acids—200–400 mg/24 h (14–29 nmol/24 h)
Amylase—6.5–48.1 U/h
Calcium—100–300 mg/day (2.5–7.5 mmol/day) on unrestricted diet
Chloride—80–250 mEq/day (80–250 mmol/day) (varies with intake)
Copper—0–100 μg/24 h (0–1.6 μmol/day)
Coproporphyrin—50–250 μg/24 h (76–382 nmol/day)
Creatine—Male: 4–40 mg/24 h (30–305 mmol/24 h); female: 0–100 mg/24 h (0–763 mmol/h)
Creatine clearance—Male: 97–137 mL/min; female: 88–128 mL/min

Creatinine—15–25 mg/kg per 24 h (133–221 mmol/kg per 24 h)
Creatinine clearance—90–140 mL/min (0.09–0.14 L/min)
5-hydroxyindoleacetic acid (5-HIAA)—2–9 mg/24 h (10.4–46.8 μmol/day)
Osmolality (Medicine)—38–1,400 mosm/kg H_2O
Osmolality (Ob/Gyn)—50–1,400 mOsmol/kg
Phosphate, tubular resorption—79–94% (0.79–0.94) of filtered load
Potassium—25–100 mEq/24 h (25–100 mmol/24 h) (varies with intake)
Protein (Medicine)—<100 mg/24 h
Proteins, total (Ob/Gyn)—< 150 mg/24 h
Sodium (Medicine)—100–260 mEq/24 h (100–260 mmol/24 h) (varies with intake)
Sodium (Ob/Gyn)—Varies with diet
Uric acid—250–270 mg/24 h (1.48–4.43 mmol/24 h) (varies with diet)
Urobilinogen—0.05–2.50 mg/24 h (0.08–4.22 μmol/24 h)

Blueprints
Q&As for Step 3

Section

1 Medicine

SETTING 1: COMMUNITY-BASED HEALTH CENTER

You work at a community-based health facility where patients seeking both routine and urgent care are encountered. Many patients are members of low-income groups; many are ethnic minorities. Several industrial parks and local businesses send their employees to the health center for treatment of on-the-job injuries and employee health screening. There is a facility that provides x-ray films, but CT and MRI scans must be arranged at other facilities. Laboratory services are available.

1. A previously healthy 20-year-old man presents to your clinic with a complaint of "coca-cola"–colored urine that he noticed this morning. Since the first episode, he has had two more episodes of dark urine. Yesterday, he developed upper respiratory symptoms of clear rhinorrhea, sore throat, and nonproductive cough. On physical examination, he has a normal BP and temperature is 99°C. HEENT examination reveals clear rhinorrhea with erythematous and slightly swollen nasal turbinates. There is minimal pharyngeal erythema without any tonsillar exudates. Results of abdominal and GU examinations are normal. Urinalysis is positive for 100 RBCs/HPF and 2+ protein. Serum complement levels are normal. Which of the following is the most likely diagnosis?

   A. Poststreptococcal glomerulonephritis
   B. IgA nephropathy
   C. Systemic lupus erythematosus (SLE)
   D. Cryoglobulinemia
   E. Membranoproliferative glomerulonephritis

The next two questions (items 2 and 3) correspond to the following vignette:

A 76-year-old woman who resides in a nursing home presents to your clinic with watery stools every 2 to 3 hours for the past 4 days. Her prior medical history includes hypertension and coronary artery disease. She has recently completed a course of amoxicillin for bronchitis. She is afebrile with an HR of 100, and BP is 112/75 mm Hg lying and 90/70 mm Hg standing. Laboratory values are as follows: sodium 142 mEq/L, chloride 115 mEq/L, bicarbonate 17 mEq/L, BUN 41 mg/dL, and creatinine 1.9 mg/dL. Her creatinine in the past was 0.8 mg/dL. Urinalysis reveals hyaline casts and urine sodium is <10. Urine eosinophils are negative.

2. This patient's acute renal failure is most likely due to:

   A. Prerenal azotemia
   B. Amoxicillin
   C. Hypertension
   D. Cholesterol emboli
   E. Postinfectious glomerulonephritis

3. The most appropriate next step in the patient's management would be:

   A. Renal ultrasonography
   B. Place a Foley catheter
   C. Further laboratory evaluation
   D. Hydration with intravenous fluids
   E. Dialysis

End of Set

4. A 25-year-old man comes to the clinic with a complaint of a skin rash. You take a complete medical history and note that he has significant risk factors for HIV, including unprotected sexual intercourse with high-risk persons and IVDA. You know that there are several skin diseases that are associated with AIDS. Which of the following skin disorders is pathognomonic for AIDS?

   A. Seborrheic dermatitis
   B. Molluscum contagiosum
   C. Pustular psoriasis
   D. Bacillary angiomatosis
   E. Oral candidiasis

5. A 35-year-old woman comes to the clinic with complaints of right-sided chest pain and shortness of breath that began suddenly that morning while she was cleaning up after her toddler at home. Physical examination reveals a woman who is in mild respiratory distress speaking in short sentences. Vital signs include a BP of 140/90 mm Hg, HR of 100, RR 22, temperature of 98.6, and O_2 saturation of 92% on room air. On examination, her right lung exhibits decreased breath sounds and hyperresonance to percussion. The chest x-ray reveals a 30% pneumothorax of the right lung. Which of the following diseases or patient populations are associated with a spontaneous pneumothorax?

   A. Lymphangioleiomyomatosis
   B. *Mycoplasma* pneumonia
   C. Hypersensitivity pneumonitis
   D. Mesothelioma
   E. Menopausal women

6. A 56-year-old African-American woman presents to your clinic with complaints of shortness of breath. She has a past history of hypertension for which she takes hydrochlorothiazide, and depression for which she takes paroxetine. She has no allergies. She does not smoke tobacco or drink alcohol. She has worked for many years in a ceramics laboratory that makes dental appliances and prosthetics. On examination, her temperature is 98.7°C, HR 86, RR 16, and BP 140/84 mm Hg. Heart examination results are unremarkable. Lung examination reveals fine, late, inspiratory crackles in the upper lobes bilaterally. Chest radiograph shows prominent interstitial markings in the upper lobes with bilateral hilar adenopathy. Laboratory evaluation reveals a calcium of 10.9 mg/dL but is otherwise normal. What is her diagnosis?

   A. Sarcoidosis
   B. Silicosis
   C. Berylliosis
   D. Tuberculosis (TB)
   E. Congestive heart failure (CHF)

7. A 15-year-old Native-American boy who usually lives on a reservation presents to the clinic with complaints of fever and "funny movements of his arms and legs." He has been staying with an aunt and uncle off the reservation for the past week and was usually in good health except for a severe sore throat that occurred approximately 3 weeks ago. He was treated on the reservation with a special tea given to him by his grandmother with gradual resolution of his symptoms. On examination, he is febrile to 101°C, BP 105/70 mm Hg, HR 90, and RR 16. He appears ill, and the rest of his examination is significant for a tachycardia with a rub and a swollen left knee and right ankle with evidence of synovitis. He also is moving his hands and arms in a writhing, snakelike movement that he is unable to control. You are suspicious for acute rheumatic fever. Which of the following is considered a major diagnostic (Jones) criterion for rheumatic fever?

   A. ECG changes such as a prolonged PR interval
   B. Chorea
   C. Fever
   D. Erythema nodosum
   E. Recent streptococcal infection as manifested by elevated ASO titer

8. A 65-year-old white woman presents to your clinic with complaints of dysphagia for approximately 1 year. She notes difficulty with swallowing of liquids and solids that is not progressive in nature, and says that she feels as if the food and liquid is getting "stuck." She notes a minimal weight loss of approximately 2–3 pounds over the past year. She denies any history of tobacco or alcohol abuse. She denies any history of heartburn in the past. Vital signs are stable and physical examination findings are within normal limits. Which diagnostic modality will help you make the likely diagnosis?

   A. Endoscopy
   B. 24-hour pH recording
   C. Manometry
   D. CT scan
   E. Video fluoroscopy

9. A 65-year-old African-American man comes to your clinic with complaints of heartburn. He describes the pain as a burning sensation located substernally that radiates to his mouth. He has noted the symptoms for approximately 1 year. He notes that it gets worse with spicy and fatty foods. He usually eats dinner at 10 P.M., and goes to bed at 11 P.M., and he often has the sensation while in bed. He denies any dysphagia or weight loss. He also denies any tobacco or ETOH abuse. He has never tried any medications to relieve his symptoms. Examination is significant only for obesity. The treatment option most likely to relieve this patient's symptoms is:

   A. Weight loss
   B. Fundoplication
   C. H2 blockers
   D. Proton pump inhibitors
   E. Cutting out spicy and fatty foods, elevating the head of the bed, and not lying down for at least 3 hours after each meal

10. A 40-year-old woman comes to your clinic with symptoms of heartburn and dyspepsia for the past month. She states she had this discomfort approximately 5 years ago. The doctor at that time told her she had an ulcer with a bacterial infection. She remembers taking medications for 2 weeks and improving significantly. She states that the symptoms that she is having now are similar to her previous symptoms. You are debating treating her for *Helicobacter pylori* again. What is the incidence of reinfection of *H. pylori* in the United States?

   A. 30%
   B. <1%
   C. 50%
   D. 10%
   E. 25%

11. A 29-year-old white woman presents to your clinic with a 2- to 3-week history of left lower quadrant abdominal pain. She states that the pain was intermittent, but has now progressed to constant in nature. She denies experiencing any nausea, vomiting, diarrhea, fever, or chills. The pain does not radiate. She is not sexually active and is currently menstruating. These pains do not remind her of her menstrual cramps. She states that she has bowel movements one to two times per week and that her stools are hard and often difficult to pass. On past medical history she states that she had an appendectomy at age 12. Physical examination is significant only for fullness in the left lower quadrant with some tenderness to palpation. There is no rebound or peritoneal signs. Your next step is:

   A. KUB radiography
   B. CT of abdomen and pelvis
   C. Barium enema
   D. Increase water and fiber intake along with daily exercise
   E. Abdominal and pelvic ultrasonography

12. A 22-year-old woman presents to your clinic with a 2- to 3-week history of nausea, vomiting, and right upper quadrant pain. She also notes that her skin has begun to turn yellow. Preliminary laboratory values show an elevated AST at 2000 U/L and an ALT of 2700 U/L with a total bilirubin of 2.5 mg/dL. She denies having any sexual activity or IVDA. She recently returned from a church group trip to Ecuador where they worked on building latrines for coastal towns. You order hepatitis serologies. Which of the following do you expect?

   A. Anti-HCV positive
   B. HBsAg positive, anti-HBc IgM positive
   C. Anti-HAV IgM positive, anti-HAV IgG negative
   D. Anti-HAV IgM negative, anti-HAV IgG positive
   E. HBsAg negative, anti-HBc negative, HBsAb positive

13. A 55-year-old man with a history of chronic hepatitis C presents to your clinic with complaints of abdominal swelling. This has never happened before and he says that he feels pregnant. His wife is with him, and she says that he has not "been himself" lately. He denies having any fever, chills, or abdominal pain. On physical examination, the patient is afebrile with the following vital signs: BP 110/70 mm Hg, HR 90, and RR 16. In general, he is in no acute distress. Mucous membranes are moist, and scleral icterus is noted. Chest is clear to auscultation, and heart is regular without murmurs or gallops. His abdomen is distended, and there is a notable fluid wave with shifting dullness. There are spider angiomata across his chest and palmar erythema of the hands. He has asterixis and 2+ pitting edema of the lower extremities to the knees. You order basic laboratory studies and do a diagnostic paracentesis to evaluate the ascites fluid. You plan to calculate the Child-Pugh criteria for this patient to determine the severity of his hepatic disease. Which one of the following choices are included in the Child-Pugh criteria?

A. Direct bilirubin
B. aPTT
C. Ascites albumin content
D. Encephalopathy
E. Creatinine

14. A 30-year-old woman comes to your clinic with complaints of palpitations. She says that since she was a teenager she remembers having episodes of palpitations in which she would feel as if her heart was racing. These episodes would last for several seconds to a minute or so, and then go away spontaneously. Sometimes she would feel slightly short of breath with the episode. She denies chest pain or dizziness. She says that the episodes are becoming more frequent, and this is why she is coming to you for evaluation. She is single and does not smoke or drink alcohol or use illicit drugs. She has no other significant past medical history. Her physical examination is normal. ECG is obtained (Figure 1-14). Which of the following statements is true regarding her diagnosis?

A. The arrhythmia present during her episodes of palpitations is likely a narrow-complex PSVT due to increased automaticity.
B. If she presented with a wide-complex tachycardia, the treatment of choice would be IV verapamil.
C. She should be referred to cardiology for an electrophysiology study.
D. Treatment of atrial fibrillation with rapid ventricular response or atrial flutter should be with digitalis.
E. Patients with WPW should not be placed on chronic oral verapamil therapy because of the risk for ventricular fibrillation.

15. A 32-year-old white woman presents to your clinic with amenorrhea for the past 4 months. She states that she is not sexually active. She has had regular periods for most of her life until recently. She denies any history of headaches or visual changes. Past medical history is significant for depression treated with fluoxetine. She occasionally drinks alcohol and smokes marijuana on a regular basis. Physical examination results are essentially normal. A pregnancy test result is negative, and prolactin level is 75 ng/dL and TSH 2.5 mU/L. The most likely cause of her hyperprolactinemia is:

A. Fluoxetine
B. Marijuana
C. Pregnancy
D. Prolactinoma
E. Hypothyroidism

16. A 24-year-old woman who has been previously healthy presents to your clinic complaining of diarrhea, sweaty skin, and irritability for the past couple of months. She has been having up to three bowel movements a day and they are somewhat

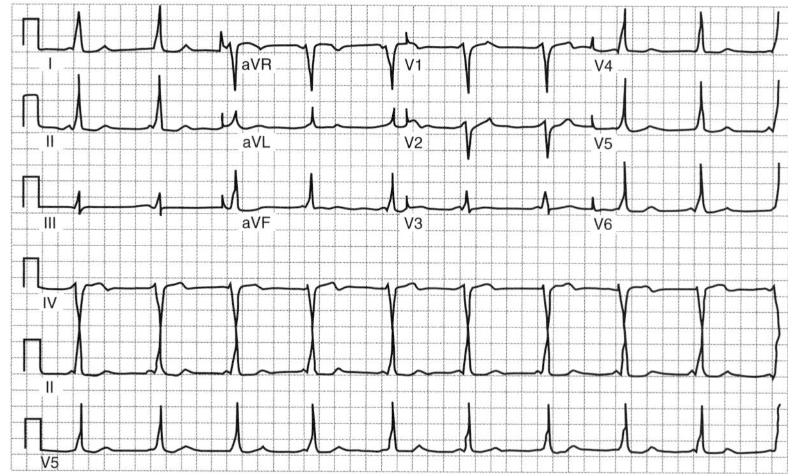

Figure 1-14 • Image Courtesy of Dr. Brenda Shinar, Banner Good Samaritan Medical Center, Phoenix, Arizona.

loose and without blood or mucus. She has noticed that she is warm and sweaty when others in her family are comfortable or even cool. She has been getting in more arguments with her boyfriend and feels extremely irritable. She denies using tobacco, alcohol, or drug. She currently takes no medications or herbs, and family history is noncontributory. On physical examination, the patient is afebrile and thin appearing with stable vital signs. HEENT examination is notable for bilateral lid lag, and her neck examination is notable for diffuse thyromegaly without bruits or obvious nodules. Heart and lung examination results are within normal limits. Neurologic examination is significant for hyperreflexia throughout. Her skin is warm and smooth, and you note that her palms are warm and sweaty. This patient's TSH is 0.03 mU/L and free T_4 is 10 ng/dL. You order RAIU and thyroid scintigraphy. You expect the following results:

A. High uptake on RAIU, single cold nodule
B. Low uptake on RAIU, single hot nodule
C. Normal uptake on RAIU, normal scintigraphy
D. High uptake on RAIU, homogeneous uptake
E. Low uptake on RAIU, normal scintigraphy

17. A 19-year-old white man is brought to your clinic by his parents. They are concerned that he has become more "distant." He has lost 20 pounds in the past 4 months and has intermittent abdominal pain and headaches. He has also complained of increasing fatigue. He denies having any past medical problems, pr using tobacco, alcohol, or drugs. HR is 110, RR is 18, BP is 90/60, and oxygen saturations are 99% on room air. On examination he appears thin and withdrawn, and his skin has a tanned appearance noted in the skin folds, palmar creases, and along the dentate line of the gums. Lungs are clear, and heart is tachycardic without murmur. Abdomen is soft without hepatosplenomegaly. You order basic laboratory studies that show a normal CBC and a BMP with the following values: sodium 130 mEq/L, potassium of 6.0 mEq/L, chloride 107 mEq/L, bicarbonate 20 mEq/L, BUN 18 mg/dL, creatinine 0.8 mg/dL. What other laboratory study would be the best to help confirm the diagnosis?

A. Random cortisol
B. A.M. serum cortisol
C. P.M. serum cortisol
D. Cosyntropin stimulation test
E. Serum glucose

18. A 65-year-old Hispanic woman comes to your clinic with complaints of irritability and depression for the past several months. She also notes an intermittent sensation of numbness around her mouth. She has a history of anxiety disorder and chronic renal insufficiency secondary to poorly controlled hypertension. Past surgeries include an appendectomy and thyroidectomy 1 year ago secondary to a large goiter. On physical examination the patient appears anxious. Vital signs are within normal limits, with the exception of a BP of 190/79 mm Hg. As you recheck her BP, you note carpal spasm. This patient's problem is most likely caused by:

A. Renal failure
B. Pseudohypoparathyroidism
C. Vitamin D deficiency
D. Malignancy
E. Hypoparathyroidism

19. A 35-year-old woman presents to your clinic with complaints of headache and muscle weakness. She notes that she just recently checked her BP at the drug store and it read "high." She denies having any other medical problems or using any medications. She also denies using any tobacco, drug, or alcohol. The patient is afebrile, HR is 88, RR is 12, and BP is 180/90 mm Hg. Results of her examination are otherwise noncontributory. Basic laboratory studies reveal the following: sodium 145 mEq/L, potassium 2.5 mEq/L, bicarbonate 30 mEq/L, BUN 10 mg/dL, creatinine 1.0 mg/dL, renin (upright posture) 0.1 ng/mL, and aldosterone (upright posture) 200 ng/dL. What is the likely cause of her symptoms?

A. Cushing syndrome
B. Licorice ingestion
C. Conn syndrome
D. Renal artery stenosis
E. Renal hypoperfusion

20. A 40-year-old white male kindergarten teacher presents to your clinic with 3 weeks of fatigue and pallor. He denies having fever, chills, or weight loss, but has noted gum bleeding while brushing his teeth. Physical examination reveals normal vital signs with the exception of an HR of 100. He has pale conjunctiva and mucous membranes, but otherwise normal cardiovascular and pulmonary examination results. There is no palpable lymphadenopathy. Abdominal examination results are benign, without evidence of hepatosplenomegaly.

A CBC is obtained with the following results: WBC count 2,600 (60% neutrophils, 30% lymphocytes, 6% monocytes, remainder eosinophils and basophils), hemoglobin 8.0 g/dL, hematocrit 26%, MCV 85 fL, platelet count 32,000/μL, reticulocytes 0.7%. Choose the test and result that is consistent with his diagnosis:

A. Iron studies—low iron, increase total iron binding capacity, low ferritin
B. Iron studies—low iron, low total iron binding capacity, high ferritin
C. Bone marrow biopsy—hypocellularity of bone marrow with increase fat cells
D. Bone marrow biopsy—hypercellularity of bone marrow with dysplasia of cell lines
E. Bone marrow biopsy—hypercellularity of bone marrow with >30% blasts

21. A 63-year-old man presents to the clinic with generalized fatigue and a 10-pound weight loss over the past month. He denies having fevers, chills, weakness, or abdominal pain. Vital signs show an HR of 95, BP 123/78 mm Hg, and RR 16, with oxygen saturations of 98% on room air. Physical examination reveals pale mucous membranes without lesions and no scleral icterus. Cardiac examination shows a regular rhythm with mild tachycardia. Lungs are clear to auscultation bilaterally. Abdomen is soft, nontender, nondistended, and without hepatosplenomegaly. Results of initial laboratory studies are remarkable for hemoglobin of 10.1 g/dL, hematocrit 27%, MCV 71 fL, and RDW 16 (high). The peripheral smear is shown (Figure 1-21). Which of the following is the next most appropriate step in this patient's care?

A. Start iron therapy
B. Bone marrow biopsy
C. Transfusion of packed RBCs
D. Colonoscopy
E. Hemoglobin electrophoresis

22. A 65-year-old man presents to your clinic with headaches, dizziness, and blurred vision for the past month. He also notes pruritus after hot showers. He has a 50 pack/year history of smoking and denies using alcohol or drugs. There is no other significant medical history and he takes no medications. Vital signs include HR 86, RR 16, oxygen saturation 98% on room air, and BP 128/85 mm Hg. Physical examination is remarkable for ruddiness of the face. Spleen is enlarged and palpable well below the left costal margin. Cardiovascular and pulmonary examination results are normal. Laboratory values are as follows: hemoglobin 20 g/dL, hematocrit 58%, WBC count 13,000 with a normal differential, and platelet count 480,000/μL. Which of the following tests should be performed next in the evaluation of this patient?

A. Bone marrow biopsy
B. Iron studies
C. Erythropoietin level
D. Leukocyte alkaline phosphatase
E. Coagulation studies

23. You are seeing several patients in the clinic and have laboratory studies performed on many of them. The laboratory calls you about a tube of blood that was sent without a label on it and you are unsure which patient the blood belongs to. The laboratory studies are run, and a smear is obtained (Figure 1-23):

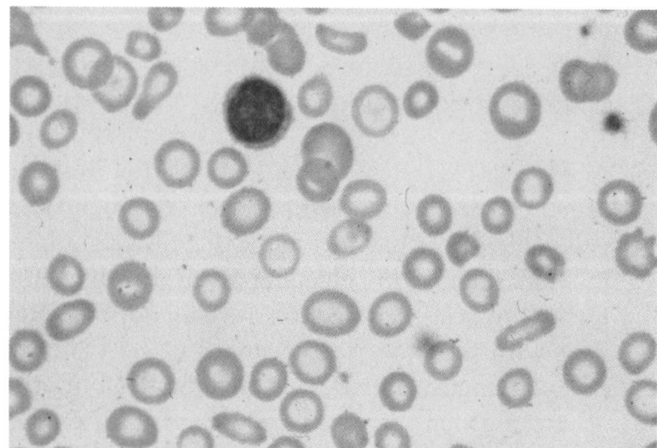

Figure 1-21 • Image Courtesy of Dr. Brenda Shinar, Banner Good Samaritan Medical Center, Phoenix, Arizona.

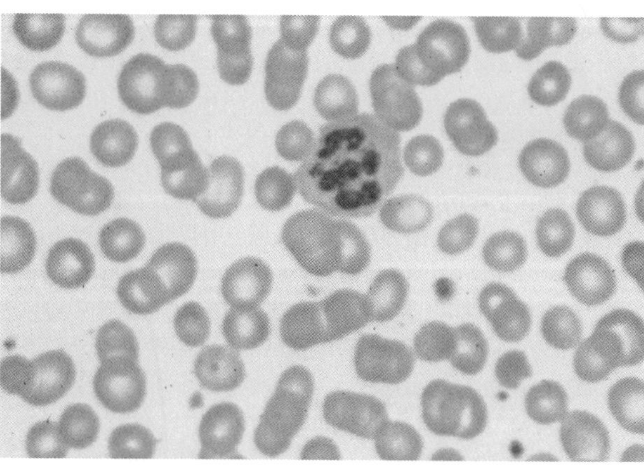

Figure 1-23 • Image Courtesy of Dr. Brenda Shinar, Banner Good Samaritan Medical Center, Phoenix, Arizona.

hemoglobin 10.2 g/dL, hematocrit 31%, and MCV 110 fL. To which of the following patients does this most likely belong?

A. A 23-year-old woman with heavy menses
B. A 57-year-old man with chronic alcoholism
C. A 48-year-old woman with rheumatoid arthritis on NSAIDs
D. A 43-year-old man with history of radiation exposure
E. A 25-year-old man who presents with right upper quadrant pain, splenomegaly, and scleral icterus

24. A 35-year-old moderately obese Hispanic woman comes to your clinic with complaints of irregular menstrual cycles. Her menses began at age 11 and she had initial "mostly" regular cycles, but for the past 10 years they have been irregular, occurring every 30–50 days and lasting anywhere from 3 to 8 days in length. She has been trying to get pregnant for years without success. Her last period was 45 days ago. On physical examination, her BMI is 32 and you note that she has terminal hairs on her upper lip and on the sides of her face. She says that the hair growth has been present since around the time of puberty, but that it seems to have increased over the past several years. Of note, the patient has gained approximately 50 pounds in the past 3 years. The rest of the examination, including pelvic, is otherwise normal. Urine pregnancy test results are negative. Laboratory testing yielded the following results: serum testosterone 95 ng/dL, serum DHEAS 3 mg/mL, serum prolactin 15 ng/mg, LH 35 mIU/mL, FSH 10 mIU/mL, estradiol 60 pg/mL, and fasting glucose 130 mg/dL. What is the most likely cause of her hirsutism?

A. A testosterone-secreting tumor of the ovary
B. A virilizing tumor of the adrenal gland
C. Polycystic ovary syndrome (PCOS)
D. Congenital adrenal hyperplasia (CAH)
E. Normal ethnic variation

25. You are seeing a 20-year-old female medical student in the clinic for a complaint of a new vaginal discharge. You ask her about her gynecologic history and specifically if she has ever had a Pap smear. You go into a lengthy discussion about screening tests. A screening test that detects a disease before the onset of symptoms, with treatment that does not affect survival, may *appear* to improve survival by increasing the amount of time from diagnosis to death. This is an example of:

A. Selection bias
B. Length bias
C. Overdiagnosis
D. Lead time bias
E. Effective screening test

26. A 42-year-old white woman presents to your clinic after finding a lump in her right breast. She has no significant medical history and takes no medications. She is G3P2. She began menses at age 14 and she gave birth to her first child at age 28. She has regular periods and her last menses were 2 weeks ago. There is no family history of breast cancer. On physical examination, there is a palpable mass in the upper outer quadrant of the right breast. No axillary nodes are palpable. Mammography confirms a 2-cm mass. A biopsy reveals a well-differentiated ductal cell carcinoma. Which of the following statements regarding treatment for this patient is true?

A. Breast-conserving therapy has been shown to have the same survival rates as mastectomy in randomized control trials.
B. A radical mastectomy is indicated for patients with a history of breast irradiation.
C. Radiation therapy is optional after surgery if a lumpectomy is done.
D. Adjuvant chemotherapy does not reduce the risk of recurrence if the patient has lymph nodes positive for metastatic disease.
E. Tamoxifen decreases recurrence if estrogen receptors are negative.

27. A 78-year-old man presents to your clinic with hemoptysis for 2 weeks. His history is significant for smoking one and a half packs of cigarettes per day for the past 60 years. He denies having a fever or purulent sputum. He also reports a weight loss of 20 pounds over the past 2 months and increasing dyspnea. On physical examination BP is 165/90 mm Hg, and the rest of his vital signs are normal. The patient appears to have a full, round face with truncal obesity, and there is wasting and bruising of the extremities. Cardiovascular and pulmonary examination results are normal. A chest x-ray is obtained and shows an enlargement of the right hilum. Laboratory studies reveal a fasting serum glucose of 200 mg/dL. What is the most likely diagnosis?

A. Adenocarcinoma of the lung
B. Small cell carcinoma of the lung
C. Large cell carcinoma of the lung
D. Squamous cell carcinoma of the lung
E. Non-Hodgkin lymphoma

28. A 55-year-old man with a history of prostate cancer presents to your clinic with new-onset back pain. He complains of numbness in both upper thighs. On physical examination there is tenderness to palpation over the lumbosacral spine. There is saddle anesthesia. Strength is diminished in both lower extremities. Patellar and Achilles reflexes are 3+ and toes are upgoing. What should be the next step in this patient's management?

A. MRI of the lumbosacral spine
B. Administration of dexamethasone IV
C. Determine the serum prostate-specific antigen level
D. Radiation therapy
E. Pain management

The next 2 questions (items 29 and 30) correspond to the following vignette:

A 25-year-old man presents to your clinic with complaints of a rash. He states that the rash began 1–2 days prior to his visit. He denies any recent travel, medication use, illicit drug use, change in laundry detergent, or use of topical creams. The rash is somewhat pruritic and involves the palms and soles. He is otherwise healthy and denies any past medical history. Physical examination reveals a temperature of 99.0°C, HR of 76, RR of 14, and BP of 128/86 mm Hg. Head and neck examination reveals a nearly healed cold sore on his upper lip. Heart, lung, and abdominal examination results are all normal. Skin examination reveals the rash depicted (Figure 1-29). There is no mucous membrane involvement.

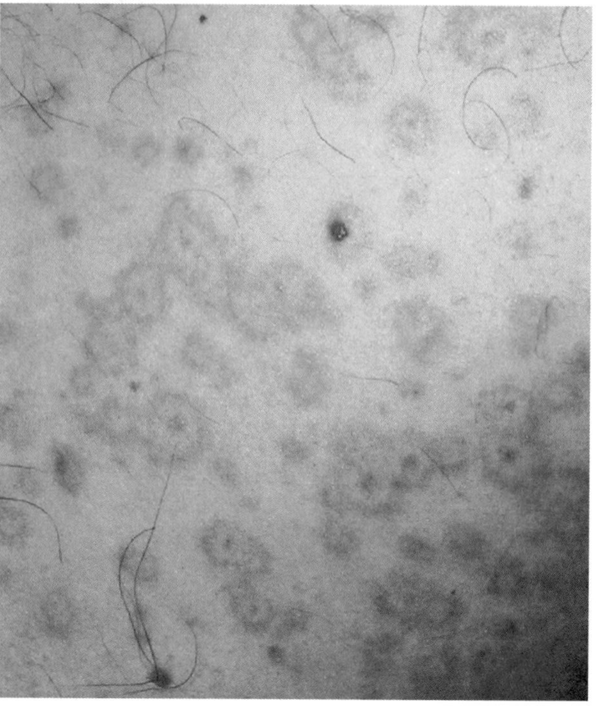

Figure 1-29 • Image Courtesy of Dr. Brenda Shinar, Banner Good Samaritan Medical Center, Phoenix, Arizona.

29. What is the most likely diagnosis?

A. Stevens-Johnson syndrome
B. Rocky Mountain spotted fever
C. Secondary syphilis
D. Erythema nodosum
E. Erythema multiforme

30. What is the most likely cause of his rash?

A. *Treponema pallidum* infection
B. Herpes simplex virus infection
C. Idiosyncratic drug reaction
D. *Rickettsia rickettsiae* infection
E. Sarcoidosis

End of Set

The next two questions (items 31 and 32) correspond to the following vignette:

A 60-year-old man with a history of diabetes mellitus type 2 presents to your clinic with complaints of a skin rash for the past month. The rash is located on the flexor surfaces of the arms and abdomen. He has no oral involvement. Initially, it began as erythematous annular lesions with some pruritus, and then it evolved into firm, bullous lesions that are not easily broken (Figure 1-31). You perform a skin biopsy of the normal-appearing perilesional skin, which shows a sparse perivascular leukocytic infiltrate with some eosinophils. The direct immunofluorescence microscopy shows linear deposits of IgG and C3 in the epidermal basement membrane.

31. Which of the following is the likely diagnosis?

A. Dermatitis herpetiformis
B. Bullous pemphigoid
C. Pemphigus vulgaris
D. Pemphigoid gestationis
E. Nikolsky disease

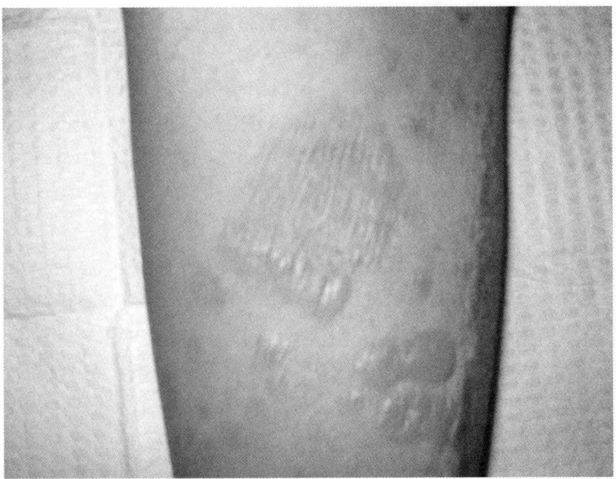

Figure 1-31 • Image Courtesy of Dr. Brenda Shinar, Banner Good Samaritan Medical Center, Phoenix, Arizona.

32. Which of the following statements best describes the patient's disease?
    A. The mainstay of treatment is glucocorticoids.
    B. In the absence of treatment, the mortality rate is very high.
    C. Patients with this disease never have oral mucosal involvement.
    D. Patients with high circulating antibody titers that bind the epidermal basement membrane have more severe disease.
    E. The bullous lesions usually heal with scarring.

End of Set

33. A 30-year-old man presents to your clinic with complaint of headache for the past 30 minutes. He describes the pain as an "ice-pick" stabbing pain behind his left eye. He has been having these attacks three to four times daily for the past 3 days. The headaches come on suddenly and usually resolve within 90 minutes. Vital signs and physical examination results are normal. What would be the most appropriate next step for diagnosis or treatment of this patient?
    A. Ibuprofen 800 mg PO
    B. CT scan of the head
    C. Lumbar puncture
    D. 100% oxygen
    E. Sumatriptan PO

34. A 60-year-old man comes to your clinic complaining of a symmetric burning and tingling in his feet for the past year. The discomfort in his extremities is worse at night when he is going to sleep. On physical examination, he has normal vital signs. His neurologic examination reveals normal cranial nerves and cerebellar function. He has decreased sensation to pinprick and light touch in a stocking pattern with diminished Achilles reflexes. There is some weakness of dorsiflexion of the great toes bilaterally. There is diminished proprioception and vibratory sensation in the feet as well, and the patient has a positive Rhomberg test result. Laboratory studies reveal a fasting glucose of 80 mg/dL. Which of the following laboratory studies should be ordered next to evaluate the cause of his peripheral neuropathy?
    A. Vitamin B_{12} level
    B. Serum immunoelectrophoresis
    C. Serum lead level
    D. Serum folate level
    E. CSF analysis

The following two questions (items 35 and 36) relate to the same clinical scenario:

A 29-year-old woman comes to your clinic with complaints of diffuse weakness for the past 3 months that seems to be getting worse. She has been in good health, but over the past year has noted subtle changes in her ability to exercise to her usual capacity, and she has had to have her husband do more for her during the day. When they realized that she needed his assistance to climb the stairs in their home, they decided to seek medical attention. Her weakness appears to worsen toward the end of the day. She has had occasional diplopia and difficulty chewing and swallowing her evening meals. She denies numbness or tingling or pain. On physical examination, the patient has normal vital signs. Her neurologic examination reveals normal cranial nerves. Her weakness is not apparent initially, but her muscles fatigue easily. She has no shoulder or thigh tenderness. Her sensation, reflexes, and cerebellar examination results are normal, as are the rest of her physical examination results.

35. Which of the following tests are the most sensitive and specific for making the diagnosis in this patient?
    A. Anticholinesterase (tensilon) test
    B. Repetitive nerve stimulation testing
    C. Anti-acetylcholine receptor antibodies
    D. Single-fiber EMG
    E. Muscle biopsy

36. After confirming your diagnosis, what is the most important next test to evaluate for conditions known to be associated that may affect the patient's treatment?
    A. MRI of the mediastinum
    B. Colonoscopy
    C. Thyroid function tests
    D. DEXA scan
    E. Urinalysis

End of Set

The next two questions (items 37 and 38) correspond to the following vignette:

A 35-year-old man with a history of recent head trauma develops generalized tonic-clonic seizures. He is started on phenytoin therapy. Two weeks later, he develops fever and an erythematous skin eruption and comes to your clinic. On physical examination, he is febrile to 102°C and appears uncomfortable and ill. His physical examination is unremarkable except for diffuse axillary and inguinal lymphadenopathy and an erythematous cutaneous eruption that does not blanch. His laboratory studies reveal a WBC count of 18,000 with a left shift. His AST and ALT are elevated to 95 and 100 U/L, respectively.

37. Which of the following is the most likely diagnosis?
    A. Acute HIV infection
    B. Phenytoin hypersensitivity reaction
    C. CMV
    D. Bacillary angiomatosis
    E. B-cell lymphoma

38. Which of the following antiepileptic drugs is safe to use in this patient?
    A. Carbamazepine
    B. Phenobarbital
    C. Valproic acid
    D. Phosphenytoin
    E. Felbamate

End of Set

39. A 65-year-old man comes to the clinic after stepping on an old nail while working in his garage. The nail went through the bottom of his tennis shoe and into the soft tissue of his foot. He is unsure if he has ever received his primary series of tetanus immunization, and he does not recall any booster immunization for tetanus. You remove the nail and order an x-ray of the foot to look for any remaining radiopaque material. You clean the puncture wound thoroughly. Which of the following describes the appropriate management for the prevention of tetanus in this patient?
    A. Give tetanus toxoid IM now, and have the patient follow up with his primary care doctor for the rest of the primary series.
    B. Give tetanus immune globulin IM now, and have the patient follow up with his primary care doctor for the primary series.
    C. Give tetanus immune globulin IM now and the tetanus toxoid IM in two separate sites. He does not need follow up for the primary series.
    D. Give tetanus immune globulin IM now and the tetanus toxoid IM in two separate sites. He should follow up with his primary doctor for the rest of the primary series.
    E. He does not need any tetanus immunization or immune globulin. The wound has been cleaned appropriately, and he just needs follow up to make sure that it doesn't become infected.

40. A 24-year-old female medical student presents to your clinic after developing a malar rash several days ago. She has no medical problems, but is currently taking isoniazid therapy after being told that her recent PPD test result was positive. In addition to the rash, she has had subjective fevers and malaise. She denies having arthralgias or myalgias, headaches, visual changes, or respiratory complaints. There is no history of autoimmune disease in her family. You are concerned that she has developed drug-induced SLE. You order laboratory tests to help confirm your suspicion. Which of the following would you expect to find if she has drug-induced lupus from the isoniazid?
    A. Positive antihistone antibodies with hypocomplementemia
    B. Positive antihistone antibodies with positive anti-dsDNA antibodies
    C. Positive antihistone antibodies with negative anti-dsDNA antibodies
    D. Negative antihistone antibodies with hypocomplementemia
    E. Negative antihistone antibodies with positive anti-dsDNA antibodies

The next two questions (items 41 and 42) correspond to the following vignette:

A 28-year-old woman with well-controlled SLE presents to your clinic with complaints of increasing fatigue, fevers, arthralgias, and malar rash. She is concerned she is having a lupus flare-up. She is in her 32nd week of her first pregnancy, which has been uneventful thus far. Her regular medications, which include hydroxychloroquine and prednisone, were stopped prior to her becoming pregnant. On examination, you find her to be afebrile with normal vital signs. She has a faint malar rash and mild synovitis in her hands bilaterally. Her heart and lung examination results are normal. Her abdomen is gravid, with the uterus easily palpated to approximately 32 cm above the pubic symphysis. Fetal heart tones are normal. Urinalysis reveals no evidence of infection or hematuria. You concur with her and are worried that she is having an exacerbation of her SLE.

41. Which of the following could be assessed to help confirm an exacerbation of her disease?

    A. ANA and anti-SSA (Ro) levels
    B. Anti-dsDNA and anti-SSA (Ro) levels
    C. Anti-dsDNA and complement levels
    D. ANA and complement levels
    E. Anti-ds DNA and ANA levels

42. The presence of which of the following markers increases the likelihood of her baby developing neonatal lupus with complete heart block?

    A. Anti-Smith antibodies
    B. Anti-SSA (Ro) antibodies
    C. Speckled pattern on ANA
    D. Antihistone antibodies
    E. Anti-dsDNA antibodies

End of Set

The following three questions (items 43 to 45) relate to the same clinical scenario:

A 32-year-old woman presents to your clinic with complaints of arthralgias, subjective fevers, and hair loss. She has not noticed any rashes, but states she gets sunburned more easily than normal. On examination, her vital signs are normal, including her BP. She appears well nourished and well developed. Results of her HEENT examination are unremarkable, with the exception of patchy alopecia. There is no evidence of a malar rash. Her lungs are clear to auscultation and her heart examination results are normal. She has normal bowel sounds without peritoneal signs. There is no clubbing, cyanosis, or edema present. Her skin examination results are unremarkable. There is no evidence of synovitis or arthritis on examination. Based on her history, you are concerned she may have SLE. You order a CBC, which shows a normocytic, normochromic anemia. A basic metabolic panel and urinalysis results are normal. ANA testing is positive.

43. The presence of which of the following antibodies would help confirm your diagnosis of SLE?

    A. Anti-SSA (Ro) and antihistone antibodies
    B. Anti-dsDNA and anti-SSB (La) antibodies
    C. Anti-SSA (Ro) and anti-SSB (La) antibodies
    D. Anti-dsDNA and anti-Smith antibodies
    E. Anti-dsDNA and anti-SSA (Ro) antibodies

44. You discuss the diagnosis with the patient and choose to start her on corticosteroid therapy. Before beginning therapy, you have a detailed discussion with her about the many possible adverse effects of prednisone. Included in these are which of the following?

    A. Hypotension
    B. Retinal detachment
    C. Glaucoma
    D. Hypoglycemia
    E. Interaction with oral contraceptives reducing their effectiveness

45. You start your patient on therapy for SLE, which includes daily oral prednisone. She fails to keep her 1-month follow-up appointment with you because she is feeling so well. She returns after 3 months with complaints of pain in her right hip. She says the pain had a gradual onset and has been getting worse over the past 4 weeks. She describes it as a deep, achy pain that is worse with weight bearing and motion. The pain also wakes her up at night. There are no other joints involved. She denies fevers or trauma. On examination, she is afebrile with normal vital signs. Results of her examination are unremarkable except for her right hip pain. She is uncomfortable with motion of her hip but there is no limitation to range of motion, no crepitance, and no effusion noted. You are concerned that she may have developed AVN because of her steroid therapy. Which of the following tests should you order to help you make the diagnosis?

A. Plain film x-rays of the hip
B. MRI of the hip
C. Technetium-99m bone scan of the hip
D. Joint aspiration with synovial fluid analysis
E. Bone biopsy

End of Set

46. A 36-year-old man presents to your clinic for evaluation of a productive cough. He has also noted some blood-streaked sputum. He has had some intermittent fevers. His symptoms have been present for 1–2 weeks. His past medical history is significant for several episodes of severe pneumonia as a child. Since that time he has had a recurrent cough productive of purulent sputum. On physical examination he is in no distress. His temperature is 100.8°C, HR is 86, RR is 18, and BP is 138/86 mm Hg. Lung examination reveals crackles and rhonchi in multiple areas of both lung fields. Chest radiography shows areas of dilated airways with thickened walls. What organism is most likely to be responsible for his current symptoms?

    A. *Pseudomonas aeruginosa*
    B. *Streptococcus pneumoniae*
    C. *Mycoplasma pneumoniae*
    D. *Staphylococcus aureus*
    E. *Aspergillus fumigatus*

47. A 26-year-old woman, G1P0, presents to the clinic for evaluation of an itchy rash. She is 28 weeks pregnant. The rash began approximately 2 days ago. It started on her trunk. The lesions are extremely pruritic vesicles and pustules on an erythematous base. On evaluation you note lesions in several different stages of evolution. She has never had chicken pox. You diagnose varicella infection. Which complication are you most concerned about?

    A. Hepatitis
    B. Pneumonia
    C. Cellulitis
    D. Shingles
    E. Postherpetic neuralgia

48. A 20-year-old man comes to your clinic with complaints of a cough that he says he has had for the past month. He is usually in good health and is taking no medications. He says that the cough is nonproductive, but it is worse at night and often keeps him awake. He denies having fever or other constitutional symptoms. On physical examination, he appears well nourished, with normal vital signs and a room air oxygen saturation of 98%. You review in your mind the differential diagnosis for a chronic cough as you prepare to examine him. Which of the following is the most common cause of a chronic cough?

    A. Asthma
    B. Gastroesophageal reflux disease (GERD)
    C. Use of an ACE inhibitor
    D. Postnasal drainage
    E. TB

The next two questions (items 49 and 50) correspond to the following vignette:

A 20-year-old man with no significant past medical history presents to the clinic with complaints of headache and nausea for the past 24 hours. He says the headache is getting progressively worse and is global in nature. He also complains of subjective fevers and neck pain. He states that lights hurt his eyes and make his headache worse. He denies any trauma, recent travel, or ill contacts. He is currently enrolled in college and plays on the varsity football team. He has been taking ibuprofen every 3–4 hours for low back pain that resulted from a football injury. He uses alcohol on a recreational basis, but denies any other drug or tobacco use. On examination, he has a temperature of 100.4°C and is ill appearing. His HEENT examination reveals photophobia but no papilledema. He has mild nuchal rigidity but no focal neurologic changes. The remainder of his examination is unremarkable. You are concerned that your patient has meningitis, so a lumber puncture is performed and the CSF is sent to the laboratory for analysis.

49. Which of the following CSF results would support the diagnosis of aseptic meningitis in this patient?

    A. Elevated WBC count, normal glucose, high protein, positive culture
    B. Elevated WBC count, normal glucose, normal protein, negative culture
    C. Elevated WBC count, low glucose, high protein, positive culture
    D. Normal WBC count, normal glucose, normal protein, negative culture
    E. Normal WBC count, low glucose, high protein, negative culture

50. Which of the following statements regarding the different causes of aseptic meningitis is true?
    A. Enterovirus is responsible for the majority of cases of aseptic meningitis in the fall and winter.
    B. Ibuprofen may induce an aseptic meningitis picture, especially in patients with rheumatoid arthritis.
    C. White populations from northern latitudes are at increased risk for disseminated *coccidioides immitis* to the CNS.
    D. Primary HIV infection presents with aseptic meningitis in 50% of cases.
    E. Aseptic meningitis with a history of exposure to rodents suggests the possibility of LCMV infection as a cause.

End of Set

A Answers and Explanations

1. B
2. A
3. D
4. D
5. A
6. C
7. B
8. C
9. D
10. B
11. D
12. C
13. D
14. C
15. A
16. D
17. D
18. E
19. C
20. C
21. D
22. C
23. B
24. C
25. D
26. A
27. B
28. B
29. E
30. B
31. B
32. A
33. D
34. A
35. C
36. A
37. B
38. C
39. D
40. C
41. C
42. B
43. D
44. C
45. B
46. A
47. B
48. D
49. B
50. E

1. **B. This patient is presenting with a history most consistent with IgA nephropathy. Serum complement levels are normal in IgA nephropathy. Patients are usually young adults who present with hematuria *immediately following or concomitant with* an upper respiratory infection. (This distinguishes it from poststreptococcal glomerulonephritis that occurs approximately 2 weeks after the pharyngitis or skin infection.) Proteinuria may or may not be present.**

   A. Poststreptococcal glomerulonephritis presents 10–14 days after an acute streptococcal pharyngitis. Serum complement levels are decreased. Patients may present with hematuria, proteinuria, or nephritic syndrome.
   C. Lupus erythematosus may present with nephritic syndrome or glomerulonephritis. Other findings consistent with lupus should be evident. Clinical manifestations of lupus include a malar rash, photosensitivity, mucus ulcerations, serositis, and seizures. None of these findings are present in this patient.
   D. Cryoglobulinemia is associated with infections such as hepatitis C and collagen vascular disease. Serum complement levels are low.
   E. Most patients with membranoproliferative glomerulonephritis present with nephrotic syndrome. Serum complement levels are usually low.

2. **A. This patient's history and physical examination results are consistent with prerenal azotemia. She has large volumes of water loss diarrhea, tachycardia, and orthostatic hypotension, all of which point to volume loss as a cause of her acute renal failure.**

   B. Aminoglycosides are most likely to be associated with antibiotic-induced nephrotoxicity. In these cases, urine sodium should be high due to intrinsic renal damage. Amoxicillin and other penicillins have been associated with acute interstitial nephritis. This can also progress to acute renal failure. However, the urine should reveal an active sediment including blood, protein, and eosinophils. None of these are present in this patient.
   C. Although the patient has a history of hypertension, the history suggests volume depletion as the cause of the acute renal failure.
   D. Cholesterol emboli usually occur in patients who have had recently undergone an invasive cardiovascular procedure. Other signs and symptoms found in this disease include fever, livedo reticularis, petechiae, and digital ischemia. None of these are present in our patient.
   E. In cases of postinfectious glomerulonephritis, the urine sediment should be active and include blood and protein.

3. **D. The treatment of prerenal azotemia is correction of volume status. Initial fluid should be normal saline. Fluid status and urine output should be monitored carefully, especially if the patient is oliguric.**

   A. Renal ultrasonography should be performed to evaluate for any structural abnormalities if renal function does not improve after optimizing volume status.
   B. There is no evidence for obstructive or postrenal causes in this patient. History and examination clearly point to a prerenal cause. A Foley catheter could be placed to monitor urine output accurately after fluids were started.
   C. Further laboratory evaluation may be needed if the patient's renal function does not correct. However, at this time fluids can be started without further evaluation.
   E. This patient has no indications for dialysis. Indications for dialysis include uncorrectable acidemia, hyperkalemia refractory to treatment, intoxication with methanol or ethylene glycol, volume overload refractory to diuretic management, and uremia causing pericarditis or encephalopathy.

4. **D. Bacillary angiomatosis is a systemic disorder characterized by vascular tumors in patients with HIV and AIDS. When the tumors are seen in the skin, it is called bacillary angiomatosis and in the liver or spleen it is called bacillary peliosis hepatis. In the skin it looks like Kaposi sarcoma, but unlike Kaposi sarcoma, it is caused by the infectious organism *Bartonella henselae.* In hosts with normal immunity, *Bartonella* infection causes cat scratch fever.**

   A. Seborrheic dermatitis is a chronic inflammatory disorder of the skin characterized by a base of erythema with a yellow-white "greasy" scale in the areas of the body with highly active sebaceous glands. This includes the scalp, nasolabial folds, eyebrows, and parasternal area. It is seen commonly in patients with normal immunity, but patients with HIV and AIDS may have severe disease.

B. Molloscum contagiosum is a skin lesion that is caused by a pox virus. It can be seen in children and adults of normal immunity, but when it is extensive and about the face, HIV should be considered. (Before HAART, 10% of patients with HIV were found to have molluscum contagiosum, and 30% of patients with CD4 counts of <100 had the disease.) It is characterized by skin-colored, umbilicated-appearing, pearly papules or nodules. In HIV, the lesions may regress with antiviral therapy.

C. Psoriasis is a chronic inflammatory disorder of the skin that is seen in both immunocompetent patients and in patients with HIV and AIDS. Psoriasis manifests in many different forms, including plaque, guttate, pustular, and scalp forms. Patients with severe psoriasis that is new in onset should be questioned regarding HIV risk factors, and should be checked for HIV disease if they are present.

E. Oral candidiasis is characterized by the presence of white, milklike removable plaques on the oral mucosa. In the setting of HIV, oral candidiasis correlates with a moderate degree of immunodeficiency, but it is not pathognomonic for HIV disease, and is commonly seen in patients who are on steroid-containing inhaler medications who do not rinse their mouths.

5. **A. Lymphangioleiomyomatosis is a disease that occurs among women of childbearing age caused by an abnormal proliferation of immature smooth muscle cells involving the alveolar septa and airway walls. Chest radiographs reveal reticulonodular infiltrates and "honeycombing" throughout the lung fields. Spontaneous pneumothorax and chylous pleural effusions are complications of lymphangioleiomyomatosis.**

B. PCP causes a spontaneous pneumothorax in approximately 2% of cases. Pneumothorax is more common in patients who were prophylaxed with aerosolized pentamidine or who have had PCP in the past. The mortality of pneumothorax with PCP is 10% and aggressive treatment is required. There is no increased risk for pneumothorax in patients with *Mycoplasma* pneumonia, however.

C. The most common cause of secondary peumothorax is COPD. Pneumothorax occurs when a bleb ruptures, and it can be dangerous because COPD patients rarely have good pulmonary reserves. Patients with COPD who develop sudden chest pain or shortness of breath need to be evaluated for a possible pneumothorax. Patients with severe, end-stage pulmonary fibrosis, cystic fibrosis, and other bullous lung diseases are all more likely to have secondary spontaneous pneumothorax. Hypersensitivity pneumonitis is not associated with this entity.

D. Patients with mesothelioma usually present with pleuritic chest pain secondary to the inflammation of the pleura surrounding the lesion. There is no association, however, with mesothelioma and spontaneous pneumothorax.

E. Premenopausal women, not postmenopausal, may have a secondary spontaneous pneumothorax during their menses. This is called catamenial pneumothorax and is due to ectopic endometrium in the lung tissue that bleeds at the time of menstruation because of the usual hormonal influence. Other presentations of thoracic endometriosis include hemoptysis and pulmonary nodule.

6. **C. Berylliosis is remarkably similar in presentation to sarcoidosis. It has a tendency to cause a chronic interstitial pneumonitis of the upper lobes. The disease is granulomatous in nature and essentially indistinguishable from sarcoidosis. It is a result of chronic exposure to beryllium that occurs in occupations involving high-tech electronics, alloys, and dental ceramics. This patient is a middle-aged African-American woman and has an elevated calcium level and bilateral hilar adenopathy consistent with sarcoidosis, but she has had occupational exposure to beryllium, which makes berylliosis more likely. The beryllium lymphocyte transformation test may be used to diagnose berylliosis, and the disease is treated with corticosteroids and usually responds.**

A. Sarcoidosis. This patient certainly has signs and symptoms consistent with sarcoidosis and is in the right age and ethnic group to have sarcoidosis, but her exposure to beryllium makes berylliosis the more likely etiology.

B. Silicosis is an interstitial lung disease caused by occupational exposure to silica. It, too, affects the upper lobes of the lungs. The exposure to silica, however, occurs in occupations such as quartz mining, glassmaking, and sandblasting. In addition, the latency period between exposure and onset of illness may be 20 to 30 years. It is important to note that patients with silicosis have an increased susceptibility to TB and should be monitored periodically with PPD skin tests.

D. TB also affects the upper lung lobes, but patients with TB usually have a clinical presentation more consistent with infection. They will often have fevers, weight loss, and hemoptysis. In addition, they should have risk factors for TB infection, such as exposure to someone with the disease, HIV infection, or a history of spending time in prison.

E. CHF may present with shortness of breath, but this patient has no prior history of heart disease. The crackles noted on physical examination in patients with CHF are heard early in inspiration and are more coarse sounding. The radiographic findings are of cephalization of the vasculature and pulmonary edema.

7. **B. Chorea is a major criterion. With rheumatic fever reemerging, the modified Jones criteria were established in 1992 to help make the diagnosis simpler. In order to make the diagnosis of rheumatic fever, a patient must have two major criteria as outlined in the table below, or have one major and two minor criteria (and evidence of a preceding GAS infection).**

A, C. ECG changes such as prolonged PR interval and fever are minor criteria (see Table 1-7 for all criteria).

TABLE 1-7 Modified Jones Criteria

Major Criteria	Minor Criteria
Carditis	Previous rheumatic fever
Polyarthritis	Arthralgias
Chorea	Fever
Erythema marginatum	Acute phase reactants (high ESR or WBC)
Subcutaneous nodules	ECG changes: prolonged P-R interval

D. Erythema nodosum is a rash characterized by tender, erythematous to violaceous subcutaneous nodules most commonly seen on the anterior shins. The microscopic findings on biopsy are inflammation of the septal fascia in the subcutaneous fat. It is associated with poststreptococcal infections, granulomatous infections, disorders such as sarcoidosis and coccidioidomycosis, and autoimmune disorders such as Crohn disease.

E. See explanation for B. Evidence of a preceding GAS infection is defined as a positive streptococcal test result or elevated (ASO >250 Todd units) or rising ASO titers.

8. **C. This patient most likely has achalasia, a motor disorder of the esophagus that has lack of peristalsis and increased LES pressure. Manometry is the gold standard for diagnosis.**

A. Endoscopy is indicated in people with dysphagia, primarily for the diagnosis of Barrett esophagus and carcinoma. Although endoscopy may have helped with the diagnosis, the patient's risk factors for esophageal adenocarcinoma are minimal.

B. Twenty-four-hour pH recording is the first-line objective test to evaluate for reflux disease. Often, however, patients with a good history for reflux are treated with histamine blockers or PPIs empirically, and diagnosis is confirmed when symptoms improve.

D. CT scan is used to look for extrinsic causes of dysphagia.

E. Video fluoroscopy is used in the evaluation of oropharyngeal dysphagia associated with hoarseness, cough, and nasopharyngeal regurgitation.

9. **D. PPIs have been shown to have the best efficacy and provide the most rapid and complete symptom relief in GERD.**

A. Weight loss is often recommended, although there are no evidence-based studies showing its efficacy in improving the symptoms of GERD.

B. Fundoplication is usually performed after a 24-hour pH probe proving GERD in patients who fail medical management.

C. H2 blockers are often used first line secondary to their easy accessibility, but they often do not offer as complete relief as a PPI.

E. Lifestyle modifications are recommended, although similar to weight loss, there are no evidence-based studies showing its efficacy in improving symptoms of GERD.

10. **B. *H. pylori* colonization usually occurs in youth through fecal-oral and oral-oral routes. Infection is lifelong unless given appropriate therapy. Reinfection later in life after treatment occurs in <1% of people per year in the United States. It is unlikely that recurrent** H. pylori **is responsible for her symptoms, and you should not treat her again.**

A, C, D, E. See explanation for B.

11. **D. This patient is constipated, by both physical examination and by definition. Constipation is defined as stooling less than two to three times per week. Patients will describe having to strain to have bowel movements, and the bowel movements are hard and difficult to pass. The best initial therapy would be to increase water and fiber intake along with daily exercise.**

A. KUB radiographs can be checked, but is not essential in making the diagnosis of constipation.
B. Her physical examination does not suggest an acute abdomen. CT of the abdomen would help assess intraabdominal pathology, although the patient has no significant past medical history or examination findings to warrant this examination at present.
C. Barium enema would help to assess rectosigmoid pathology and would be indicated if colorectal carcinoma were on the differential diagnosis.
E. Abdominal and pelvic ultrasonography would aid in the initial evaluation of abdominal pain and would help exclude ovarian cyst and appendicitis as possible etiologies for pain, although in this patient the appendix is already gone and she is currently menstruating.

12. **C. This patient most likely has acute hepatitis A, which is transmitted by the fecal-oral route and is more common in areas of poor sanitation. Her laboratory studies will show a positive IgM antibody to HAV, and in the acute infection, she will not have yet made IgG antibodies.**

A. Anti-HCV-positive laboratory studies are suggestive of hepatitis C with anti-HCV-positive titers. Hepatitis C is transmitted by blood exposure, most often by used needles in tattoos or IVDA. The acute form is most often asymptomatic.
B. HbsAg-positive, anti-HAV IgG–negative laboratory studies are suggestive of an acute hepatitis B infection with a positive HBsAg detected as well as an IgM antibody to the HBc portion of the virus. Hepatitis B is transmitted by body fluids such as blood, semen, and cervical fluids. Risk factors include sexual exposure and blood exposures.
D. Anti-HAV IgM–negative, anti-HAV IgG–positive laboratory values suggests an old hepatitis A infection, with IgG positivity, but not an acute infection, because the IgM is negative.
E. HbsAg-negative, anti-HBc-negative, HBsAb-positive laboratory values are consistent with immunization for hepatitis B. The serologies indicate that there is immunity to the hepatitis B virus because of the antibody to the surface antigen. However, this person was immunized rather than recovered from an acquired infection because of the lack of hepatitis core antibody. If the person had actually "seen" the virus, they would have an IgG antibody to the core portion of the virus.

13. **D. The Child-Pugh criteria are used to determine the severity of a patient's liver disease. The criteria include the following: total bilirubin, PT, serum albumin, the presence of ascites, and the presence of encephalopathy. One to three points are assigned for each category. A score of 5–6 is considered grade A (well-compensated disease), 7–9 is grade B (significant functional compromise), and 10–15 is considered grade C (decompensated disease.) These grades correlate with patient survival statistics.**

E. Creatinine is not used in the calculation of the Child-Pugh classification, but it is a factor in the MELD (Model for End Stage Liver Disease) score that is used to follow patients awaiting liver transplantation. It is a score calculated by plugging the serum bilirubin, INR, and creatinine into a formula. Scores can range from 6 to 40.
A, B, C. See explanation for D.

14. **C. This patient has Wolff-Parkinson-White syndrome, or WPW. It is characterized by patients with both preexcitation on their ECG and paroxysmal tachycardias. Her ECG has a short PR interval and a slurred upstroke to the QRS, called a delta wave. In WPW, conduction starts in the sinus node with the sinus impulse. After the**

depolarization of the atria, the conduction can follow three possible paths: (1) the impulse can be conducted strictly through the bypass tract and stimulate the ventricles early, resulting in a short PR interval and a slurred upstroke to the QRS as the ventricles are depolarized; (2) the impulse can be conducted normally through the AV node–His-Purkinje system, resulting in a normal PR interval and QRS morphology; or (3) the impulse can be conducted through both pathways and form a fusion complex, which results in a short PR interval and variable slurring of the QRS. Patients with preexcitation on ECG and symptomatic tachycardias should be referred for electrophysiology studies and possible ablation of their accessory pathway.

A. Patients with WPW are at high risk for arrhythmias, and the most common is a paroxysmal supraventricular tachycardia due to reentry (not increased automaticity as in multifocal atrial tachycardia). This results in a narrow-complex QRS as the impulse is conducted through the AV node system in an anterograde direction, then moves in a retrograde direction through the bypass tract. The conduction continues to circle around and around this circuit until it is terminated, either spontaneously or with drugs that slow conduction through the AV node (such as verapamil).

B. In about 5% of cases, the tachycardia occurs in the opposite direction, with anterograde conduction through the bypass tract (preexciting the ventricles) and retrograde conduction through the AV node. This results in a wide-complex tachycardia. It must be terminated with antiarrhythmic drugs that slow conduction through the bypass tract, such as procainamide or quinidine.

D, E. If you give a patient IV verapamil or digitalis, which slows conduction through the AV node, to terminate an atrial fibrillation, flutter, or a wide-complex tachycardia, you may precipitate a ventricular arrhythmia. (Note that chronic PO verapamil therapy is not associated with this complication.)

15. **A. Various medications can cause hyperprolactinemia. Dopamine secreted by the hypothalamus acts to inhibit the secretion of prolactin from the pituitary gland. Therefore, any medication that works to decrease dopamine levels in the brain such as phenothiazines and metaclopramide, or medications that alter other neurotransmitters such as SSRIs (like fluoxetine) or MAO inhibitors and tricyclics can be associated with elevated prolactin levels. These levels are usually <150 ng/dL. If the levels are >150 ng/dL, there is a higher likelihood that a prolactinoma is responsible.**

B. Marijuana use is typically thought to correlate with gynecomastia, but not hyperprolactinemia.

C. This patient had a negative pregnancy test result and denies sexual activity, so pregnancy is an unlikely cause of her hyperprolactinemia.

D. Prolactinomas are the most common pituitary subtype, often presenting in women with oligomenorrhea, amenorrhea, and galactorrhea. They are not necessarily the most common cause of hyperprolactinemia. Microadenomas are defined as lesions <1 cm in size and macroadenomas >1 cm in size. Treatment usually begins with dopamine agonists that help to decrease tumor size and normalize serum prolactin.

E. Primary hypothyroidism can also cause elevated prolactin levels secondary to alteration of the hypothalamic-pituitary axis. This patient has a normal TSH level, making this unlikely.

16. **D. This patient likely has Graves disease as a cause of her hyperthyroidism. RAIU is high in Graves disease, indicating that the thyroid gland is avidly taking up iodine for the production of thyroid hormone. The RAIU is reported as a number, and it is the first test to order when evaluating a cause for hyperthyroidism. The RAIU helps to distinguish between high uptake causes of hyperthyroidism, such as Graves disease and toxic multinodular goiter, and low uptake causes of hyperthyroidism, which include thyroiditis and factitious hyperthyroidism. The thyroid scintigraphy is reported as a picture. Thyroid scintigraphy is used to evaluate a pattern of uptake within the thyroid gland, and helps to define any nodules and whether they are "cold" (with less uptake) or "hot" (with more uptake.) A person with Graves disease alone as a cause of hyperthyroidism would have diffuse uptake on scintigraphy without evidence of nodules. Graves disease is typically seen in women 20–40 years of age. Clinical presentation includes signs and symptoms of hyperthyroidism such as tachycardia, diarrhea, and tremulousness. Clinical findings include a diffuse, nontender goiter, ophthalmopathy (to include lid lag, lid retraction, proptosis, extraocular muscle weakness), and**

pretibial myxedema (but patients don't have to have all three or even two of the three components to have Graves disease). Treatment is medical, with the drugs that decrease the production of thyroid hormones such as methimazole or PTU, or with radioactive iodine ablation or surgery. Patients treated with radioactive iodine ablation may eventually become hypothyroid and require thyroid supplementation.

A, B, C, E. These results would not be expected. See explanation for D.

17. **D. The cosyntropin stimulation test is felt to be the most sensitive test in detecting adrenal insufficiency. Cortisol levels are checked at 0 hour, 30 minutes, and 60 minutes after a dose of ACTH (cosyntropin) is given to assess whether or not the adrenal glands are able to respond to ACTH stimulation. A peak value of less than 18–20 is considered inadequate and suggestive of primary adrenal insufficiency.**

A. Random cortisol is not measured secondary to overlap with the normal values from the diurnal nature of the hormone. It is thought to be helpful in determining insufficiency in the critically ill because it should be maximal at all times in a high-stress environment, such as the intensive care unit.

B. An A.M. serum cortisol level is only considered useful if it is <3 (insufficient) or >18 (normal). Levels between 3 and 18 do not help to make a diagnosis.C.

C. A P.M. serum cortisol is not indicated because it would have little clinical value.

E. Checking serum glucose would be helpful to determine quickly if hypoglycemia were the cause of this patient's symptoms. However, his symptoms have been ongoing and his electrolyte abnormalities do not correlate with hypoglycemia.

18. **E. This patient is exhibiting signs and symptoms of hypocalcemia. Clinical manifestations include perioral paresthesias, cramps, Chvostek sign (tapping of facial nerve to illicit contraction of facial muscles), and Trousseau sign (inflation of BP cuff eliciting carpal spasm). Other manifestations include irritability, depression and seizures. Hypoparathyroidism can be isolated, secondary to hypomagnesemia, or can be evident status postthyroidectomy, in which case the parathyroids are accidentally removed or their blood supply is disrupted. Diagnosis is made by checking calcium, albumin, PTH, vitamin D, and other basic electrolytes. Treatment is with calcium replacement. Vitamin D replacement may also be required.**

A. Renal failure can cause hypocalcemia by way of decreased vitamin D production and decreased phosphorus excretion leading to increased calcium deposition in the soft tissue. Clinical manifestations include renal osteodystrophy that can consist of osteomalacia, osteitis fibrosa cystica, and osteoporosis.

B. Pseudohypoparathyroidism is defined as PTH end organ resistance. This syndrome is also associated with skeletal abnormalities and retardation. Consequently, serum calcium levels are low, serum phosphate levels are elevated, and serum PTH levels are elevated.

C. Vitamin D deficiency can be caused by decreased intake, inadequate production in the skin, or renal failure. In renal failure there is decreased hydroxylation of calcidiol to calcitriol, the end product of vitamin D. The function of vitamin D is to increase absorption of calcium and phosphate at the level of the intestine. In deficiency, there is reduced absorption of both calcium and phosphate, which leads to increased production of parathyroid hormone (secondary hyperparathyroidism) to improve serum calcium levels, which then lowers serum phosphate levels.

D. Hypercalcemia of malignancy can be secondary to production of a PTH-rP or local osteoclastic activity at the level of bone. Calcium levels are elevated and phosphate levels can be variable depending on the etiology for the elevated calcium. Endogenous parathyroid hormone levels will be low in response to feedback inhibition from the elevated serum calcium.

19. **C. Conn syndrome is caused by an increase in aldosterone levels secondary to an adrenal adenoma. Symptoms of hyperaldosteronism include diastolic hypertension, headaches, muscle weakness (from hypokalemia) and polyuria. Laboratory findings include hypokalemia, hypernatremia and metabolic alkalosis. Aldosterone levels are typically elevated secondary to the adenoma and renin levels are low in response to a negative feedback loop. With those laboratory values, a CT or MRI should be ordered to determine the presence of an**

adenoma. If no adenoma is found, adrenal vein aldosterone sampling should be obtained. If there is no localization of aldosterone, the elevated aldosterone levels are thought to be secondary to hyperplasia.

A. Cushing syndrome is defined as cortisol excess. Clinical signs of cortisol excess include central obesity, buffalo hump, easy fatigability, and easy bruising. Hypertension can also be present. Etiologies include a pituitary adenoma (Cushing disease), adrenal tumor, or ectopic ACTH production from a cancer. This patient does not have any examination findings suggestive of cortisol excess. Renin and aldosterone levels are low in Cushing syndrome.

B. Licorice ingestion is a nonaldosterone, exogenous cause of apparent mineralocorticoid excess. Renin and aldosterone levels will be low in this case.

D. Renal artery stenosis can result in secondary hyperaldosteronism, with an elevated renin and aldosterone level. This patient did not have an abdominal bruit on physical examination, and she had normal renal function. Patients with renal artery stenosis may have both of these findings, but the lack of these findings does not rule out the disease.

E. This patient gives no story to suggest renal hypoperfusion, which would lead to elevated renin and aldosterone levels in response to low flow states. This is also referred to as secondary hyperaldosteronism.

20. **C. The clinical presentation of aplastic anemia can include fatigue and pallor due to anemia, mucosal bleeding due to thrombocytopenia, and recurrent infections due to neutropenia. Peripheral blood counts will reveal pancytopenia with a normocytic anemia and poor reticulocyte count. Bone marrow aspirate shows all cell lines to be hypocellular, with increase in bone marrow fat cells. The causes of aplastic anemia include chemicals such as benzene and arsenic; drugs such as chloramphenicol and carbonic anhydrase inhibitors; and viral infections including CMV, EBV, and parvovirus. In many cases of aplastic anemia, a cause is never established. Ultimate cure is a bone marrow transplant.**

A. These iron studies are characteristic of iron deficiency anemia. This patient has a normocytic anemia, which is not consistent with that diagnosis. In addition, iron deficiency does not cause pancytopenia.

B. These iron studies are characteristic of anemia of chronic disease. Anemia of chronic disease does not cause pancytopenia.

D. This bone marrow aspirate is typical of a myelodysplastic syndrome. Myelodysplastic syndromes have a similar clinical presentation to aplastic anemia because both cause pancytopenia. However, myelodysplastic syndromes cause abnormal features of the cells that can be seen on the peripheral smear. Bone marrow aspirate will usually reveal hypercellularity with dysplasia of marrow precursor cells.

E. This bone marrow aspirate is typical for an acute leukemia. Acute leukemia can present with pancytopenia, but there are often blasts on peripheral smear.

21. **D. This patient has a microcytic anemia, as evidenced by the low MCV and microcytosis on peripheral smear. There is also a variable RDW, which is revealed by a high value, indicating that this is not a thalassemia. Iron deficiency would be the most likely cause in this patient. It is not enough, however, to say the patient is iron deficient. A reason for the iron deficiency must be found. Gastrointestinal bleeding from a malignancy would be a possible and likely source. Colonoscopy should be performed to rule out this possibility prior to the initiation of iron therapy.**

A. Iron supplementation will likely be needed, but a cause for the anemia should be sought. In addition, iron studies would be helpful to confirm the diagnosis prior to therapy.

B. Bone marrow biopsy is not indicated in this patient. Microcytic anemia should be evaluated with additional studies, including iron studies and hemoglobin electrophoresis. If iron deficiency is confirmed, a source for blood loss should be pursued. Bone marrow biopsy is usually not needed unless other diagnostic studies fail to produce a diagnosis.

C. This patient does not have any indications for transfusion therapy at this time. Indications to transfuse would include cardiac or pulmonary symptoms secondary to the anemia.

E. Hemoglobin electrophoresis can be used to evaluate for thalassemia, which is in the differential diagnosis for a microcytic anemia. However, it is a much less likely etiology, especially at this age of presentation, and the high RDW also points to iron deficiency as the diagnosis rather than thalassemia.

22. **C. Erythropoietin level can be used to differentiate polycythemia vera from secondary polycythemia. In polycythemia vera, erythropoietin will be low, and in secondary polycythemia, erythropoietin will be elevated. RBC mass studies can also be useful in confirming the diagnosis of polycythemia vera. RBC mass will be elevated in polycythemia vera, but not in other myeloproliferative disorders. It cannot distinguish polycythemia vera from secondary erythrocytosis because RBC mass can be elevated in both.**

    A. Bone marrow biopsy will show hypercellularity with decreased iron stores. Bone marrow biopsy would be indicated if the serum erythropoietin is normal or an underlying malignancy is suspected.

    B. Iron studies would not be the next test indicated in this patient. They may be obtained at some point in the workup and to monitor treatment. The treatment of polycythemia vera consists of phlebotomy once or twice weekly until the patient is iron deficient and hemoglobin is <14 g/dL.

    D. LAP can be elevated on polycythemia vera. This is a nonspecific finding and is not useful for diagnostic purposes.

    E. This patient has hyperviscosity from polycythemia. It is not a hypercoagulable state due to a defect in the coagulation pathway.

23. **B. This patient has a macrocytic anemia as noted on the peripheral smear and by the hypersegmented neutrophils. This can be seen in patients with vitamin B_{12} and folate deficiency from chronic malnutrition or malabsorption.**

    A. Iron deficiency anemia would be more likely in this clinical setting. This would produce a microcytic anemia.

    C. This patient's history is consistent with anemia of chronic disease, which can be normocytic or microcytic.

    D. Radiation exposure would predispose this patient to aplastic anemia, which is normocytic. It produces a pancytopenia.

    E. This patient has hemolytic anemia secondary to spherocytosis. Patients with this diagnosis often have gallstones due to the breakdown of the RBCs. Splenomegaly is also a common physical examination finding.

24. **C. This patient has PCOS. Criteria for diagnosis include menstrual irregularity as a result of anovulation or oligoovulation and evidence of hyperandrogenism. Laboratories may reveal a high LH to FSH ratio (2–3:1 in PCOS). Women with PCOS also have a slightly elevated testosterone level (rarely >100 ng/dL), with a normal DHEAS level. Treatment for PCOS includes weight loss and drugs that improve insulin resistance. Both of these modalities have been shown to reduce ovarian androgen production and in turn lead to regular ovulatory menstrual cycles. A low-dose estrogen/progestin oral contraceptive can be used to help protect the endometrium from chronic, unopposed estrogen secretion if the patient does not desire pregnancy. Spironolactone is used for improvement of the hirsutism, which decreases both androgen secretion and action. Dilation and curettage are performed in patients in whom there is a high suspicion of endometrial cancer, but in whom an office endometrial biopsy sample is either inconclusive or difficult to obtain. Patients with PCOS are at higher risk than the general population for endometrial cancer because of unopposed estrogen stimulation. However, it is not routine to perform biopsies on women solely because they are diagnosed with PCOS.**

    A. This patient has some evidence of hirsutism on physical examination by the terminal hair growth on the upper lip and sides of the face. This is associated with menstrual irregularity; therefore, it requires workup. (If she had normal menstrual cycles, no workup would be required.) The physical examination does not reveal male pattern baldness, acne (obviously not specific), male musculature, deepening of the voice, or clitoromegaly, all of which would point to more severe virilization. The testosterone is minimally elevated, which is consistent with PCOS. (Much higher values are seen in testosterone-secreting tumors.) Therefore, a testosterone-secreting tumor of the ovary is not likely.

    B. This patient has a normal DHEAS level, which is the testosterone precursor hormone secreted by the adrenal gland. It should be significantly elevated in patients with adrenal tumors that are responsible for virilizing symptoms.

    D. CAH usually manifests in infancy as ambiguous genitalia or salt wasting, and is due to enzyme deficiencies in the normal synthesis of adrenal hormones. Late-onset adrenal hyperplasia does exist, however, due to partial enzyme deficiencies that may manifest after adolescence. Late-onset adrenal hyperplasia may account for 5% to 25% of women who present with hirsutism and oligomenorrhea, depending on the population. Patients may have normal or mildly elevated DHEA levels and urinary 17-ketosteroids. This is probably the second most likely choice, but PCOS is a much more common diagnosis. To completely rule out late-onset CAH in this patient, levels of precursors of cortisol synthesis, such as 17-hydroxyprogesterone and 17-hydroxypregnenolone, should be checked. These levels will increase substantially after an ACTH challenge, which confirms the diagnosis.

E. Some patients have ethnic predispositions to hairiness, such as Mediterranean populations. Drugs such as phenytoin and minoxidil may cause hypertrichosis, but it is usually diffuse and not in a male pattern distribution. It is important to ask patients about the timing of onset of hirsutism and whether or not they have patterns of hair growth similar to their female relatives. Sudden, new onset of hirsutism that is not around the time of puberty is suspicious for adrenal or ovarian tumor. This patient had the onset of her hirsutism around the time of puberty and it worsened with significant weight gain, which is often seen in PCOS disease.

25. **D. Lead time bias occurs when a screening test increases the length of time from diagnosis to death, but does not affect survival outcomes.**

A. Selection bias occurs when screening participants do not reflect the characteristics of the whole population to be screened.

B. Length bias occurs when screening tests preferentially detect disease in asymptomatic cancers. This may cause misleading outcome comparisons of screened versus nonscreened cancers.

C. Overdiagnosis is an extreme form of length bias. This refers to a phenomenon by which some asymptomatic cancers that are detected by screening have a slow enough course that patients would die from other causes prior to becoming symptomatic from their cancer.

E. Effective screening tests are ones that detect diseases that have an acceptable form of treatment, which will modify the disease outcome.

26. **A. Breast-conserving lumpectomy followed by radiation therapy has been shown to have the same survival rates as modified radical mastectomy in several randomized trials. This has changed the approach to breast cancer treatment.**

B. If mastectomy is indicated, then a modified radical mastectomy is done. Indications for mastectomy would include a tumor that is >7 cm in size (or smaller if the breast is smaller, which makes it harder to obtain clean margins,) two or more primary tumors, or history of breast irradiation. Radical mastectomy (removal of the pectoralis muscles in addition to the breast tissue) is no longer performed.

C. Radiation therapy is part of the breast-conserving approach. It always follows lumpectomy.

D. Chemotherapy has been shown in several randomized trials to decrease incidence of recurrence in the same breast. The decision to have adjuvant chemotherapy is based on tumor size, nodes affected, and estrogen receptor susceptibility.

E. Tamoxifen is a selective estrogen receptor modulator. Use of tamoxifen has improved survival and rates of recurrence in patients with estrogen receptor–positive tumors.

27. **B. Small cell carcinoma can produce Cushing syndrome by ectopic production of ACTH. It can also produce SIADH by ectopic production of ADH. Small cell carcinoma is heavily associated with smoking and is one of the lung cancers that is usually centrally located, along with squamous cell cancer. The patient displays evidence of excess cortisol: moon facies, truncal obesity with extremity wasting, easy bruising, hypertension, and diabetes mellitus.**

A. Adenocarcinoma of the lung is associated with digital clubbing and can also cause SIADH. It does not produce Cushing syndrome. It is the most common lung cancer in women and nonsmokers. It is usually peripheral in location.

C. Large cell carcinoma can produce ectopic secretion of hCG. This can produce gynecomastia and nipple discharge.

D. Squamous cell carcinoma can cause hypercalcemia due to ectopic production of PTH-rP. It can also be associated with SIADH. It is not associated with Cushing syndrome.
E. Non-Hodgkin lymphoma can present with a hilar mass, but it is not associated with the production of ACTH as a paraneoplastic syndrome.

28. **B. This patient has evidence of spinal cord compression, which is a medical emergency and should be treated immediately with high-dose steroids. MRI should also be performed, but steroids should be given immediately.**

A. An MRI of the spine should be obtained and a neurosurgeon consulted. However, administration of steroids should not be delayed due to the MRI.
C. A serum PSA may be helpful to detect reoccurrence of the prostate cancer, but is not the next step in management.
D. Radiation therapy may be part of the treatment regimen in this patient, and it is reasonable to consult radiation oncology urgently; however, steroids should be started while you are arranging for radiation treatment.
E. Pain management is important in patients with cancer. This should be addressed in this patient after the emergent issues of spinal cord compression are evaluated.

29. **E. Erythema multiforme is a rash that is usually characterized by target-shaped plaques. The center of the target may blister because of necrosis. The rash often involves the palms and soles. This rash may be seen with mycoplasma infections, acute coccidioidomycosis, and reactions to drugs.**

A. Stevens-Johnson syndrome is a severe form of erythema multiforme and is fairly rare. In extreme cases, it is known as toxic epidermal necrolysis. It involves the skin and mucous membranes. It usually involves more body surface area than erythema multiforme. It may also have internal organ involvement and constitutional symptoms. Like erythema multiforme, it is self-limited, but it does have a high mortality rate.
B. Rocky Mountain spotted fever may present with a rash that involves the palms and soles. However, these patients usually have a travel history as well as fevers, chills, myalgias, headache, and other constitutional symptoms. These systemic complaints usually precede the rash. The lesions are usually red, blanchable macules and not target shaped like those of erythema multiforme.
C. Secondary syphilis is another one of the few rashes that may involve the palms and soles. Patients will usually have a history of a painless chancre 3–12 weeks prior to the rash. Not all patients, however, will recall this primary phase. The lesions are usually symmetric but are not target shaped like the lesions of erythema multiforme.
D. Erythema nodosum is a rash characterized by tender nodules usually affecting the knees, shins, and ankles. It may be seen with acute coccidioidomycosis, sarcoidosis, and inflammatory bowel disease.

30. **B. Herpes simplex virus infection is the most common etiology for erythema multiforme. It usually occurs after the herpes simplex virus eruption. In this patient, the healing cold sore on his lip was likely a stomatitis due to herpes simplex virus. This stomatitis probably incited the eruption of erythema multiforme. Interestingly, despite the close relationship between herpes simplex virus and varicella zoster virus, neither varicella nor herpes zoster is associated with erythema multiforme.**

A. *Treponema pallidum* is the etiologic agent for syphilis. This rash is not syphilis.
C. Idiosyncratic drug reactions may result in Stevens-Johnson syndrome, which is the more severe form of erythema multiforme.
D. *Rickettsia rickettsiae* is the etiologic agent for Rocky Mountain spotted fever, which this patient does not have.
E. Sarcoidosis is associated with erythema nodosum, and not erythema multiforme.

31. **B. Bullous pemphigoid is an autoimmune disorder that presents as a chronic bullous eruption most commonly in patients over the age of 60. It often starts as an erythematous lesion that resembles urticaria, and has variable pruritus. The lesions then evolve into firm bullae that are not easily ruptured. The diagnosis is made clinically and confirmed by biopsy. The lesions show the described histopathology and immunopathology.**

A. Dermatitis herpetiformis is an intensely pruritic "burning" vesicular rash that occurs on the extensor surfaces and buttocks. It is associated with celiac sprue disease. Immunofluorescence detects IgA deposits.
C. Pemphigus vulgaris is an autoimmune bullous skin disease that involves the oral mucosa in 90% of patients. Immunofluorescence shows deposits of IgG on the surface of keratinocytes.
D. Pemphigoid gestationis is a rare, subepidermal blistering disease of women during pregnancy and around the time of delivery.
E. Nikolsky *sign* (not disease) is seen in many bullous skin diseases. It consists of putting manual pressure to the skin and eliciting a separation of the epidermis. This will induce or extend a bullous lesion.

32. **A. The mainstay of treatment for bullous pemphigoid is glucocorticoids. These are usually given systemically, although patients with minimal disease can sometimes be treated with topical glucocorticoids.**

B. Although the disease may be diffuse and cause loss of significant skin integrity, the mortality rate is low, even in the absence of treatment.
C. Oral mucosal lesions are found in 10%–40% of patients.
D. Approximately 70% of these patients have circulating antibodies that bind the epidermal basement membrane, but there is no correlation between the titer of the autoantibody and the disease activity.
E. The bullous lesions usually heal without scarring unless they are traumatized or infected.

33. **D. This patient has a cluster headache. Cluster headaches are more commonly seen in males than females. Typical age of onset is in the twenties and thirties. The headaches are characterized by recurrent unilateral headaches that come on suddenly and intensely. The pain is usually around or behind the eye and reaches very high intensity shortly after onset of the headache. Many patients describe an intermittent sharp or stabbing quality. Often the patient will have rhinorrhea and tearing on the same side of the face as the headache. The headaches can occur daily or several times daily for a number of weeks (thus the name *cluster*) and last 1–2 hours. The headaches can be triggered by alcohol. The only treatment that has been useful to abort the headache is oxygen. Most medications by mouth are not helpful because the headache is usually over by the time the medication is absorbed.**

A. Ibuprofen and other NSAIDs are not helpful in cluster headaches.
B. The patient has symptoms consistent with cluster headache and normal physical examination results. There is no evidence of an intracranial lesion and therefore no indication for a CT of the head.
C. This patient does not a have a fever or any other associated symptoms to indicate meningitis. A lumbar puncture is not indicated.
E. Sumatriptan is used in treatment of migraine headache. This patient has a cluster headache.

34. **A. The neurologic symptoms associated with vitamin B_{12} deficiency usually begin with paresthesias of the feet, which may be distressing to patients as they persist. Over time, there is a loss of vibration sense greater in the legs than arms, and eventual proprioception loss due to involvement of the large nerve fibers. At an early stage, the Achilles reflex may be diminished or absent, but it also may be increased. Motor deficits most often involve the legs and may include weakness and spasticity. Neurologic symptoms may occur without any hematologic abnormality. This patient has involvement of the peripheral nerves of the feet with sensory symptoms and mild motor weakness as well as involvement of the posterior columns of the spinal cord (as evidenced by the positive Rhomberg test result), resulting in loss of proprioception. A vitamin B_{12} level is the next most appropriate test to evaluate this patient's complaints. If the vitamin B_{12} level is in the low normal range, a methylmalonic acid and total serum homocysteine level should be ordered. If these two values are elevated, it can help to confirm a relative vitamin B_{12} deficiency that is the source of his neuropathy.**

B. Polyneuropathies secondary to paraproteinemias are similar to diabetic polyneuropathy in that they are usually slowly progressive over 5–10 years. There are two specific chronic demyelinating neuropathies that you should know about: (1) Monoclonal IgM protein that reacts with a myelin-associated glycoprotein in peripheral nerve myelin. This neuropathy is more sensory than motor and should not affect the dorsal columns, as in our patient. (2) Monoclonal IgG or IgA antibodies that do not react with a myelin-associated glycoprotein in the peripheral nerve myelin. This neuropathy is predominantly motor, and may eventually produce severe limb wasting. Sensory and autonomic findings are rare in this neuropathy. It is good to realize that paraproteinemias may cause peripheral neuropathies, but in our patient, vitamin B_{12} deficiency is the most likely cause.

C. The peripheral neuropathy associated with chronic lead toxicity in adults is a motor neuropathy resulting in a paralysis of the wrist and foot extensors. This results in a "wrist and foot drop" scenario. Patients also may develop abdominal pain, headache, irritability, fatigue, and a normocytic, normochromic anemia with basophilic stippling.

D. Unlike vitamin B_{12} deficiency, folate deficiency does not cause any neurologic sequelae, but rather a megaloblastic anemia, diarrhea, cheilosis, and glossitis. It is seen most commonly in alcoholics because of their generally poor nutrition and because alcohol itself interferes with the metabolism of folate.

E. The appropriate workup when evaluating a patient with a peripheral neuropathy is to do blood work to evaluate for diabetes, vitamin B_{12} deficiency, paraproteinemia, or a microscopic nerve-related vasculitis. The tests ordered should include a fasting blood sugar, serum vitamin B_{12} level (with eventual methylmalonic acid and homocysteine levels), serum immunoelectrophoresis and quantitative immunoglobulins, and a sedimentation rate, respectively. The next test to order is EMG and a nerve conduction study. These tests can help to determine if the neuropathy is due to myelin degeneration or axonal problems. There is no need to evaluate the CSF in the usual workup of a peripheral neuropathy.

35. **C. MG is a relatively common disorder occurring in approximately 1 in 7500 persons. It is more common in women than men, with a 3:2 predominance. Classically, myasthenia presents with complaints of muscle weakness and fatigability. In MG, the patient is producing antibodies that destroy the acetylcholine receptor at the muscle side of the neuromuscular junction. These antibodies are approximately 85% sensitive and 100% specific for the diagnosis of MG. It is the best single test to evaluate for MG, but because of the 85% sensitivity, it is possible that approximately 15% of patients who do not have positive antibodies still have the disease. It is therefore a diagnosis made by a combination of tests, including EMG and repetitive nerve stimulation and tensilon testing.**

A. A tensilon test is done by giving the patient an acetylcholinesterase inhibitor and looking for improvement in the muscle strength. Acetylcholinesterase inhibitors allow the acetylcholine to be in the neuromuscular junction longer, which causes a better muscle contraction. This test can be subjective and can be difficult to interpret. It is usually done in combination with other more objective tests to make the diagnosis of MG.

B. A nerve conduction study with repetitive nerve stimulation can be helpful to see the decrease in muscle contraction amplitude with repetitive stimulation of the nerve, which is classic for MG. This test may be negative in patients with myasthenia that affects ocular muscles only.

D. A single-fiber EMG is an extremely sensitive test for the diagnosis of MG, but it is not specific for myasthenia. This test can be abnormal in patients with neuropathies, ALS, and other nervous system disorders, in addition to myasthenia.

E. A muscle biopsy is not done in the evaluation of MG.

36. **A. Thymic abnormalities occur in 75% of patients with MG. Neoplastic change (thymoma) occurs in approximately 15% of patients, with a higher incidence in patients over age 40. It is important to do imaging of the anterior mediastinum in patients who are diagnosed with MG to evaluate for that possibility.**

B. There is no reason to order a colonoscopy in patients who are diagnosed with MG, because there is no associated risk for colon cancer.

C. Approximately 3%–8% of patients with MG will have associated hyperthyroidism that may exacerbate their problem of muscle weakness. Thyroid function tests should be ordered in patients who are diagnosed with MG to evaluate for that possibility.

D. A DEXA scan is also a reasonable test to order in a patient who is diagnosed with MG (but it is not the first test to order), because the treatment will involve placing the patient on prolonged courses of glucocorticoids. This will put the patient at risk for osteopenia and osteoporosis. According to the American College of Rheumatology, a baseline DEXA scan should be ordered on all patients who are going to be on >10 mg of prednisone per day for 3 months or longer. She should also be placed on appropriate calcium and vitamin D supplementation when she begins the steroid regimen.

E. There is no correlation with urinalysis abnormalities and MG except that some patients with MG will also have other autoimmune diseases such as rheumatoid arthritis and lupus. A thorough history and physical examination should be performed with a good review of systems to evaluate for that possibility.

37. **B. Phenytoin hypersensitivity reaction is a cutaneous reaction that usually occurs 1–3 weeks after starting the drug. It manifests with fever, a diffuse erythematous cutaneous eruption that may eventually become purpuric, lymphadenopathy, leukocytosis, hepatitis, and sometimes nephritis. It resolves with cessation of the drug and the administration of systemic glucocorticoids. It is important to identify this syndrome, because patients will have recurrence upon drug rechallenge, and there is significant cross-reactivity with other antiepileptic drugs.**

A. Approximately 50%–70% of patients with HIV have an acute clinical syndrome 1–3 weeks after the primary infection. This syndrome is composed of, but not limited to, the following symptoms: fever, pharyngitis, lymphadenopathy, arthralgia and myalgia meningitis, a blanchable, erythematous maculopapular rash, and mucocutaneous ulceration. These symptoms are similar to those seen with mononucleosis, and to our described patient. However, the proximity of his symptoms to the initiation of dilantin therapy, and the characteristics of the rash (the nonblanchable component), should make you worry about hypersensitivity to dilantin.

C. CMV is a herpes virus that causes variable clinical presentations depending on the age and immune status of the person infected. In late adolescence or early adulthood, CMV is often transmitted sexually, and patients with normal immune systems may present with a mononucleosis type syndrome, similar to EBV infection. The hallmark of both CMV and EBV infection (although not specific for it) is the presence of atypical lymphocytes in the peripheral smear, which are activated CD8 T lymphocytes. Again, the proximity of the phenytoin use should make you more suspicious of a drug reaction.

D. Bacillary angiomatosis is an infection in immunocompromised patients (usually those with AIDS) that is caused by the same organism that causes catscratch disease in immunocompetent patients: *Bartonella henselae.* Bacillary angiomatosis of the skin usually presents as a lesion that is nodular, violet to red-brown, and ulcerated. It resembles Kaposi sarcoma. Patients with disseminated disease may not have any of the skin findings. Their symptoms may include fever, abdominal pain, weight loss, and malaise. Involvement of the liver or spleen may cause bacillary peliosis hepatis, which is the same vascular nodule that involves these organs. It may be seen on CT of the abdomen.

E. B-cell lymphoma can present with fever and lymphadenopathy, but it usually does not present with a diffuse erythematous rash and an elevated WBC count with a left shift. The other mentioned choices are more likely, and the best answer is the phenytoin hypersensitivity reaction.

38. **C. Valproic acid is a nonaromatic antiepileptic drug that is safe to use in patients with hypersensitivity to phenytoin. The phenytoin hypersensitivity reaction is seen in patients with an inherited deficiency of an enzyme called epoxide hydrolase. This enzyme is required for the breakdown of a toxic metabolite formed by the metabolism of phenytoin.**

A, B, E. There is cross-reactivity with other aromatic anticonvulsants such as carbamazepine, phenobarbital, and felbamate, and these drugs should not be used in patients with the hypersensitivity.

D. Phosphenytoin is phosphorylated, water-soluble form of phenytoin that can be given intravenously. It is metabolized into phenytoin and is therefore obviously contraindicated.

39. **D. This patient has an unknown immune status against *Clostridium tetani,* because he is unsure if he has ever received a tetanus primary series. (Most people have received their primary series as children.) The wound is high risk because it is a puncture wound. Other high-risk wounds include lacerations or abrasions that occur outdoors and are contaminated with organic materials, or necrotic-appearing wounds. Every patient who presents with such a wound should be asked about tetanus vaccinations. If the patient has never had a primary series, then it should be begun at that visit. However, it will take too long for the patient to develop antibodies if he currently has an infection with *C. tetani.* Therefore, he must also receive tetanus immune globulin as well, in a separate IM site. The primary series for adults consists of three doses: the first and second doses are given 4–8 weeks apart, and the third dose is given 6–12 months after the second dose. If the patient has had a tetanus primary series in the past, then immune globulin does not need to be given. If it has been >10 years since the patient had a booster tetanus toxoid immunization, then it must be repeated at this visit.**

A, B, C, E. See explanation for D.

40. **C. This patient has drug-induced lupus secondary to INH therapy. Other drugs that can cause this include hydralazine, phenothiazines, procainamide, and beta blockers. Patients with drug-induced lupus usually have antibodies to histone. The absence of antihistone antibodies virtually excludes the diagnosis of drug-induced lupus (i.e., they are good for ruling out drug-induced lupus). Patients who have drug-induced lupus usually have no CNS or kidney involvement. They also usually do not have other serologic markers consistent with SLE, such as hypocomplementemia and anti-dsDNA antibodies.**

A, B, D, E. These results would not be expected. See explanation for C.

41. **C. Of all the serologic markers that are associated with SLE, most do not correlate with the level of disease activity. However, levels of anti-dsDNA antibodies are usually increased, and complement levels are decreased during acute exacerbations of SLE. Therefore, elevated levels of anti-dsDNA antibodies with hypocomplementemia would be suggestive of an acute flare-up of SLE.**

A, B, D, E. Levels of ANA, as well as anti-Ro and anti-La antibodies, do not correlate with disease activity. Levels of anti-ss DNA are elevated in many diseases and are not useful for measuring disease activity. ANA, Anti-SSA (Ro), and anti-SSB (La) levels may be useful in the initial workup of a suspected case of SLE, but they do not warrant repeat analysis during acute flare-ups.

42. **B. Anti-SSA (Ro) antibodies have been associated with the development of neonatal lupus syndrome. The most frightening complication associated with this is congenital complete heart block. These antibodies are passively transferred to the fetus in utero and may persist in the fetal circulation for up to 6 months after birth. As the circulating antibodies are cleared from the infant, the symptoms associated with them also decrease.**

A, E. Anti-dsDNA and anti-Smith antibodies can be helpful in the initial workup of a patient with suspect SLE, but their presence does not incur an increased risk for developing neonatal lupus.

C. ANA with speckled pattern is nonspecific and has no association with the development of neonatal lupus.

D. Antihistone antibodies are helping in distinguishing SLE from drug-induced lupus, but are not associated with the development of neonatal lupus.

43. **D. This patient has several clinical features consistent with SLE. In order to make the diagnosis, a patient must have 4 or more of the following 11 criteria: photosensitivity, hematologic changes (anemia, neutropenia, thrombocytopenia), kidney disease, symmetric arthritis, malar rash, discoid rash, oral lesions, serositis, positive ANA, anti-dsDNA or anti-Smith antibodies, or CNS involvement (seizures or psychosis). She already has three of these criteria before doing any further testing (photosensitivity, anemia, ANA positivity). Of all the antibodies that can be tested for in the workup of SLE, ANA has the highest sensitivity (95%–97%). However, it has a low specificity. (In other words, when it is negative, you have practically excluded the diagnosis. However, its presence does not rule in the diagnosis.) Anti-dsDNA and anti-Smith antibodies are both very specific (near 100%) for SLE**

(i.e., if they are positive, your patient most likely has SLE). Yet, they are not very sensitive—as many as 25%–60% of patients with SLE will be negative for these antibodies. So, the ANA is a good screening test for SLE, and the anti-dsDNA and anti-Smith are good tests for confirming the diagnosis. Anti-SSA (Ro) and anti-SSB (La) antibodies have low sensitivity and low specificity for SLE, but are good for prognostic reasons and should be checked. Antihistone antibodies are usually found in drug-induced lupus, not in SLE.

A, B, C, E. See explanation for D.

44. **C. Before starting a patient on any new medication, the health-care provider should be familiar with the possible adverse effects associated with that drug. There are numerous adverse effects associated with chronic or frequent corticosteroid use. These include, but are not limited to, skin thinning with purpura, acne, striae, hypertrichosis, weight gain, buffalo hump, moon facies, hirsutism, truncal obesity, cataracts, glaucoma, premature atherosclerosis, peripheral insulin resistance, hyperinsulinemia, gastritis, ulcer formation, GI bleeding, pancreatitis, fatty liver, fluid retention, hypertension, kaliuresis, azotemia, metabolic alkalosis, menstrual irregularities, infertility, osteoporosis, AVN, muscle weakness, psychosis, euphoria, depression, immunosuppression, growth retardation (children), and hyperglycemia.**

    A, B, D, E. These are not adverse effects of prednisone. See explanation for C.

45. **B. Patients on chronic corticosteroid use are at increased risk for developing AVN of the femur and humerus. Trauma and alcohol use have both been implicated in the development of AVN as well. As many as one in three patients on chronic steroid therapy will develop AVN, so one should have a low threshold for imaging these patients when they present with joint pain. The sensitivity of MRI (near 90%) is much superior to that of plain x-rays or bone scan, making it the best choice for the diagnosis of AVN.**

    A. Although the initial imaging test to perform in a case of suspected AVN is plain film x-rays (AP and frog-leg lateral) of the hip, they are often normal early in the course of the disease. It may take several months before any changes are seen on plain x-rays.

    C. A bone scan can be useful in patients with unilateral symptoms and negative plain films; however, it is not nearly as sensitive as MRI.

    D. Joint aspiration with synovial fluid analysis would be indicated if there was concern for septic arthritis. Although she may be at risk for developing septic arthritis since she is relatively immunosuppressed from her steroid therapy, septic arthritis does not usually present with insidious onset and such an indolent course. In addition, patients with septic arthritis classically have pain with passive midrange motion of the joint.

    E. Bone biopsy is the gold standard but it is invasive and should not be required to make the diagnosis because of the sensitivity and specificity of MRI in a symptomatic patient.

46. **A. This patient fits the clinical presentation of a patient with bronchiectasis. Bronchiectasis is a consequence of inflammation and destruction of the bronchial wall. It results in dilated airways. These airways often are filled with thick, purulent material. Bronchiectasis has many possible inciting causes that may be infectious or noninfectious. Recurrent pulmonary infections may occur in patients with bronchiectasis, and these patients are particularly susceptible to *Pseudomonas aeruginosa*.**

    B. *Streptococcus pneumoniae* is not usually an organism causing infections in patients with bronchiectasis, although these patients may be colonized with this organism. In addition, *S. pneumoniae* is not one of the more common organisms associated with inciting bronchiectasis.

    C. *Mycoplasma pneumoniae* is not an organism associated with infections in patients with bronchiectasis, nor is it an organism associated with causing bronchiectasis.

    D. *Staphylococcus aureus* is not commonly associated with recurrent infections associated with bronchiectasis. It is, however, a potential cause of bronchiectasis due to its necrotizing nature.

    E. *Aspergillus* organisms are not commonly associated with infections in bronchiectasis. *Aspergillus* organisms may incite bronchiectasis. The mechanism, however, is not destruction from infection. Rather, it is an immune response to the fungus, which results in inflammation and destruction of bronchial walls.

47. **B. Pregnant women who develop varicella infection after 20 weeks' gestation are at risk for developing varicella pneumonia. Therefore, it is recommended that pregnant women at 20 weeks' gestation or more be treated with antiviral medications for varicella infection if they present within 24 hours of onset.**

A. Varicella virus may result in hepatitis and other manifestations of visceral dissemination, but this is not usually seen in pregnancy. Rather, it is seen in patients, usually children, with hematologic malignancies or with solid tumors being treated with chemotherapy.

C. Cellulitis is a possible complication that may occur with varicella. It results from a superinfection of a lesion with skin flora. This complication, however, may occur in any patient with varicella infection, and not just pregnant women.

D. Shingles is a late complication of varicella virus, which may occur in anyone who develops the infection. It results from reactivation of the virus, which, after primary infection, persists in the neurons of sensory ganglia in a dormant state. It is not a complication unique to pregnancy.

E. Postherpetic neuralgia is a complication of shingles or reactivated varicella virus. It is not a complication of primary varicella infection.

48. **D. Postnasal drainage. Postnasal drainage is the most common cause of a chronic cough. A chronic cough is one that lasts at least 3 weeks. It is usually not productive and is usually not associated with other symptoms. Patients may complain of postnasal drainage or rhinorrhea but not always. Treatment is with decongestants. If no improvement is seen, evaluation for other causes of chronic cough should be undertaken.**

A. Cough variant asthma is the second most common cause of chronic cough. Patients may not note any wheezing or shortness of breath. The cough is worse at night. Definitive diagnosis is made with a methacholine challenge test. Treatment is with inhaled corticosteroids and bronchodilators.

B. GERD is the third most common cause of a chronic cough. It may be difficult to diagnose, because patients may not complain of heartburn or other symptoms of gastroesophageal reflux. Like asthma, the cough caused by GERD is worse at night in the supine position. Treatment is with lifestyle modification (avoiding chocolate and other relaxants of the LES, raising the head of the bed, avoiding large meals before bedtime, etc.) and PPIs. Patients with atypical symptoms of GERD such as a chronic cough often require a higher dose and longer duration of treatment with PPIs than patients who simply have heartburn.

C. Use of ACE inhibitors may result in a chronic cough. It is not one of the most common causes of chronic cough but it may occur in 3%–20% of patients taking ACE inhibitors. It is a class effect, so if a patient develops a cough on one ACE inhibitor, all ACE inhibitors will have the same effect. Patients with a chronic cough who are on an ACE inhibitor should discontinue the medication for several weeks. It may take up to 4 weeks for the cough to resolve. If the cough does not resolve after 4 weeks, evaluation for other causes of a chronic cough should be performed.

E. TB may cause a cough that lasts longer than 3 weeks. However, this is usually a productive cough and is associated with other symptoms such as fevers, night sweats, and weight loss, which prompt the patient to seek medical attention. A chronic cough is not usually productive and is not usually associated with other symptoms.

49. **B. Aseptic meningitis is used to describe the condition in which a patient has evidence of meningeal irritation, but cultures from the CSF fail to reveal an organism. There are many causes of aseptic meningitis, with viral etiologies being one of the most common. Other causes, such as medications, fungal infections, malignancies, and autoimmune processes, can also cause aseptic meningitis. The CSF analysis can often give the examiner an initial idea as to whether or not the patient actually has meningitis and if it is bacterial or nonbacterial in nature. The parameters that are routinely tested on CSF are cell count with differential, protein, and glucose levels, Gram stain, and culture. Meningitis is characterized by the appropriate clinical findings and an elevated WBC count in the CSF. The differential can be helpful in sorting out bacterial versus possible viral causes. A high proportion of neutrophils raises concern about a potential bacterial cause, and a predominance of lymphocytes is usually**

suggestive of viral causes. However, these findings are not absolute. Protein levels may be normal or mildly elevated in aseptic meningitis, but are usually markedly elevated in bacterial causes. Glucose, which is a major fuel source for bacteria, gets depleted in the CSF in the presence of bacterial infections. With aseptic meningitis, the CSF glucose levels are usually normal. Finally, results of the Gram stain and culture may be positive in bacterial meningitis, but should be negative in aseptic meningitis. This patient had been taking too much ibuprofen, which contributed to his development of aseptic meningitis. His CSF should have showed an elevated WBC count with normal glucose and either normal or slightly elevated protein. Results of his Gram stain and culture should be negative.

A, C, D, E. These results would not support the diagnosis. See explanation for B.

50. **E. Patients with aseptic meningitis should be asked about their exposure to rodents. Approximately 10%–15% of cases of aseptic meningitis may be related to LCMV infection. The virus lives in the urine and feces of rodents, including rats, mice, and hamsters, and is transmitted to humans by direct contact with infected animals or by contaminated surfaces.**

A. Enteroviruses such as coxsackieviruses A and B, echoviruses, and polioviruses are the cause of the majority of cases of aseptic meningitis. The viruses are acquired most commonly in the summer months and are transmitted through the fecal-oral route and respiratory secretions. The majority of cases occur in children and young teenagers, but any age may be affected.

B. NSAIDs are a common drug-related cause of aseptic meningitis. Patients with lupus erythematosus are at higher risk for this complication of NSAID use than other populations.

C. Certain populations such as Filipino and African-American populations are at higher risk than white populations for dissemination of coccidioidomycosis infection. The fungus lives in the soil of endemic areas in the southwest United States and is inhaled. Most patients are able to contain the organism and experience a mild respiratory infection. The above-mentioned ethnicities or those who are immunosuppressed because of steroids or HIV disease are at risk for the fungus becoming disseminated. The organism likes to disseminate to skin, bones, and meninges.

D. Primary HIV may manifest as aseptic meningitis in 10%–25% of patients who are symptomatic.

SETTING 2: OFFICE

Your office is in a primary care generalist group practice located in a physician office suite adjoining a suburban community hospital. Patients are usually seen by appointment. Most of the patients you see are from your own practice and are appearing for regular scheduled return visits, with some new patients as well. As in most group practices, you will often encounter a patient whose primary care is managed by one of your associates; reference may be made to the patient's medical records. You may do some telephone management, and you may have to respond to questions about articles in magazines and on television that will require interpretation. Complete laboratory and radiology services are available.

The next two questions (items 51 and 52) correspond to the following vignette:

A 57-year-old white man presents to your office for a follow-up visit. He has a history of DM for which he is on oral hypoglycemic medications. He has been following his BP at home and reports to you that the readings have been 150–160 mm Hg systolic and 80–90 mm Hg diastolic. On examination today he is found to have a BP of 148/90 mm Hg. There are no other abnormalities on examination. His urine is negative for microalbumin and he has a normal BUN and creatinine.

51. What is the best initial management of this patient?

    A. Advise weight loss and follow-up in 3 months for a recheck of the BP.
    B. Advise a low-salt diet and follow-up in 1 month for a recheck of the BP.
    C. Continue to follow BP as an outpatient without any intervention.
    D. Advise lifestyle modifications including weight loss, exercise, low-salt diet, and start a beta blocker.
    E. Advise lifestyle modifications including weight loss, exercise, low salt diet, and start an ACE inhibitor.

52. What should the target BP be in this patient?

    A. <150/90 mm Hg
    B. <140/90 mm Hg
    C. <130/80 mm Hg
    D. <125/75 mm Hg
    E. There is no defined goal

End of Set

53. A 40-year-old woman recently diagnosed with autosomal-dominant polycystic kidney disease (ADPKD) presents to your office inquiring about other associated risks with this disease. Which of the following is associated with ADPKD?

    A. Cerebral arteriovenous malformations
    B. Hepatic adenomas
    C. Diverticular disease of the colon
    D. Abnormalities of the ocular lens
    E. Bicuspid aortic valve

54. A 31-year-old with lupus nephritis presents to your office following a renal biopsy to discuss the biopsy results. Her BP today is 141/90 mm Hg. On physical examination, a malar rash is noted over her face. She has 1+ pedal edema. Her previous laboratory studies include ANA titer of 1:640 and anti-dsDNA titer of 1:320, and a 24-hour urine protein of 3.2 g. The biopsy reveals diffuse proliferative glomerulonephritis. The treatment option that has been shown to have the most benefit for preserving her renal function is:

    A. Glucocorticoids
    B. Cyclophosphamide
    C. Plasmapheresis, cyclophosphamide, and glucocorticoids
    D. Cyclophosphamide with glucocorticoids
    E. Azathioprine

The next two questions (items 55 and 56) correspond to the following vignette:

A 45-year-old man presents for routine well care. His only complaint is chronic back pain for the past year. He takes atenolol for hypertension and ibuprofen 800 mg three times a day for the back pain. He has no known drug allergies. His examination is notable for BP of 138/77 mm Hg and tenderness to palpation over the lumbosacral paraspinous muscles. Laboratory values are as follows: BUN 27 mg/dL, creatinine 1.7 mg/dL, sodium 135 mEq/L, chloride 110 mEq/L, bicarbonate 18 mEq/L, and urinalysis 0 protein, 25 RBCs, 0 WBCs, and no eosinophils.

55. Which of the following is the most likely diagnosis?

    A. Glomerulonephritis
    B. Acute interstitial nephritis
    C. Nephrotic syndrome
    D. Analgesic nephropathy
    E. Nephrolithiasis

56. Which of the following medications is most associated with tubulointerstitial nephritis?

A. Ibuprofen
B. Atenolol
C. Gentamicin
D. Vancomycin
E. Amphotericin B

End of Set

57. A 55-year-old man with liver disease secondary to chronic hepatitis C comes to your office as a new patient. Baseline laboratory studies reveal a sodium of 128 mEq/L. Which of the following is true regarding the evaluation and treatment of hyponatremia?

A. In hyponatremia caused by SIADH, urine osmolality is typically lower than the serum osmolality.
B. In hyponatremia caused by psychogenic polydipsia, the urine osmolality is inappropriately high.
C. Correction of chronic hyponatremia at a rate of >3 mEq/L per hour may lead to central pontine myelinolysis.
D. Causes of hyponatremia can be divided into volume depleted, euvolemic, and volume expanded.
E. Shifts in water from intracellular to extracellular space do not affect measured sodium levels.

58. A 67-year-old man presents to you for a routine physical examination. He denies any current complaints except that he cracked a tooth and will be going to the dentist tomorrow for repair. His past medical history is significant for hypertension for which he takes hydrochlorothiazide, aortic valve replacement for bicuspid aortic valve, and chronic low back pain for which he uses Tylenol. He is allergic to penicillin. On examination, his BP is 132/74 mm Hg. Prior to going to the dentist the patient should:

A. Take an extra dose of hydrochlorothiazide to lower his BP before the dental procedure.
B. Take clindamycin 600 mg PO 1 hour prior to the dental procedure.
C. Take amoxicillin 2 g PO 1 hour prior to the dental procedure.
D. Avoid Tylenol prior to the dental procedure to decrease the risk for bleeding.
E. Do nothing; the patient is low risk for any complications from the dental procedure.

The next two questions (items 59 and 60) correspond to the following vignette:

During a routine office visit, a new patient asks you about her risks for having a heart attack and what she can do to prevent one. She is a 50-year-old woman with no prior history of known CAD. Her medical problems include hypertension and DM, which have been treated with an ACE inhibitor and metformin. She denies having a history of tobacco abuse or any illicit drug use. Her family history is remarkable only for her father having his first MI at 57 years of age. Two of her sisters have been diagnosed with breast cancer. On examination, she has a BP of 120/80 mm Hg. Her physical examination results are completely within normal limits.

59. According to the NCEP, which of the following are risk factors for the development of CAD in this patient that help you to calculate her LDL goal?

A. Fasting triglycerides >200 mg/dL
B. Age of 50 years
C. BP 120/80 mm Hg on treatment
D. Family history of father with first MI at age 57 years
E. BMI >30

60. You advise her to quit smoking, encourage her to maintain good BP and diabetes control, and order a fasting lipid profile. Her total cholesterol is 232 mg/dL, HDL is 63 mg/dL, triglycerides are 151 mg/dL, and LDL is 138 mg/dL. Which of the following statements is correct regarding her LDL level?

A. Although her total cholesterol is elevated, her LDL is at goal and does not require treatment.
B. An HDL level of >60 mg/dL counts as a "negative" risk factor, and its presence removes one risk factor from the total count. Therefore, her LDL level is at goal.
C. Her LDL should be <130 mg/dL and requires treatment with medication.
D. Her LDL should be <100 and requires treatment with medication.
E. Her LDL should be <100 and requires dietary and lifestyle changes.

End of Set

61. A 28-year-old white woman comes to your office with complaints of 5–6 days of loose stools. The stools are watery in nature without any blood. She is having approximately four to five bowel movement per day, and occasionally awakens at night to have diarrhea. She notes intermittent abdominal cramping with the episodes. She denies any recent travel or sick contacts. She was recently treated for a sinus infection with a course of antibiotics. This type of diarrhea is most likely:

A. Osmotic
B. Toxin mediated
C. Inflammatory
D. Dysmotility
E. Secondary to parasites

62. A 26-year-old white man comes for a repeat visit to your office. He is a medical student who was seen previously for a 2- to 3-month history of abdominal pain, fever, and anorexia. At that time he also had noted intermittent diarrhea with weight loss. He was seen by a gastroenterologist who performed a colonoscopy. After the procedure the GI doctor said to the medical student that the findings on colonoscopy looked like Crohn disease, but that they would wait for the biopsy for a confirmatory diagnosis. The pathologic findings suggestive of Crohn disease correlate best with which of the following:

A. Villous flattening, infiltration of lymphocytes
B. Noncaseating granulomas, transmural inflammation, skip lesions
C. Periodic acid-Schiff–positive macrophages
D. Superficial ulcerations from rectum to colon, crypt abscesses
E. Eosinophillic infiltration

63. A 40-year-old white woman comes to your office for a preventative care visit. In general she is doing well without any complaints. She takes no medications. She is active, playing tennis three times weekly. She is trying to cut down on red meats, but finds this difficult when cooking for her husband. She does not smoke, but does enjoy three to four glasses of wine weekly. Her father was diagnosed with colon cancer at age 60. What is (or would have been) the appropriate colon cancer screening recommendation for her?

A. Colonoscopy every 3–5 years, starting at age 30
B. FOBT annually, sigmoidoscopy every 3–5 years, or colonoscopy every 10 years, starting at age 40
C. FOBT and sigmoidoscopy every 3–5 years, colonoscopy every 10 years, starting at age 50
D. Sigmoidoscopy every 1–2 years, starting at age 12
E. FOBT every year, no need for sigmoidoscopy or colonoscopy

64. A 45-year-old African-American woman is referred to your office for elevated liver function test results (AST 75 U/L, ALT 85 U/L, normal albumin, alkaline phosphatase, and bilirubin) without symptoms. She denies any recent travel or IVDA. She denies having any history of autoimmune disorders. She does not take any medications or herbs and denies having any history of tobacco or alcohol abuse. She is not sexually active. Review of systems is otherwise negative. On physical examination the patient is afebrile, with HR of 95, RR of 16, BP of 145/90 mm Hg, and BMI of 35. In general she is notably obese, but in no acute distress. There is no scleral icterus. No jaundice is noted. Lungs are clear and heart sounds are regular. Abdomen is obese, nontender, without appreciable hepatosplenomegaly. The remainder of the examination results are within normal limits. This patient most likely has:

A. Hemochromatosis
B. Wilson disease
C. Nonalcoholic steatohepatitis (NASH)
D. Hepatitis C
E. Autoimmune hepatitis

65. A 35-year-old man comes to your office for initiation of medical care, because he recently moved to the community. On his physical examination, you notice an abnormality of his fingernails, especially of the second and third fingers of both hands (Figure 1-65). The angle between the nailbed and the base of the finger is approximately 190 degrees. When you push down on the distal nailbed and, simultaneously, feel the proximal nailbed with the other hand, the proximal nail "floats" upward. Which of the following disease states is known to be associated with this physical finding?

A. COPD
B. Cystic fibrosis
C. Adenocarcinoma of the colon
D. Hypothyroidism
E. Hemochromatosis

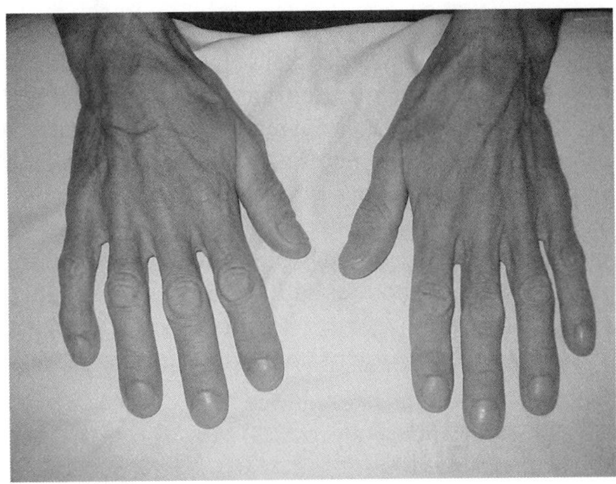

Figure 1-65 • Image Courtesy of Dr. Brenda Shinar, Banner Good Samaritan Medical Center, Phoenix, Arizona.

The following two questions (items 66 and 67) relate to the same clinical scenario:

A 55-year-old man without any known medical problems comes to your office with his wife, complaining of daytime sleepiness. He will fall asleep while watching TV, and has almost gotten into a car accident because of falling asleep at the wheel of the car in the middle of the day. He tells you that he goes to bed at approximately 10 P.M. each night and sleeps a good 8 hours on a regular basis. His wife tells you that he snores so badly that she sleeps in the guest bedroom. She also tells you that she has often witnessed episodes where her husband seemed to stop breathing and then began to struggle for air. He is not taking any medications or herbs and denies any tobacco or alcohol abuse. He also denies having any feelings of sadness or anhedonia. On examination you note the patient is moderately obese with a BMI of 30. Vital signs are within normal limits with the exception of his BP, which is elevated at 150/90 mm Hg. The physical examination is significant for obesity with a neck circumference of 17.5 inches. When the patient opens his mouth, you are able to see only the tongue without visible tonsillar pillars or uvula. The thyroid is not palpable. The rest of the physical examination results are within normal limits.

66. What is the most likely diagnosis?

    A. Hypothyroidism
    B. Narcolepsy
    C. Obstructive sleep apnea (OSA)
    D. Major depressive disorder
    E. Central sleep apnea

67. You send the patient for a formal sleep study evaluation, which confirms your diagnosis. Which of the following treatments should you recommend next?

    A. CPAP
    B. Tracheostomy
    C. Uvulopalatopharyngoplasty
    D. Weight loss
    E. Dental appliance to keep the patients jaw thrusted forward

End of Set

68. A 66-year-old white woman in your practice calls you over the weekend, stating that she lost her prescription eye drops. She was diagnosed with glaucoma 1 month ago. She cannot remember the name of her medication but asks you to call in a prescription. She denies having any current symptoms, including eye pain, nausea, vomiting, or halos. Therapy for glaucoma usually begins with:

    A. Topical beta blockers
    B. Topical ACE inhibitors
    C. Oral carbonic anhydrase inhibitors
    D. Topical calcium channel blockers
    E. Topical cholinergic agonists

69. A 35-year-old white woman who was recently diagnosed as HIV positive comes to your office for her gynecology care. Her menstrual periods began at the age of 12 and she has regular periods. She is currently sexually active and is monogamous, using condoms for birth control. She first had sexual intercourse at the age of 15 and has had eight sexual partners since then. She smokes one pack per day of cigarettes and drinks socially on the weekends. She has had chlamydia once and had genital warts, treated with cautery approximately 2 years ago. Of all the following risk factors, which one puts her at highest risk for cervical neoplasia?

    A. Multiple sex partners
    B. Early age at onset of intercourse
    C. Infection with HPV
    D. HIV positivity
    E. Tobacco use

70. A 60-year-old woman with a history of breast cancer diagnosed 3 years ago comes to your office for her gynecology care. Her cancer was

confined to the breast and she has undergone lumpectomy and radiation therapy and is currently on tamoxifen. Her gynecologic history is significant for menarche at age 14. She had four pregnancies with three live births and one spontaneous miscarriage. She underwent menopause approximately 9 years ago. On physical examination, her BMI is 24. Her vital signs are within normal limits. She has a well-healed scar at the site of her lumpectomy and there are no appreciable breast masses. Her pelvic examination reveals a small amount of dark blood in the vaginal vault, and she tells you that she has had some new spotting that started approximately a week ago. Which of the following is this patient's most significant risk factor for endometrial cancer?

A. Obesity
B. Multiparity
C. Tamoxifen use
D. Late menopause
E. Late menarche

71. A 40-year-old white woman comes to your office for routine physical examination. She is fairly active and reports no history of medical problems. She does not drink, smoke, or take any medications. She has questions regarding her risks for breast cancer and what she can do to screen for it. The patient states that her mother was diagnosed with breast cancer at age 68. She states that she has never had a mammogram and rarely does regular breast self-examinations. Her examination results are within normal limits. Which of the following screening recommendations has been shown to reduce mortality from breast cancer?

A. Annual clinical breast examination and bilateral screening mammography starting at age 40
B. Annual bilateral screening mammography and monthly breast self-examination starting at age 50
C. Only annual bilateral screening mammography starting at age 50 until age 69
D. Only bilateral diagnostic mammography every 2 years until age 69
E. Annual clinical breast examination and bilateral screening mammography every year until the patient has three consecutive negative examination results; then decrease the frequency to every 3 years

72. A 65-year-old Hispanic man comes to your office with concerns over erectile function. He states he had no difficulty obtaining erections until recently. He denies having any recent psychosocial stressors and notes that he will wake up with an erection. He has a past medical history significant for hypertension, which is controlled on a thiazide diuretic. Physical examination is essentially within normal limits, including normal testicular size and positive cremasteric reflex. What is the best treatment option for this man?

A. Vacuum-assisted device
B. Intraurethral alprostadil
C. Sildenafil
D. Testosterone replacement
E. Penile prosthesis

73. A 30-year-old woman comes to your office with complaints of a skin rash on her lower legs that she has noticed for the past 3 weeks while shaving. She has also noted a few nosebleeds, which have occurred spontaneously and have been difficult to stop over the same time period. She has no other complaints of fever or fatigue. On physical examination, her vital signs are normal. She has petechiae on her soft palate and conjunctivae are pink. Her heart, lung, and abdominal examination results are normal. Her lower extremities reveal a nonblanching petechial rash. You suspect ITP. Which of the follow statements is true regarding ITP?

A. Peak age of occurrence is in the third decade.
B. First-line therapy is splenectomy.
C. IVIG has been shown to increase platelet counts in 60%–70% of patients.
D. It is caused by a membrane defect of the platelets.
E. Persistence of thrombocytopenia for more 3 months is considered chronic autoimmune thrombocytopenia.

74. A 35-year-old man comes to your office for a preoperative physical examination. On history he notes easy bruising and gum bleeding. He has no significant prior medical or surgical history and takes no medications. The patient's father required transfusion following a routine hernia repair due to excessive bleeding. Physical examination results are unremarkable. Laboratory values are as follows: hemoglobin 13.8 g/dL, Hematocrit 39%, platelet count 280,000/μL,

PT 11 seconds, aPTT 43 seconds, and bleeding time 20 minutes. Which of the following should be requested for further evaluation?

A. Factor VIII
B. Factor IX
C. Ristocetin cofactor assay
D. Anticardiolipin antibody
E. Fibrinogen level

75. A 55-year-old African-American woman comes to your office with questions regarding her risk factors for osteoporosis. Her past medical history is only significant for hypertension that is well controlled with hydrochlorothiazide. She is postmenopausal and is not on hormone replacement therapy. She has smoked approximately one pack of cigarettes a day for the past 30 years. On physical examination, her BMI is 25 and BP is 120/75 mm Hg. The rest of her physical examination results are within normal limits. Which factor, in addition to her postmenopausal state, puts her at risk for osteoporosis?

A. Ethnicity
B. Tobacco use
C. Hydrochlorothiazide
D. BMI
E. Hypertension

76. A 53-year-old man presents to your office for a routine examination. He was last seen 5 years ago. He has a history of hypertension, but is otherwise well and without complaints. His family history is positive for a father with CAD diagnosed at age 64. There is no family history of colon cancer. Physical examination results are unremarkable. Which of the following is a true statement regarding colon cancer screening for this patient?

A. His colon cancer screening should have started at age 40.
B. A negative FOBT result on rectal examination in the office is adequate for screening, as long as the patient has a normal hemoglobin and iron parameters on blood testing.
C. Colonoscopy every 10 years beginning at age 50 is one accepted form of colon cancer screening—the patient is overdue for screening.
D. If a benign polyp is found on colonoscopy, the patient can be reassured and resume cancer screening with colonoscopy in 10 years.
E. CEA levels are a useful screening tool for colon cancer.

77. A 47-year-old African-American man is referred to your office for further evaluation of an elevated PSA of 8 ng/mL found on a preemployment physical. He is otherwise healthy and has no urinary complaints. A digital rectal examination shows a smooth prostate without enlargement or nodules. What should be the next step in treatment and evaluation?

A. Radical prostatectomy
B. Radiation therapy
C. Transrectal ultrasound-guided biopsy
D. Repeat PSA in 6 months
E. Advise the patient to return for further evaluation if he develops urinary symptoms

78. A 54-year-old man presents to your office to establish care. On physical examination you note an abnormality of his fingernails. You have his wife, with normal nails, place her hand on top of his to reveal the comparison (Figure 1-78). All nails are involved uniformly. Which systemic disease is most commonly associated with this physical finding?

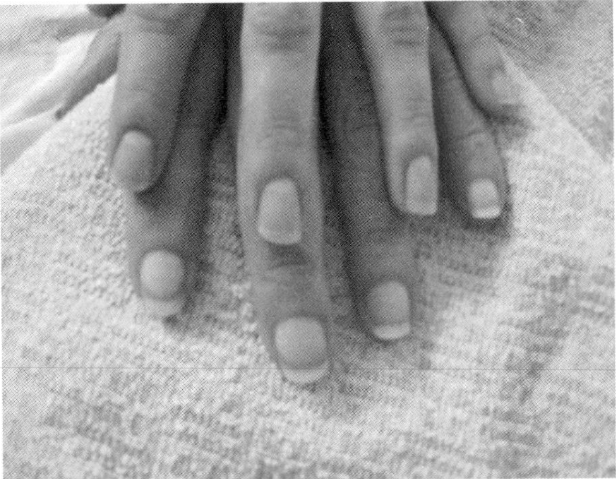

Figure 1-78 • Image Courtesy of Dr. Brenda Shinar, Banner Good Samaritan Medical Center, Phoenix, Arizona.

A. DM
B. Congestive heart failure (CHF)
C. Cirrhosis of the liver
D. Iron deficiency anemia
E. Systemic sclerosis

The next two questions (items 79 and 80) correspond to the following vignette:

A 31-year-old woman presents to your office with complaints of frequent nose bleeds and a skin rash on her lower extremities for the past 2 weeks. On physical examination, her vital signs are normal and she appears nontoxic and well nourished. She has a few petechial lesions on her soft palate and several non-blanching, macular lesions <2 mm in diameter on her lower extremities (Figure 1-79). The remainder of her examination results are normal. Her CBC reveals the following: WBC count of 6000 with a normal differential, hemoglobin of 13 g/dL, hematocrit 40%, platelet count of 30,000/μL.

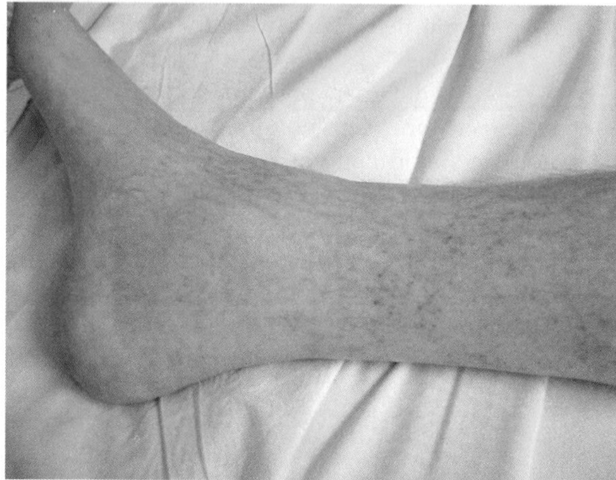

Figure 1-79 • Image Courtesy of Dr. Brenda Shinar, Banner Good Samaritan Medical Center, Phoenix, Arizona.

79. Which of the following is the most likely diagnosis?

A. Drug-induced thrombocytopenia
B. Systemic lupus erythematosus (SLE)
C. HIV infection
D. You cannot make the diagnosis without more information
E. Idiopathic thrombocytopenic purpura (ITP)

80. Once the other diseases have been ruled out and your suspected diagnosis is confirmed, which of the following courses of action is appropriate?

A. Follow the platelet count every month. No intervention unless the patient develops significant bleeding or a platelet count of <10,000/μL.
B. Admit for IVIG therapy now.
C. Refer the patient for splenectomy.
D. Start prednisone 60 mg PO daily for 4–6 weeks, then taper over several weeks.
E. Start a combination of prednisone 20 mg PO daily and a steroid-sparing agent, such as azathioprine, to avoid the steroid side effects.

End of Set

81. A 14-year-old girl comes to your office with complaints of headaches that began approximately 2 months ago and often awake her from sleep. Her mother took her to the emergency room a week ago for the headache and a CT scan was done at that time that was negative for any intracranial pathology. On examination, the patient has normal vital signs. She is obese. Neurologic examination results are normal, but there is papilledema noted on funduscopic examination. You are concerned about possible pseudotumor cerebri. Pseudotumor cerebri is associated with which of the following?

A. Pregnancy and menopause
B. Diplopia with normal funduscopic examination results
C. Normal cerebral spinal fluid opening pressure
D. Medications including vitamin A, tetracycline, and oral contraceptive pills
E. Ventriculomegaly on CT of the head

82. A 36-year-old woman comes to your office with complaints of unusual forgetfulness over the past month. She has episodes where she is in the middle of a sentence and forgets the correct word that she wants to use; or, in the middle of writing a sentence, she will forget how to write the word she plans to use. This has never happened to her before. She has also noted some recent headaches, and has been taking over-the-counter pain relievers. She denies having nausea or vomiting or weight loss. Her neurologic examination results are normal, with the exception of occasional word-finding problems. You order an MRI of the brain that reveals a 5-cm, heterogenous mass in the left temporoparietal lobes. What is the most common primary brain tumor found in adults?

A. Meningioma
B. Pituitary tumor
C. CNS lymphoma
D. Astrocytoma
E. Craniopharyngioma

83. A 31-year-old woman comes to your office telling you that she awakened with a feeling as if her left foot had gone to sleep 3 days ago and the sensation has remained since then. She has no significant past medical history and has never had anything like this happen before. She had her second child 5 months ago after a normal pregnancy and delivery. Her physical examination results are normal, with the exception of decreased sensation to pinprick on the plantar and dorsal surfaces of her foot in a nondermatomal distribution. Reflexes and strength are normal. You order an MRI of the brain, which reveals one gadolinium-enhancing lesion, which is ovoid in shape and approximately 5 mm in size in the periventricular white matter. Which of the following statements is true regarding the diagnosis of this patient?

A. She currently meets criteria for the diagnosis of MS.
B. She would meet criteria for MS if she also had a lumbar puncture that showed oligoclonal IgG bands in the CSF.
C. She would meet criteria for MS if 1 year later she developed transient hemiparesis with a new gadolinium-enhancing lesion on repeat MRI.
D. She would meet criteria for MS if she had oligoclonal bands in the CSF and a delayed wave on visual evoked potentials testing.
E. MS should not be considered in her diagnosis.

84. A 52-year-old woman comes to your office for a new patient visit. She has a history of hypertension that has been well controlled on a thiazide, and hyperlipidemia which is controlled with diet. She has been postmenopausal for the last year and is not on HRT. Her mother, who is 82 years old, has developed Alzheimer dementia over the past 5 years, which has required her to be placed in an assisted-living environment for her safety. Your new patient would like to know what she can do to prevent herself from developing dementia. Which of the following statements is true regarding the prevention of dementia?

A. She should be on estrogen replacement, which has been shown in randomized, controlled trials to prevent dementia.
B. Randomized controlled trials show that statins may help to prevent dementia in addition to their lipid-lowering effects, and she should be placed on one immediately.
C. Prospective cohort studies have reported that higher dietary intake of vitamin E may be associated with a lower risk for Alzheimer disease—you recommend 400 IU of vitamin E every day.
D. Long-term NSAID use has been shown to decrease the risk for Parkinson disease, but doesn't have any effect on the prevention of Alzheimer dementia—you recommend avoidance of NSAIDs.
E. You recommend that the patient begin a strict exercise program, because physical activity has been shown to decrease the risk for Alzheimer dementia.

85. A 65-year-old man with a history of CHF and ventricular tachycardia requiring an implanted defibrillator comes to your office with the complaint of dyspnea on exertion. The dyspnea has been gradual over the past 8 to 10 months, and has been interfering with his usual activities. He used to be able to climb a flight of stairs, and is now only able to walk a short distance in his home. He denies having orthopnea, paroxysmal dyspnea, lower extremity edema, or chest pain. He has had an occasional nonproductive cough. His medications include carvedilol, lisinopril, lasix, digoxin, and amiodarone. Physical examination shows BP 120/70 mm Hg, HR 65, and RR 18, and he is afebrile. He can speak in full sentences at rest and does not appear dyspneic. He has a normal jugular venous pressure. His heart sounds are regular without murmurs or gallops, and his lungs reveal coarse crackles in the bilateral bases on inspiration. His abdomen is benign, and his extremities show no edema or clubbing. Chest x-ray reveals cardiomegaly with diffuse reticulonodular markings in the lower lobes bilaterally. His oxygen saturation is 95% on room air at rest, but as he ambulates around the office, his saturation drops to 85% and he becomes dyspneic. Which of the following tests would be most helpful in making the diagnosis?

A. Left heart catheterization
B. High resolution CT scan of the chest
C. CT angiogram of the chest
D. VQ scan
E. Lower-extremity Doppler scans

The following two questions (items 86 and 87) relate to the same clinical scenario:

A 68-year-old woman presents to your office today to discuss her concerns about developing osteoporosis. She is worried because she remembers her mother's problems with frequent fractures and a "hunch-back" appearance. Her past medical history includes well-controlled hypertension, a recent left calf DVT, and ongoing tobacco abuse. She is postmenopausal and no longer has any vasomotor symptoms such as hot flashes. She has no prior history of fractures. In addition to her mother's osteoporosis and fractures, her family history is significant for a sister with breast cancer. You discuss appropriate diet and exercise, as well as smoking cessation, and you order DEXA to assess her bone mineral density.

86. Which of the following would be most consistent with the diagnosis of osteoporosis in this patient?

    A. T-score of 0
    B. Z-score of −1.0
    C. T-score of −1.5
    D. Z-score of −2.0
    E. T-score of −2.5

87. The DEXA scan you ordered above is consistent with osteoporosis. In addition to smoking cessation, appropriate calcium and vitamin D supplementation, and weight-bearing exercise, which of the following would be the best choice of treatment for this patient?

    A. Alendronate 35 mg once a week
    B. Raloxifene 60 mg daily
    C. Estrogen-progestin replacement
    D. Intranasal calcitonin
    E. Parathyroid hormone 40 µg daily

End of Set

The next three questions (items 88-90) correspond to the following vignette:

A 25-year-old woman presents to your office complaining of dyspnea with exertion. She had a baby 2 years ago without complications and says that for the past year or so, she has noticed a worsening shortness of breath when playing with her son and doing household chores. In the past month, she felt short of breath when doing minimal activities. She denies having cough, fever, night sweats, orthopnea, or weight loss. She has no other medical problems and takes no medications or herbs. She smoked a few cigarettes in high school, but does not currently smoke. She drinks a glass of wine approximately three times a week and has never used drugs. On physical examination, she appears well. Her vital signs are as follows: BP 130/80 mm Hg, HR 90, and RR 15; she is afebrile, and her oxygen saturation is 91% on room air. Her examination results are remarkable for elevated jugular venous pressure, a right ventricular heave, and a loud S_2 heart sound. She has a systolic murmur at the left lower sternal border that increases with inspiration. Her lungs are clear. Her abdomen is benign, and her pulses are equal in all four extremities. ECG (Figure 1-88A) and chest x-ray (Figure 1-88B) are performed.

88. Which of the following is the most likely diagnosis?

    A. Atrial septal defect (ASD)
    B. Primary pulmonary hypertension (PPH)
    C. Idiopathic pulmonary fibrosis
    D. Ventricular septal defect (VSD)
    E. Cardiac tamponade

89. You order an echocardiogram that reveals a pulmonary artery systolic pressure of 90 mm Hg, right atrial and ventricular enlargement, and 3+

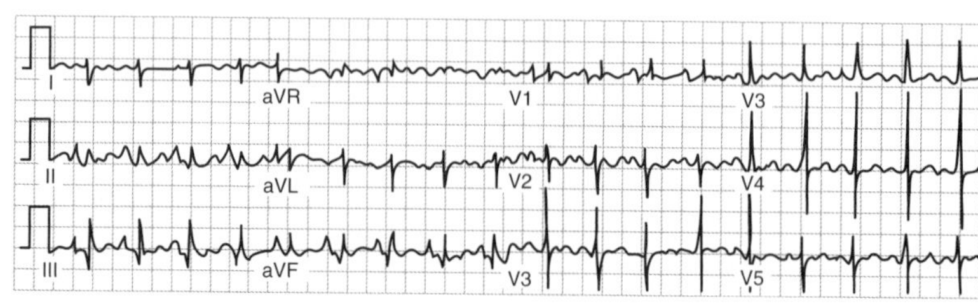

Figure 1-88A • Image Courtesy of Dr. Brenda Shinar, Banner Good Samaritan Medical Center, Phoenix, Arizona.

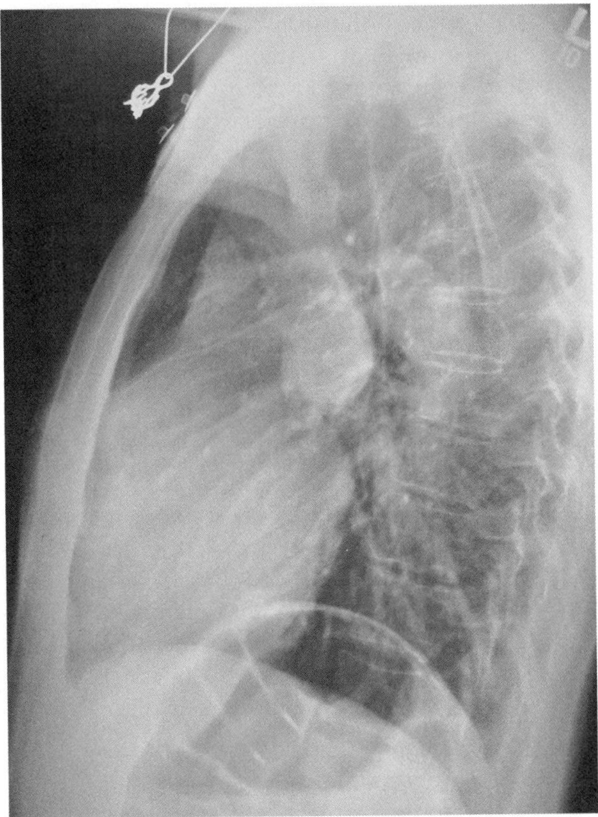

B

Figure 1-88B • Image Courtesy of Dr. Brenda Shinar, Banner Good Samaritan Medical Center, Phoenix, Arizona.

tricuspid regurgitation. There is no evidence of an atrial or ventricular septal defect. Which of the following tests should you order next to evaluate the cause of her disorder?

A. Rheumatoid factor (RF)
B. HIV serology
C. Spirometry
D. Lower-extremity Doppler scans
E. ABG

90. Which of the following statements is true regarding treatment of this patient's disorder?

A. All patients with this disorder should be evaluated with right heart catheterization to assess their response to vasodilator therapies.
B. Oral verapamil is the calcium channel blocker of choice to treat this disorder.
C. Epoprostenol therapy is superior to calcium channel blocker therapy only in patients who are nonresponders to vasodilators on right heart catheterization.
D. Patients with this disorder should be given supplemental oxygen therapy at the time of diagnosis regardless of their oxygen saturation to prevent worsening of their disease.
E. Patients with this disorder should be anticoagulated with warfarin to a goal INR of 3.

End of Set

91. A 42-year-old woman presents to your office with complaints of pain in her fingers when they are exposed to cold. She reports that her fingers turn various colors, including blue, white, and intensely red during these times of exposure. A thorough review of systems is negative, with the exception of some difficulty swallowing. She says she occasionally has the sensation that food is getting stuck in her chest when she tries to swallow. She has no other medical history and takes no medications. Her family history is unremarkable. On examination, you find a well-nourished and well-developed woman in no acute distress. Her vital signs are completely normal. HEENT examination results are unremarkable. Lungs are clear to auscultation, and cardiac examination results are normal. Her abdomen is benign, with no masses, organomegaly, or peritoneal signs. You do not appreciate any color changes in her fingers as she has reported to you. However, the skin covering her fingers does have a tight and shiny appearance. She has no evidence of synovitis on examination. You are suspicious that she has Raynaud disease and may have CREST syndrome. Which of the following antibodies would be most helpful in making the diagnosis?

A. Anti-Jo1 antibodies
B. Anti–smooth muscle antibodies
C. Antimitochondrial antibodies
D. Anti–topoisomerase 1 antibodies
E. Anticentromere antibodies

92. A 25-year-old man comes to your office with complaints of diarrhea, which has been going on for the past week. It is associated with abdominal cramping and bloating and foul-smelling stools. He has not noticed any blood in the stool and has not had fever. Physical examination is normal. Stool studies reveal no occult blood or white cells. Which of the following pathogens is most likely the cause of his diarrhea?

A. *Campylobacter jejuni*
B. *Giardia lamblia*
C. *Salmonella typhi*
D. *Shigella sonnei*
E. *Clostridium difficile*

93. A 28-year-old man was diagnosed with chronic ITP 3 years ago. He has undergone multiple treatments for this illness. He was initially treated with prednisone but did not respond. He was then treated with IVIG, which resulted in some improvement of his platelet counts, but the effects did not last. He is now being referred for splenectomy. Which of the following vaccines should he receive before his splenectomy?

A. Hepatitis A and B
B. *Pneumococcus, Meningococcus,* and *Haemophilus influenzae*
C. Influenza, *Pneumococcus,* and hepatitis A and B
D. *Pneumococcus, Meningococcus,* and hepatitis A and B
E. *Pneumococcus* only

94. A 42-year-old man from Arizona presents to your office with a 9-month history of intermittent cough, chest tightness, and wheezing. His symptoms have become progressively more frequent. The only symptom-free period he can remember was a week-long trip that he took to Hawaii 2 months ago. He thought his symptoms must be due to the dry air since they improved in Hawaii. He has no past medical history. He does not smoke. He is married and works as a baker. His family history is noncontributory. His wife reports he keeps her awake at night with his coughing but that she notices the cough does not seem to be as bad on the weekends. He wants to know if he should buy a humidifier or if he should relocate to a more humid climate. On physical examination his vital signs are normal. Lung examination reveals expiratory wheezes, but the physical examination results are otherwise normal. Chest radiograph is normal. What is the most likely etiology for his symptoms?

A. OSA
B. Emphysema
C. Occupational asthma
D. Chronic pulmonary emboli
E. Coccidioidomycosis

95. A 37-year-old nurse presents for evaluation of an abnormal chest radiograph. Chest radiography was performed as part of an evaluation for a positive TB skin test. The radiograph revealed elevation of the left hemidiaphragm. The patient is healthy and asymptomatic and questions you as to the need for further evaluation. What should you recommend as the next step in evaluation of this finding?

A. CT scan of the thorax
B. Ventilation/perfusion scan
C. Fluoroscopic sniff test
D. Abdominal ultrasonography to look for splenomegaly
E. Thoracentesis

96. A 24-year-old man is seen in your office for complaints of a chronic nonproductive cough for the past 3 months. His vital signs and physical examination results are within normal limits. Chest x-ray reveals a posterior mediastinal mass. Which of the following is the most likely diagnosis?

A. Lymphoma
B. Neurogenic tumor
C. Teratomy
D. Thymoma
E. Thyroid tumor

The next two questions (items 97 and 98) correspond to the following vignette:

A 61-year-old woman presents to your office with complaints of urinary incontinence. She states that over the past several weeks she has had four episodes where she lost control of her bladder. She said that these episodes happened at random times, but thinks they happen more often when she coughs or sneezes. She has not had any other symptoms associated with her incontinence, including fevers, abdominal pain, dysuria, or hematuria. She has no significant medical problems and takes no regular medications. She has only had one surgery, which was a cesarean section for the birth of her fifth child (the others were delivered vaginally). The episodes of incontinence are now affecting her quality of life and she is afraid to go out into public for fear of have incontinence while in a public place. On examination, you find a healthy-appearing woman in no acute distress. Her vital signs are normal and she is afebrile. Her examination results are completely unremarkable, including her genitourinary examination results.

97. What is the most likely cause of her incontinence?

    A. Urge incontinence
    B. Stress incontinence
    C. Overflow incontinence
    D. Urinary tract infection
    E. DM

98. Which of the following is an appropriate approach to her therapy?

    A. Behavioral therapy
    B. Intermittent clean catheterization
    C. Antihyperglycemic therapy
    D. Antibiotic therapy
    E. Pelvic floor muscle exercises

End of Set

99. A 64-year-old man presents to your office with complaints of progressive lower extremity weakness. He first noticed his symptoms about 4 years earlier, but simply thought it was "old age." The weakness has progressively worsened since that time, and now he has difficulty standing from a seated position on occasion. He was evaluated by your partner approximately 3 months ago for similar complaints. At that time he also had nonspecific complaints of myalgias and malaise. Your partner ordered laboratory studies, the results of which showed a CK level of 438 U/L, ESR <20 mm/h, normal CBC, and normal electrolytes. The patient was started on an empiric trial of prednisone at that visit and did not return for follow-up as directed. He is now stating that the prednisone is not helping his weakness, but the myalgias are better. He denies having any skin changes or rashes. He has had no fevers. Social history reveals that he drinks approximately 10 beers every day, but does not smoke or use illegal drugs. He takes no medications except for the prednisone. He has no other significant past medical history. On examination, he is afebrile with normal vital signs. His HEENT examination reveals no abnormalities. His lungs are clear and his heart examination results are normal. Abdominal examination results are benign, and his skin shows no rashes or other lesions. Neurologically, he has marked weakness in the proximal muscle groups (hips and shoulders) with muscle atrophy. He has diminished, symmetric deep tendon reflexes. His cranial nerves are intact. You send him for a muscle biopsy to further evaluate his condition. The biopsy report shows basophilic-rimmed vacuoles within the sarcoplasm of the muscle fibers. What is the most likely diagnosis?

    A. Dermatomyositis
    B. Polymyositis (PM)
    C. Inclusion body myositis (IBM)
    D. Alcohol-induced myopathy
    E. Duchenne muscular dystrophy

100. A 36-year-old Hispanic woman presents to your office with complaints of diffuse itching. She states that this has been a chronic problem. She notes that her skin becomes red and itchy. She has tried a number of detergents and soaps over the past 15 years without improvement of symptoms. She notes that it gets worse with exercise, stress, and hot showers. Physical examination results are within normal limits. What is the cause this patient's itchiness?

    A. Urticaria pigmentosa
    B. Cholinergic urticaria
    C. Familial cold urticaria
    D. Delayed pressure urticaria
    E. Contact dermatitis

A Answers and Explanations

51. E
52. C
53. C
54. D
55. D
56. A
57. D
58. B
59. C
60. D
61. B
62. B
63. B
64. C
65. B
66. C
67. A
68. A
69. D
70. C
71. C
72. C
73. C
74. C
75. B
76. C
77. C
78. C
79. D
80. D
81. D
82. D
83. C
84. C
85. B
86. E
87. A
88. B
89. B
90. A
91. E
92. B
93. B
94. C
95. C
96. B
97. B
98. E
99. C
100. B

51. E. According to the JNC-VII guidelines, both lifestyle modification and pharmacologic therapy are recommended for a patient with stage I hypertension and diabetes. Lifestyle recommendations include weight loss, a low-salt diet, exercise, and reduction of alcohol intake. The preferred initial therapy for a patient with hypertension and diabetes is an ACE-inhibitor due to the renal protective effects.

A. Although it is estimated that weight loss may reduce BP by 5–7 mm Hg for patients who are 10% above an ideal body weight, it is not adequate for management in this patient with diabetes.

B. A low-salt diet may have some effect on lowering BP, but again it is inadequate management in a patient with diabetes and hypertension.

C. This patient has already established that he has hypertension on multiple readings. Pharmacologic therapy should be initiated at this time.

D. A beta blocker is not the preferred initial antihypertensive drug of choice in patients with diabetes. A beta blocker can mask the beta-adrenergic symptoms of hypoglycemia, such as diaphoresis, and should be used with caution in patients with tendencies toward hypoglycemic events.

52. C. According to JNC-VII guidelines, the goal BP in a patient with diabetes should be <130/80 mm Hg to reduce the cardiovascular complications associated with hypertension.

A, B. These values are above the current recommended guidelines.

D. This BP goal is to be used in patients with renal insufficiency or significant proteinuria (>1 g/24 hours) secondary to their diabetes.

E. There are defined goals for optimum BP, as in the explanation for C.

53. C. ADPKD is the fourth most common cause of end-stage renal disease. It is a systemic disorder, not just a disorder of the kidneys. Mitral valve prolapse is seen in 26% of patients with ADPKD, as opposed to 2% in a non-ADPKD control group. Diverticular disease of the GI tract is more frequent and severe in ADPKD patients, especially in those with end-stage renal disease.

A, B, E. Other manifestations of ADPKD include hypertension, cerebral aneurysms (not arteriovenous malformations), hepatic cysts (not adenomas), and mitral valve prolapse (not bicuspid aortic valve).

D. Abnormalities of the ocular lens and deafness are associated with Alport syndrome, not ADPKD.

54. D. Cyclophosphamide and glucocorticoids in combination have been shown to have the most effect on preserving renal function.

A. Pulsed dosing of glucocorticoids can be used for treatment of lupus nephritis, but has not been shown to be as effective as cyclophosphamide alone or in combination with steroids.

B. Cyclophosphamide can be used alone, but combination therapy with glucocorticoids has more benefit.

C. Plasmapheresis does not have additional advantage to combination therapy with cyclophosphamide and glucocorticoids. Plasmapheresis is used to remove large molecular substances from the plasma, such as autoantibodies, immune complexes, and cryoglobulins.

E. Azathioprine alone does not have the benefit seen with combination therapy. Azathioprine is used in renal transplants, rheumatoid arthritis refractory to other treatments, and other autoimmune conditions.

55. D. Chronic interstitial inflammation and papillary necrosis are the two primary lesions of AN. Originally this was described in patients taking phenacetin, which was removed from the market in the 1980s. Now AN may be seen in patients who take NSAIDs and/or acetaminophen. The risk for AN appears to be greater with larger amounts of drugs ingested and with combinations of the drugs. Patients may have improvement of their renal function if the offending medication is discontinued. RBCs may be seen on urinalysis if papillary necrosis is present.

A. Glomerulonephritis will present with hypertension and hematuria with red cell casts on urinalysis. There may also be proteinuria with acute glomerulonephritis. This patient does not have these findings.

B. Acute interstitial nephritis is most commonly caused by drugs such as NSAIDs, sulfonamides, penicillins, and cephalosporins. Eosinophils, WBCs, and WBC casts can be found on urinalysis, which are not seen in this patient.
C. Nephrotic syndrome presents with proteinuria, hyperlipidemia, edema, and hypoalbuminemia. This patient has no proteinuria or findings consistent with this diagnosis.
E. Nephrolithiasis typically presents with colicky flank pain that may radiate to the groin. RBCs are usually present on urinalysis.

56. **A. Ibuprofen and other NSAIDs, penicillins, especially methicillin, sulfonamide derivatives, rifampin, hydrochlorothiazide, and furosemide, as well as phenytoin, cimetidine, and allopurinol are the drugs most commonly associated with tubulointerstitial nephritis. Tubulointerstitial nephritis presents as a range from a mild, self-limited disease to oliguric renal failure. It is often reversible if caught early, especially with drug-induced nephritis, and prognosis is often good if the offending agent is discontinued. Microscopic findings on urinalysis may include microscopic hematuria, mild proteinuria (which can reach nephrotic range with NSAID-induced AIN), and urine eosinophilia (but this is only 72% specific for AIN).**

B. Atenolol is metabolized renally, so it should be used with caution in patients with renal insufficiency. It has no specific renal toxicities and is not associated with AIN.
C. Gentamicin is directly toxic to the kidneys as well as to the vestibular and auditory nerves. Both of these toxicities occur with greater frequency in patients with preexisting renal disease. There is not an association with AIN, however.
D. Vancomycin has been rarely reported to cause AN, but ibuprofen is much more commonly associated with the disease. Vancomycin in high doses can cause renal insufficiency and levels should be monitored carefully, especially in patients with preexisting renal disease. Other toxicities of vancomycin include neutropenia and ototoxicity.
E. Amphotericin B is toxic to the kidneys and commonly causes renal tubular damage in the form of a distal type 1 renal tubular acidosis. This manifests by a hyperchloremic nongap metabolic acidosis with significant hypokalemia (from potassium wasting). Amphotericin B is not associated with AN.

57. **D. Hyponatremia is first evaluated by measuring the serum osmolality. Most patients with hyponatremia will also be hypoosmolar, but an exception is a patient who has hyponatremia related to another significant highly osmolar substance, such as mannitol, or elevated blood glucose. In this case, the hyponatremia is "pseudohyponatremia" because the osmolar substance in the vascular space is pulling water from the intracellular space into the vascular space and "diluting" the sodium in the vascular space. In the case of hyperglycemia, the sodium can be corrected for the degree of elevated blood sugar by the following formula: *Corrected Na = 0.016 (measured glucose − 100) + measured Na.* Once you have determined that the patient is hypoosmotic, the next step is evaluation of the patient's volume status: is he hypervolemic, euvolemic, or hypovolemic? This will help you determine therapy. The last step in the evaluation is looking at the patient's urine osmolality and urine sodium.**

A. SIADH is the inappropriate secretion of ADH. This hormone works on the collecting duct of the kidney to allow resorption of water. If there is too much of the hormone, the kidneys absorb too much water and the serum osmolality is low. The patients are usually euvolemic, and the urine is inappropriately concentrated (the osmolality is too high for the degree of hypoosmolality of the serum).
B. In psychogenic polydipsia the kidneys work fine, but the patient is ingesting too much water, which overloads the kidney's capacity to remove it. In this case, the patient's serum osmolality is low and the urine osmolality is also extremely low.
C. Correcting the sodium too quickly can lead to a complication called central pontine myelinolysis. Typically, the sodium should not be corrected faster than 0.5 mEq/L per hour.
E. This statement is false. Changes in the composition of extracellular fluid (such as increased glucose) cause a shift of water out of the cell and into the extracellular fluid. This effectively dilutes the serum sodium that is measured, an example of pseudohyponatremia, as in the explanation for D.

58. B. **This patient should take clindamycin 600 mg PO 1 hour prior to the dental procedure. The patient has a prosthetic valve and is therefore at high risk for contracting infective endocarditis from a dental procedure. Recommended oral regimens for endocarditis prophylaxis include amoxicillin 2 g, clindamycin 600 mg, cephalexin 2 g, cefadroxil 2 g, or clarithromycin 500 mg. All should be given 1 hour prior to the dental procedure. Because our patient is allergic to penicillin, the drug of choice from among those listed would be clindamycin.**

A. The patient's BP is normal on his current dose of hydrochlorothiazide. There is no reason to take an extra dose of his BP medication.

C. The patient is allergic to amoxicillin. See explanation for B.

D. There is no reason to avoid Tylenol prior to the dental procedure, because it does not increase the risk for bleeding. Had he been taking aspirin or NSAIDs for his back pain, consideration should be given to discontinuing them for a week prior to the dental procedure to avoid bleeding complications.

E. Doing nothing is not an appropriate option for this high-risk patient. Other conditions associated with a high risk for endocarditis include prior infective endocarditis, surgically constructed systemic pulmonary shunts, and complex cyanotic congenital heart disease. These patients should all receive endocarditis prophylaxis prior to any dental procedure.

59. C. **According to the NCEP, the following are all major risk factors for CAD that modify LDL goals: (1) cigarette smoking, (2) hypertension (BP ≥140/90 mm Hg or on antihypertensive medical therapy), (3) low HDL cholesterol (<40 mg/dL), (4) family history of premature CAD (CAD in a male first-degree relative <55 years of age or in a female first-degree relative <65 years of age), (5) personal age (men ≥45 years; women ≥55 years.) Conversely, an HDL cholesterol level of ≥60 mg/dL counts as a "negative" risk factor and allows for the removal of one risk factor from the total count. The presence of DM is considered a CAD "equivalent"; therefore, patients with DM have the same LDL goal as those patients with known CAD.**

A, E. Triglycerides and obesity are not considered in the major risk factors by the NCEP when calculating a patient's LDL goal.

B, D. See explanation for E.

60. D. **She has numerous risk factors for the development of CAD; however, the presence of DM is considered a risk "equivalent." Therefore, patients with known CAD or CAD risk equivalents should be managed aggressively as outlined in Table 1-60. The goal LDL for this patient is <100 mg/dL. Her level of 138 mg/dL requires treatment with a lipid-lowering agent. Of note, the LDL value is calculated using the following formula: *LDL = Total Cholesterol − HDL − (1/5 Triglycerides)*.**

A. Total cholesterol is used in the calculation of the LDL level; however, it has no bearing on determining the goal LDL level for a patient.

B. Although her HDL level is over 60 mg/dL and counts as a "negative" risk factor (and its presence removes one risk factor from the total count), the presence of DM is still a CAD equivalent. Therefore, her LDL level is not at goal.

C, E. See explanations for A, B, D, and Table 1-60.

TABLE 1-60 CAD Management Guidelines

Risk Category	Goal LDL Level (mg/dL)	LDL Level at Which to Initiate Lifestyle Changes	LDL Level at Which to Consider Drug Therapy
CAD or CAD risk equivalent (e.g., DM)	<100	≥100	≥130
2+ Risk Factors	<130	≥130	≥160
0–1 Risk Factor	<160	≥160	≥190

61. **B. This patient likely has diarrhea caused by *Clostridium difficile.* Toxin-mediated diarrhea is secretory in nature. Toxins increase the cAMP, which inhibits absorption and promotes secretion in the gut. Diagnosis in this patient is made by finding toxin in the stool. Initial treatment is with metronidazole. This may be repeated with recurrence or the patient can be started on vancomycin.**

A. Osmotic diarrhea is seen more commonly in those with malabsorption or lactase deficiency and can be differentiated from secretory diarrhea by stool electrolytes and a fecal osmotic gap [280 − 2(Na+K)] of >50. In general, osmotic diarrhea gets better when patients are fasting, such as at night while sleeping, whereas secretory diarrhea is more likely to awaken a patient at night.
C. Inflammatory forms of diarrhea include Crohn's disease and ulcerative colitis. Enteroinvasive infections can also cause an inflammatory diarrhea. Neutrophils can be found in the stool.
D. Diarrhea caused by dysmotility is usually seen in irritable bowel syndrome, diabetes, or in cases of bacterial overgrowth. These patients will have a negative stool examination result and a positive glucose breath test result.
E. It is unlikely that this patient's diarrhea is secondary to a parasite, because she has not had any recent travel or ingestion of contaminated foods.

62. **B. Noncaseating granulomas, transmural involvement, and skip lesions are characteristic of Crohn's disease.**

A. Villous flattening is seen with celiac disease.
C. Periodic acid-Schiff-positive macrophages are seen in Whipple disease.
D. Superficial ulcerations with crypt abscesses are seen with ulcerative colitis.
E. Eosinophils are seen in eosinophilic enteritis.

63. **B. This patient has a first-degree relative with colorectal cancer, so it is advised that she undergo FOBT annually with sigmoidoscopy every 3–5 years or colonoscopy every 10 years to begin at age 40.**

A. There are no recommendations for the general population to begin colonoscopy at age 30.
C. The screening recommendation for the average patient without any risk factors is FOBT annually and sigmoidoscopy every 3–5 years or colonoscopy every 10 years starting at age 50.
D. Patients with a risk for familial adenomatous polyposis should have sigmoidoscopy every 1–2 years starting at age 12.
E. There are no recommendations for just fecal occult blood testing without sigmoidoscopy or colonoscopy.

64. **C. This patient most likely has NASH given patient history (no alcohol use, no IVDA, no constitutional symptoms) and presence of obesity. Other risk factors for NASH include diabetes, hyperlipidemia, and total parenteral nutrition. Ultrasonography can be used to evaluate for the presence of fatty liver disease. Treatment for this patient includes weight loss.**

A. A patient with hemochromatosis might complain of arthralgias, bronzing of the skin, and diabetes.
B. Wilson disease is associated with young adults and a psychiatric presentation.
D. This patient does not have any hepatitis C risk factors.
E. This patient has no history of any autoimmune disorders, and although autoimmune hepatitis is still in the differential diagnosis, the more common reason for the patient's abnormal liver enzymes is NASH.

65. **B. Clubbing is a finding of the distal extremities that is an early part of the spectrum of HOA. The pathophysiology of clubbing has recently been attributed to platelet fragmenting and their interaction with endothelial cells in the distal extremities. This causes a low-grade inflammation in the periosteum and new bone formation, which makes the distal finger enlarge. The findings of true clubbing are verified by the described physical examination written in the question. Primary HOA is rare and is characterized by clubbing, periosteal inflammation and elevation, and unusual skin features. It is transmitted in an autosomal-dominant pattern, but effects boys nine times more often than girls.**

A, C, E. Secondary HOA may be due to many different disease states, including pulmonary, gastrointestinal, and cardiovascular diseases, such as bronchogenic carcinoma (not usually COPD alone), cystic fibrosis, inflammatory bowel diseases (not colon adenocarcinoma), cyanotic heart diseases, and infective endocarditis.

D. Clubbing is also seen in Graves' disease (not hypothyroidism), where the term *thyroid acropachy* has been used.

66. **C. This patient's history and physical examination are both consistent with OSA as the cause of his daytime sleepiness. OSA is the most common sleep disorder in the United States, affecting 3 million men and 1.5 million women. Patients develop obstruction of the pharynx during sleep, which they struggle to overcome, causing partial arousal into wakefulness. This contributes to nonrestful sleep and daytime sleepiness. Patients with OSA are usually obese, but may not be. They often have hypertension, which may improve with treatment of the OSA. A large neck circumference (>17.5 inches) and pharyngeal "crowding" are physical findings to look for in a patient suspected of OSA. Patients may have bed partners that notice loud snoring, occasional apneic episodes, and restless legs, which can be helpful clues to the diagnosis. Patients themselves may complain of early morning headaches and falling asleep with minimal sensory deprivation, such as when sitting down to watch TV or while driving.**

A. Hypothyroidism may be associated with OSA because of resulting weight gain that may predispose to obesity and myxedematous features that may result in redundant pharyngeal tissue. It is important to check patients with OSA for hypothyroidism, but correction of the hypothyroidism is not enough to treat the sleep apnea. Other systemic diseases associated with OSA include acromegaly, amyloidosis, and neuromuscular disorders.

B. Narcolepsy is a central nervous system sleep disorder characterized by daytime sleepiness with cataplexy, hypnagogic hallucinations, and sleep paralysis. It is the second most common sleep disorder in the United States after OSA. Cataplexy is a sudden episode of bilateral weakness that may result in collapse, brought on by intense emotion, such as laughing. There is no loss of consciousness. A hypnagogic hallucination is a vivid, often frightening hallucination that occurs while a patient is going to sleep. It is probably an intrusion of REM sleep dreaming into wakefulness. Sleep paralysis occurs when a patient is awakening and is unable to move for a short period of time. None of the features of narcolepsy are present in our patient.

D. Depression can manifest as insomnia or hypersomnolence. It is important to ask patients questions about their general sleep habits and their mood when they complain about any change in sleep pattern. Our patient denied having depression or anhedonia, which makes this less likely.

E. Central sleep apnea can be combined with OSA in patients with pickwickian syndrome. This syndrome is also referred to as obesity-hypoventilation syndrome. The difference between central and OSA is whether or not effort is made to breathe. Our patient had occasional apneic episodes with efforts to breathe, according to his wife, which makes his apnea obstructive in nature. A formal sleep study can determine if he has components of both forms of apnea, but the most likely diagnosis is OSA.

67. **A. Treatment for OSA usually starts with the use of a nasal mask that provides CPAP to splint the airway open during sleep. The mask can be uncomfortable and produces sensations of claustrophobia in some people, which limits its use. Overall, the compliance of CPAP mask treatment is poor, with 20%–40% of patients refusing to use the mask at all, and other patients using the mask for less time than that which is recommended. Once the CPAP mask is initiated, patients must undergo further sleep studies to make sure that the seal is adequate and the pressure is adequate to appropriately treat the sleep apnea. Patients who are compliant with their CPAP will often report improvement in their symptoms of daytime sleepiness, and increased quality of life.**

B. Tracheostomy is the only definitive treatment for sleep apnea. It should be pursued in patients who are unable to tolerate CPAP and for which weight loss and uvulopalatopharyngoplasty are unsuccessful. Tracheostomy effectively bypasses the obstruction wherever it occurs from the soft palate to the glottis, but its invasiveness and social implications make it unattractive for patients. The seriousness of OSA should be explained to patients when counseling them on their treatment options.

C. Uvulopalatopharyngoplasty has been used as a surgical treatment for OSA with variable results. It may be difficult to know where the obstruction is occurring in the airway in any given patient, although the most common area of obstruction is in the nasopharynx at the level of the soft palate. Therefore, making a wider opening in the area of the soft palate may or may not correct the disorder. Another sleep study should be obtained after the operation to determine its effectiveness. It is recommended that patients have a trial of CPAP before they undergo uvulopalatopharyngoplasty, because they may have more difficulty tolerating CPAP with the postsurgical anatomic changes.

D. Weight loss should always be recommended to the patient with OSA who is overweight; however, it should not be the sole intervention. A patient whose sleep study results show evidence of OSA needs to be started on CPAP in addition to the recommendation of weight loss. It is possible that a patient who loses a significant amount of weight may improve to such an extent, as evidenced by repeat sleep study, that he no longer needs CPAP (or another treatment), but a clinician should not wait for the patient to lose weight to intervene.

E. There actually are several oral devices that are custom made by dentists to try to keep the lower jaw in a jaw-thrust position during sleep to keep the airway open. Other devices hold the tongue in an anterior position to try to decrease airway obstruction. Some studies have evaluated the efficacy of the appliances, and although promising, they are not currently first-line therapy for OSA.

68. **A. Glaucoma is a disease of the eye that ultimately causes damage to the optic nerve. It is the leading cause of blindness in the world, and the second leading cause of blindness in the United States after diabetic retinopathy. There are four major categories of glaucoma: (1) acute angle closure, (2) secondary, (3) congenital, and (4) primary open-angle. The most common type of glaucoma is primary open-angle glaucoma. Patients usually have elevated intraocular pressure, >21 mm Hg (normal is 8–20 mm Hg), but up to half of patients may have only high-normal intraocular pressures. Patients are usually asymptomatic and should be screened for the disease if they have risk factors such as a family history of glaucoma or systemic hypertension. The incidence of glaucoma also increases with age and is five times more common in African-Americans than in whites. Topical beta blockers work by reducing aqueous humor production, therefore lowering intraocular pressure, and are usually first-line treatment for glaucoma.**

B. Oral ACE inhibitors are used in the treatment of systemic hypertension and have not been used in the treatment of glaucoma. There are no topical ACE inhibitors.

C. Oral carbonic anhydrase inhibitors decrease aqueous humor production, but their use has declined secondary to their side effects and newer topical agents, such as prostaglandins. Topical prostaglandins are usually used in addition to topical beta blockers in patients who do not have adequate reduction of intraocular pressure with beta blockers alone. They work by increasing aqueous outflow.

D. Oral calcium channel blockers are used in the treatment of systemic hypertension, and not in the treatment of glaucoma. There are no topical calcium channel blockers.

E. Cholinergic agonist medications are usually second-tier drugs, secondary to their ocular side effects of small pupils, myopia, and some subjective visual disturbances.

69. **D. Multiple sex partners, young age at onset of intercourse, infection with human papilloma virus (resulting in genital warts in this patient,) tobacco use, and low socioeconomic status are all risk factors. Immunosuppressed women with HIV are also at risk for early or more aggressive cervical cancer and require more frequent screening. The American College of Obstetrics and Gynecology recommends Pap smears every 6 months in patients with HIV.**

A, B, C, E. See explanation for D.

70. **C. The risk for developing endometrial cancer is directly proportional to the amount of estrogen stimulation of the endometrium. Estrogen stimulates the endometrial cells to proliferate dominating the first half of the menstrual cycle. During the second half of the menstrual cycle, after ovulation, the corpus luteum produces progesterone that limits the growth of the endometrium and allows it to become secretory in preparation for a fertilized egg. When there is no ovulation, there is continued growth of the endometrium without the opposing effects of progesterone. This predisposes to hyperplasia and the possibility of malignancy. Therefore, anything that increases the amount of unopposed estrogen stimulation of the endometrium increases the risk for the development of malignancy. Tamoxifen is a competitive inhibitor of estrogen, but it also has partial agonist activity. There is a two- to threefold risk for endometrial cancer associated with tamoxifen, and this increase was seen almost exclusively in women over the age of 50.**

A. Obesity increases the exposure to estrogen because the fat cells convert androstenedione to estrone and convert androgens to estradiol, but this patient is not obese with a BMI of 24.

B. Nulliparity is a risk factor for breast cancer, and multiparity, especially if the first baby was born before the mother was 30 years old, is actually a negative risk factor for breast cancer. There is not a direct association between parity and endometrial cancer.

D, E. Early menarche and late menopause both increase a woman's lifetime exposure to estrogen and have been associated with an increased risk for endometrial cancer. Oral contraceptive pills decrease the risk for both endometrial and ovarian cancer. The benefit of oral contraceptives is most likely related to the progestin component, which suppresses endometrial proliferation.

71. **C. According to the American College of Physicians, women should begin screening for breast cancer with yearly mammography at age 50. Other societies such as the American Cancer Society, American College of Radiology, and American College of Obstetrics and Gynecology recommend starting routine screening at age 40. There is, however, no proven benefit in mortality to warrant screening women between the ages of 40 and 50, and this is what causes the discrepancy in the recommendations of the above-mentioned societies. Women should decide with their physician when to start their mammograms, whether at age 40 or 50. After age 50, they should have bilateral screening mammography every year (some groups may allow up to 2 years) until age 69. Even though the prevalence of breast cancer increases with age, mortality from all causes also increases, and there is no statistical benefit in mortality to warrant screening women for breast cancer with mammography over the age of 70. It is probably reasonable to continue breast cancer screening in women as long as they have a life expectancy of at least 10 years.**

A. Clinical breast examination may detect about 10% of breast cancers that are missed by mammography, whereas approximately 40% of breast cancers are detected by mammography and missed on physical examination. Clinical examinations are probably of more benefit if they are performed with the appropriate technique and time allowance. They are recommended by some groups and not by others. There is no proven mortality benefit seen with doing annual clinical breast examinations. (Also see answer "C" regarding the age to start mammograms.)

B. Breast self-examination is not proven to be of benefit, and may increase the number of biopsies done on benign lesions. There are no official recommendations for monthly breast self-examinations even though it is encouraged by many physicians and breast cancer awareness groups. There is no mortality benefit seen from breast self-examinations.

D. A diagnostic mammogram is not the same as a screening mammogram. Diagnostic mammography is done when there is already an abnormality noted on breast examination or on a prior mammogram that was done for screening purposes.

E. Mammography for breast cancer screening are continued annually even if the patient has three consecutively normal examination results. Pap smears can be decreased in frequency to every 3 years in patients who have had three consecutive normal Pap smear results and who are low risk for cervical neoplasia (monogamous, HIV negative, etc.).

72. **C. Sildenafil is the first oral medication created for the treatment of erectile dysfunction. Given approximately 1 hour before sexual intercourse, it acts by increasing nitric oxide, which in turn vasodilates the penile vessels, allowing for erection. It is contraindicated in patients with CAD. Side effects are similar to those experienced by patients who take nitrates, including headache and hypotension. This is likely the best option for this patient.**

A. Vacuum-assisted devices work by increasing arterial inflow and prohibiting venous outflow at the level of the penis. Satisfaction is mixed secondary to difficulty in its use.

B. Intraurethral alprostadil relaxes smooth muscle trabeculae in the penis, allowing for the inflow of blood to engorge the penis. Intraurethral alprostadil is much less invasive than penile self-injections and has a success rate of 60%. Side effects are minimal because it is locally acting. Its use does require a significant amount of education.

D. Testosterone replacements are given to men with signs and symptoms of hypogonadism. This patient does not appear hypogonadal by physical examination. Testosterone levels, thyroid hormone levels, and prolactin levels should be checked prior to administration of testosterone for erectile dysfunction.

E. Penile prostheses have become less common since the discovery of sildenafil. Complications of this surgery include local wound infections, anesthesia, and the need to remove the implant later in life.

73. **C. IVIG has been shown to play a role in the treatment of ITP. First-line therapy is high-dose steroids. Over 50% of patients respond to this treatment with increased platelet counts. Patients who do not respond to high-dose steroids can receive IVIG. Another 60% to 70% of patients respond to this treatment with increased platelet counts. The exact mechanism of IVIG is uncertain, but it appears to inhibit removal of antibody bound platelets.**

A. Peak age of onset for ITP is during childhood between ages 2 and 6. This ITP is usually acute and follows a viral illness. Most children recover spontaneously or require a short dose of treatment with steroids. Adults with ITP are more likely to experience a chronic and refractory course than children.

B. First-line therapy for ITP is high-dose steroids. Splenectomy is indicated for patients who have been refractory to other treatments and suffer bleeding complications from low platelet counts. All patients should be immunized against *Streptococcus pneumoniae, Haemophilus influenzae b,* and *Neisseria meningitidis* prior to splenectomy.

D. ITP is caused by IgG and IgM antiplatelet antibodies that attack membrane platelet glycoproteins, leading to platelet destruction.

E. Chronic ITP is defined as persistence of thrombocytopenia for longer than 6 months.

74. **C. This patient has a history consistent with a primary hemostasis problem. Patients with primary hemostasis problems have mucosal bleeding, such as gingival bleeding, epistaxis, and menorrhagia. The problem is in the initial platelet plug formation, which occurs secondary to platelet insufficiency, platelet dysfunction, or vWF deficiency. VWF combines with factor VIII, and deficiency of vWF can cause a "pseudodeficiency" of functional factor VIII, which may cause a prolongation of aPTT, such as is seen in this patient. Von Willebrand disease is the most common inherited bleeding disorder. Patients usually have easy bruising, nosebleeds, menorrhagia, or prolonged bleeding with trauma. vWF plays a critical role in platelet function. A ristocetin cofactor assay determines the activity of vWF. Additional tests include vWF antigen and factor VIII level. Treatment with desmopressin, which mimics antidiuretic hormone, increases factor VIII and vWF levels.**

A, B. Factor VIII levels would evaluate for hemophilia A, and factor IX levels would evaluate for hemophilia B. This patient does not present with clinical bleeding consistent with these diseases, such as spontaneous hemarthrosis.

D. Anticardiolipin antibody would be elevated in patients with antiphospholipid antibody syndrome. These patient are predisposed to clot formation, not prolonged bleeding.

E. A fibrinogen level will not be affected by vWF deficiency. This level would be useful in patients with DIC. A fibrinogen level would be low in DIC.

75. **B. Current tobacco use has been associated with low bone mineral density. This is our patient's only additional risk factor for osteoporosis other than her postmenopausal status.**

A. Whites are at highest risk for osteoporosis. Asians, because of their small frames, are second in line for osteoporosis. African Americans are actually somewhat protected from osteoporosis based on their relatively higher peak bone mass.

C. The most commonly used drug that adversely affects BMD is glucocorticoids. It is recommended that patients who are to be started on steroids for chronic use of 3 months or greater at a dose of 5 mg a day or more obtain a baseline DEXA scan and be started on bone-protective medications as well as optimal calcium and vitamin D. Other drugs that adversely affect BMD include phenytoin, cyclosporine, and supratherapeutic doses of thyroid supplement. Hydrochlorothiazide does not affect BMD.

D. A BMI of <22 or weight <127 pounds is a risk factor for osteoporosis. Our patient's BMI is 25; therefore, her BMI is not a risk factor.

E. Hypertension is not associated with low BMD. Other systemic diseases such as celiac disease, cystic fibrosis, and inflammatory bowel disease are associated with increased risk for fracture secondary to osteoporosis because of malabsorption of calcium and vitamin D. Patients with these diagnoses should be considered for DEXA scan to evaluate their need for treatment of osteopenia or osteoporosis.

76. **C. Colon cancer screening should start at age 50 unless there is a history of colon cancer in the individual or family. Acceptable screening includes annual FOBTs with at least three cards to be used on 3 separate days to improve the sensitivity of the test; a flexible sigmoidoscopy every 5 years in addition to a double-contrast barium enema to visualize the complete colon; double contrast barium enema every 5–10 years; or colonoscopy every 10 years.**

A. Screening for colon cancer should start at age 50 unless there is a family history of colon cancer. If there is a family history, then it is recommended that screening begin when the patient is 10 years younger than the youngest relative was when they were diagnosed.

B. A negative FOBT result on rectal examination is not adequate screening.

D. Colonoscopy should be repeated every 3–5 years after a benign polyp is found.

E. CEA and other tumor markers are not effective screening tools.

77. **C. A PSA level of >4 ng/mL is suspicious for malignancy; >10 ng/mL is highly probable for malignancy. A biopsy should be pursued to determine if further treatment is needed. In addition, African-American men are at a higher risk for prostate cancer than other ethnic groups, and you should be more worried about this patient because of this fact.**

A. Prostatectomy may not be indicated depending on the findings of the biopsy. Some stages of prostate cancer can be treated with radiation or hormonal therapy. It would be premature to proceed with this step.

B. Radiation therapy may be indicated in this patient, but that should be determined after pathology of biopsy is performed.

D. Further evaluation should not be deferred until a definitive diagnosis has been obtained.

E. Prostate cancer may not be symptomatic at presentation. Therefore, further workup should not be delayed based on the lack of symptoms.

78. **C. This is an example of Terry's nails. The normal lunula of the nail (the white semicircle at the proximal portion of the nail) now appears to extend to almost the tip of the fingernail. This is thought to be due to severe hypoalbuminemic states, and the most common disease that this finding is associated with is cirrhosis of the liver.**

A. Terry's nails may be seen in DM, but is most commonly associated with liver cirrhosis.

B. Terry's nails may be seen in CHF, but is most commonly associated with liver cirrhosis.

D. Iron deficiency anemia may cause nail changes, but, classically, iron deficiency causes koilonychias (spoon-shaped nails) and brittle nails, not Terry's nails.

E. Patients with systemic sclerosis may have Terry's nails, but the usual disease associated with this finding is liver cirrhosis.

79. **D. Thrombocytopenia can be classified into three categories: (1) a production problem, (2) a sequestration problem, or (3) a destruction problem. ITP is a disorder of autoantibody production against platelet receptors which causes the platelets to be destroyed. It is a likely diagnosis in a 31-year-old woman, but other disorders must be considered and ruled out before diagnosis can be made. A thorough medication history must be elicited to evaluate for a drug-induced thrombocytopenia. In young women, especially, thrombocytopenia may be a result of lupus, and it is important to check an ANA and evaluate for other symptoms such as joint pain, photosensitivity, and mouth ulcers. Finally, thrombocytopenia may be a result of many different viral infections such as EBV, CMV, and HIV. Thrombocytopenia may be the presenting initial manifestation of HIV infection.**

    A, B, C, E. See explanation for D.

80. **D. Symptomatic patients with chronic ITP are usually placed on glucocorticoids. Fifty percent will normalize their platelet count on 60 mg of prednisone per day.**

    A. If a patient is not bleeding and maintains a platelet count of greater than 20,000/μL then consideration should be given to withholding therapy; however, our patient is having frequent nosebleeds. Therefore, treatment is warranted.
    B. IVIG is an effective form of therapy, but it is expensive and should be reserved for patients with severe thrombocytopenia who are clinically bleeding and have not responded to other measures. It is also only transiently effective, but can be used to temporarily raise the platelet count to support a patient before surgery or childbirth.
    C. Emergency splenectomy is indicated in patients who are acutely ill and bleeding without response to other medical measures. Elective splenectomy is used in patients who are steroid responsive, but unable to wean off steroids without a decline in their platelet counts. It is effective in 70% of patients. Occasionally, splenectomy is helpful in patients who do not respond to steroids.
    E. Patients who are still thrombocytopenic after steroids or splenectomy may be tried on other immunosuppressive therapies such as azathioprine and cyclophosphamide. These are not routinely used, however, due to their serious side effects.

81. **D. The exact cause of pseudotumor cerebri or benign intracranial hypertension is not known. However, it does have a known association with some medications, including vitamin A, tetracycline, oral contraceptives, and glucocorticoids.**

    A. Pseudotumor cerebri is seen mostly in premenopausal obese women. There is a known association with pregnancy, but not with menopause.
    B. Patients usually present with headache and diplopia. Funduscopic examination will show papilledema. Pseudotumor cerebri must be treated because the patient is at risk for irreversible visual loss. Most patients will have peripheral visual field loss. Treatment includes acetazolamide, furosemide, and repeat lumbar punctures with CSF drainage. If these treatments fail, a lumboperitoneal shunt can be placed.
    C. Opening pressure will be elevated on lumbar puncture. Usually, the pressure is greater than 250 mm water.
    E. CT of the head will show small or normal ventricles.

82. **D. Gliomas, particularly astrocytomas, account for over half of adult primary brain tumors. Clinical presentation of brain tumors is highly variable, and depends on the region of the brain that is involved. Symptoms may include headache, nausea, vomiting, seizure, focal weakness, impaired cognitive function, behavior changes, or any number of other neurologic symptoms.**

    A. Meningiomas account for 25% of adult primary brain tumors. Most meningiomas are benign in nature.
    B. Pituitary tumors comprise 10% of primary brain tumors. Patients present with pituitary dysfunction.
    C. CNS lymphomas are the etiology of 5% of primary brain tumors. They are seen most often in AIDS patients.
    E. Craniopharyngiomas comprise only 2% of primary brain tumors. This tumor arises along the path from the nasopharynx to the diencephalon, mostly in the pituitary stalk. Patients with this tumor often present with headache, pituitary dysfunction, and visual impairment.

83. **C. Approximately 33% of women with MS and 25% of men with MS will present with complaints of sensory changes in their limbs. Visual loss is the second most common complaint on presentation. Therefore, MS should be on the differential diagnosis of this patient's complaint. Her physical examination does not reveal numbness in a single nerve distribution, and therefore excludes a compressive neuropathy from the diagnosis. MS is often difficult to diagnose. Its definite criteria require there to be at least two separate clinical attacks with some degree of symptom resolution between the attacks over time (30 days) and two or more lesions that are consistent with MS that are separated by time or space on the MRI. (Remember: "Two lesions separated by time and space.") Our patient presents with one complaint in time, and one finding in space on the MRI. Therefore, she does not currently meet the criteria for diagnosis of MS. If she develops another attack in a different distribution after 30 days have elapsed, and if she develops a new lesion on MRI after 3 months (McDonald WI, Compston A, Edan G, Goodkin D, et al. Recommended diagnostic criteria for multiple sclerosis: guidelines from the International Panel on the Diagnosis of Multiple Sclerosis. *Ann Neurol* 2001;50:121–127), then she will meet the criteria for MS. If the CSF showed oligoclonal bands at the time of the first "attack" with the one MRI finding, or if she had oligoclonal bands and positive delayed waves on visual evoked potential testing with the MRI finding, then this means that she may have MS, but the diagnosis is still not yet confirmed.**

A, B, D, E. See explanation for C.

84. **C. Prospective cohort studies have reported that a higher dietary intake of antioxidants, and vitamin E in particular, may help to lower the risk for Alzheimer dementia. [Englehart MJ, Geerlings MI, Ruitenberg A, et al. Dietary intake of antioxidants and risk of Alzheimer disease. *JAMA* 2002;287(24):3223–3229]. As yet, there are no randomized-controlled trials looking at the primary prevention of Alzheimer disease with antioxidants such as vitamin E, but since therapy with vitamin E supplement is simple and without harm, it is reasonable to recommend it to patients with family histories of Alzheimer disease.**

A. Initially, epidemiologic studies seemed to suggest that estrogen replacement would help to prevent dementia. However, the Women's Health Initiative Memory Study, which was an ancillary study of the Women's Health Initiative, showed that women on hormone replacement therapy (both estrogen and progesterone) were at increased risk for developing dementia. (The effects of unopposed estrogen use, or HRT use in younger postmenopausal women was not studied.) However, because of this study, HRT is not recommended for the prevention of dementia.

B. There have been no randomized controlled trials evaluating the use of statins to prevent Alzheimer disease. Two large trials using other methods of study such as case control and a cross-sectional analysis have suggested that statins may have an effect in the prevention of Alzheimer disease; however, more studies need to be done to confirm this.

D. A metanalysis of cohort and case control studies [Etminan M, Gill S, Samii A. Effect of non-steroidal anti-inflammatory drugs on risk of Alzheimer disease: systematic review and meta-analysis of observational studies. *BMJ* 2003;327(7407):128–131] showed that there was a pooled relative risk reduction in the development of Alzheimer dementia in NSAID users, with more benefit seen the longer the patient was on the drug. There also may have been a reduction in the development of Parkinson disease, which is another important cause of dementia. A randomized, controlled trial is currently underway, but patients at high risk for Alzheimer disease may benefit from ibuprofen 200 mg daily.

E. It is difficult to be certain of the relationship between exercise, physical fitness, and dementia. Some observational studies have shown a correlation and others have not. Therefore, we recommend exercise based on the health benefits that we already know exist because of it (reducing hypertension and obesity, among others), and not particularly for the prevention of dementia.

85. **B. This patient most likely has pulmonary fibrosis, which is a known complication of amiodarone use. The clues to this diagnosis lie in his physical examination findings. He has no evidence of**

systolic heart failure, because his jugular venous pressure is normal, he has no gallop, and he has no peripheral edema. However, he does have bilateral inspiratory crackles. The nature of the inspiratory crackles is important to note, especially when they are heard without any other manifestation of left heart failure. Crackles associated with pulmonary edema and pulmonary fibrosis start in the first half of the inspiratory cycle and continue into late inspiration. Crackles associated with pulmonary fibrosis have a dry, "Velcro-like" quality, unlike those associated with pulmonary edema or pneumonia, which often sound "wet." The fact that this patient desaturates quickly with ambulation implies a diffusion problem, such as pulmonary fibrosis. The best test to evaluate this patient for fibrosis is a high-resolution CT scan. Pulmonary function tests (spirometry and DLCO) also may be helpful. Therapy for the condition consists of discontinuing the amiodarone. If there appears to be active inflammation, as evidenced by a "ground glass" appearance on the high-resolution CT scan, then sometimes glucocorticoids are used.

A. Dyspnea on exertion can be a sign of cardiac ischemia, but patients usually present more acutely and may have associated chest pain. Our patient gives a history of slowly progressive dyspnea on exertion over several months. The chest x-ray also gives clues that something is going on in the parenchyma of the lung, with the reticulonodular markings. Therefore, left heart catheterization is not likely to give us the correct diagnosis in this patient.

C, D, E. CT angiography, VQ scan, and lower extremity Doppler scans are all tests to look for acute or chronic thromboembolic disease as a cause for this patient's symptoms. Chronic thromboembolic disease can be an etiology for slowly progressive dyspnea on exertion, but the chest x-ray and the physical examination finding of inspiratory crackles do not fit with that particular diagnosis. Most people with pulmonary emboli have normal chest x-rays or x-rays with small amounts of volume loss, such as plate atelectasis. Patients with peripheral pulmonary infarcts may have a noticeable plural rub on physical examination, but not bilateral inspiratory crackles.

86. **E. There are three main tests for determining BMD: quantitative CT, dual photon absorptiometry, and DEXA. Of the three, DEXA is the simplest, the cheapest, and the most accurate. Therefore, it is the preferred test in evaluating for osteoporosis. There are two values that are usually reported with the various BMD tests: the T-score and the Z-score. The T-score is a value that represents the difference between the patient's bone density and that of healthy young bone density (i.e., age and gender is not considered). The scores assigned are numbers of standard deviations away from normal. So, a score of −1.0 would be one standard deviation less than normal. A score between −1.0 and −2.5 is suggestive of osteopenia, whereas a score less than −2.5 is diagnostic of osteoporosis. The Z-score is a comparison of the patient's bone density to that of age- and gender-matched people. The Z-score gives you an idea if the patient's bone density is worse than what you would expect for a person of that age and gender (i.e., if there is a secondary cause that is giving the patient accelerated loss of bone density).**

A, B, C, D. These scores would not be consistent. See explanation for E.

87. **A. Bisphosphonates are effective at preventing and treating bone density loss by inhibiting bone resorption. This effect seems to be increased when used in combination with HRT. The two main bisphosphonates are alendronate and risedronate. They can be taken on a daily basis or their dose can be compiled into a weekly dose. Regardless of the dose, precautions must be taken to prevent esophagitis from the medication (e.g., taking the medicine on an empty stomach with plenty of fluids and sitting upright for 30 minutes afterward).**

B. Raloxifene and tamoxifen are selective estrogen-receptor modulators (SERMs). Raloxifene, which is FDA approved for the prevention and treatment of osteoporosis, works by inhibiting bone resorption, similar to estrogen. However, this effect is less than estrogen and presumably less than bisphosphonates. Tamoxifen is not currently FDA approved for the treatment and prevention of osteoporosis. The incidence of DVT in patients taking SERMs is comparable with that seen in patients on HRT. Because it is likely less effective than bisphosphonates and has an associated risk for DVT, raloxifene would not be the best choice for initial therapy in this patient.

C. Although estrogen-progestin replacement may help reverse bone density loss by inhibiting bone resorption, it is no longer a first-line drug in the treatment of osteoporosis because of increased risk for stroke, DVT, and breast cancer. It would not be advisable in this patient for several reasons. She has minimal to no vasomotor symptoms that are affecting her quality of life (which is one of the reasons to consider using HRT in postmenopausal patients). More importantly, her prior history of DVT, ongoing tobacco abuse, and strong family history of breast cancer make this a poor choice for treatment.

D. Because it is less effective than the bisphosphonates, has an unfavorable route of administration, and has a risk of tachyphylaxis, intranasal calcitonin is not a first-line drug in the treatment of osteoporosis. Calcitonin does have an analgesic quality and should be considered for use in patients who have pain from fractures that have resulted from osteoporosis.

E. Parathyroid hormone therapy may seem paradoxic because it stimulates bone resorption. However, it actually stimulates increased calcium absorption from the gut and results in a higher serum calcium level, which leads to new bone formation. Although some studies have suggested that PTH is more effective than bisphosphonates at increasing spine density and decreasing nonvertebral fractures, the FDA recommends using it only in patients who are high risk (e.g., prior fractures or increased risk of fracture from osteoporosis or patients who have failed other forms of treatment). It is expensive and is given as a daily injection, which also makes it a less attractive choice for first-line therapy.

88. **B. Patients with primary pulmonary hypertension classically present with a history of shortness of breath, which gradually worsens over 1 to 2 years. It is more common in women, with a ratio of 1:1.7. The disease typically presents in young women in their twenties and thirties. The pathophysiology includes three separate components: (1) injury to the pulmonary vascular endothelium, (2) medial hypertrophy and intimal proliferation resulting in a narrowed lumen, and (3) a localized procoagulant state within the endothelium, leading to thrombosis. These changes result in increased resistance to pulmonary arterial flow and eventual right heart hypertrophy and resulting tricuspid regurgitation. The patient's physical examination reveals a right ventricular heave (because of the enlarged right ventricle); a loud P_2 component of the S_2 heart sound (because of the high pressure in the pulmonary artery "slamming" the pulmonary valve shut); and a systolic murmur of tricuspid regurgitation (which increases with inspiration, as all right-sided murmurs do). The patient also may have a diastolic murmur of pulmonary valvular insufficiency and a right-sided S_3 or S_4 heart sounds secondary to systolic failure or poor compliance of the hypertrophied right ventricle, respectively. The ECG shows evidence of right axis deviation and right atrial enlargement. The chest x-ray reveals large pulmonary arteries, clear lung fields, and a small retrosternal air space on the lateral view, because the right heart hypertrophy has filled that space. All other causes of pulmonary hypertension are ruled out before the diagnosis of primary pulmonary hypertension is made, but the physical examination and story, as well as the fact that the patient tolerated a pregnancy and delivery 2 years ago without difficulty, point to a diagnosis of primary pulmonary hypertension in this patient.**

A. ASD can present in adults who are asymptomatic earlier in life. The ASD causes a left-to-right shunt in the heart that eventually can cause a volume overload in the right heart with elevation of right heart pressures. Patients usually present in their fourth decade with evidence of elevated right heart pressures. Physical examination shows a right ventricular heave, but they usually have an S_2 that is widely split and fixed throughout the respiratory cycle. They may have a midsystolic ejection murmur of increased blood flow going across the pulmonic valve (which sounds like a pulmonic stenosis murmur). As the pressure increases in the right heart, the shunt from left to right decreases, and the systolic murmurs of tricuspid regurgitation and "relative" pulmonary stenosis may become softer. Our patient did not have the "wide fixed split S_2" that is classic for an ASD.

C. Pulmonary fibrosis may present as insidious shortness of breath with exertion. Patients are usually in their fifties and sixties, and on physical examination they have inspiratory "Velcro" crackles, which this patient did not have. Patients with significant pulmonary fibrosis and hypoxemia may develop pulmonary hypertension secondary to their lung disease.

D. VSDs are usually found in childhood because of their left-to-right shunt and possible complications of pulmonary vascular obstruction, endocarditis, and aortic regurgitation. Small VSDs often close spontaneously in childhood. Patients may have a holosystolic murmur that does not increase with inspiration (like tricuspid regurgitation would). This patient is not likely to have had an undetected VSD as an adult with her uneventful pregnancy 2 years ago.

E. Cardiac tamponade may present acutely such as after a Q-wave MI with a free wall rupture, or it may present insidiously over time in a more chronic presentation (usually associated with metastatic lung or breast cancer). Patients complain of shortness of breath and orthopnea. They may have distant heart sounds on examination and a low-voltage ECG with electrical alternans (swinging of the heart in the effusion can cause variable alternating voltages of the QRS). On chest x-ray, they have a boot-shaped cardiac silhouette that may appear different from prior, even recent, x-rays. On physical examination, the heart sounds are distant. The patient usually has elevated jugular venous pressure, hepatomegaly, and peripheral edema from the "back up" of blood flow. The patient should be evaluated for pulsus paradoxus, which is a sign of tamponade. This is a weakening of the arterial pulse during the inspiratory phase of the respiratory cycle that occurs because of the inability of the right heart to fill (as it usually does during inspiration). Put simply, the septum of the heart shifts to the left side during inspiration in tamponade, and decreases the cardiac output, resulting in a weakened pulse. (The maneuver is done with a BP cuff, and you should know how to perform the technique of a pulsus paradoxus evaluation.)

89. **B. This patient may have PPH as the cause of her symptoms, but diagnosis of PPH is made by exclusion; you must rule out all other causes of secondary pulmonary hypertension. Patients with connective tissue diseases such as scleroderma or lupus may develop pulmonary hypertension, and an ANA screens for this possibility (not an RF). HIV disease also can also be associated with pulmonary hypertension and should be ruled out. Pulmonary function test results are classically normal, with a decreased DLCO in patients with primary pulmonary hypertension, and significantly abnormal in patients with pulmonary hypertension related to lung disease such as COPD or pulmonary fibrosis.**

A. See explanation for B.

C. Spirometry alone is not sufficient, and full pulmonary function tests with DLCO should be ordered.

D. Pulmonary angiography can be helpful to look for pulmonary venoocclusive disease, or chronic pulmonary embolic disease as a source of the pulmonary hypertension. Angiography has a characteristic "pruned" tree pattern in PPH. (Doppler scans are not sufficient.)

E. An ABG analysis can be helpful to determine the degree of her hypoxia, but it is not helpful for making the diagnosis. When secondary causes of pulmonary hypertension are eliminated, the diagnosis of PPH can be made.

90. **A. All patients with the diagnosis of PPH should undergo a right heart catheterization to determine if they are vasodilator responders or nonresponders. Approximately 30% of patients are considered responders. This is defined as a person who has a >20% reduction in pulmonary artery pressure and pulmonary vascular resistance with increased or unchanged cardiac output, and a minimally reduced or unchanged systemic BP. Patients who are responders can be tried on oral calcium channel blockers. There is significant benefit in 5-year survival rates of patients who are responders that were given calcium channel blockers as opposed to nonresponders.**

B. The calcium channel blockers of choice to treat PPH are nifedipine and diltiazem, not verapamil. Verapamil is not recommended because of its significant negative inotropic effects. Patients often require high doses; up to 240 mg a day of nifedipine, and up to 900 mg a day of diltiazem. The dose is started low and titrated to the highest dose that is tolerated by the systemic BP and HR.

C. Epoprostenol is a prostaglandin that is given by continuous IV infusion through a central line. It is superior to calcium channel blockers in efficacy in both responders and nonresponders to vasodilator therapy. Side effects include jaw pain, diarrhea, arthralgias, and flu-like symptoms. Complications include those related to a chronic central line, including thrombosis and infections. Patients who stop the therapy suddenly (such as in pump failure) may have significant rebound pulmonary hypertension, which can be fatal.

D. Oxygen therapy should be given to patients who are hypoxemic at rest or with exertion with saturations less than 88%. There is no benefit in oxygen therapy prior to becoming hypoxemic.

E. Because of the propensity to thrombosis in the pulmonary arteries, warfarin is recommended with a goal INR of 2. Warfarin has shown to improve survival in patients with PPH and is considered standard of care.

91. **E. CREST syndrome, considered by many to be a limited form of scleroderma, is characterized by calcinosis cutis (C), Raynaud phenomenon (R), esophageal dysfunction (E), sclerodactyly (S), and telangectasias (T). The anticentromere antibody is highly specific for CREST, but not very sensitive (near 80%). In other words, a positive anticentromere antibody test is good at ruling in the diagnosis, but a negative test does not exclude it.**

A. Anti-Jo1 antibodies are typically associated with inflammatory myositis (polymyositis, dermatomyositis, etc.), not with CREST syndrome.

B. Anti-smooth muscle antibodies are classically seen in patients with autoimmune hepatitis.

C. Antimitochondrial antibodies are most often associated with PBC. Of note, PBC may develop in up to 15% of patients with systemic sclerosis (not CREST syndrome).

D. Anti-topoisomerase 1 antibodies are most frequently seen in systemic sclerosis (scleroderma).

92. **B. *Giardia lamblia* is a protozoan parasite that inhabits the small intestine. It is one of the most common intestinal protozoal parasites in the United States, along with *Cryptococcus*. It is transmitted by the fecal-oral route or as a food-borne or waterborne illness. It results in watery diarrhea, abdominal cramping, and gas. It also may result in fat malabsorption. It does not cause an inflammatory diarrhea. The treatment for the infection is with metronidazole.**

A. *Campylobacter jejuni* is the most common cause of bacterial gastroenteritis in the United States. It is most often seen in children, but its incidence is also increased in patients with HIV infection. It usually occurs after the ingestion of contaminated food such as undercooked chicken. Infection with *Campylobacter jejuni* may be complicated by Guillain-Barré syndrome or postinfectious arthritis. The mechanism of infection involves bacterial invasion; therefore, it results in an inflammatory diarrhea. The incubation period is from 2 to 4 days. Symptoms include abdominal pain and profuse watery diarrhea, which may or may not be bloody. Treatment is with erythromycin.

C. *Salmonella typhi* is usually a food-borne illness, but may be acquired from pets (reptiles and birds). It may be contracted from eating undercooked eggs. It is unusual in the United States, but seems to occur with more frequency in patients with HIV. It results in nausea, vomiting, diarrhea, and abdominal cramps. It does not cause bloody stools, but it is a cause of inflammatory diarrhea. Patients should have WBCs in their stool. Treatment is supportive.

D. *Shigella sonnei* is the most common *Shigella* species in the United States. It is acquired via the fecal-oral route. A very small inoculum is required to infect the host. *Shigella* infection results in fevers, abdominal cramps, and diarrhea that includes blood or mucus. It may be associated with tenesmus. A reactive arthritis can develop after infection with this organism.

E. *Clostridium difficile* is a nosocomial infection that most commonly occurs after antibiotic use. It may also be transmitted person to person via spores. A potentially lethal complication of *Clostridium difficile* infection is toxic megacolon. The diarrhea caused by this organism is an inflammatory diarrhea and should be suspected in anyone who has recently taken antibiotics or has recently been hospitalized. The treatment for this infection is metronidazole.

93. **B. The most serious consequence of splenectomy is increased susceptibility to bacterial infections, particularly those bacteria with capsules such as *Streptococcus pneumoniae, Neisseria meningitidis,* and *Haemophilus influenzae.* There is no increased risk for viral infections in patients without a spleen. The susceptibility to bacterial infections relates to the inability to remove opsonized bacteria from the bloodstream and a defect in making antibodies to T cell-independent antigens such as staphylococcal components of bacterial capsules. Patients who have undergone splenectomy also have increased susceptibility to babesiosis.**

A. Hepatitis A and B vaccines are not indicated because splenectomized patients do not have an increased risk for viral infections.

C, D, E. See explanation for B.

94. **C. Occupational asthma is asthma caused by prolonged exposure to a specific inhaled substance in the workplace. It differs from asthma exacerbated by exposure to certain irritant dusts in that the asthma is not present until there is exposure to the agent. The symptoms consist of wheezing, coughing, and chest tightness, primarily while the patient is at work. Symptoms may resolve somewhat when the patient leaves work only to recur the next time the patient returns to the job. Symptoms may go undiagnosed for months or years. Many different substances may induce occupational asthma. A common one is wheat or rye flour seen in bakers. Diagnosis is usually suspected on history but may be confirmed by having the patient inhale the suspected offending substance and subsequently undergo pulmonary function testing for several hours. If symptoms are mild they can be treated with inhaled corticosteroids or bronchodilators. The patient may be cured by eliminating exposure to the agent altogether.**

A. Patients with OSA also often keep their bed partner awake. However, this is usually due to snoring and apneic episodes rather than coughing and wheezing. In addition, symptoms don't usually improve intermittently unless the patient makes some lifestyle changes, such as weight loss or decreasing alcohol or other sedating agents.

B. Emphysema may result in some of the symptoms this patient has, such as coughing, wheezing, and chest tightness. However, the symptoms of emphysema are usually chronic and progressive, not intermittent. In addition, this patient does not smoke, which is the biggest risk factor for emphysema. Emphysema may develop in the absence of tobacco abuse in patients with alpha-1 antitrypsin deficiency, but these patients will often have a family history of early emphysema or liver disease (ours does not).

D. Pulmonary emboli will usually be asymptomatic or have symptoms of pulmonary hypertension rather than of airway obstruction. Symptoms of pulmonary hypertension include fatigue, dyspnea, or syncope on exertion (our patient has none of these symptoms).

E. Although at risk for coccidioidomycosis by living in Arizona, the usual manifestation of the infection in immunocompetent hosts is either an asymptomatic infection or a very mild upper respiratory illness. Pneumonia may also occur. Chronic pulmonary infection may occur with coccidioidomycosis, but this is usually seen in older patients with emphysema and diabetes. The manifestations of the illness are similar to those of TB. Chronic infection does not usually occur in young, healthy patients, and his symptoms are not consistent with coccidioidomycosis.

95. **C. An elevated hemidiaphragm in an asymptomatic patient may indicate unilateral diaphragmatic paralysis. To confirm the diagnosis, a fluoroscopic sniff test is administered. This test shows that with forceful inspiration, the diaphragm ascends further into the thorax. This is the opposite of what normally occurs, and is caused by the increase in intraabdominal pressure and decrease in intrathoracic pressure that occur on forceful inspiration.**

A. CT scan of the thorax will eventually need to be performed if unilateral diaphragm paralysis is diagnosed. This is because most causes of unilateral diaphragmatic paralysis are neoplastic in nature, resulting in invasion of the phrenic nerve. Other structures such as enlarged lymph nodes or aneurysms may also encroach on the phrenic nerve and may be seen on CT scan. Besides compression, damage to the nerve from surgery or trauma as well as idiopathic types may occur. Unfortunately, these may not be diagnosed by CT scan, but may be suspected on the basis of history.

B. A ventilation/perfusion scan is a test that may be necessary in the evaluation of a patient with a hemidiaphragm elevation because pulmonary embolism may sometimes present with hemidiaphragm elevation. However, this patient is asymptomatic and has no known predisposition for pulmonary embolus.

D. Splenomegaly might cause left hemidiaphragm elevation because hepatomegaly may cause right hemidiaphragm elevation. However, this patient has no known predisposing conditions to splenomegaly and is asymptomatic, making this unlikely.

E. Thoracentesis is not at all indicated in cases of simple hemidiaphragm elevation. Occasionally, however, a pleural effusion may mimic hemidiaphragm elevation. In this case, lateral decubitus views would confirm the etiology of the hemidiaphragm elevation and subsequently, thoracentesis should be performed. Again, however, this patient has no reason to have a pleural effusion nor is she symptomatic.

96. **B. Neurogenic tumors, such as paragangliomas or schwannomas, cause posterior mediastinal masses. Other etiologies for a posterior mediastinal mass include gastroenteric cysts, esophageal lesions. and aortic aneurysms.**

A, C, D, E. Lymphoma usually causes an anterior mediastinal mass. Other etiologies for anterior mediastinal masses include thymomas, thymus gland, teratomas, parathyroid tumors, thyroid tumors, aortic aneurysms, endocrine tumors, and lipomas. Lymphadenopathy from granulomatous disease may be seen in the mediastinum, but this usually causes a middle mediastinal mass. Other etiologies of a middle mediastinal mass include vascular masses and pleuropericardial and bronchogenic cysts.

97. **B. The patient described above has symptoms that are classic for stress incontinence. Incontinence can be broken down into two categories: transient (or isolated) and persistent (or established). Transient urinary incontinence is usually the result of an underlying reversible process. There are a multitude of causes, but problems such as urinary tract infections, volume overload, metabolic problems (e.g., diabetes), postoperative states, delirium, and medications are all known to cause transient incontinence. Of the persistent or established causes of incontinence, there are three main types: stress, urge and overflow. Stress incontinence develops when the abdominal pressure is greater than the sphincter pressure, and leakage of urine results. In this setting, any situation that increases intraabdominal pressure (laughing, coughing, sneezing, bending over, etc.) will cause leakage of urine. The patients who develop stress incontinence most often are women who have had children by vaginal delivery because of the resulting weakening of the pelvic floor muscles.**

A. Urge incontinence is usually the result of detrusor muscle instability and overactivity. Patients with urge incontinence typically feel the sudden urge, hence the name, to urinate and experience leakage of urine without much warning.

C. Overflow incontinence occurs as a result of detrusor muscle weakness and bladder outlet obstruction, which leads to overfilling of the bladder. This is a more common type of incontinence in men and is often associated with persistent dribbling of urine, spontaneous leakage of urine and can be worsened by maneuvers that increase intraabdominal pressures. The patient described above is a woman (and women rarely have bladder outlet obstruction) who has leakage of urine with sneezing, which is highly suggestive of stress incontinence.

D, E. These are causes of incontinence, but are not the most likely. See explanation for B.

98. **E. The treatment of stress incontinence in women consists of doing pelvic floor muscle exercises (Kegel exercises) to help increase muscle tone. In addition, pessaries can be used to provide**

additional support for women who have uterine or bladder prolapse. Drugs such as estrogens and alpha-receptor agonists (imipramine) have been used in patients with some benefit. Surgical maneuvers such as bladder neck suspensions or slings have the highest cure rates in patients with stress incontinence, but they also have higher inherent risks associated with them. In men with stress incontinence (usually occurs after prostatectomy), treatment can be very difficult.

A. Behavioral therapy is used in urge incontinence as a means to attempt to "retrain" the detrusor muscle. This is done by having the patient void at regular intervals, which can gradually be increased.

B. Intermittent clean catheterization is sometimes helpful in patients who have overflow incontinence due to bladder outlet obstruction.

C. Antihyperglycemic therapy would be indicated if she had transient incontinence cause by diabetes that was poorly controlled, resulting in an osmotic diuresis.

D. Antibiotic therapy is indicated in the treatment of urinary tract infections in elderly women who are symptomatic (including incontinence).

99. **C. IBM is classified as one of the idiopathic inflammatory myopathies along with dermatomyositis and PM. There are several clinical features that help distinguish dermatomyositis and PM from IBM. Patients with all of these diseases often present with complaints of muscle weakness. However, patients with dermatomyositis and PM usually have more skin involvement, which include the Gottron sign (a violaceous, nonscaling rash covering extensor surfaces of the fingers) and a heliotrope rash affecting the chest and face. This latter rash is usually described as being a violaceous rash that involves the eyelids with swelling and a v-shaped pattern on the neck. Patients with IBM often do not have skin involvement. Women are afflicted with dermatomyositis and PM twice as often as men. However, men are much more likely to develop IBM. Patients with dermatomyositis and PM usually have a more abrupt onset of symptoms, whereas IBM is more insidious. The laboratory studies are also different. CK levels are often markedly elevated (>10 times normal) in dermatomyositis and PM, but are usually only mildly elevated in IBM. Another distinguishing feature between these diseases is their response to steroid therapy. PM and dermatomyositis typically show marked improvement on therapy, whereas IBM often does not. IBM usually affects the proximal muscle groups in the patients who have the disease. Muscle biopsy often reveals the vacuoles within the sarcoplasm of the muscle fiber, but this is not specific. Eosinophilic inclusions are sometimes seen adjacent to the vacuoles, and these are much more specific for IBM.**

A, B. See explanation for C.

D. Alcohol abuse can cause both a chronic and an acute form of myopathy, but the findings on muscle biopsy are different from IBM. The biopsy of the muscle fibers reveals necrosis with degeneration and regeneration, not vacuoles or inclusions.

E. Duchenne muscular dystrophy is an X-linked disorder that affects people in their toddler years and progresses to early death.

100. **B. Urticaria can be a debilitating symptom, disrupting a person's ability to sleep and work. It typically presents as raised erythematous, well-circumscribed lesions that are pruritic and that subsequently coalesce. Symptoms are secondary to cutaneous mast cell release. This patient is suffering from cholinergic urticaria that commonly occurs after exposure to warm water and hot weather. Anithistamines and refraining from extremes in temperature can help with symptoms.**

A. Urticaria pigmentosa is a skin finding in mastocytosis, which is a series of disorders with proliferation of superficial mast cells. A patient with urticaria pigmentosa has multiple pigmented papules that exhibit Darier sign, or a wheal when subjected to minor trauma. This patient has no skin lesions on examination.

C. Familial cold urticaria is an inherited disorder that leads to the development of fever, leukocytosis, rash with urticaria, and muscle tenderness after exposures to cold. Our patient has reactions to warmth so this is unlikely the etiology of her urticaria.

D. Delayed pressure urticaria presents with burning, rather than itching. It typically occurs after holding heavy items for some time and presents with swelling of the hands. It can also occur on the soles of the feet after spending a long time standing.

E. Contact dermatitis typically presents with an intensely pruritic rash that is secondary to an allergen exposure, including detergents and plants, to name a few. The reaction is a delayed hypersensitivity type reaction. This patient does not give a history of any exposures and has no skin findings suggestive of contact dermatitis.

SETTING 3: INPATIENT FACILITIES

You have general admitting privileges to the hospital. You may see patients in the critical care unit, the pediatrics unit, the maternity unit, or recovery room. You may also be called to see patients in the psychiatric unit. A short-stay unit serves patients who are undergoing same-day operations or who are being held for observation. There are adjacent nursing home/extended-care facilities and a detoxification unit where you may see patients.

101. You are admitting a 50-year-old man with end-stage renal disease who presents with altered mental status secondary to uremia and fluid overload. The patient is indigent and was not receiving medical care prior to his arrival in the ER. Your medical student asks you about the cause of the patient's renal failure. What is the most likely cause of his renal failure because it is the most common cause of end-stage renal disease in the United States?

    A. Diabetes mellitus (DM)
    B. Cystic renal disease
    C. Hypertension
    D. Obstructive uropathy
    E. Chronic glomerulonephritis

102. An 18-year-old woman is admitted to the medical floor with complaints of fever, nausea, vomiting, and back pain. She had felt well until approximately 1 week ago when she developed dysuria and urinary frequency. She developed fever and nausea this morning, as well as bilateral flank pain. On physical examination, she appears ill. Her vital signs show a BP of 105/65 mm Hg and an HR of 100. She has a fever to 102.5°C, and her RR is 16. Her examination is significant for a regular tachycardia without murmur and diffuse abdominal tenderness to deep palpation without guarding or rebound. She has bilateral costovertebral angle tenderness, left greater than right. Her laboratory studies reveal a WBC count of 15,000 with a left shift, a BUN of 20 mg/dL, and a creatinine of 1.0 mg/dL. Her urine reveals 3+ bacteria (gram-negative rods), 50–100 WBCs, 5–10 RBCs, and WBC casts. You begin her on IV ceftriaxone with an empiric diagnosis of pyelonephritis, after the blood and urine cultures are sent. After 72 hours of appropriate IV antibiotics, she is still spiking temperatures to 101.5°C and has persistent left costovertebral angle tenderness. What is the most appropriate next step in management of this patient?

    A. Repeat blood and urine cultures; await culture results before starting any new antibiotics.
    B. Perform renal ultrasonography to evaluate for an abscess formation.
    C. Repeat blood and urine cultures; add better coverage of gram-positive and anaerobic organisms with vancomycin and flagyl until the culture results return.
    D. Perform CT scan with contrast to evaluate for an abscess formation.
    E. Continue the same antibiotics, no need for cultures or imaging; wait another 24 hours before reevaluation.

103. You are taking care of a new admission, a 67-year old man with COPD admitted for bright red blood per rectum. You order a baseline ABG analysis on your patient to assess his respiratory status. Soon, the laboratory calls to tell you that the specimen may have been mislabeled. Which of the following ABG results would you expect to see in a 67-year-old male with COPD and a 60 pack/year history of tobacco use at his baseline?

    A. pH 7.16/pCO_2 71/bicarbonate 20
    B. pH 7.35/pCO_2 70/bicarbonate 32
    C. pH 7.4/pCO_2 40/bicarbonate 24
    D. pH 7.45/pCO_2 25/bicarbonate 16
    E. pH 7.10/pCO_2 20/bicarbonate 7

104. A 48-year-old man is admitted through the ER with a possible left lower extremity cellulitis. The patient says that he has been having fever, swelling, and redness of his left lower extremities that comes and goes spontaneously over the past couple of months. He also tells you about an episode in which he lost vision in his left eye for several minutes a couple of weeks ago, but the vision returned without incident. He had a urologic evaluation for penile trauma 3 months ago. On physical examination, his BP is 125/80, HR 70, RR 14, and he is currently afebrile. His examination is significant for a 3/6 systolic murmur heard at the left lower sternal border without radiation while lying supine. Blood cultures return positive results for *Enterococcus* species, and an echocardiogram reveals a large mitral vegetation. You review treatment for enterococcal endocarditis. Which of the following antibiotics always misses enterococcal infections?

A. Ampicillin-sulbactam
B. Nitrofurantoin
C. Cefipime
D. Vancomycin
E. Linezolid

The next two questions (items 105 and 106) correspond to the following vignette:

A 36-year-old type 1 diabetic is admitted to the ICU with DKA. He is confused and unable to give much history. An initial evaluation does not reveal a cause for his DKA. You appropriately treat the patient with IV fluids, an insulin drip, and replacement of the appropriate electrolytes. The following morning, he is noted to have a left facial droop. This prompts you to do a closer nasal and oral examination and you find a black eschar on his nasal mucosa.

105. What is the likely cause of his DKA?

A. *Nocardia* infection
B. Cerebrovascular accident (CVA)
C. Bell palsy
D. Coccidioidomycosis
E. Mucormycosis

106. What is the treatment of choice for the above patient?

A. Trimethoprim-sulfamethoxazole
B. Warfarin
C. Amphotericin B
D. Fluconazole
E. Prednisone

End of Set

107. You are getting ready to discharge a patient from the hospital who came in with a COPD exacerbation. Prior to his hospitalization, he was not on supplemental oxygen therapy. He asks you if he can get oxygen to take home with him. You discuss with him the criteria for continuous home oxygen therapy. Which of the following patients with COPD meets criteria for continuous home oxygen therapy?

A. A patient with a room air oxygen saturation of 86% on ambulation and 90% at rest
B. A patient with a resting room air paO_2 of 57 mm Hg
C. A patient with a resting room air paO_2 of 58 mm Hg and evidence of cor pulmonale
D. A patient with a resting room air paO_2 of 57 who feels symptomatic improvement with oxygen therapy
E. A patient with a room air oxygen saturation of 91% while awake who desaturates to 86% while asleep

108. A 70-year-old woman with a history of type 2 DM and CAD with a known left bundle branch block on ECG is admitted to the ICU with sepsis from a urinary source. She is fluid resuscitated, and empiric broad-spectrum antibiotics are begun after the appropriate cultures are obtained. Despite what appears to be adequate resuscitative efforts with volume replacement, the patient has had minimal urine output over the past couple of hours. You decide to place a pulmonary artery catheter to help to determine the patient's hemodynamic situation. Which of the following complications of pulmonary artery catheter placement is the patient at increased risk for because of her past medical history?

A. Pulmonary artery perforation
B. Pulmonary infarction
C. Complete heart block
D. Pneumothorax
E. Ventricular tachycardia

109. You are rotating on the cardiology service, and have been reviewing the various cardiomyopathies with your attending physician. He asks you the following question: What do hemachromatosis, amyloidosis, sarcoidosis, and eosinophilic endomyocardial disease (Loeffler's syndrome) have in common?

A. They can cause a restrictive cardiomyopathy.
B. They can cause a dilated cardiomyopathy.
C. They can cause a constrictive pericarditis.
D. They can cause a hypertrophic obstructive cardiomyopathy (HOCM).
E. The can cause a diffuse myocarditis.

The next three questions (items 110–112) correspond to the following vignette:

A 71-year-old woman is admitted to the hospital with complaints of shortness of breath and fatigue that have progressively worsened over the past 2 weeks. She states that she is now short of breath even while watching television. She normally sleeps in a supine position, but has had to sleep on two pillows for the past week. She also frequently awakens gasping for air.

She has had mild lower extremity edema, but denies having cough, fevers, or chills. Her past medical history is significant for poorly controlled hypertension and hypothyroidism for which she takes prinivil and levothyroxine. On examination, her BP is 172/94 mm Hg, with an HR of 78. She is afebrile and has an RR of 22. You note mild jugular venous distention, and no thyromegaly. Bibasilar rales are noted on lung examination. Cardiac examination reveals a regular rate with a prominent gallop that occurs immediately after S_2. There are no murmurs. There is mild bilateral lower extremity edema present. An ECG reveals normal sinus rhythm with no acute ST-segment or T-wave changes. Her ECG does show left-axis deviation with Q-waves in leads V_2, V_3, and V_4. A chest x-ray reveals cardiomegaly with bilateral pleural effusions and Kerley B lines. You diagnose her with CHF and order an echocardiogram that shows left ventricular enlargement with an EF of 25%. The pulmonary artery systolic pressure is estimated at 25 mm Hg.

110. Her CHF can best be described as primarily:

A. Right-sided, diastolic dysfunction likely caused by pulmonary hypertension
B. Right-sided, systolic dysfunction likely caused by hypothyroidism
C. Left-sided, diastolic dysfunction likely caused by hypertensive heart disease
D. Left-sided, systolic dysfunction likely caused by ischemic heart disease
E. Biventricular, diastolic dysfunction likely caused by an infiltrative process

111. She meets criteria for which NYHA functional classification?

A. She does not meet criteria for any class
B. Class I
C. Class II
D. Class III
E. Class IV

112. Which of the following medications have been shown to reduce mortality in patients with CHF?

A. Spironolactone
B. Furosemide
C. Digoxin
D. Dobutamine
E. Brain-natriuretic peptide

End of Set

The next two questions (items 113 and 114) correspond to the following vignette:

113. You are called to see a patient on telemetry who is hypotensive with a BP of 70/35 mm Hg and has an HR of 35. The patient was admitted with a diagnosis of syncope and has no prior cardiac history. ECG reveals second-degree AV block. You place transcutaneous pacer pads and begin pacing while you put a call in to the cardiologist on call. After your patient is stabilized, you review indications for pacemaker placement and you review the different types of pacers. Which of the following is an indication for transvenous dual-chamber pacemaker placement?

A. Sinus bradycardia in the forties while asleep
B. Mobitz type I second-degree heart block
C. New Mobitz type I second-degree heart block that develops post-MI
D. Hypertrophic cardiomyopathy with severe outlet obstruction
E. Systolic dysfunction with an EF of <35% and intraventricular conduction delay

114. In the classification of permanent pacemakers, a series of letters are commonly used to characterize a particular pacemaker. You are told that your patient had a VVI pacemaker placed. What does the second "V" in VVI stand for?

A. The chamber that is sensed
B. The chamber that is paced
C. The mode of response of the pacemaker
D. The type of modulation of the pacemaker
E. The manufacturer of the pacemaker

End of Set

115. A 64-year-old man is admitted with complaints of a fever that has been persisting for the past month. He also has noted painful nodules on the distal ends of two of his fingers and a 10-pound weight loss over this time period. On examination, he has a temperature of 100.8°C and an HR of 88. His BP is normal. Examination of his fundi reveal a right-sided retinal hemorrhage with a pale center. Although his posterior pharynx appears normal, there are several petechiae on his palate. His cardiac examination reveals a new regurgitant murmur over the apex. His hands reveal tender nodules on the pads of two of his fingers. There are also splinter hemorrhages present in his nailbeds. Concerned about endocarditis, you order an

echocardiogram and obtain blood cultures from three different sites. The echocardiogram confirms the presence of a vegetation on the mitral valve. The laboratory calls to report that all three sets of blood cultures are positive for *Streptococcus bovis.* Which of the following is the most likely predisposing factor for this patient's endocarditis?

A. Ongoing IVDA
B. Recent genitourinary instrumentation
C. A prosthetic heart valve
D. Colon cancer
E. Indwelling venous catheter

The following three questions (items 116–118) relate to the same clinical scenario:

Your fellow resident calls you from his rotation in the ER to tell you about an admission. He presents to you the following case: A 40-year-old woman came to the ER with complaints of a sudden onset of dyspnea. She has been feeling poorly for the past several months with complaints of fatigue, occasional palpitations, and unintentional weight loss of approximately 10 pounds. She is a smoker and has been for the past 20 years. She denies having orthopnea, paroxysmal nocturnal dyspnea, cough, or fever. On physical examination, BP is 120/85, HR is 130, temperature is 99.7°C, RR is 18, and room air oxygen saturation is 98%. In general, she is thin and is able to speak in full sentences. Her pupils are 4 mm and reactive. Her hands are warm and moist and she has a fine postural tremor bilaterally. Her heart is irregularly irregular and is without murmur or gallop. Her lungs are clear and her abdominal examination results are unremarkable. An ECG is obtained, which shows atrial fibrillation with a rapid ventricular response. You are admitting her with this diagnosis. As you go to the ER to see the patient, you begin thinking about conditions associated with atrial and ventricular arrhythmias.

116. Which of the following conditions is commonly associated with the development of a ventricular arrhythmia?

A. Thyrotoxicosis
B. Acute alcohol intoxication
C. Hypertension
D. Long QT syndrome
E. Wolff-Parkinson-White (WPW) syndrome

117. You present the patient to your attending physician, who asks, "What is the first test to order to help determine the cause of hyperthyroidism in a patient who presents with classic symptoms and a low TSH?" She gives you some choices:

A. Thyroid scintigraphy
B. Thyroid ultrasonography
C. Radioactive iodine uptake (RAIU) scan
D. Thyroid MRI
E. Fine-needle aspiration (FNA)

118. When you go to the patient's bedside, you notice something that your fellow resident failed to mention (Figure 1-118). The patient tells you that she has noticed a mass in her neck for the past year. The mass is smooth, symmetric, and has a "rubbery" consistency. It is not tender. Upon auscultation, you hear a bruit over the mass. You also note an area of thickened, hyperpigmented skin over the patient's right tibia. You obtain additional social history that the patient is from Mexico and has not sought medical care until now. The laboratory study results return, and her TSH level is virtually undetectable. Which of the following is the most likely cause of the patient's neck mass?

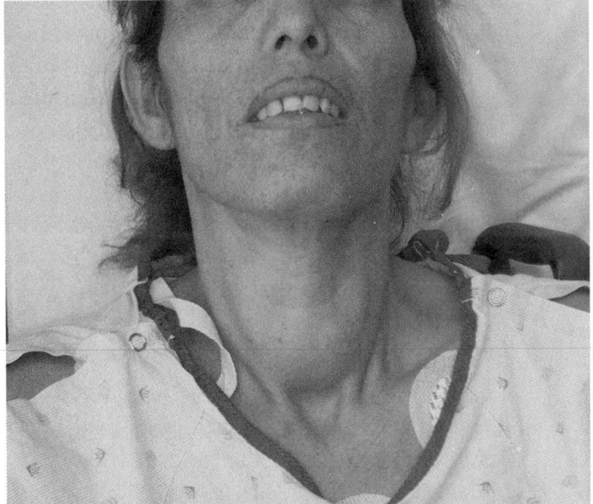

Figure 1-118 • Image Courtesy of Dr. Brenda Shinar, Banner Good Samaritan Medical Center, Phoenix, Arizona.

A. Simple goiter
B. Toxic multinodular goiter
C. Subacute thyroiditis
D. Graves disease
E. Iodine deficiency

End of Set

119. A 55-year-old man is hospitalized in the ICU with pneumonia and sepsis requiring mechanical ventilation. He has now developed DIC and requires blood product transfusion. You must obtain consent from the wife of the patient. She inquires about the risks of transfusion. Which of the following is a true statement?

   A. This patient will likely require transfusion with packed RBCs only.
   B. Acute hemolytic transfusion reactions occur primarily in patients who have had many transfusions.
   C. Hepatitis B is the most common viral infection that can be acquired from a transfusion.
   D. The risk for acquiring hepatitis C from a blood transfusion is approximately 1 in 100 units of blood transfused.
   E. Delayed transfusion reaction is usually due to ABO incompatibility.

120. A 65-year-old woman who has never smoked is brought to the ER by paramedics because of a generalized tonic-clonic seizure. She has never had a seizure before. Her family reveals that she has also had an unintentional weight loss of 10–15 pounds over the past few months. A head CT done in the ER reveals multiple lesions in the brain, most likely metastatic disease, and she is admitted for workup of the lesions and evaluation for a primary cancer. She has a history of diabetes and hypertension that has been reasonably well controlled and has always tried to take good care of herself, and her family is distraught when you explain to them that there is a strong possibility that this is cancer. Which of the following cancers is seen commonly in nonsmokers?

   A. Squamous carcinoma of the head and neck
   B. Squamous carcinoma of the esophagus
   C. Adenocarcinoma of the lung
   D. Carcinoma of the pancreas
   E. Carcinoma of the urinary bladder

121. A 25-year-old man is admitted with shortness of breath for the past four weeks. He complains of dyspnea on exertion, palpitations, weight loss of 10 pounds, fever, and night sweats. On examination, his HR is 110, RR 18, and oxygen saturation 98% on room air. A fixed, matted, 3-cm left supraclavicular node is palpable. His lungs are clear to auscultation bilaterally, and no hepatosplenomegaly is present. The results of the remainder of the examination are normal. A chest x-ray reveals a large left hilar mass. A CT scan is obtained and it confirms a large mass in the anterior mediastinum. The most appropriate next step to make the diagnosis would be:

   A. Open thoracotomy
   B. Bronchoscopy with biopsy
   C. Bone marrow biopsy
   D. Excisional biopsy of the supraclavicular lymph node
   E. Obtain a high-resolution CT scan to further characterize the mass

The next two questions (items 122 and 123) correspond to the following vignette:

A 58-year-old man is admitted with complaints of severe fatigue. He says that for the past 2 months he has experienced fatigue, fevers to 101°C, and night sweats. On physical examination the patient is afebrile with normal vital signs. Cardiovascular and pulmonary examination results are normal. Abdominal examination reveals splenomegaly. Laboratory results show a peripheral blood leukocyte count of 48,000/μL with 3% blasts as well as many leukocyte precursors, such as metamyelocytes and myelocytes. The platelet count is elevated at 600,000/μL. The patient is anemic, with a hemoglobin of 9.8 g/dL and a normal MCV.

122. Which of the following is the most likely diagnosis?

   A. Chronic lymphocytic leukemia (CLL)
   B. Chronic myelogenous leukemia (CML)
   C. Acute myelogenous leukemia (AML)
   D. Richter's syndrome
   E. A leukemoid reaction with a reactive thrombocytosis.

123. Which of the following statements is true regarding CML?

   A. The LAP score is elevated.
   B. The natural history of the disease is characterized by one phase.
   C. The Philadelphia chromosome or translocation 9:22 is present in 90% of patients.
   D. A bone marrow transplantation should be delayed as long as possible and is not usually curative.
   E. Median age of onset for CML is 20–30 years.

End of Set

124. A 66-year-old man with a history of well-controlled hypertension is admitted through the ER because of severe fatigue and a refractory nosebleed. He says that for the past 10 days or so he has noticed bleeding gums, fatigue, and easy bruising. These symptoms, along with the nosebleed, prompted him to come to the ER. On physical examination he is afebrile with normal vital signs except for a regular tachycardia of 105. His conjunctivae are pale and he has notable gingival bleeding as well as a packing in his nose which has stopped the epistaxis. There is no palpable adenopathy. Liver and spleen are enlarged. The results of the remainder of the examination are normal. Laboratory values are as follows: WBC 30,000 with 85% blasts, hemoglobin 8.7 g/dL, and platelet count 20,000/µL. A bone marrow biopsy is done and shows greater than 40% blasts. Myeloperoxidase is positive on cytochemistry testing. The diagnosis that is most consistent with this patient's history, physical, and laboratory findings is:

A. Acute lymphocytic leukemia (ALL)
B. AML
C. CLL
D. CML
E. Hodgkin's lymphoma

125. A 60-year-old man is admitted with lower GI bleeding. He has been appropriately fluid resuscitated and stabilized. You consult a gastroenterologist, who concurs that the patient needs a colonoscopy to evaluate the source of bleeding. The patient is taken to the endoscopy suite where he is to have his procedure performed. As you are seeing your other patients, a "code arrest" is called in the endoscopy suite. Upon arrival, you find your patient is minimally responsive and has agonal respirations. As you secure his airway and begin providing bag-valve-mask ventilation, the nurse informs you that he was given 10 mg of midazolam in preparation for the procedure. The most important next step in the stabilization of your patient is to administer which of the following?

A. Nalaxone
B. *N*-acetylcysteine
C. Flumazenil
D. Deferoxamine
E. Sodium bicarbonate

The next two questions (items 126 and 127) correspond to the following vignette:

You are called to the bedside of a 48-year-old man because of cyanosis. The nursing staff reports that the patient was just brought back to his room after undergoing esophagogastroduodenoscopy evaluation for hematemesis. The patient was given 5 mg of midazolam and cetacaine throat spray for the procedure, which went well without complications. Upon her postprocedure assessment, the nurse noticed he appeared cyanotic. Upon arrival, you find a well-developed man with mild shortness of breath. He is alert and responsive and has a slate blue appearance. His vital signs reveal a BP of 128/76 mm Hg, HR of 78, RR of 22, and temperature of 98.7°C. Room air oxygenation saturation is 97%. On examination, his lungs are clear to auscultation with good air exchange. His cardiac examination results are normal. There is no swelling, pain, erythema, or edema in his lower extremities. You order chest radiography and some immediate laboratory studies. While the phlebotomist is drawing the patient's blood, you notice that it has a chocolate brown appearance. ABG analysis is performed while the patient is breathing room air, yielding the following results: pH = 7.41, pCO_2 = 39, pO_2 = 92, HCO_3^- = 23, saturation = 97%.

126. Which of the following tests will be most helpful in confirming your diagnosis?

A. Helical CT of the chest
B. ABG cooximetry
C. Chest x-ray
D. Serum hemoglobin level
E. B-natriuretic peptide level

127. Which of the following is the best choice for initial treatment of this patient?

A. Intravenous heparin therapy
B. Intravenous loop diuretic
C. Transfusion of packed RBCs
D. Insertion of chest tube
E. IV methylene blue

End of Set

The following three questions (items 128–130) relate to the same clinical scenario:

A 28-year-old man with HIV is admitted with a 3-day history of cough and progressive shortness of breath. His cough is productive of minimal white secretions. He has also been having fevers to 102.5°C. Physical examination results are unremarkable, including normal lung examination results. A CBC reveals a leukocyte count of 18,500/μL with a left shift. A basic metabolic panel is normal. His LDH level is elevated at 550 U/L. His CD4 count is 56/μL. ABG analysis performed on room air shows a pH of 7.25, pco_2 of 50, and po_2 of 61. A chest x-ray is obtained (Figure 1-128). Analysis of sputum is ordered but the results are not helpful because the sample is full of epithelial cells.

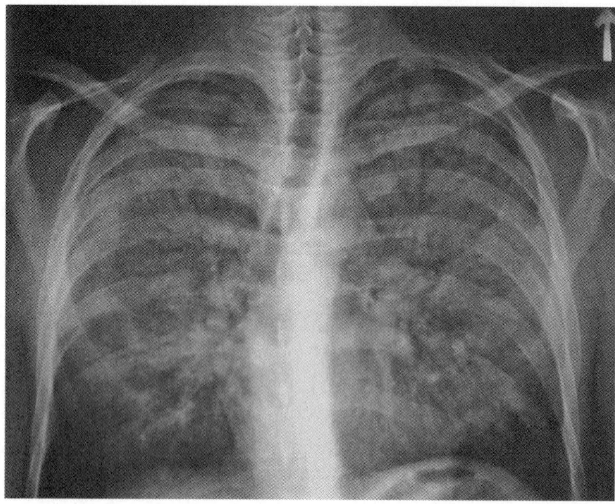

Figure 1-128 • Image Courtesy of Dr. Robert Raschke, Banner Good Samaritan Medical Center, Phoenix, Arizona.

128. What should you order next to make the diagnosis in this patient?
    A. CT scan of the chest
    B. Pulmonary consult for bronchoscopy
    C. Angiography of the chest
    D. Transtracheal aspirate
    E. PPD skin test

129. The bronchoscopy shows evidence of PCP organisms. You order him to be started on IV trimethoprim-sulfamethoxazole. Which of the following is an indication for also starting corticosteroid (prednisone) therapy in this patient?
    A. pao_2 <70 mm Hg
    B. WBC count >15,000
    C. $paco_2$ >45 mm Hg
    D. Fever >101.0°C
    E. CD4 count <200/μL

130. The patient becomes tachypneic with increased work of breathing and requires intubation for hypoxemic respiratory failure. After being ventilated for an hour on assist control mode at a rate of 14 with a tidal volume of 550 cc, PEEP of 5 cm H_2O and 80% Fio_2, you obtain an ABG analysis result that shows the following: pH = 7.22, $paco_2$ = 62, pao_2 = 88, HCO_3^- = 24, saturations = 97%. Which of the following actions would be appropriate to try to correct the above abnormality?
    A. Increase the Fio_2
    B. Increase the PEEP
    C. Decrease the tidal volume
    D. Decrease the rate
    E. Increase the rate

End of Set

The next two questions (items 131 and 132) correspond to the following vignette:

A 64-year-old man with no significant past medical history is admitted for a left hip fracture after falling while playing tennis. He undergoes open reduction with internal fixation without complications. Postoperatively he is given DVT prophylaxis with low-molecular-weight heparin, and his pain is managed with IV morphine sulfate. His postoperative course is uneventful, with the exception of a precipitous drop in his platelet count. At admission, his platelet count was 184,000/μL and dropped to 102,000/μL on postoperative day 4 and then to 48,000/μL on postoperative day 5. The remainder of his CBC was within normal limits.

131. What is the most likely cause of his thrombocytopenia?
    A. Hypersplenism
    B. Bone marrow suppression
    C. Iron deficiency
    D. Morphine sulfate
    E. Heparin

132. What is a common complication that results from his new problem?
    A. Anaphylaxis
    B. Bleeding diathesis
    C. Thrombosis
    D. Anemia
    E. Splenomegaly

End of Set

133. You are called to evaluate a 35-year-old Hispanic man in the trauma ICU. He was admitted 4 days ago following an unrestrained motor vehicle accident where he sustained significant injuries. He has remained unresponsive since admission and has received no sedatives. On physical examination, the patient is intubated, with otherwise normal vital signs. He does not respond to voice, tactile, or other vigorous stimulation. Pupils are midpoint and unreactive. Doll's eyes are not present, and the patient is unreactive to ice water calorics. His face is symmetric. Deep tendon reflexes appear intact and toes are downgoing. When you hold mechanical ventilation, the patient's respirations are ataxic. All laboratory values obtained are normal. Which of the following is a true statement?

A. Ataxic respirations describe a respiration pattern of hyperventilation alternating with apnea.
B. The presence of doll's eyes indicates a midbrain lesion.
C. The cause of this patient's coma is most likely metabolic.
D. The physical examination is not helpful in determining a cause for coma in this patient.
E. Physical examination findings indicate a midbrain injury as a cause for coma for this patient.

The next two questions (items 134 and 135) correspond to the following vignette:

A 28-year-old white man is admitted to the hospital because of a new onset of progressive lower extremity weakness and numbness in his hands and feet that has occurred over the past 3 days. He describes a tingling sensation in his hands and feet and cannot feel his fingertips. He describes difficulty with gait due to the weakness and inability to feel where his feet are being placed on the ground. He is now unable to walk. He has no significant past medical history, but reports having diarrhea and vomiting for 3 days, 2 weeks ago. He denies having fever, chills, headache, visual changes, shortness of breath, bowel or bladder incontinence, or any other symptoms. Vital signs are within normal limits. Cardiopulmonary examination results are normal. Neurologic examination reveals normal mental status, intact cranial nerves, and 1/5 strength in proximal and distal lower extremities bilaterally and 3/5 in all upper extremity muscle groups. Sensation is diminished in the hands and feet, but otherwise intact. Patellar and heel reflexes are absent. Upper extremity reflexes are 1+/4.

134. The diagnosis that best fits this patient is:

A. Charcot-Marie-Tooth disease
B. Alcoholic neuropathy
C. Myasthenia gravis (MG)
D. Guillain-Barré syndrome
E. Multiple sclerosis (MS)

135. Which of the following is true regarding this patient?

A. Nerve conduction studies will be unaffected.
B. CSF will show an elevated protein without pleocytosis.
C. Clinical course will be progressive without recovery of function.
D. Patients with a vital capacity of less than 50 cc/kg should be intubated.
E. Treatment includes pyridostigmine and thymectomy.

End of Set

136. You admit a 75-year-old woman with right-sided weakness that is new in onset. The weakness is worse in the arm than in the leg. The patient's vital signs reveal a BP of 170/90 mm Hg, with an HR of 78 and normal RR and temperature. She is saturating at 95% on room air. Her neurologic examination is significant for weakness of the right upper extremity (3/5) and right lower extremity (4/5) with decreased sensation. There is no abnormality of cranial nerves. Reflexes are hyperactive on the right-sided extremities, and the right toe extends when you stroke the bottom of her foot. You try to localize the site of the presumed stroke in this patient. Which of the following symptoms is suggestive of a stroke in the vertebrobasilar distribution rather than in the carotid distribution?

A. Syncope
B. Transient aphasia
C. Transient loss of vision in one eye "as if a shade is being pulled down"
D. Motor and sensory loss of one extremity
E. Headache

137. You are a hospitalist called to admit a 70-year-old man to the ICU. His wife states that he was sitting at the table eating breakfast with her when he dropped his fork and had difficulty speaking. Within a couple of minutes he was unable to move his right side. She called the paramedics, who brought him to the hospital. Now in the ICU, his vital signs are as follows: BP 200/98 mm Hg, HR 100, RR 10, O_2 saturation 94% on room air. He is afebrile. On physical examination he is lethargic and unable to speak. His pupils are equal and round but sluggish. He has flaccid paralysis of the right arm and leg with a Babinski sign present on the right. His heart is irregularly irregular, and an ECG confirms atrial fibrillation. A CT of the head shows a large bleed in the left frontoparietal area with mass effect and midline shift. You decide to intubate the patient to protect his airway. What is the next most appropriate step in the treatment of this patient while you are awaiting your urgent neurosurgical consult?

A. Hyperventilate the patient to a goal pCO_2 of 20 mm Hg
B. Give a bolus of IV mannitol
C. Give a bolus of IV dexamethasone
D. Give sublingual nifedipine to decrease the BP
E. Anticoagulate with IV heparin because of the atrial fibrillation

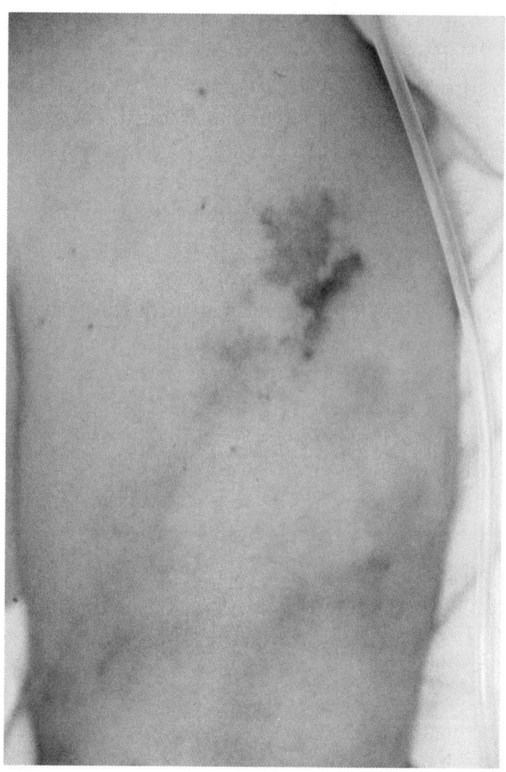

Figure 1-138 • Image Courtesy of Dr. Brenda Shinar, Banner Good Samaritan Medical Center, Phoenix, Arizona.

138. An 18-year-old woman presents with a 1-day history of fever, headache, and a rash on her right shoulder. She is usually in good health. Her mother brought her to the hospital because the patient was difficult to arouse and had obvious altered mental status. On physical examination, her BP is 70/40 mm Hg, with an HR of 140. Her RR is 16, and she is febrile to 103°C. In general she is lethargic. Pupils are equal, round, and reactive at 4 mm. She has positive Kernig and Brudzinski signs, and her neck is stiff. Her heart is tachycardic and without murmur. Her abdomen is soft and has normal bowel sounds. Her right shoulder has a lesion (Figure 1-138). It appears to be growing larger. You tell the family that the patient is going to be admitted to the ICU, and that she very likely has a bacterial meningitis. Her mother says that the patient has a 16-year-old sister that had "the same thing" 2 years ago. Which immunodeficiency state should you evaluate the patient and her siblings for?

A. Chronic granulomatous disease
B. Agammaglobulinemia
C. IgA deficiency
D. Thymic aplasia
E. Terminal complement deficiency

The next two questions (items 139 and 140) correspond to the following vignette:

A 31-year-old woman is admitted to your service with an acute DVT in her right leg. She has no identifiable risk factors that predisposed her to developing this DVT. She has no past medical history and takes no regular medications. Review of systems is unrevealing, with the exception of three prior spontaneous abortions. You are worried that she has an underlying hypercoagulable condition, specifically APLA syndrome.

139. Which of the following statements is true regarding APLA syndrome?

A. The pregnancy loss associated with APLA syndrome can occur at any time during gestation, but it usually happens early in the first trimester.
B. The lupus anticoagulant is identified by a prolonged aPTT that does not correct with a mixing study but normalizes when a preparation of phospholipids is added to the patient's plasma.
C. Antiphospholipid antibodies are a type of anticardiolipin antibody.
D. Patients with positive antibodies but no evidence of thrombosis should be empirically anticoagulated.
E. APLA syndrome is characterized by venous or arterial thrombosis, pregnancy loss, and/or thrombocytosis.

140. Which of the following is true regarding anticoagulant therapy in this patient?

A. Lifelong anticoagulation is needed with a goal INR of 1.5–2.5.
B. Lifelong anticoagulation is needed with a goal INR of 2.0–3.0.
C. Lifelong anticoagulation is needed with a goal INR of >3.0.
D. Anticoagulation with a goal INR of 2.0–3.0 is only necessary for 6 months following a clotting event.
E. Anticoagulation with a goal INR of >3.0 is only necessary for 6 months following a clotting event.

End of Set

141. You admit a 35-year-old woman with complaints of shortness of breath and occasional chest pains, which have been going on for the past week. Her chest x-ray and lung examination are unrevealing, so you order complete PFTs to try to evaluate the cause of her complaints. Her PFTs reveal a normal FVC and FEV_1, but a low DLCO that is 30% of predicted. Which of the following is the most likely cause for an isolated low DLCO level on PFTs?

A. Pulmonary edema
B. Pulmonary hemorrhage
C. Pulmonary infarction
D. Pulmonary embolism
E. Idiopathic pulmonary hemosiderosis

142. A 75-year-old man is admitted for shortness of breath with minimal exertion and lower extremity edema that has developed over the past couple of weeks. It has been a year since he saw his doctor, and he is noncompliant with his medicines, which include a sulfonylurea for DM and NSAIDs for osteoarthritis. He does not drink alcohol. He has smoked two packs of cigarettes per day for the past 52 years and was told at his last examination that he likely has emphysema. He refused to undergo PFTs at that time. He is married and lives in a retirement community with his wife. On examination, his vital signs are as follows: temperature 98.4°C, HR 89, RR 18, and BP 128/78 mm Hg. He has jugular venous distention approximately 2 cm above the sternal angle at 30 degrees elevation. Heart examination reveals a right ventricular heave and a short, high-pitched systolic murmur at the left lower sternal border. His lung examination reveals diminished breath sounds bilaterally, and his abdominal examination reveals mild hepatomegaly with positive hepatojugular reflux. Examination of the extremities reveals mild clubbing and pitting edema from the foot to the knee. You order laboratory tests and an ECG. Which of the following findings are the most likely to be seen on his ECG?

A. rSR complex in V_1, QRS complex in V_6
B. Widened QS complexes in V_1, notched R wave in V_6
C. Wide, notched P wave in II, tall R wave in V_6, and left axis deviation
D. Tall P wave in II, tall R wave in V_1, deep S wave in V_5, right axis deviation
E. Short PR interval, wide QRS complex with delta wave

143. A 54-year-old previously healthy woman is admitted to the hospital for chest pain, cough, and fever that began 4 days ago. She initially had an episode of shaking chills and then developed a cough productive of green sputum. She had fevers at home as high as 102.5°C. She went to an urgent care center 2 days ago and had a chest x-ray performed (Figure 1-143). She was given azithromycin for empiric antibiotic coverage for community-acquired pneumonia. After she went home, she began to feel short of breath and had some left-sided pleuritic chest pain that prompted her to come to the hospital. On physical examination her temperature is 101.4°C, HR is 88, RR is 22, and BP is 130/85 mm Hg. She has bronchial breath sounds and egophany of the left lower lobe. What is the appropriate treatment of this patient?

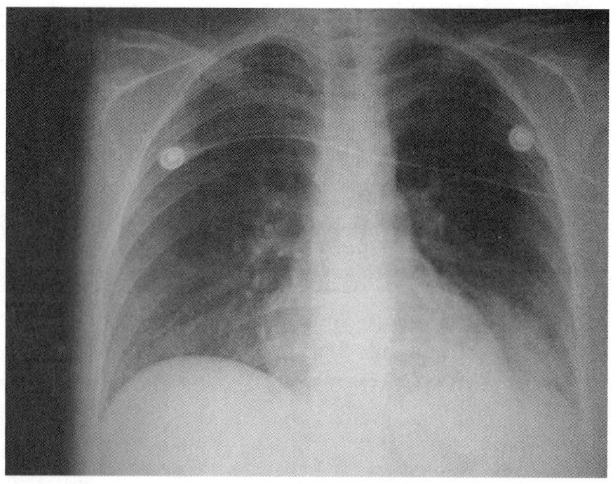

Figure 1-143 • Image Courtesy of Dr. Robert Raschke, Banner Good Samaritan Medical Center, Phoenix, Arizona.

A. Start IV azithromycin and ceftriaxone
B. Start IV vancomycin
C. Continue the patient on oral antibiotics
D. Start IV azithromycin and ceftriaxone and evaluate for an effusion with decubitus films
E. Start IV vancomycin, azithromycin, and ceftriaxone, and evaluate for an abscess with a CT scan

144. You and the critical care attending physician admit a 65-year-old woman from the ER with probable sepsis due to a urinary source. She is hypotensive and requires pressors to keep her systolic BP in the mid-eighties to mid-nineties. You obtain appropriate cultures and treat her with broad-spectrum antibiotics. You continue IV fluids and pressors and note that her urine output has been minimal for the past 2 hours. As you prepare to place a pulmonary artery catheter, the critical care attending physician asks you about the pathophysiology of septic shock. Which of the following patients meet the definition of SIRS?

A. A 24-year-old woman with a history of paroxysmal supraventricular tachycardia who presents with an HR of 175 and RR of 28. Her temperature is normal. Laboratory evaluation is normal.
B. An 18-year-old man with a history of ulcerative colitis who recently had a large lower GI bleed. His HR is 120, and his BP is 80/40 mm Hg. Temperature is normal. WBC count is 12,000.
C. A 65-year-old woman with a productive cough and pleuritic chest pain. Her temperature is 102.3°C, HR is 110, RR 26, and BP is 100/70 mm Hg. Her sputum culture shows gram-positive diplococci. Her WBC count is 14,000.
D. A 28-year-old woman with dysuria and hematuria for 2 days. Her temperature is 100.2°C, HR is 80, and BP is 120/80 mm Hg. Urinalysis reveals leukocyte esterase, nitrite, and bacteria. CBC reveals a WBC count of 11,000.
E. A 42-year-old man with shortness of breath. He has a history of viral myocarditis that has left him with an EF of 15%. His HR is 110, RR is 28. Lung examination reveals diffuse crackles.

145. A 24-year-old woman with a history of Crohn's disease is admitted to the hospital with a history of abdominal pain and bloody bowel movements for the past 2 weeks. She had been placed on a prednisone burst by her gastroenterologist as an outpatient, but her flare-up of Crohn's disease was refractory to outpatient management and she was admitted for IV therapy. After 3 days in the hospital, you note that her peripheral IV site appears erythematous and tender and that she has tenderness and some swelling up the vein to her shoulder. You order that the IV site be changed, and because of the swelling, you order a Doppler scan to be performed to rule out DVT. The result of the Doppler scan reveals a superficial vein thrombosis without evidence of deep vein involvement. Which of the following is a true statement regarding superficial vein thrombosis?

A. Spontaneous superficial vein thrombosis may be a marker for cancer.
B. Superficial vein thrombosis may result in pulmonary embolism.
C. It is difficult to differentiate superficial vein thrombosis from DVT.
D. Varicose veins are not an etiology for superficial vein thrombosis.
E. The treatment of superficial vein thrombosis is anticoagulation.

146. A 62-year-old man is admitted with shortness of breath and fever. For approximately 1 week he has had fevers, chills, headache, diarrhea, cough, and pleuritic chest pain. On examination, he is in mild distress. His temperature is 101.5°C, HR is 98, RR is 22, and BP is 100/72 mm Hg. Lung examination reveals diffuse inspiratory rales. Heart examination results are normal. The patient is not oriented to person, place, or time. Laboratory evaluation reveals a WBC count of

11,500, sodium of 128 mEq/L, and phosphorous of 2.0 mg/dL. Remaining laboratory values are within normal limits. Chest radiography reveals multiple patchy infiltrates. What is the best test to order to make the diagnosis in this patient?

A. Sputum culture
B. Lumbar puncture
C. CT scan of the thorax
D. Organism serology
E. Direct immunofluorescence antibody

147. You are admitting a 62-year-old woman to the ICU from the ER because of difficulty protecting her airway. Four days ago she was seen by her primary care doctor for an infected-looking laceration on her left calf, which she had sustained while gardening. The primary doctor cleaned the wound and gave the patient oral cephalexin for a presumed infection. The next day the patient noted severe muscle cramping in the leg, but she placed a heating pad on the area and took over-the-counter ibuprofen for the pain. The spasms worsened over the next 24 hours to include the muscles of the patient's jaw and face, and her husband brought her to the hospital. On evaluation, her vital signs are normal and she is alert and oriented appropriately, although it is hard for her to speak because of trismus. Heart and lung examination results are normal. Neurologic examination reveals hyperactive reflexes. A spasm of the left calf muscles is present. A superficial laceration is noted on her left knee. The patient's electrolytes, including calcium and ionized calcium, are normal. What is the most likely diagnosis?

A. Botulism
B. Tetany
C. Guillain-Barré syndrome
D. Hepatic encephalopathy
E. Acute dystonic reaction

148. Choose the patient who best matches the pulmonary function test results as seen in Figure 1-148.

A. A 60-year-old man with an 80 pack/year history of smoking who coughs up white sputum every morning
B. A 25-year-old woman with a history of uncontrolled asthma since age 8
C. A 57-year-old nonsmoking woman who presents with a year-long history of progressively worsening dyspnea on exertion and a nonproductive cough
D. A 30-year-old man with a history of alpha-1 antitrypsin deficiency and a 10 pack/year history of smoking
E. A 40-year-old man with a history of cystic fibrosis and recurrent *Pseudomonas aeruginosa* infections

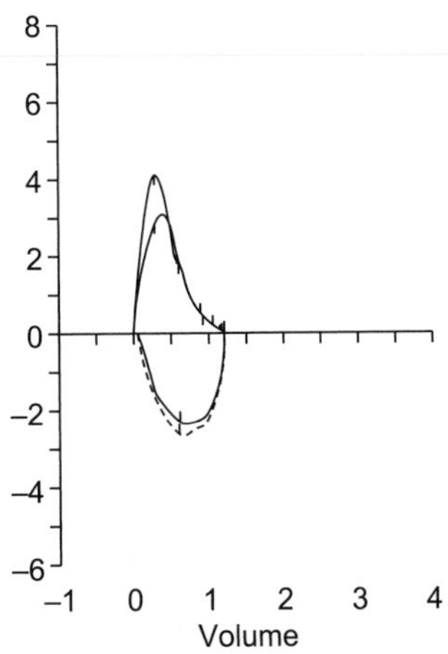

A

Spirometry

		Ref	Pre Meas	Pre %Ref	Post Meas	Post %Ref
FVC	Liters	2.54	1.24	49	1.22	48
FEV1	Liters	2.03	1.06	52	1.06	52
FEV1/FVC	%	83	86		87	
FEF25-75%	L/sec	2.14	1.32	62	1.42	66

Figure 1-148 • *(Continued)*

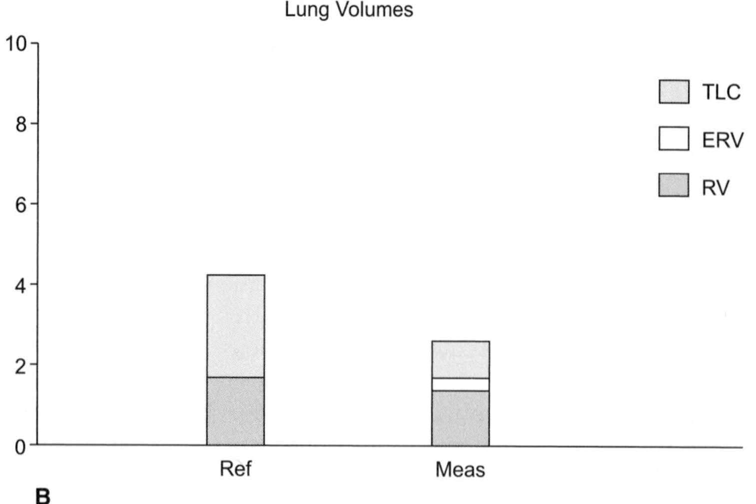

Lung Volumes				
		Ref	**Pre Meas**	**Pre %Ref**
TLC	Liters	4.23	2.62	62
VC	Liters	2.54	1.24	49
RV	Liters	1.67	1.39	83

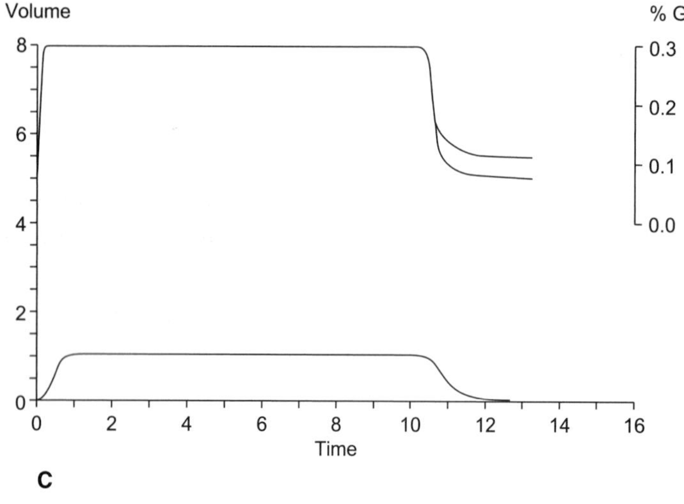

Diffusion				
		Ref	**Pre Meas**	**Pre %Ref**
DLCO	mL/mmHg/min	15.6	5.7	36

Figure 1-148 • Images Courtesy of Dr. Brenda Shinar, Banner Good Samaritan Medical Center, Phoenix, Arizona.

149. Choose the patient who best matches the pulmonary function tests seen in Figure 1-149.

A. A 30-year-old woman who presents with ascending weakness, hyporeflexia, and shortness of breath after a recent diarrheal illness

B. A 65-year-old man who is on amiodarone for 2 years for atrial fibrillation who develops gradual onset of worsening dyspnea on exertion

C. A 55-year-old woman with a 60 pack/year history of tobacco abuse who is continuing to smoke and develops increasing shortness of breath with exertion over the past year

D. A 25-year-old woman who develops gradual dyspnea on exertion over the past 2 years and is now short of breath at rest; physical examination reveals a right ventricular heave and a loud P_2 with clear lungs

E. A 55-year-old woman with a history of chronic urinary tract infection who has been on nitrofurantoin suppression for 1 year develops dyspnea with exertion and coarse inspiratory crackles on lung examination

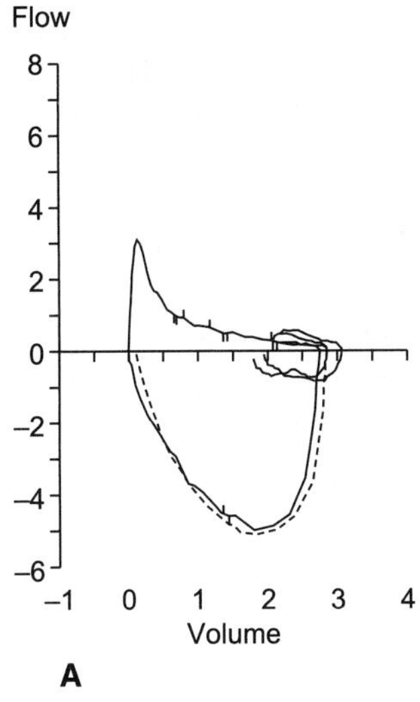

Spirometry							
		Ref	Pre Meas	Pre %Ref	Post Meas	Post %Ref
FVC	Liters	4.16	2.77	67	2.88	69
FEV1	Liters	3.28	1.19	36	1.19	36
FEV1/FVC	%	78	43		41	
FEF25-75%	L/sec	3.25	0.52	16	0.50	15

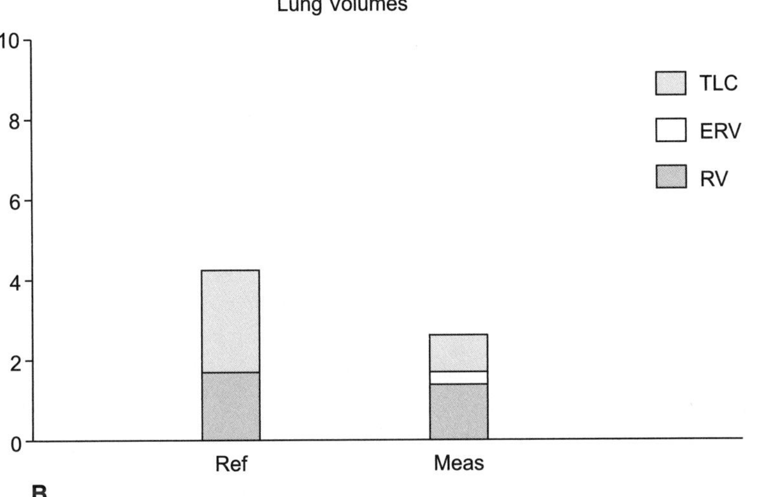

Lung Volumes				
		Ref	Pre Meas	Pre %Ref
TLC	Liters	6.51	8.34	128
VC	Liters	4.16	3.49	84
RV	Liters	2.54	4.85	191

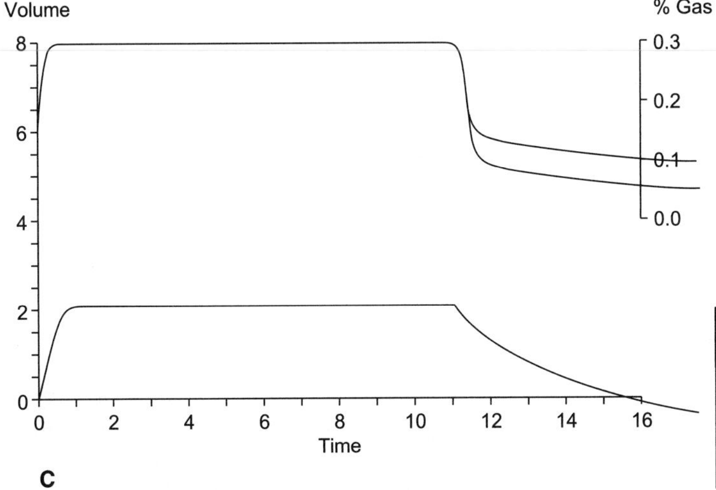

Diffusion				
		Ref	Pre Meas	Pre %Ref
DLCO	mL/mmHg/min	21.5	12.7	59

Figure 1-149 • Images Courtesy of Dr. Brenda Shinar, Banner Good Samaritan Medical Center, Phoenix, Arizona.

150. A 50-year-old man with a history of cirrhosis secondary to hepatitis C is admitted with complaints of shortness of breath. It has been worsening over the past week and is associated with some right-sided chest pain that is pleuritic in nature. He denies having cough, fever, hemoptysis, or lower extremity edema. On physical examination, his BP is 105/65 mm Hg, HR is 80, RR is 20, and oxygen saturation is 92% on room air. He is afebrile. His HEENT examination reveals mild scleral icterus and normal jugular venous pressure. His lungs reveal decreased breath sounds on the right side, half way up his back, with dullness to percussion. His heart sounds are regular without murmurs, rubs, or gallops. His abdomen is soft with a palpable spleen tip. There is no shifting dullness or fluid wave. His lower extremities have trace edema bilaterally. Chest x-ray reveals a large, right-sided pleural effusion which layers on decubitus view. You tap the fluid and remove 1 L of clear, yellow fluid that reveals a protein of 1.5 g/dL (serum protein is 5.4 g/dL) and an LDH of 45 U/L (serum LDH is 120 U/L.) The cell count is unimpressive, and the cytology is negative. Which of the following statements is true regarding this pleural effusion?

A. It cannot be a hepatic hydrothorax, because the patient does not have any ascites.
B. It cannot be a hepatic hydrothorax, because it is on the right side.
C. It is likely a hepatic hydrothorax.
D. You are unable to determine if it is a hepatic hydrothorax by the information given.
E. It cannot be a hepatic hydrothorax because it is an exudate by Light's criteria.

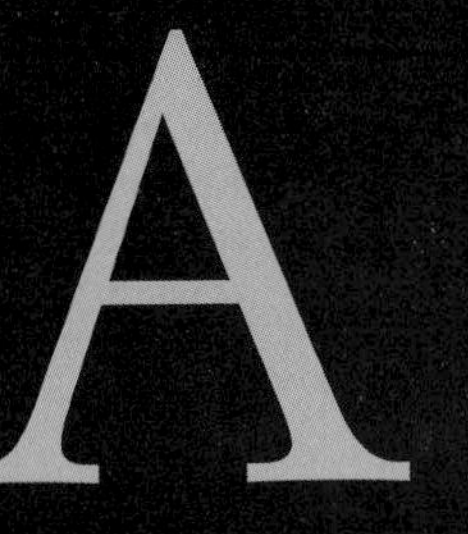

Answers and Explanations

101. A
102. D
103. B
104. C
105. E
106. C
107. C
108. C
109. A
110. D
111. E
112. A
113. D
114. A
115. D
116. D
117. C
118. C
119. C
120. C
121. D
122. B
123. C
124. B
125. C
126. B
127. E
128. B
129. A
130. E
131. E
132. C
133. E
134. D
135. B
136. A
137. B
138. E
139. B
140. C
141. D
142. D
143. D
144. C
145. A
146. E
147. B
148. C
149. C
150. C

101. **A. Nearly 500,000 people in the United States are receiving dialysis, and DM is the most common cause of end-stage renal disease in this population, accounting for 40% of cases. Controlling hypertension is the most important factor for halting progression of renal disease in a diabetic. Goal BPs for diabetics are <130 mm Hg systolic and <80 mm Hg diastolic. If the patient has significant proteinuria, the BP goal should be even lower.**

B. Cystic renal diseases, including ADPKD, cause only 3%–4% of end-stage renal disease.
C. Hypertension is responsible for 30% of patients with end-stage renal disease. Optimal BP control is imperative in halting disease progression.
D. Obstructive uropathy comprises 10% of patients with end-stage renal disease.
E. Chronic glomerulonephritis also comprises 10% of patients with end-stage renal disease.

102. **D. A patient with pyelonephritis who has not defervesced within 72 hours of antibiotic therapy should undergo imaging of the kidneys to evaluate for an abscess formation. A CT scan with contrast is the most sensitive test to evaluate for this. If the patient has contraindications to CT scans (such as pregnancy) or IV contrast (such as renal failure), then ultrasonography should be performed. Ultrasonography, however, may miss abscesses that are <2 cm. This imaging modality is operator dependent and varies in its sensitivity because of patient body habitus (e.g., it is harder to see findings in obese patients).**

A. A patient with pyelonephritis who has not defervesced after 72 hours on appropriate antibiotics should have a CT scan with IV contrast. Repeat cultures are unlikely to be helpful on antibiotics, and even a repeat urinalysis may not show WBCs despite the formation of an abscess if the abscess does not communicate with the collecting system.
B. Renal ultrasonography is not as sensitive as CT, and should be used only if a CT scan with contrast is contraindicated.
C. Adding more antibiotics is not the appropriate response, because this patient requires imaging.
E. Patients with pyelonephritis who have not improved after 72 hours need an imaging study as described above.

103. **B. This patient has a chronic respiratory acidosis with a compensatory metabolic alkalosis. The pH in chronic respiratory acidosis should decrease by 0.03 units for each increase in 10 mm Hg by pCO_2. The predicted change in bicarbonate can be calculated by using the following formula: *increase in bicarbonate = change in pCO_2 × 0.4*.**

A. This blood gas result is consistent with an acute respiratory acidosis such as you might see in an acute asthma exacerbation.
C. This is a normal blood gas result.
D. This blood gas result is consistent with a chronic respiratory alkalosis.
E. This blood gas result is consistent with a metabolic acidosis and a respiratory alkalosis that is appropriately compensated.

104. **C. The cephalosporins are universally inactive against enterococcal infection. Enterococci can be difficult to treat because of resistance to many antibiotics as well as because of their often confusing results on in vitro susceptibility tests. In vitro tests may report susceptibility to cephalosporins; however, in vivo, these drugs are not useful.**

A. Ampicillin-sulbactam is useful for treatment of enterococcal infections. Enterococci can produce beta-lactamase, so the penicillins alone are not always sufficient. With the addition of sulbactam, a beta-lactamase inhibitor, enterococci are usually susceptible. A penicillin in combination with an aminoglycoside is also appropriate therapy.
B. Nitrofurantoin can be effective against enterococci, but is not first-line treatment.
D. Vancomycin is effective against enterococci and may be used in the case of penicillin allergy or resistance to penicillin. Unfortunately, an increasing number of vancomycin-resistant strains of enterococci are being discovered. Vancomycin resistance often goes along with penicillin resistance. Vancomycin-resistant enterococcus is a nosocomial infection that can be spread by health-care workers, causing outbreaks in hospitals and nursing homes.
E. Linezolid is a newer antibiotic with strong activity against gram-positive bacteria. It is used for the treatment of vancomycin-resistant enterococcus infections in addition to another drug called quinupristin/dalfopristin.

105. E. The mucormycoses are a group of fungal organisms that cause infection primarily in immunocompromised hosts. The clinical scenario frequently resembles invasive aspergillosis. There are multiple forms of illness. For example, cutaneous infections may occur in patients with severe trauma. Diabetes, and particularly DKA, increase the risk for disseminated infection with the molds. Classically, on examination, a black eschar will be present on the nasal or palatal mucosa, indicating rhinocerebral disease. This can then lead to cranial nerve palsies, particularly cranial nerve VII, cavernous sinus thrombosis, and possibly proptosis.

A. *Nocardia* is a gram-positive rod that forms branching filaments. Infection with the organism is rare but occurs in immunosuppressed patients, particularly those with impaired cell-mediated immunity such as those on corticosteroids. Although *Nocardia* can affect the CNS, the most common manifestation of infection is pulmonary infection. The black eschar characteristic of infection with mucormycosis is not seen with *Nocardia* infection.

B. A CVA is possible in a 36-year-old diabetic, but it would not likely lead to DKA, and a black eschar on the nasal mucosa would not likely be seen.

C. Bell palsy results in an isolated, peripheral, seventh cranial nerve palsy. Occasionally, this can be a result of diabetic neuropathy or Lyme disease, but more often it is idiopathic. In either case, it would not result in DKA, and patients with this condition would not likely have a black eschar on the nasal mucosa.

D. Coccidioidomycosis may cause a wide variety of clinical manifestations. Usually these patients are from or have spent time in the Southwestern United States, and we have no information indicating that this applies to our patient. The usual CNS manifestation of coccidioidomycosis is meningitis that may result in headache and cranial nerve palsies. Again, the classic black eschar of mucormycosis is not seen in coccidioidomycosis.

106. C. Amphotericin B is the antifungal medication of choice for patients with infections due to the mucormycoses. Treatment may be necessary for up to 12 weeks. In addition to antifungal treatment, surgical débridement of any masses found must also be performed on a regular basis until the débrided tissue is culture negative.

A. Trimethoprim-sulfamethoxazole is the treatment of choice for *Nocardia* infection.

B. Warfarin could be useful if the patient suffered a CVA that was due to atrial fibrillation. However, this was not the cause of his clinical syndrome.

D. Fluconazole is an antifungal medication that could be used for less severe fungal infections. It may be used to treat coccidioidomycosis in some patients, but patients with severe disseminated infection with coccidioidomycosis often require amphotericin B.

E. Prednisone would not be appropriate for this patient. It may sometimes be effective for patients with Bell palsy. However, in this patient with a disseminated fungal infection, it would most likely worsen his condition.

107. C. Indications for continuous home oxygen therapy include the following: (1) a room air resting $pa O_2$ of ≤55 mm Hg, (2) a room air resting saturation of ≤88%, or (3) a room air resting $pa O_2$ of <59 mm Hg with evidence of cor pulmonale ("P pulmonale" on ECG, lower extremity edema secondary to right heart failure, and/or hematocrit >55%.) Home oxygen therapy is the only treatment for COPD that prolongs survival. It is most effective when used as close to 24 hours per day as possible, because intermittent use does not prolong survival in those who require continuous use.

A. This patient would qualify for oxygen with exercise, but does not qualify for oxygen therapy that is continuous at rest based on the above criteria.

B. This patient's $pa O_2$ is >55 mm Hg; therefore, he doesn't meet criteria for continuous home oxygen therapy.

D. Requirement for continuous home oxygen therapy relies on resting $pa O_2$ of 55 mm Hg or less, as outlined above. Unfortunately, it doesn't matter that the patient feels symptomatically better with oxygen; he doesn't meet criteria for the oxygen to be paid for by insurance.

E. This patient should be evaluated for OSA because he may require treatment with CPAP or other modalities. He may respond to oxygen therapy while sleeping, but he doesn't meet criteria for continuous oxygen.

108. C. **Complications of pulmonary artery catheters (also called Swan-Ganz catheters) are either associated with the placement of the catheter, the "floating" of the catheter, or the maintenance of the catheter. Patients with a preexisting left bundle branch block may develop a new right bundle branch block while the catheter is being "floated," which can put them into complete heart block. This complication should be prepared for in patients who are going to have a Swan-Ganz catheter placed with availability of pacer pads at the bedside.**

A, B. Pulmonary artery perforation is a complication that has a mortality rate of 30% and necessitates urgent cardiothoracic surgery consultation for repair. It may occur during the initial placement of the catheter, or later, after the catheter has been left in too distal a position. After the Swan numbers have been obtained, the catheter should have the balloon deflated and the catheter should always be pulled back slightly from where it wedges, to avoid the possibility of perforating the artery, forming a pseudoaneurysm in the artery, or causing a pulmonary infarction.

D. Complications such as the development of a pneumothorax or hemothorax can occur when one is trying to cannulate the central veins in the initial placement of the catheter. Our patient is not at increased risk for either of these complications.

E. Atrial and ventricular arrhythmias can occur as the balloon is inflated and the catheter is "floated" through the right side of the heart into the pulmonary artery, where it eventually wedges. They are usually transient during the floating of the catheter. Antiarrhythmic medical therapy is not indicated for prophylaxis prior to the placement of the catheter.

109. A. **Restrictive cardiomyopathy is characterized by decreased ventricular filling due to decreased compliance of the ventricle. This decrease in compliance can be caused by a variety of processes, such as infiltrative diseases (hemachromatosis, sarcoidosis, amyloidosis, etc.), myocardial fibrosis, such as in Loeffler's syndrome, metastatic disease, radiation therapy, and scleroderma. Restrictive cardiomyopathy also may be idiopathic.**

B. Dilated cardiomyopathies are caused by many different etiologies: postinfectious (viral, HIV, Chagas' syndrome), toxic (alcohol, adriamycin), tachyarrhythmic induced, pregnancy related, catecholamine induced (cocaine, pheochromocytoma), and metabolic (hypothyroidism, and vitamin B_1 deficiency). Ischemic heart disease, hypertension, and valvular heart disease are often considered causes of dilated cardiomyopathy, but they are not technically cardiomyopathies because they are not primary diseases of the heart muscle, per se.

C. Constrictive pericarditis may present very similarly to restrictive cardiomyopathy. Patients have diminished filling capacity due to the constriction of the pericardium around the heart; however, unlike restrictive cardiomyopathy, the septum of the heart can shift toward the left side to accommodate more preload. This allows for some respiratory variation of the ventricular filling velocity, which is not seen in restrictive cardiomyopathy. (This physiology can be seen on Doppler echo, which helps to make the diagnosis. The physical examination is not helpful in distinguishing between the two problems.) Patients with constrictive pericarditis may have a history of pericarditis or a disease that is known to infiltrate the pericardium, such as TB or connective tissue disease. Calcification of the pericardium seen on chest x-ray is strongly suggestive of constrictive pericarditis.

D. HOCM is a disorder that may be inherited in an autosomal-dominant pattern. It consists of left ventricular and septal enlargement with abnormal myocytes arranged in a "pinwheel" pattern. The hypertrophy of the septum and other areas of the left ventricle in addition to the abnormally large and displaced anterior mitral valve leaflet may cause a dynamic (not fixed) obstruction of the outflow tract. Certain conditions make the obstruction worse, such as decreased preload, increased contractility, and decreased afterload states.

E. Myocarditis usually has an infectious etiology but may be a result of drugs or radiation. In the United States, myocarditis is usually related to coxsackie B virus when it is of an infectious etiology. It may progress to a dilated cardiomyopathy. It is not related to the infiltrative agents that are mentioned in this question.

110. **D. There are several ways to categorize a patient with CHF. Two of the most common ways are to divide the patients into right versus left heart failure, and into diastolic versus systolic dysfunction. Right-sided heart failure typically presents with increased jugular venous pressure, congestive hepatomegaly, and peripheral edema. In addition, pure right-sided heart failure should not cause pulmonary congestion on examination. Left-sided heart failure most often presents with symptoms consistent with pulmonary edema (shortness of breath, orthopnea, cough, paroxysmal nocturnal dyspnea, etc.). The echocardiogram is useful in distinguishing between systolic and diastolic dysfunction. Decreased EF or abnormally increased chamber sizes suggest systolic dysfunction, whereas hypertrophy or abnormal flow across the mitral valve suggests diastolic dysfunction. The patient in this vignette had clinical signs and symptoms of primarily left-sided heart failure with mild right-sided involvement as well. Her echocardiogram showed left ventricular dilatation with a decreased EF, suggesting systolic dysfunction. Ischemic heart disease is the most common cause of left-sided heart failure with systolic dysfunction. This diagnosis is supported by the presence of Q waves on ECG, which suggest an old anteroseptal infarct. Other known causes of left-sided systolic dysfunction include coarctation of the aorta, aortic stenosis, dilated cardiomyopathy, chronic aortic insufficiency or mitral regurgitation, and sepsis.**

A. Pulmonary hypertension can cause right-sided heart failure with diastolic dysfunction. Although our patient had some evidence of mild right-sided heart failure, her echocardiogram was consistent with systolic dysfunction. In addition, her pulmonary artery systolic pressure was normal, which does not support the diagnosis of pulmonary hypertension.

B. As noted above, the patient had more left-sided heart failure symptoms. In addition, the thyroid disease usually associated with CHF is thyrotoxicosis, not hypothyroidism, causing high-output CHF.

C. Hypertension is a common cause of left-sided heart failure with diastolic dysfunction. Aortic stenosis and hypertrophic cardiomyopathy are other known causes.

E. Infiltrative processes (such as hemochromatosis, amyloidosis, and sarcoidosis) can cause decreased ventricular compliance, leading diastolic dysfunction and ultimately biventricular failure. However, these patients present more commonly with right-sided heart failure symptoms. Our patient had only slight evidence of right-sided involvement, had systolic dysfunction and no evidence of an infiltrative process.

111. **E. Although there are several schemes used to classify the severity of CHF, the NYHA functional classification (Table 1-111) is one of the most widely used. It is based on historical information obtained from the patient regarding their symptoms. The classification can then be used to help determine prognosis, with the higher classes having poorer prognoses. This patient had symptoms even at rest, which meets criteria for NYHA class IV CHF.**

A, B, C, D. See explanation for E.

TABLE 1-111 NYHA Functional Classification

Class	Definition
I	No limitations with normal physical activity. Symptoms are only present with greater than normal activity.
II	Minimal limitation of physical activity. Symptoms are present with ordinary activity.
III	Marked limitation of physical activity. Symptoms are present with minimal activity.
IV	Unable to carry on physical activity. Symptoms are present even at rest.

112. A. Several medications have been shown to decrease mortality rates in patients with CHF. ACE inhibitors have been shown to decrease mortality rates from 16% to 40% in various trials (CONSENSUS and SOLVD trials) depending on the NYHA classification. Hydralazine in combination with nitrates has also been shown to decrease mortality (V-HeFT I trial), but the combination is not as effective as ACE inhibitor therapy (V-HeFT II trial). Therefore, the hydralazine/nitrate combination is used as an afterload reducer only when a patient is unable to tolerate an ACE inhibitor. Beta blockers have been shown to decrease mortality rates in patients with CHF (MDC, CIBIS-II, and MERIT trials) but must be used with caution and titrated carefully in patients who are not acutely decompensated. The RALES trial proved that spironolactone was effective in decreasing mortality by 30% in patients with NYHA class III and IV CHF.

B, C, D. Digoxin, dobutamine, and furosemide do not improve mortality rates in CHF, although digoxin therapy may decrease the number of hospitalizations. Dobutamine appears to improve patients' quality of life, but actually may increase mortality rates.

E. BNP is a hormone produced by the dilated ventricles in systolic heart failure. It is useful in the setting of systolic heart failure in two ways. First, the serum level of BNP correlates with the NYHA class of heart failure and can help in the diagnosis of less clinically obvious presentations of failure. Second, infusions of BNP (also called nesiritide) can help to decrease the volume load in heart failure by effective diuresis and improve symptoms of failure without the risks for dangerous rhythm disturbances (like the risks that occur with dobutamine). The drug appears promising in many ways for the diagnosis and treatment of systolic heart failure, but there are no randomized, controlled trials to confirm a mortality benefit yet.

113. D. There are several indications for the use of dual-chamber pacemakers. (Dual-chamber pacers have electrodes placed in both the right atrium and the right ventricle and depend on a stable atrial rhythm for proper function. If the atrial rhythm is fibrillation, flutter, or multifocal atrial tachycardia, then a single-chamber ventricular-inhibited device should be implanted instead.) Indications for dual-chamber pacemaker include Mobitz type II second-degree and third-degree AV block, symptomatic bradycardia, bradycardia of <40 beats/min or with pauses of >3 seconds while awake, hypersensitive carotid sinus syncope with documented asystole of >3 seconds, and symptomatic hypertrophic cardiomyopathy with significant outflow obstruction. Also, there are several arrhythmias that may develop post-MI that require a pacemaker. These include symptomatic sinus bradycardia, asystole, or any new Mobitz type II second-degree or third-degree AV block. Also, any patient who develops a bifascicular block after an MI should be considered for pacing.

A, C. See explanation for D.

B. Mobitz type I second-degree block (Wenckebach) does not usually require a pacemaker, unless it is symptomatic, which rarely happens.

E. Biventricular pacing is helpful in patients with symptomatic heart failure with systolic dysfunction (EF <35%) and intraventricular conduction delay (QRS interval ≥130 msec). Biventricular pacing reduced hospitalizations and decreased symptoms in patients according to the MIRACLE trial. Biventricular pacing differs from the usual dual-chamber pacer by helping to synchronize the ventricles to contract together; the term *cardiac resynchronization therapy* has been used.

114. A. Three or four letters usually are used in the classification of permanent pacemakers. Each of these letters represents a particular characteristic of the pacemaker and is usually reported in a particular order. The first letter stands for the chamber that is paced. This is usually designated by the letter V, A, or D (ventricle, atrium, or double). The second letter, which represents the chamber that is sensed, is usually a V, A, D, or O (ventricle, atrium, double, or nOne). The third letter indicates the mode of response of the pacemaker. This can be either triggered, inhibited, double, or nOne (T, I, D or O). The fourth letter, which may or may not be noted, indicates whether the pacemaker is programmable or rate modulated. Because most pacemakers are rate modulated, this fourth letter is often omitted. For example, the VVI pacemaker mentioned above is a pacemaker that has a single lead in the right ventricle. This pacemaker senses the ventricle and paces the ventricle.

Spontaneous ventricular beats are sensed and subsequently inhibit ventricular pacing. VVI pacemakers are often used in the treatment of chronic atrial fibrillation and symptomatic bradycardia.

B, C, D. See explanation for A.

E. There is no single letter that represents a particular manufacturer.

115. **D. Although a variety of clinical conditions may predispose a person to developing endocarditis, there are several correlations between the causative organism and the underlying predisposing condition. Because many of these infectious agents can be seen in a variety of hosts, their presence on a blood culture is by no means pathognomonic, but rather it should raise concern for possible underlying causes. For example, *Streptococcus bovis* is often associated with GI malignancy in elderly patients. A colonoscopy is indicated in any older patient with documented *S. bovis* endocarditis.**

A. *Streptococcus viridans, Staphylcoccus aureus, Staphylococcus epidermidis* (coagulase-negative *Staphylococcus*), and gram-negative endocarditis are seen more commonly in IV drug users and patients with prosthetic heart valves. Our patient had no history of IV drug use or prosthetic heart valve placement.

B. Enterococcal endocarditis is found in older men with a history of GU disease or recent GU instrumentation or surgery. The patient listed above had neither of these risk factors.

C. See explanation for A.

E. Indwelling venous catheters put patients at risk for the development of endocarditis with organisms similar to those seen in IV drug users (i.e., normal skin flora). Please refer to answer A above.

116. **D. Long-QT syndrome is a familial syndrome that is the result of unequal cervical sympathetic input to the heart. This results in widely divergent repolarization states throughout the heart, and predisposes to a polymorphic ventricular tachycardia known as torsade de pointes. Patients with long-QT syndrome may have a normal resting QT interval that lengthens in response to sympathetic stimulation such as exercise or fright. This diagnosis should be considered in young patients without overt heart disease who present with ventricular tachycardia or syncope. Atrial arrhythmias are not associated with long-QT syndrome.**

A. Atrial fibrillation may be precipitated because of thyrotoxicosis. Hyperthyroidism needs to be ruled out when patients present with new-onset atrial fibrillation, especially in elderly patients whose sole manifestation of thyrotoxicosis may be atrial fibrillation.

B. Acute alcohol intoxication may precipitate atrial fibrillation, and this entity has been named "holiday heart syndrome." Atrial fibrillation may occur in up to 60% of binge drinkers, and they do not have to have alcohol-induced cardiomyopathy to develop atrial fibrillation.

C. Hypertension increases the risk for developing atrial fibrillation by approximately 1.42-fold. Although this risk is not enormous, the prevalence of hypertension makes it the most commonly associated disorder in patients with atrial fibrillation.

E. WPW syndrome is a type of ventricular preexcitation syndrome. In preexcitation syndromes, there is an accessory pathway of conduction tissue called an atrial bypass tract, which allows anterograde conduction to stimulate the ventricle ahead of the usual pathway. The PR interval is shortened because of the early ventricular depolarization, and the fusion between the accessory pathway and the normal AV node conduction pathway produces a slurred upstroke to the QRS. WPW syndrome predisposes to many different arrhythmias, including atrial fibrillation, flutter, and paroxysmal supraventricular tachycardia. In addition, ventricular responses during atrial flutter or fibrillation may be unusually rapid and may cause ventricular fibrillation.

117. **C. An RAIU scan is a test that helps to determine if a patient has hyperthyroidism due to a thyroid gland that is avidly taking up iodine (high uptake) or a different cause in which the thyroid is not avidly taking up iodine (low uptake). It is a test that results in a number value (whereas scintigraphy results in a picture). The two most common causes of hyperthyroidism with high RAIU are Graves' disease and toxic multinodular goiter. Causes of hyperthyroidism with low RAIU include thyroiditis (in which the thyroid gland is injured, unable to take up iodine, and leaking hormones into the circulation) and factitious thyroid hormone ingestion.**

A. Thyroid scintigraphy is a nuclear test used in the evaluation of a thyroid nodule, usually in a euthyroid patient. (It also may be used in patients with hyperthyroidism to determine if there is a nodular component to their disease, and whether the nodules are functioning or not.) A radioactive isotope (usually of iodine) is injected into the patient, and the thyroid is scanned, yielding an image that reflects where the iodine was taken up within the thyroid. A "cold nodule" that did not take up the radioactive iodine is nonfunctioning and may represent thyroid cancer. All cold nodules require workup with FNA for cytology. A "hot nodule" is functional; the radioactive iodine is taken up by the thyroid tissue and incorporated into thyroglobulin. These nodules are rarely cancerous and can often be followed.

B. Thyroid ultrasonography is an excellent modality to evaluate the anatomy of the thyroid gland. It may be used when a nodule is palpated to better determine the size of the nodule and whether it is cystic or solid. Ultrasonography can be used to guide FNA. It does not help with the evaluation of thyroid physiology, and it is not the first test to order when evaluating a person with hyperthyroidism.

D. There is little need for evaluation of the thyroid by MRI scanning. It is definitely not the first test to order when evaluating a patient with clinical hyperthyroidism.

E. FNA of the thyroid gland is done for cytology when there is a palpable thyroid nodule of >1 cm on physical examination or ultrasonography, and it appears "cold" on scintigraphy. FNA should not be done in a patient who is clinically hyperthyroid without nodules.

118. **D. Graves' disease consists of three clinical manifestations: (1) hyperthyroidism with diffuse goiter, (2) ophthalmopathy, and (3) dermopathy. In order to be termed Graves' disease, only one of the manifestations needs to be present. This patient has two of the manifestations, namely, hyperthyroidism with diffuse goiter, and pretibial myxedema, or dermopathy. The hyperthyroidism of Graves' disease is caused by autoantibodies that bind to the TSH receptor and stimulate the thyroid gland to produce thyroid hormone. The ophthalmopathy is thought to be from cytokine-mediated stimulation of fibroblasts and the deposition of glycosaminoglycans in the periorbital tissue. The patient develops proptosis and sometimes ophthalmoplegia. The "frightened stare" is another component of the ophthalmopathy and is due to sympathetic stimulation of the levator palpebrae muscle of the upper eyelid. This component of the eye disease may reverse with treatment of the thyrotoxicosis, whereas the proptosis may require surgical correction. The dermopathy is also called pretibial myxedema, and the mechanism is unclear. It is important to remember that pretibial myxedema is associated with hyperthyroidism, not hypothyroidism.**

A. A simple goiter is an enlargement of the thyroid gland that is not caused by an inflammatory process or neoplastic process, and in which the patient is euthyroid. It occurs when the thyroid's ability to secrete enough hormone to meet the needs of the peripheral tissue is impaired. You would think that this would cause an elevated TSH and clinical hypothyroidism, but this is usually not the case, and most patients have a normal TSH. Simple goiter may progress to goitrous hypothyroidism over time. Our patient is manifesting symptoms of hyperthyroidism, and also has the dermopathy associated with Graves' disease.

B. Toxic multinodular goiter is the second most common cause of hyperthyroidism after Graves' disease. It results from a long-standing simple goiter that becomes multinodular. Eventually the nontoxic nodules develop independence from TSH stimulation and become autonomous. When this happens, the result is a "toxic" (autonomous) multinodular goiter (TMG) and clinical hyperthyroidism. The presentation of TMG differs from Graves' disease in a few significant ways. First, TMG occurs in elderly patients (because it takes time to progress from a simple goiter, to nontoxic, to toxic), whereas Graves' disease is mostly a disease of women in their thirties and forties. Second, the hyperthyroidism is often not as severe in TMG as in Graves' disease. Third, the ophthalmopathy is rarely seen in TMG, and if present, should suggest another diagnosis. And lastly, although both TMG and Graves' disease can be treated with radioactive iodine ablation, the dose required for TMG is often much larger than that required for Graves' disease.

C. Subacute thyroiditis is usually a virally mediated inflammatory disorder of the thyroid gland. Synonyms for subacute thyroiditis include granulomatous thyroiditis and de Quervain's thyroiditis. The gland is usually tender to palpation, which was not the case in our patient. Patients with subacute thyroiditis may develop hyperthyroidism because the injured thyroid gland leaks thyroid hormone into the circulation.

E. Iodine deficiency may cause goiter in patients from endemic areas. Our patient is from Mexico and, theoretically, she could have a goiter from iodine deficiency. Patients with iodine deficiency resulting in goiter often have a low T_4 and T_3 that causes an increase in TSH and stimulation of the gland. This results in a growth of the gland, and a goiter. Initially the goiter is diffuse, but over time it becomes nodular because some of the follicles proliferate more than others. Therefore, in endemic areas, most goiters in children are diffuse and most adults have nodular goiters. Our patient had a smooth, diffusely enlarged thyroid. It is important to realize that some of the nodules in an iodine-deficient gland may mutate their TSH receptor and, in effect, become continuously stimulated. These patients can actually present with hyperthyroidism if their iodine deficiency is not severe, or if they are given large doses of iodine (jodbasedow phenomenon).

119. **C. Hepatitis B is the most common viral infection acquired from transfusion, with a risk of 1 per 60,000 units transfused. Hepatitis C is the second most common viral infection that can be acquired from blood transfusion. Risk of HIV transmission is 1 per 500,000 units transfused. Although all blood is screened for infection, current screening methods do not detect early stages and some subclinical infections.**

A. This patient could require transfusion with fresh frozen plasma, cryoprecipitate, blood, and platelets. Transfusion of these products is mainly supportive and given in an attempt to stop bleeding.

B. Acute hemolytic transfusion reactions are serious, life threatening, and can occur in any patient receiving a blood transfusion. Acute hemolytic transfusion reactions are due to ABO incompatibility. Symptoms include fever and back pain with development of renal failure.

D. Risk of acquiring Hepatitis C from transfusion is 1 in 100,000 units transfused.

E. Delayed transfusion reactions are seen in patients who have developed autoantibodies due to prior transfusion or pregnancy. Rh, Kidd, Duffy, and Kell are the typical antigens to which the antibodies are directed. Onset of delayed transfusion reaction can vary by 5 to 10 days after transfusion and manifests with fever, jaundice, and anemia due to extravascular hemolysis.

120. **C. Adenocarcinoma is the most common type of lung cancer in women and in nonsmokers. There is not nearly the correlation with tobacco use in adenocarcinomas of the lung when compared with squamous cell carcinoma and small cell carcinoma of the lung, which have a very obvious correlation with smoking. Adenocarcinomas also often metastasize to the brain.**

A. Squamous carcinomas of the head and neck are definitely associated with tobacco use, and in fact, the precancerous dysplasias of the oral cavity and larynx may regress following the cessation of smoking. Alcohol use has also been implicated in these cancers.

B. Squamous cell carcinoma of the esophagus has been linked to tobacco use and alcohol use. It is important to distinguish that adenocarcinoma of the esophagus is not related to the same risk factors as squamous cell cancer, but is related to chronic gastroesophageal reflux disease.

D. Pancreatic cancer is associated with tobacco use. The risk for pancreatic cancer among heavy smokers is at least 1.5 times that of nonsmokers. Additionally, patients who have undergone a partial gastrectomy have two to five times the risk for acquiring pancreatic cancer over the long term.

E. Cigarette smoking is clearly the most important risk factor in the development of urinary bladder carcinoma, increasing the risk by three to seven times.

121. D. An excisional biopsy of the supraclavicular lymph node is the least invasive technique to establish a tissue diagnosis in this patient. This patient most likely has Hodgkin lymphoma based on the history, symptoms, and radiographic findings. These patients will usually present with palpable lymphadenopathy, and they may also have mediastinal adenopathy. An excisional biopsy is usually preferred over FNA so that the pathologist can appreciate the architecture of the whole node.

A. Open thoracotomy or mediastinoscopy to obtain the lymph node in the chest for diagnosis should be done if there is not a more accessible lymph node to biopsy. In this case, there is a very accessible node to biopsy in the supraclavicular region, and thoracotomy is not needed.
B. Bronchoscopy could be used to obtain a tissue biopsy if the nodes were accessible by bronchoscopy and there was not another more easily accessed lymph node available.
C. Bone marrow biopsy is not indicated at this time. It may be needed later for staging of the malignancy, but not as a next step in workup.
E. There would be no more information gained to do a high-resolution CT scan. What is needed now is tissue for pathologic diagnosis, not more imaging tests.

122. B. CML usually begins insidiously. Patients may be asymptomatic or may develop fatigue, weight loss, or left upper quadrant pain because of splenomegaly. Ten percent to 15% of patients present with an acceleration of their disease with unexplained fever, significant weight loss, bone and joint pain, bleeding, or thrombosis. The WBC count is usually elevated, with various degrees of immature white cells seen in the peripheral blood, and usually there are <5% circulating blasts. Patients may have a mild normocytic anemia and elevated platelets.

A. CLL may present with only a predominance of lymphocytes on a WBC differential. It may progress to an extremely elevated WBC count, but again it is lymphocyte predominant and there is not the early myelocyte lineage seen on the differential. Eventually, there are resulting cytopenias, either as a result of bone marrow infiltration of the monoclonal cell line, or as a result of autoimmune destruction, such as autoimmune hemolytic anemia. The patient may have extremely bulky adenopathy as well as an enlarged spleen.
C. AML presents with a more acute onset. It classically presents with a 1- to 2-week onset of fatigue, fever, bone pain, and various bleeding manifestations. The laboratories reveal a marked anemia, granulocytopenia, and thrombocytopenia.
D. Richter's syndrome is the transformation of CLL into a more aggressive, usually diffuse histiocytic B cell lymphoma.
E. A leukemoid reaction is seen in instances of acute severe illness often due to infection or stress and, by definition, the WBC should go above 50,000. There is a significant left shift, and early WBC precursors such as metamyelocytes (also called "bands") may be seen in circulation. This must be distinguished from CML. Our patient did not present with a severe illness or stress that would suggest a leukemoid reaction. The splenomegaly is also a clue that this is most likely CML. A bone marrow will show normal development of the myeloid precursors in leukemoid reaction and can be helpful in situations where the diagnosis is unclear.

123. C. The Philadelphia chromosome has a known association with CML. The translocation activates the abl protooncogene and brings it into contact with the bcr (breakpoint cluster region). The combination bcr-abl allows induction of CML.

A. The LAP level is low in CML. A high LAP score indicates normal maturation of the neutrophils and does not indicate CML as a diagnosis. A high LAP score can help distinguish a leukemoid reaction from CML.
B. The natural history of CML is characterized by three phases. The chronic phase is usually asymptomatic, but may have some generalized symptoms, including fevers, night sweats, and fatigue. Splenomegaly may be noted on examination. The accelerated phase has an elevated peripheral WBC count with bone marrow hypercellularity. The blastic phase is consistent with acute leukemia and a severely elevated WBC count.

D. Bone marrow transplantation is the only curative treatment for CML. Patients who undergo transplantation earlier in the course of their illness have a higher long-term disease-free survival. Bone marrow transplantation should be undertaken prior to the patient entering the blast phase.
E. Median age of onset for CML is 50–60 years.

124. **B. AML typically presents with symptoms related to depression of all cell lines. These include fatigue secondary to anemia, easy bleeding secondary to decreased platelet count, and recurrent infections from neutropenia. Laboratory evaluation shows a pancytopenia with half of patients showing a leukocytosis and half showing a normal WBC count or leukopenia at time of presentation. Circulating blasts should be present. Bone marrow biopsy will have >30% blasts. Further morphologic and cytochemistry testing will show granules and myeloperoxidase.**

A. ALL also presents with fatigue, infection, and bleeding secondary to pancytopenia. It can also present with bone pain and a mediastinal mass. ALL is much less common than AML in adults. It does not contain myeloperoxidase.
C. The neoplastic cell in CLL is a small-appearing lymphocyte, not peripheral blasts. The patient may present with fatigue, night sweats, and weight loss. Lymphadenopathy is usually present.
D. CML can present in three different phases. Symptoms include bleeding, infection, fever, and night sweats. A leukocytosis can be found on CBC. The cells can be in varying degrees of maturation, but usually there is not a large predominance of blasts.
E. In Hodgkin lymphoma the typical presenting symptom is lymphadenopathy. Other symptoms may include fever, night sweats, and weight loss. Laboratories may show an anemia and thrombocytopenia. A leukocytosis is usually not observed.

125. **C. The patient in this scenario was given a generous dose of benzodiazepine and subsequently developed respiratory failure. As with any poisoning, the proper treatment is dependent on knowing the appropriate antidote. Flumazenil is a competitive inhibitor of the GABA/benzodiazepine receptor. Its half-life is quite short, so additional dosages of the medication may be necessary in cases of overdose with medium- or long-acting benzodiazepines.**

A. Naloxone is a pure opioid antagonist that not only competes with, but replaces, narcotics at the opioid receptor site. Again, the half-life of naloxone is quite short, so repeated dosing may be necessary in cases of overdose with a long-acting narcotic. Naloxone should be used very judiciously in patients on chronic narcotic treatment because it can precipitate acute withdrawal symptoms.
B. *N*-acetylcysteine is an antidote that is used in acetaminophen toxicity. Its mechanism of action is not well understood, but it is thought to act by binding the toxic metabolite of acetaminophen.
D. Deferoxamine is used in the treatment of acute and chronic iron toxicity. It acts by binding with ferric ions (trivalent ions) to form ferrioxamine, which is cleared by the kidneys.
E. Sodium bicarbonate is used in the treatment of toxic ingestions where alkalinization of the urine is necessary to increase excretion of the chemical from the body. Examples of this include tricyclic antidepressant and aspirin overdose.

126. **B. The patient described above has methemoglobinemia. Hemoglobin is composed of two pairs of chains of globin. Each chain of globin has a heme group attached to it, which is bound to a single ferrous (Fe^{2+}) ion. Methemoglobinemia is a condition in which the ferrous (Fe^{2+}) form of iron attached to heme is oxidized to the ferric (Fe^{3+}) state. The ferric form of iron is unable to bind oxygen and as a result the ferrous forms develop a higher affinity for oxygen (i.e., the oxygen-dissociation curve is left-shifted and there is impaired oxygen delivery to the tissue). In methemoglobinemia, the patient's hemoglobin is not all available for oxygen binding, therefore the patient has a relative anemia. Methemoglobinemia should be suspected in any patient who has a cyanotic or slate blue appearance yet has normal oxygen saturation on pulse oximetry or a normal paO_2. The patient appears cyanotic because of the different absorbance spectrum of methemoglobin compared with oxyhemoglobin. To understand why pulse oximetry can be normal in these patients, it helps to understand how pulse oximetry works.**

Pulse oximetry functions by spectrophotometric absorption analysis of deoxyhemoglobin (spectrum of 600–750 nm) and oxyhemoglobin (850–1000 nm) by using two diodes—one emitting light at 660 nm and the other at 940 nm. A detector reads the amount of light absorbed during pulsatile and nonpulsatile flow and feeds the information into a microprocessor, which then uses an algorithm to calculate the ratio of oxyhemoglobin to the sum of oxyhemoglobin plus deoxyhemoglobin. This ratio is then reported as the percentage saturation. In other words, pulse oximetry only measures deoxyhemoglobin and oxyhemoglobin—not methemoglobin—levels. Methemoglobin absorbs light at 631 nm; therefore, it is not detected by normal pulse oximetry, nor does it affect the measurements or calculations involved in pulse oximetry. In order to diagnose this, you must perform an ABG analysis with cooximetry. Measurements are taken in the entire 630-nm range, and a percentage of methemoglobin is reported. There are several drugs that can cause methemoglobinemia, such as nitrites, dapsone, and local anesthetic agents (such as the benzocaine spray that the patient received).

A. Helical CT of the chest may be beneficial in assessing a patient for a pulmonary embolus, but not for methemoglobinemia.
C. Chest x-ray will be normal and of no benefit in the diagnosis of methemoglobinemia.
D. Total serum hemoglobin levels are not affected by methemoglobinemia. The total amount of hemoglobin will not change—it's the portion of heme units in the ferric state that will increase.
E. BNP level may be useful in helping distinguish between pulmonary and cardiac causes of dyspnea, but it is of no use in the diagnosis of methemoglobinemia.

127. **E. Intravenous methylene blue is the treatment of choice for patients with acquired methemoglobinemia. When given intravenously (1–2 mg/kg), methylene blue acts as an electron receptor and allows for the reduction of methemoglobinemia. This causes a rapid clinical response with improvement in symptoms. Occasionally the dose will need to be repeated in 1 hour. The reduction of methemoglobin occurs through a pathway that is dependent on NADPH, which is generated by G6PD. Therefore, in patients with G6PD deficiency, methylene blue should not be given. Not only will it not work, but it can also act as a possible oxidant and cause further hemolysis in this subset of patients.**

A. Intravenous heparin therapy is the treatment of choice for a pulmonary embolus, not methemoglobinemia.
B. Intravenous loop diuretic therapy is indicated in the treatment of fluid overload states such as pulmonary edema and CHF. It will not help with methemoglobinemia.
C. Methemoglobinemia is not a deficiency in the amount of circulating RBC mass or hemoglobin mass. Transfusing a patient with packed RBCs will increase their hemoglobin mass, but the amount of heme in the ferric state will not change.
D. Insertion of a chest tube is indicated for the treatment of symptomatic pneumothorax. Our patient's chest x-ray was normal, making this answer incorrect.

128. **B. This patient most likely has PCP because of his immunocompromised status, his nonproductive cough and fever, his chest x-ray findings, and his elevated LDH. An early bronchoscopy is needed to make the diagnosis because the patient is immunocompromised, making several opportunistic infections possible. If sputum is obtainable and shows classic findings of PCP on silver stain, then a bronchoscopy is not necessary. However, if the sputum is unrevealing, the most appropriate next test is a bronchoscopy with broncheoalveolar lavage for culture and appropriate stains for AFB, PCP, and other fungi as well as the usual bacteria. Patients with CD4 counts of <200/μL should be started on prophylaxis for PCP pneumonia. The chest x-ray findings of PCP are variable and may be normal in up to 25% of cases. Classically, there is a bilateral "bat wing"–appearing alveolar infiltrate. Pleural effusions are rare in PCP. The LDH may be elevated and clue you in to the diagnosis of PCP in a person with risk factors, but it is not sensitive or specific for this disease. PCP is an intracellular organism, and therefore may cause a release of LDH from the cells that it infects.**

A. A CT scan may help to further characterize the infiltrate, but is not indicated at this time. It would not help you make the diagnosis of PCP.
C. Pulmonary angiography is also not indicated at this time. This immunocompromised

patient presents with a constellation of symptoms that is consistent with an infectious pneumonia and he needs to have a bronchoscopy to identify the organism.

D. Transtracheal aspiration was more commonly performed in the 1970s and 1980s because it was thought to better identify the causative organisms in lower airway infection without contaminating the cultures with organisms that colonized the upper airway. It is rarely done in current medical practice.

E. It may be reasonable to place a PPD on this patient, because TB can present in myriad ways in immunocompromised patients. However, the PPD may be negative in an HIV patient with acute TB, so a negative test result would not rule out the disease. It is more appropriate to perform bronchoscopy to look for the infectious agent by stain and culture.

129. A. Although trimethoprim-sulfamethoxazole is the first-line agent in the treatment of PCP, adjunctive corticosteroid therapy has been shown to significantly decrease mortality in patients with severe infection. Severe infection has been described as that in which the patient's paO_2 is 70 mm Hg or less or the alveolar-arterial oxygen gradient (Aa gradient) is 35 mm Hg or more on room air. The WBC count, temperature, $paCO_2$, and CD4 count are all clinically relevant, but are not used for the indication to initiate corticosteroid therapy. Of note, patients have a significant decrease in mortality when steroids are initiated early in the course of the disease. Therefore, one should not wait until the patient is severely ill, but rather start steroid therapy as soon as he or she meets criteria for its use. The suggested use of prednisone in this setting is 40 mg twice daily for 5 days, then 40 mg once daily for 5 days, then 20 mg daily for 11 more days.

B, C, D. See explanation for A.

E. Patients with HIV disease who have CD4 counts of <200/μL should be started on prophylactic therapy for prevention of PCP. The CD4 count is not an indicator for the use of adjunctive steroid therapy in the treatment of PCP.

130. E. When assessing the ABG results of a patient on a mechanical ventilator, the data can be broken down into two main categories: oxygenation and ventilation. Although overly simplified, this method will make the basics of the ABG interpretation easier. First, we will look at the oxygenation that is represented by the paO_2 and the saturation. Of the basic parameters that can be adjusted on the ventilator (rate, tidal volume, FiO_2, and PEEP), the FiO_2 and PEEP will directly effect the oxygenation status of a patient. Therefore, if a patient has hypoxemia on his ABG, then you can either increase the FiO_2 or PEEP; conversely, if the paO_2 is elevated, you can wean down the FiO_2 or PEEP. The $paCO_2$ and pH are the indicators of the ventilation component of the patient on a ventilator. Remember that as the amount of dissolved CO_2 ($paCO_2$) increases, it binds with water to form carbonic acid (H_2CO_3), which then dissociates to produce bicarbonate (HCO_3^-) and hydrogen ions (H^+): $CO_2 + H_2O \leftrightarrow H_2CO_3 \leftrightarrow HCO_3^- + H^+$. As the concentration of H^+ increases, the pH decreases and the patient becomes more acidotic. The opposite of this is also true, so that if the $paCO_2$ falls, so will the H^+ concentration, and the pH will rise. Therefore, by controlling the minute ventilation (tidal volume × rate) one can correct underlying ventilation problems as evidenced by the ABG. Our patient's oxygenation status is okay. However, he has a significant respiratory acidosis present as evidenced by the high $paco_2$ and the low pH. In order to correct this, we need to increase his minute ventilation so that he exhales more CO_2. This can be accomplished by either increasing the rate or increasing the tidal volume (or both). Because increasing the tidal volume was not a choice, the correct answer is to increase the rate.

A, B, C, D. See explanation for E.

131. E. Although there are a multitude of causes of thrombocytopenia, the only identifiable risk factor listed above was the patient's exposure to heparin. HIT is an immune-mediated problem that occurs as a result of exposure to heparin. It is most often associated with unfractionated heparin, but can be associated with low-molecular-weight heparin as well. The heparin exposure induces the formation of antibodies against the heparin–platelet factor 4 complex. These antibodies then bind the factor 4 complex and cause clumping of platelets. Ultimately the clotting cascade is activated and thrombin formation occurs. As a result of the platelet clumping, thrombocytopenia develops. The classic onset of HIT is 4–10 days after exposure to heparin. If the disorder is suspected, all

heparin-containing fluids and lines should be immediately discontinued and appropriate testing should be completed. There are two basic tests that can help diagnose HIT. These include the heparin-induced platelet aggregation assay and solid-phase immunoassay to detect the presence of HIT antibodies. Once the diagnosis is made, the mainstay of treatment is the use of a thrombin inhibitor such as lepirudin or argatroban until the platelet count recovers.

A. Hypersplenism is a common cause of thrombocytopenia in patients who have splenomegaly from portal hypertension, viral infections (e.g., EBV), lymphoma or leukemia. Our patient has no evidence of these disorders, so should not have hypersplenism.
B. Bone marrow suppression is another known cause of thrombocytopenia. However, one would expect to see other cell lines, such as WBCs or hemoglobin, if he had bone marrow suppression.
C. Iron deficiency is a common cause of microcytic anemia, but not necessarily isolated thrombocytopenia. In fact, patients with iron-deficient anemia will often have a slightly elevated platelet count.
D. Morphine sulfate is not known to cause isolated thrombocytopenia.

132. **C. Thrombosis of both arterial and venous vessels is a common complication of HIT. There are several theories that exist to try to explain the paradoxic finding of thrombocytopenia and thrombosis. As suggested in the description above, patients with HIT develop antibodies to the heparin–platelet factor 4 complex. Some believe that as a result of this complex formation, particles of the platelet membrane are dislodged and then activate the clotting pathway. Regardless of the mechanism, it is important to remember that thrombosis occurs commonly in patients with HIT, which is why antithrombin medications such as lepirudin and argatroban are indicated.**

A, B, D, E. See explanation for C.

133. **E. This patient has physical examination findings consistent with a brainstem injury as a cause of his coma. Ice water calorics and doll's eyes are both tests of the vestibular-brainstem-ocular muscle pathway. Their absence indicates a brainstem lesion. The patient also has unreactive, midpoint pupils that indicate a midbrain lesion. And, finally, an ataxic breathing pattern indicates a lesion in the medulla.**

A. Cheyne-Stokes respirations consist of hyperventilation alternating with apnea. This type of breathing pattern can be seen with heart failure, uremia, some drugs, cerebral cortex damage, and brainstem lesions. Ataxic respirations describe a breathing pattern that is irregular and unpredictable. Often, breathing may stop altogether for a period of time.
B. The absence, not presence, of doll's eyes indicates a midbrain lesion. The oculocephalic reflex (doll's eye movements) is tested by holding open the upper eyelids and turning the head from side to side. (Make sure the patient doesn't have a cervical spine fracture before you do this!) If the brainstem is intact, the eyes will continue to look forward, despite turning the head to the side, just like a doll's eyes. (Doll's eyes are present.) If doll's eyes are not present, the patient's eyes will turn with the head and look to the direction the head is turned. The oculovestibular reflex can be tested with cold calorics if the doll's eyes are not present. In this test, ice water is injected into the external auditory canal. If the brainstem is intact, the eyes will move toward the ear with the cold water.
C. The patient has localizing signs on physical examination that indicate a brainstem lesion. In addition, all laboratory values are normal, which would not indicate a metabolic process.
D. Again, the physical examination has revealing evidence to indicate a brainstem injury.

134. **D. Guillain-Barré syndrome is an inflammatory polyneuropathy that presents with ascending paralysis, areflexia, and paresthesias of the fingers and toes. The syndrome is caused by segmental demyelination of peripheral nerves. Usual onset is 2–4 weeks after a respiratory or GI infection. The ascending paralysis can be rapid and involve respiratory muscles, requiring mechanical ventilation. Many patients also have autonomic dysfunction. Most patients slowly recover all function, although a few may have residual weakness.**

A. Charcot-Marie-Tooth disease is an inherited demyelinating disease of peripheral nerves. Usual presentation is in the first two decades of life. Onset is not sudden, but more insidious in nature.

B. Alcoholic neuropathy presents with numbness in the feet, usually in a stocking distribution. It is due to nutritional deficiencies. It is not rapid in onset.

C. MG is an autoimmune disease that affects the neuromuscular junction. Patients present with weakness after repetitive muscle use, ptosis, and diplopia. Onset is usually more gradual in nature.

E. MS is a demyelinating disease with onset at age 20–30 years, more common in women. Patients may present with optic neuritis, diplopia, sensory changes in the extremities, and motor weakness. Reflexes tend to be exaggerated, not diminished.

135. **B. In a patient with Guillain-Barré syndrome, the CSF protein will be elevated (>50 mg/dL), opening pressure is normal, and there should be few cells. If pleocytosis is present, an alternative diagnosis should be considered.**

A. Nerve conduction studies show slowed conduction in Guillain-Barré syndrome. This is due to demyelination of the peripheral nerves.

C. Most patients recover completely from Guillain-Barré syndrome. Less than 10% have a residual weakness.

D. Intubation should be considered at a vital capacity of <20 cc/kg. Failure of the respiratory muscles can be part of the ascending paralysis in 20%–30% of patients. Respiratory status should be monitored closely.

E. Pyridostigmine, an anticholinergic, and thymectomy are treatments for MG. Treatment for Guillain-Barré syndrome is largely supportive, but can also include plasmapheresis, IVIG, and steroids. Plasmapheresis has been the only therapy with proven benefit.

136. **A. When first evaluating symptoms of stroke, it is important to differentiate between symptoms of the anterior (carotid) circulation and the posterior (vertebrobasilar) distribution. Symptoms associated with vertebrobasilar distribution ischemia include syncope, diplopia, nausea, vomiting, and ataxia. Syncope is never a result of a stroke in the carotid distribution; therefore, ordering carotid Doppler ultrasonography is unnecessary in the workup of syncope.**

B, C, D. Symptoms associated with carotid distribution ischemia include amaurosis fugax (temporary vision loss in one eye like "a shade is being pulled down"), aphasia, motor and sensory symptoms in a single extremity, or a clumsy "bear paw" hand.

E. Headache may accompany stroke in either distribution, and does not differentiate between the two. If headache is involved in stroke, there is greater concern for a hemorrhagic component.

137. **B. This patient probably had an embolic stroke in the middle cerebral artery distribution due to his atrial fibrillation, which then became hemorrhagic. He may have high ICP secondary to the bleeding that is causing him to become obtunded. The treatment for high ICP is dependent on the cause. For instance, steroids are used to treat vasogenic edema (defined by increased vascular permeability) causing high ICP due to tumors, radiation, and neurosurgical procedures. They are not useful to treat the cytotoxic edema associated with strokes, hypoxia, or cerebral hemorrhage. In cytotoxic edema, there is swelling and damage to the neurons and glial cells, but the vascular membrane remains intact. Increased ICP related to cytotoxic edema requires treatment with mannitol, an osmotic diuretic that helps to draw fluid out of cells and into the vascular space where it can be removed.**

A. Patients with high ICP can be hyperventilated to decrease the pCO_2 to a goal of 25–30 mm Hg. This causes cerebral vasoconstriction that decreases the intracranial pressure. If the pCO_2 is decreased below 25, there is a risk for cerebral hypoperfusion due to the vasoconstriction.

C. See explanation for B. This patient needs a bolus of mannitol, not dexamethasone.

D. Patients with acute ischemia to the brain by thrombosis or hemorrhage have lost the normal autoregulatory capacity of the brain to maintain perfusion. Because of this, it is not appropriate to acutely lower the BP in a patient with an acute infarction, because it may extend an infarct into an area that was depending on the relatively high perfusion pressures associated with the high BP. It is not recommended to give sublingual nifedine to any patient with severe hypertension.

E. This patient is having an acute stroke related to hemorrhage and probable vasospasm. Anticoagulation is contraindicated in a patient with bleeding in the brain, even if the stroke originated from a cardiac source.

138. **E. Patients with terminal complement deficiency are much more susceptible to infections with *Neisseria* species in addition to other encapsulated organisms. This patient presents with signs and symptoms consistent with bacterial meningitis, and, the purpuric skin lesion clues you to the fact that this is probably *Neisseria meningitides.* Patients with *Neisseria* meningitis who have normal immune systems are usually children. Patients who present with this disorder after the age of 15 are more likely to have a terminal complement deficiency, and especially if they have a sibling who also has had the meningitis. This patient should have a CH_{50} ordered after she has recovered, because the complements may be low during the acute infection. The CH_{50} is a screening test to determine how much activity the patient's complement has, by its ability to lyse sheep RBCs. A low complement activity may indicate that the patient is missing one of the complement proteins. If the screening test returns low, then each of the complement proteins can be measured to determine which one is missing. The patient's siblings should also be tested, because they may be affected, too. All patients with terminal complement deficiency should be immunized against *Neisseria meningitides, Haemophilus. influenza, and Streptococcus pneumoniae.***

A. Chronic granulomatous disease of childhood predisposes patients to severe infections of the skin, ears, lungs, liver, and bone with catalase-positive organisms such as *Staphylococcus aureus* and *Aspergillus* species. The problem is due to an absent respiratory burst in neutrophils, monocytes, and eosinophils. The disease is transmitted in an X-linked and an autosomal-recessive pattern.

B. Agammaglobulinemia is an X-linked disorder. Most males with the disease will begin to have sinopulmonary infections late in the first year of life, after maternal antibodies have worn off. Patients are treated with episodic IVIG replacement.

C. IgA deficiency is the most frequently occurring immunodeficiency in white populations, occurring in 1 in 600 persons. Most patients appear healthy, whereas others may have respiratory infections, bronchiectasis, and chronic diarrheal disease (especially remember *Giardia* in IgA-deficient patients). Patients with IgA deficiency may have severe anaphylactic reactions to blood transfusions or blood product transfusions and should only receive washed RBCs or blood that is donated from IgA-deficient donors.

D. Thymic aplasia is also known as DiGeorge syndrome. The disease results from a defect in the embryologic development of the third and fourth pharyngeal pouches, which occurs around the 12th week of gestation. Babies with DiGeorge syndrome also have hypoparathyroidism because of the lack of development of normal parathyroid glands, and they suffer from hypocalcemia in the first 24 hours of life. They also have recurrent viral, fungal, bacterial, and protazoal infections.

139. **B. The lupus anticoagulant is identified first by a prolonged aPTT on coagulation tests in a patient who is not on heparin. To confirm its presence, a mixing study is performed to exclude a factor deficiency as a cause of the prolonged aPTT. Normal serum is mixed with the patient's serum, and the aPTT will not correct in the case of lupus anticoagulant because of its inhibitor activity. However, when phospholipids are added to the mixture, correction of the aPTT will occur because of the dependence of the inhibitor on phospholipids.**

A. Pregnancy loss from APLA syndrome can occur at any time in gestation, but classically occurs during the second and third trimester.

C. *Antiphospholipid antibodies* is the umbrella term that comprises three different types of antibodies found in APLA syndrome: (1) anticardiolipin antibodies (IgG, IgA, and IgM all may be found, but IgG at moderate to high titer with the clinical scenario is most specific for APLA syndrome), (2) lupus anticoagulant, and (3) false-positive VDRL test results.

D. Patients who have antibodies consistent with APLA syndrome who have not experienced a thrombotic event should not be anticoagulated to try to prevent an event. Many of these patients will go through life without a clinically evident thrombotic event, and the risks of anticoagulation outweigh the benefits of trying to prevent a clot.

E. APLA syndrome is characterized by venous and/or arterial thrombosis, pregnancy loss, and thrombocytopenia, not thrombocytosis. The thrombocytopenia is usually mild to moderate (100,000–150,000 platelets/μL).

140. C. Patients with APLA syndrome are at high risk for recurrent clotting events and pregnancy losses. Therefore, lifelong anticoagulation is indicated in these patients. Because of their propensity to form clots, they require higher therapeutic levels of INR than patients on anticoagulation for other reasons (such as prosthetic valves or atrial fibrillation). Although there is some controversy regarding the ideal INR range for treatment, a goal INR of >3.0 should be maintained in these patients.

A, B. See explanation for C.

D, E. Patients who have an isolated thrombotic event (e.g., DVT) without an underlying hypercoagulable state do not require lifelong anticoagulation. These patients can be anticoagulated for a period of several (usually a minimum of 6) months following the event, keeping their INR in the range of 2.0–3.0.

141. D. The DLCO, or diffusing capacity, is a pulmonary function test that measures the efficiency of gas transfer from inspired air to the pulmonary capillaries. It reflects the interaction between the surface area and thickness of the alveolar capillary membrane and the volume of blood circulating in the alveolar capillary bed, as well as the rate of transfer of inspired gas to hemoglobin. It is measured by using carbon monoxide. DLCO may be low, normal, or elevated. It is low in diseases that result in the loss of the effectiveness of the capillary–alveolar interface. Low DLCO is seen in emphysema, interstitial lung diseases, pneumonectomy, pulmonary embolism, or pulmonary hypertension. DLCO is low in anemia as well, but is corrected for the hemoglobin concentration. Normal DLCO is seen in normal lungs as well as in asthma, as asthma does not involve alveolar disease.

A, B, C, E. An elevated DLCO is seen in conditions that increase effective blood flow to the lung. These include pulmonary edema, acute pulmonary hemorrhage, pulmonary infarction, and idiopathic pulmonary hemosiderosis. DLCO may sometimes be elevated in asthma secondary to air trapping. Pulmonary embolism will usually cause a decreased DLCO unless it results in pulmonary infarction, at which point it may cause an elevated DLCO.

142. D. This patient has a history of COPD due to a long history of tobacco abuse and now presents with new onset of lower extremity edema, which should make you suspicious for cor pulmonale. The evidence of right atrial enlargement on ECG is a tall P wave in II (termed "P-pulmonale"). A tall R wave in V_1, deep S wave in V_5, and right axis deviation are evidence of right ventricular hypertrophy. All of these findings together in a patient with emphysema help to make the diagnosis of cor pulmonale. This term is used to describe right heart failure due to pulmonary hypertension that results from chronic lung diseases such as COPD. Examination findings include elevated jugular venous pressure, hepatic congestion (evidenced by hepatojugular reflux), and lower extremity edema. A right ventricular heave may be appreciated, and tricuspid regurgitation may occur due to right ventricular and right atrial enlargement. Definitive diagnosis should be made with echocardiogram.

A. An rSR complex in V_1 and a QRS complex in V_6 compose the pattern of a right bundle branch block. Right bundle branch block may be a normal variant, but also may occur in conditions that affect the right side of the heart. It is possible that our patient could have had a right bundle branch block. However, given his history of lower extremity edema and hepatic congestion, as well as the examination findings of right ventricular hypertrophy and tricuspid regurgitation, findings of cor pulmonale would be more likely.

B. A widened QS complex in V_1 and a notched R wave in V_6 is descriptive of a left bundle branch block. Left bundle branch block, unlike right bundle branch block, usually occurs in patients with organic heart disease such as longstanding hypertension or CAD. It is not a normal variant and it is not usually seen in right-sided heart disease.

C. A wide, notched P wave in II, a tall R wave in V_6, and left axis deviation describe the findings of left atrial enlargement. Left atrial enlargement may be seen in valvular disease, especially aortic stenosis, aortic regurgitation, and mitral regurgitation. It is not usually associated with right heart disease unless the right heart failure is a result of left heart failure.

E. A short PR interval and wide QRS complex with delta wave describes WPW syndrome, a conduction abnormality in which there are two pathways that depolarize the ventricles. This results in preexcitation of the ventricles when the accessory pathway is used, bypassing the AV junction. It results in a baseline ECG in which there may be a wide QRS complex, short PR interval, and a delta wave. It may also result in arrhythmias. It is not associated with cor pulmonale.

143. D. This patient presents with a classic case of *Streptococcus pneumoniae* infection, the most common bacterial etiology of community-acquired pneumonia. Typically patients with *Pneumococcus pneumoniae* (a synonym for *Streptococcus pneumoniae* species) infection have a sudden onset of rigors, cough, and fever. Often they develop effusions that may become complicated and require drainage. This patient was appropriately triaged to outpatient care on her initial assessment based on her age, lack of comorbid conditions, and vital signs. (Criteria for admission include age >65 years, significant comorbidities like renal or liver disease, inability to take oral medications, RR >30, HR >140, or systolic BP <90.) She has failed outpatient treatment, however, by not improving and, in fact, by becoming worse. This now justifies her admission, and her placement on IV antibiotics. The appropriate antibiotics for pneumonia include ceftriaxone and azithromycin, because you do not have cultures documenting *S. pneumoniae,* and you must cover empirically for atypical organisms. You should initially evaluate the patient for a possibility of an effusion with decubitus films.

A. Initiation of IV antibiotic therapy is appropriate, but you must also look for a reason why the patient did not do well with oral antibiotics despite her low risk. She may not have been compliant with her antibiotics, but another reason for her to do poorly would be due to an effusion or possible empyema, for which you should evaluate.

B. IV vancomycin alone is not appropriate therapy for community-acquired pneumonia.

C. Continuing oral antibiotics would not be appropriate in this setting because the patient is already failing oral antibiotics. Although 2 days of oral antibiotics would not necessarily completely eradicate the infection, we would expect the patient to stabilize or show some improvement. We would not expect the patient to worsen.

E. It may be appropriate to add vancomycin empirically to therapy with ceftriaxone and azithromycin in settings where there is a high prevalence of penicillin-resistant *Streptococcus pneumoniae* species. However, a CT scan would not be the first test to evaluate for an effusion, but rather decubitus films or ultrasonography. If there were evidence of an effusion, a thoracentesis would be the next step.

144. C. SIRS is an inflammatory reaction usually occurring in response to infection with an organism such as a virus, bacteria or fungus. The purpose of this physiologic response is to defend against the pathogen until more specific immunity to the organism develops. SIRS presumably develops as a result of activation of multiple protein cascades. The definition of SIRS is two or more of the following: temperature >38°C (100.4°F) or <36°C (96.8°F), HR >90, RR >20 or arterial pCO_2 <32 mm Hg, or WBC count >12,000 or <4,000 or with 10% immature band forms. These findings should occur in the absence of other known causes of these abnormalities. The patient described in C has four of these criteria and has symptoms of a productive cough and chest pain, indicating possible pneumonia. We are not given any other reason for these abnormalities, and they do appear to be in response to an infectious process.

A. This patient has two of the criteria for SIRS, which is all that is necessary to make the diagnosis. However, she also has a history of paroxysmal supraventricular tachycardia, which may account for the abnormal vital signs. This, combined with the lack of evidence pointing toward an infection, suggests that her arrhythmia is probably causing her elevated HR and RR.

B. This patient also has two criteria for SIRS: HR and WBC count. However, he has evidence of recent, significant GI blood loss and is hypotensive, which is likely the reason for his tachycardia. An elevated WBC count is not uncommon in ulcerative colitis and may also occur in response to stress.

D. This patient has evidence of an infection of the urinary tract but does not meet criteria for SIRS.

E. This patient has two criteria for SIRS but again has evidence of another reason for these abnormalities. The shortness of breath and crackles on lung examination are indicative of a possible exacerbation of CHF. The increased HR and RR are likely due to the decreased EF and the CHF, resulting in pulmonary edema.

145. A. Superficial vein thrombosis of the leg (i.e., thrombosis of the greater or lesser saphenous vein), like DVT, may be a marker for cancer. It may also be seen in patients with vasculitis. The most common reason for a superficial vein thrombosis, however, is in hospitalized patients who develop a superficial thrombophlebitis from a peripheral IV site.

B. Superficial vein thrombosis does not usually result in pulmonary embolism. Occasionally, superficial vein thrombosis may propagate and become a DVT, at which point it may result in embolization to the lung.

C. It is usually fairly easy to distinguish a superficial vein thrombosis from a DVT. Superficial vein thrombosis causes pain that localizes to the area of the thrombus that is red and warm. A tender cord may be palpated along a superficial vein. A DVT, however, may cause calf pain and examination may reveal calf tenderness, warmth and swelling, but these signs are not always present or obvious. In cases of superficial thrombosis with large amounts of swelling, it is important to perform a Doppler examination to see if there is any involvement in the deep venous structures.

D. Varicose veins do not cause superficial vein thrombosis. However, a superficial vein thrombosis may be located in a varicose vein.

E. Treatment of superficial vein thrombosis consists of applying warm compresses to the area and giving the patient antiinflammatory agents such as NSAIDs and antibiotics if there is a possibility of infection. If the superficial vein thrombosis begins to extend to the point where it is very close to the deep venous system, anticoagulation could be considered to avoid further propagation and development of a DVT.

146. E. This patient has Legionnaires disease. Legionnaires disease is caused by the organism *Legionella pneumophila,* which is an aerobic gram-negative bacillus that is flagellated. It is very difficult to grow in culture. It is found in water and is transmitted by inhalation of aerosols that contain the organism. It occurs mainly in elderly people and people with comorbidities such as COPD or cancer. Multiple serotypes exist, but most that cause disease are serotype 1. Patients will usually have a 1-day history of malaise, myalgias, and headaches that progress to a syndrome of a dry cough, pleuritic chest pain, diarrhea, and confusion. The lung examination usually reveals rales, and the radiologic examination usually reveals diffuse infiltrates that appear worse than the patient appears clinically. Diagnosis is made by direct immunofluorescence antibody of the urine. This test only identifies organisms in serogroup 1, but this is the organism that causes most disease. Treatment is with macrolides or quinolones.

A. A sputum culture is a nonspecific test that is rarely helpful even in obvious cases of pneumonia. It is frequently contaminated by oral flora. Sputum Gram stain is occasionally helpful if a dominant organism such as pneumococcus is found. Sputum culture does not play a role in the diagnosis of Legionnaires disease.

B. A lumbar puncture would be appropriate in this patient if the patient was felt to have meningitis. However, the cough, pleuritic chest pain, diarrhea, hyponatremia, and hypophosphatemia present in addition to his headache and confusion point to Legionnaires disease, which is well known for its propensity to cause multiple extrapulmonary symptoms.

C. A CT scan of the thorax would possibly further delineate the patient's radiographic abnormalities but would not provide a definitive diagnosis.

D. Organism serology would be appropriate if the pneumonia was suspected to be caused by *Mycoplasma pneumoniae* or fungal organisms. *Mycoplasma* pneumonia can on occasion mimic Legionnaires disease. However, the diarrhea, hyponatremia, and hypophosphatemia are somewhat more specific for Legionnaires disease than pneumonia cause by these other organisms.

147. B. This patient likely has tetany, a syndrome caused by a neurotoxin produced by the bacteria *Clostridium tetani.* The bacteria are found in soil, and disease is caused by wound contamination with the organism. The syndrome is rare in the United States because of widespread immunization. However, older adults who do not maintain their immunity by vaccination are at risk for developing the disease. The disease begins 1–55 days after a wound sustained outdoors. Symptoms begin with spasm at the site of the wound, which fairly rapidly progresses to spasms of the back, neck, thighs, and abdomen. Patients may note dysphagia as it occurs in about half of affected patients. Trismus develops, and the syndrome may progress to involve the respiratory muscles, requiring mechanical ventilation. Treatment is supportive in addition to antitoxin and penicillin or metronidazole to kill organisms that may produce additional toxin.

A. Botulism may occur as a food-borne illness, as contamination of a wound, or as infant botulism. Food-borne botulism usually involves a prodrome of GI symptoms prior to the development of neurologic symptoms. Our patient did not have this prodrome. Wound botulism occurs when spores of *Clostridium botulinum* contaminate a wound. Most commonly, this is due to a major crush injury or to the use of black tar heroin. The symptoms begin with cranial nerve symptoms, and then a symmetric, descending paralysis develops. The incubation period is much shorter than that of tetany, only 18–36 hours; and rather than the stiffness seen with tetany, patients with botulism demonstrate flaccid paralysis.

C. Guillain-Barré syndrome is a syndrome of acute demyelination that occurs primarily after infection with a herpesvirus or with *Campylobacter jejuni.* It results in an areflexic motor paralysis. Sensory deficit may or may not be present. The paralysis may involve the respiratory musculature, requiring mechanical ventilation. Our patient gives no history of a preceding infection and is hyperreflexic rather than areflexic, making Guillain-Barré syndrome unlikely. Treatment of Guillain-Barré syndrome is supportive in addition to plasmapheresis or administration of IVIG.

D. Patients who present with hepatic encephalopathy usually have known or obvious liver disease and are not fully conscious. The above patient has no known liver disease and she is alert on arrival to the ER. Asterixis is the classic movement seen in hepatic encephalopathy, which is a "flapping" movement of the hands seen when the patient tries to raise the arms and dorsiflex the wrists in a sustained muscle contraction.

E. An acute dystonic reaction does involve muscle stiffness and rigidity. However, it does not usually involve the entire body. In addition, it is usually precipitated by taking a medication that is a dopamine receptor antagonist.

148. C. These pulmonary function tests reveal a restrictive pattern with a decreased vital capacity (49%) and total lung capacity (62%), but with a preserved FEV_1 to FVC ratio, which indicates that there is no obstruction to air flow. In addition, her DLCO is markedly decreased at 36% predicted. This patient has a history that is compatible with pulmonary fibrosis. This disorder is usually seen in patients in their fifties and sixties who complain of dyspnea with exertion and a dry, nonproductive cough that is gradual in onset and progressively worsening. On physical examination, the patient has inspiratory "Velcro-like" crackles. PFTs reveal a restrictive pattern with a decreased DLCO. The chest x-ray may reveal interstitial infiltrates, or it may appear normal. The diagnosis can be confirmed by high-resolution CT scanning, which will reveal the fibrosis.

A, B, D, E. These patients each have a type of obstructive lung disease. The patient in "A" gives a description of COPD and tobacco abuse and would likely have changes on his pulmonary function tests that show air trapping (with increased total lung capacity and functional residual capacity) and decreased FEV_1 to FVC ratio, which reflects obstruction to air flow on expiration. The patient in "B" has a prolonged history of uncontrolled asthma. Patients with uncontrolled asthma often go on to develop a fixed obstruction on PFTs, rather than the early reversible obstruction seen in early asthma or well-controlled asthma. The patient in "D" has a history of alpha-1 antitrypsin deficiency and a minimal tobacco history. However, patients with alpha-1 antitrypsin deficiency develop emphysematous changes with only minimal tobacco abuse, and would have signs of obstruction, not restriction, on PFTs. Patients with cystic fibrosis develop bronchiectasis and lung destruction. Their PFTs usually show a combined obstructive and restrictive pattern and not a purely restrictive pattern such as seen in the PFTs displayed.

149. C. These PFTs reveal an obstructive picture with an increased total lung capacity (128% predicted) and functional residual capacity (149% predicted) due to air trapping, and a decreased FEV_1 (36% predicted) and FEV_1 to FVC ratio, which signifies obstruction to air flow with exhalation. The only patient described in the above scenarios with a history compatible with obstructive lung disease is the patient with chronic long-term tobacco abuse with a gradual increasing dyspnea with exertion. It is important to emphasize to these patients that there is a normal small decline in lung function with age, but continuing to smoke puts these patients on a different curve with a rapid decline in lung function. If they stop smoking, they can return to the usual, gradual slope and prevent significant worsening of their lung function.

A. This patient presents with probable Guillian-Barré syndrome after a *Campylobacter* diarrheal illness. These patients can develop shortness of breath secondary to neuromuscular weakness, and PFTs may show a restrictive defect (secondary to an inability to move the chest wall), not an obstructive defect, with a small total lung capacity and preserved FEV_1 to FVC ratio.

B. This patient is on amiodarone, which is known to cause pulmonary fibrosis as a side effect. Patients on amiodarone should have baseline PFTs ordered when they start the drug. If they develop any signs of dyspnea on exertion or shortness of breath, it is important to consider pulmonary fibrosis, which may develop as a complication of their amiodarone therapy. It may be difficult to determine whether the patient's shortness of breath is due to their underlying cardiac disease or lung disease, and therefore you must have a high index of suspicion. Pulmonary fibrosis due to amiodarone should be reflected in a restrictive pattern on PFTs, not an obstructive pattern.

D. This patient is a young woman who presents with complaints of dyspnea on exertion which has been gradual. Her physical examination findings are consistent with right ventricular hypertrophy, causing a right ventricular heave, and pulmonary hypertension, causing a loud P_2, and clear lung fields. She most likely has primary pulmonary hypertension. PFT results seen in pulmonary hypertension are normal, with the exception of a reduced DLCO, and not an obstructive pattern.

E. Nitrofurantoin therapy has been associated with acute, subacute, and chronic pulmonary reactions. Diffuse interstitial pneumonitis or pulmonary fibrosis can develop slowly and insidiously and is usually seen in patients who are taking the drug for >6 months. This patient has been on therapy for a year and has symptoms of dyspnea on exertion and coarse crackles on examination consistent with fibrosis. PFTs would reveal a restrictive abnormality.

150. C. Hepatic hydrothoraces are usually right-sided pleural effusions that occur in patients with cirrhosis and portal hypertension. They are transudates by Light's criteria, and if you perform a serum-ascites-albumin gradient on the fluid, it will be greater than 1.1, indicative of portal hypertension. Patients who have cirrhosis may have a hepatic hydrothorax and no evidence of ascites. The ascitic fluid is pulled into the chest cavity through defects in the diaphragm by the negative pressure in the chest cavity, especially during inspiration. Therapy of hepatic hydrothorax is difficult and usually requires recurrent thoracentesis, pleuradesis, or a TIPS procedure. The only definitive therapy is liver transplantation.

A, B, D, E. These statements are incorrect. See explanation for C.

SETTING 4: EMERGENCY DEPARTMENT

Generally, patients encountered here are seeking urgent care; most are not known to you. A full range of social services is available, including rape crisis intervention, family support, child protective services, domestic violence support, psychiatric services, and security assistance backed up by local police. Complete laboratory and radiology services are available.

The next three questions (items 151–153) correspond to the following vignette:

A 34-year-old man with a social history significant for IVDA in the past presents with complaints of severe right flank pain that began 4 hours ago. The pain is sharp and severe and radiates into the right testicle. He has some associated symptoms of nausea and vomited once with the pain. He has never had this before. He denies having fever or chills and he has not noted any gross hematuria. He is in moderate to severe distress because of the pain and is writhing and unable to lie still. On physical examination, his BP is 155/95 mm Hg, HR is 115, and he is afebrile. There is costovertebral angle tenderness over the right flank, and his genital examination results are normal. A urinalysis is positive for only blood. Other laboratory values are as follows: sodium 141 mEq/L, potassium 2.9 mEq/L, chloride 114 mEq/L, bicarbonate 15 mEq/L, BUN/creatinine 10/1.0 mg/dL, calcium 9.5 mg/dL, AST 65 U/L, ALT 70 U/L, total bilirubin 0.8 mg/dL, alkaline phosphatase 80 U/L, albumin 3.8 g/dL, and urine pH 7.0. You suspect nephrolithiasis as a cause of the patient's pain, and order a KUB x-ray that reveals a possible radiopaque stone in the area of the mid-right ureter.

151. What should you order next to evaluate the probable nephrolithiasis?

   A. Renal imaging with ultrasonography or CT
   B. Serum uric acid level
   C. Urine culture and sensitivity
   D. 24-hour urine citrate
   E. 24-hour urine for calcium

152. You astutely note that the patient has a nonanion gap hyperchloremic metabolic acidosis as well as relative hypokalemia. He does not give any history of diarrhea, and you are suspicious of a renal tubular acidosis. What type of RTA does this patient likely have?

   A. Type 1 distal RTA
   B. Type 4 distal RTA
   C. Type 3 proximal RTA
   D. Type 2 proximal RTA
   E. You are unable to tell from the information given.

153. Which of the following is a cause of type 1 distal RTA?

   A. Heavy metal poisoning
   B. Multiple myeloma
   C. Diabetic nephropathy
   D. Chronic active hepatitis
   E. Sickle cell anemia

End of Set

154. A 36-year-old woman with type 1 DM presents to the emergency department with abdominal pain, nausea, vomiting, and polyuria. She is afebrile, with an HR of 98, RR 28, and BP 110/76 mm Hg. Mucous membranes are dry, cardiovascular examination is remarkable for tachycardia, and she is diffusely tender to palpation on abdominal examination. Laboratory values are obtained: sodium 128 mEq/L, potassium 5.5 mEq/L, pH 7.3, pCO_2 25 mm Hg, chloride 82 mEq/L, bicarbonate 12 mEq/L, BUN 50 mg/dL, creatinine 1.7 mg/dL, and glucose 650 mg/dL. Which of the following statements is true regarding this patient?

   A. The patient is hyponatremic, and for this reason should be given normal saline.
   B. Initial treatment should include IV sodium bicarbonate.
   C. The sodium would be expected to decrease once glucose returns to a normal value.
   D. The potassium would be expected to decrease once the acidosis is corrected.
   E. An elevated gap metabolic acidosis is present with an underlying respiratory acidosis.

155. A 74-year-old man with CHF presents to the ER with a complaint of generalized weakness. He reports running out of his lasix 4 days ago, but continuing all other medications, including 40 mEq of potassium chloride per day. BP is 125/85, jugular venous distension is present, cardiovascular examination is notable for an S_3 gallop, lungs are clear bilaterally, and there is 1+ pedal edema. ECG is performed (Figure 1-155). The patient's potassium is found to be 6.1 mEq/L. What is the most appropriate next step in the treatment of this patient?

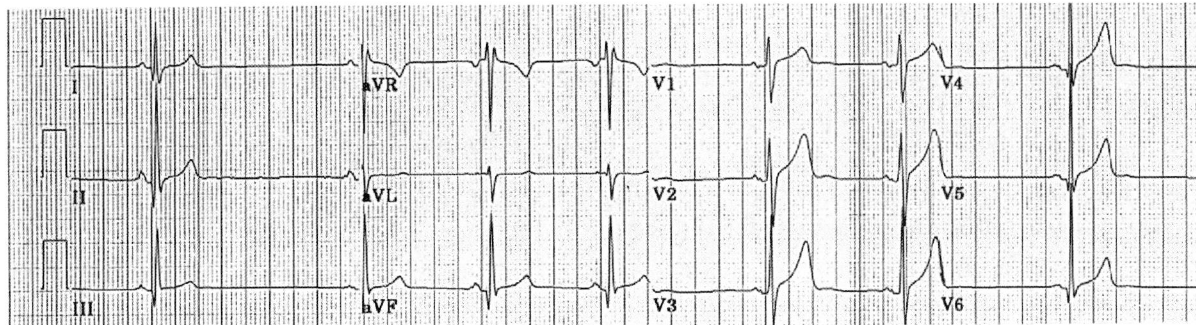

Figure 1-155 • Image Courtesy of Dr. Brenda Shinar, Banner Good Samaritan Medical Center, Phoenix, Arizona.

A. IV furosemide
B. Sodium bicarbonate
C. Glucose and insulin
D. Sodium polystyrene sulfonate
E. Calcium gluconate

156. A 21-year-old female college student with no past medical history is brought in to the ER one evening by her friends for increasing confusion. During the day she had complained of a severe headache and had also had a fever. Within the past several hours she became confused and her friends became concerned. On examination, her temperature is 102.1°C, HR 98, RR 22, and BP 100/62 mm Hg. She is confused and has nuchal rigidity on examination. You are suspicious for bacterial meningitis and wish to start antibiotics immediately prior to any further evaluation of the patient. You practice in an area with a high prevalence of penicillin-resistant *Streptococcus pneumoniae.* You begin appropriate empiric treatment for meningitis while proceeding with a lumbar puncture. Shortly thereafter, you note that the patient has a deep flush of her face and chest that blanches and leaves your fingerprints (Figure 1-156). What best explains her skin finding?

A. Infection with *Neisseria meningitidis*
B. Red man syndrome secondary to vancomycin
C. Toxic shock syndrome
D. Psoriasis
E. Staphylococcal scalded skin syndrome

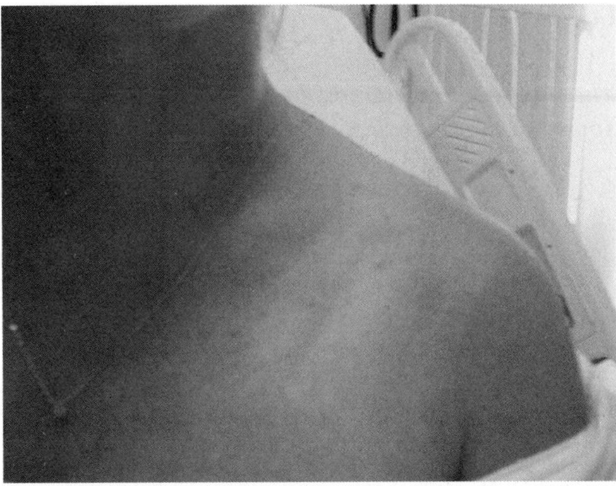

Figure 1-156 • Image Courtesy of Dr. Brenda Shinar, Banner Good Samaritan Medical Center, Phoenix, Arizona.

The next three questions (items 157–159) correspond to the following vignette:

A 75-year-old woman presents to the emergency room with complaints of shortness of breath with minimal exertion, lower extremity swelling, and orthopnea for the past week. She has no history of heart failure, but was told by her physician a few years ago that she had a heart murmur. She never had an echocardiogram evaluation. On examination, you find that she has rales in bilateral lower lung fields, slow upstroke of her carotid pulse, and a 3/6 systolic ejection murmur at the right second intercostal space with a sustained apical impulse.

157. Which of the following lesions is most likely causing her clinical presentation?

A. Aortic insufficiency
B. Pulmonary stenosis
C. Mitral regurgitation
D. Aortic stenosis
E. Mitral stenosis

158. Of the following tests, which is the best option to initially assess the severity of her valvular disease?

A. Echocardiography
B. Cardiac catheterization
C. Exercise treadmill stress test
D. ECG
E. Trial of vasodilator therapy

159. Choose the order of symptoms associated with increasing mortality in patients with this disorder.

A. Angina, exertional syncope, orthopnea
B. Exertional syncope, orthopnea, angina
C. Orthopnea, angina, exertional syncope
D. Angina, orthopnea, exertional syncope
E. Exertional syncope, angina, orthopnea

End of Set

The next two questions (items 160 and 161) correspond to the following vignette:

A very active 76-year-old woman complains of dyspnea and palpitations that started approximately 4 days prior to her arrival in the ER. She has a history of CAD, DM, and hypertension that has been well controlled. On examination, she is in no acute distress and has an HR of 142 and a BP of 132/84 mm Hg. Cardiac examination reveals an irregularly irregular tachycardia. Her lungs are clear to auscultation. The results of the remainder of her examination are unremarkable. You obtain an ECG (Figure 1-160).

160. Which of the following is the most appropriate initial step in her treatment?

A. Rate control with digoxin
B. Rate control with calcium channel blockers
C. Chemical cardioversion with amiodarone
D. Electrical synchronized cardioversion
E. Anticoagulation with warfarin

161. In regard to anticoagulation for the prevention of thromboembolic events in this patient, which of the following is true?

A. She should be emergently cardioverted and discharged home on subcutaneous low-molecular-weight heparin.
B. If TTE reveals no evidence of thrombus within the left atrium, she should be cardioverted and discharged home without further anticoagulation.
C. She should be treated with warfarin for 3 weeks, then electively cardioverted and treated with a minimum of 4 additional weeks of warfarin.
D. She does not need anticoagulation therapy because she is a low-risk patient for thromboembolic disease.
E. She should be started on IV heparin and cardioverted emergently. Afterwards, she should have an echocardiogram to assess for thrombus in the left atrium and subsequent need for anticoagulation.

End of Set

162. A 48-year-old moderately obese woman with a history of type 2 DM presents to the emergency department with 2 days of nausea and vomiting. She also notes diffuse abdominal pain as well as subjective fevers and says that she feels lightheaded when she stands. On examination the patient has a temperature of 100°C, HR 120, BP 120/70 mm Hg, RR 18, and oxygen saturation 98% on room air. On HEENT, mucous membranes are dry and there is no scleral icterus noted. Chest is clear to auscultation, and heart is tachycardic, regular, and without murmur. Abdomen has hypoactive bowel sounds and is tender to palpation in the epigastric region and the right upper quadrant. There is no hepatosplenomegaly, and the skin is without jaundice. Rectal examination reveals guaiac-negative brown stool. Laboratory studies reveal the following: WBC 18,000 with

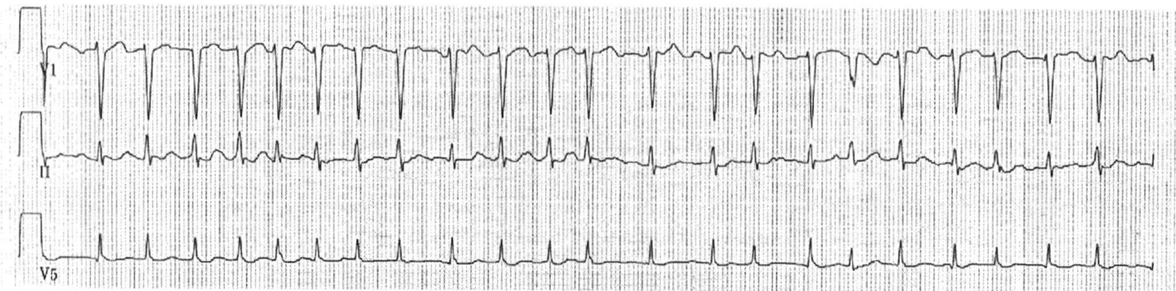

Figure 1-160 • Image Courtesy of Dr. Brenda Shinar, Banner Good Samaritan Medical Center Phoenix, Arizona.

90% segmented neutrophils, hemoglobin 14 g/dL, hematocrit 42%, sodium 143 mEq/L, potassium 4.7 mEq/L, chloride 100 mEq/L, bicarbonate 23 mEq/L, BUN/creatinine 30/1.5 mg/dL, glucose 225 mg/dL, AST 30 U/L, ALT 25 U/L, alkaline phosphotase 200 U/L, total bilirubin 1.8 mg/dL, amylase 180 U/L, and lipase 80 U/L. Urinalysis results are as follows: specific gravity 1.020; positive glucose; no blood, protein, or ketones; 0–2 WBCs/HPF, and no bacteria. Based on the above information, which of the following is the most likely diagnosis in this patient?

A. Acute pancreatitis
B. Acute cholecystitis (LDH)
C. Mesenteric ischemia
D. Perforated peptic ulcer disease
E. Diabetic ketoacidosis (DKA)

163. A 45-year-old white man with a known history of alcohol abuse presents to the emergency department with hematemesis starting suddenly this evening. On examination, the patient's temperature is 97.0°C, HR is 120, RR is 18, and BP is 100/50 mm Hg. Upon sitting, the patient's HR increases to 140 and his BP decreases to 80/46 mm Hg. Of the following, which is the first step in the treatment of this patient?

A. Call gastroenterologist immediately to schedule emergent endoscopy
B. Type and cross for 2 units of packed RBCs
C. Drop a nasogastric tube and lavage until clear
D. Place two large-bore IVs and start with 2 L of crystalloid
E. Start the patient on an octreotide drip

164. A 55-year-old man comes to the ER with complaints of severe substernal chest pain that awakened him from sleep at 5 A.M. this morning. It is associated with some diaphoresis, shortness of breath, and nausea. He states that the pain is "heavy" and "pressure-like." He has never had this before. He tried taking some Tylenol at home, but called EMS within 1 hour for transport to the hospital. He was given a total of three sublingual nitroglycerin tablets in the ambulance without relief. On presentation to the ER his vital signs are BP 110/75 mm Hg, HR 100, and RR 18. He is afebrile, and his room air oxygen saturation is 95%. He is obese and in moderate distress secondary to pain. His neck reveals some mild jugular venous distention. His heart sounds are regular with occasional ectopy, and without murmurs or gallops. His lungs are clear to auscultation, and his abdomen reveals mild hepatomegaly. His extremities reveal trace edema. ECG is performed (Figure 1-164).

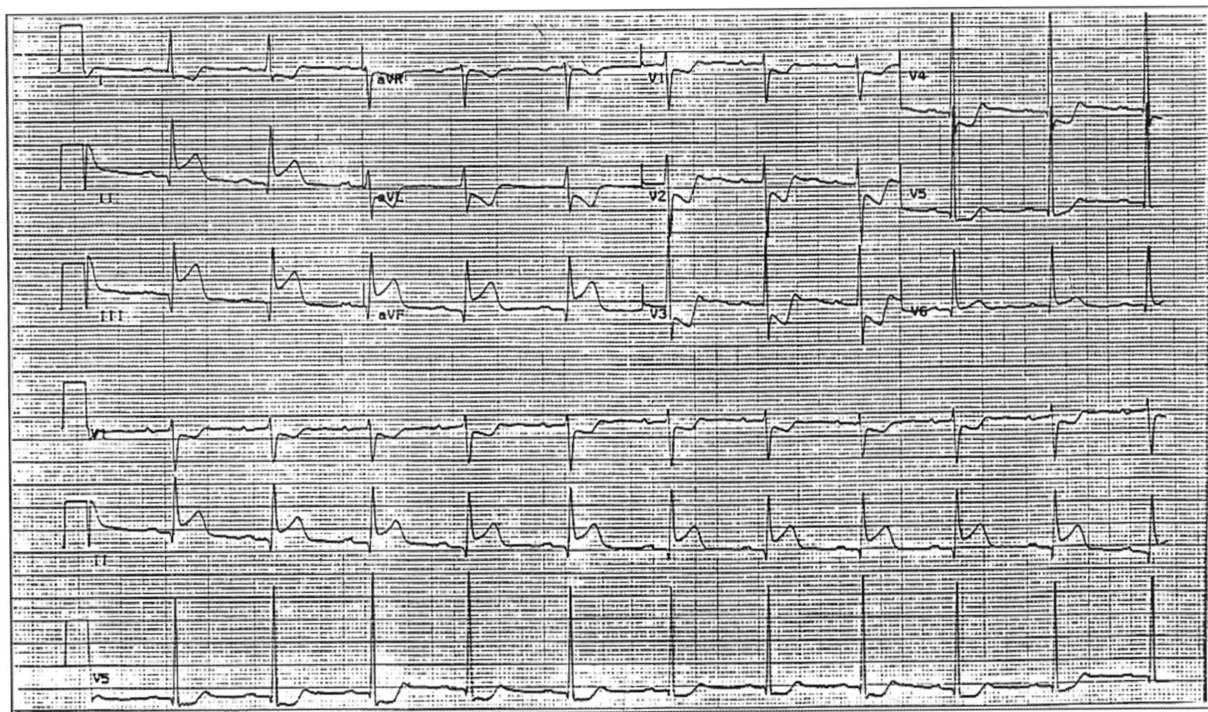

Figure 1-164 • Image Courtesy of Dr. Brenda Shinar, Banner Good Samaritan Medical Center, Phoenix, Arizona.

All of the following interventions are reasonable, but which one(s) should be undertaken with extreme caution?

A. Give the patient IV nitroglycerin
B. Give the patient thrombolytics
C. Bolus the patient with crystalloid fluids
D. Get a syringe of atropine to keep at the bedside
E. Give the patient IV morphine

165. A 28-year-old Hispanic woman presents to the ER with 1–2 days of right lower quadrant pain. The pain started suddenly, is constant, and is increasing in severity. She denies having any fever or chills. She also denies having any nausea, vomiting, anorexia, constipation, or diarrhea. She says she hasn't noticed any dysuria or hematuria. She is currently sexually active and says that she uses condoms "most of the time." Her last period was approximately 5 weeks ago. She states that her menstrual periods have always been irregular, with a cycle ranging from 28 to 40 days. On physical examination, her vital signs are stable, and she is afebrile. Her abdomen has normal bowels sounds. There is tenderness to palpation in the right lower quadrant without rebound. Pelvic examination yields a mild sanguinous discharge in the posterior fornix with some adenexal tenderness on the right, and no cervical motion tenderness. Her CBC shows a WBC count of 6,000 with a normal differential. The rest of the CBC is normal. The next step to determine the diagnosis is:

A. Culture for sexually transmitted diseases
B. Pregnancy test
C. Pelvic ultrasonography
D. Urinalysis
E. CT scan of the abdomen and pelvis

166. A 35-year-old man presents to the ER with complaints of dyspnea, lower extremity edema, and orthopnea for 3 weeks. He has also noted some skin darkening. He has no significant past medical history and takes no medications. He denies tobacco, drug, or alcohol use. Family history is significant for an uncle with liver disease. Vital signs are as follows: HR 88, BP 131/81 mm Hg, RR 18, temperature 97.3°C, and oxygen saturation 91% on room air. Physical examination is remarkable for jugular venous distention. The heart is regular with an S_3 present and no murmurs. There are bibasilar inspiratory crackles on lung examination and hepatomegaly noted on abdominal examination. The skin is diffusely hyperpigmented, most obviously in the skin folds. Which of the following statements is true for this patient's disease?

A. Transferrin saturation will be decreased.
B. Liver biopsy is not helpful in these patients.
C. Treatment includes defuroxamine and phlebotomy.
D. The most common clinical manifestations include diabetes, hyperpigmentation, and pulmonary disease.
E. Inheritance is autosomal dominant.

167. A 27-year-old black man presents to the ER with complaints of pallor, back pain, and dark urine of 2 days' duration. He denies having dysuria, nausea, vomiting, upper respiratory symptoms, or a sore throat. He was started on primaquine for malaria prophylaxis prior to travel to South America 5 days ago. Vital signs include HR 90, BP 117/77 mm Hg, RR 16, and oxygen saturation 98% on room air. Physical examination is remarkable for pallor of the mucous membranes and splenomegaly. A CBC and peripheral smear are performed (Figure 1-167). Which of the following statements is true regarding this patient's condition?

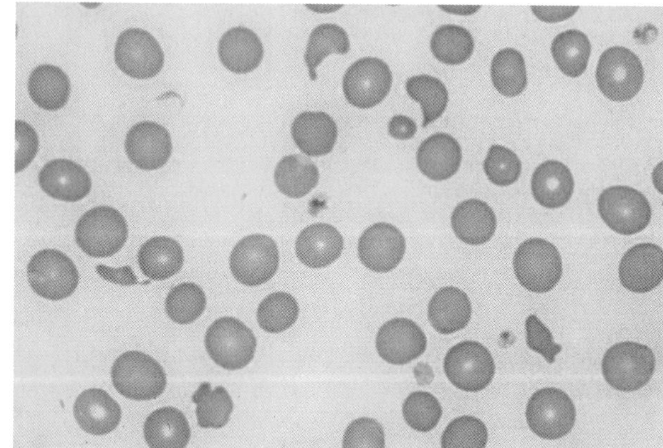

Figure 1-167 • Image Courtesy of Dr. Robert Raschke, Banner Good Samaritan Medical Center, Phoenix, Arizona.

A. It is an autosomal-recessive condition.
B. Other drugs that would trigger the same type of hemolysis include medications with sulfa, dapsone, and nitrofurantoin.
C. Splenectomy is indicated in this patient.
D. The defective enzyme in this disease catalyzes the conversion of phosphoenolpyruvate to pyruvate.
E. A reticulocyte count, if measured, would be low.

168. A 31-year-old African-American man with a history of anemia presents with 1 day of low back pain, diffuse myalgias, and bone pain. He denies having chest pain, cough, or fever. Vitals signs show mild tachycardia. Physical examination is remarkable for nonspecific tenderness over the back and extremities. Laboratory values are remarkable for hemoglobin of 6.1 g/dL with a reticulocyte count of 13%. A peripheral smear is obtained (Figure 1-168). Which of the following choices is a known complication of his disease?

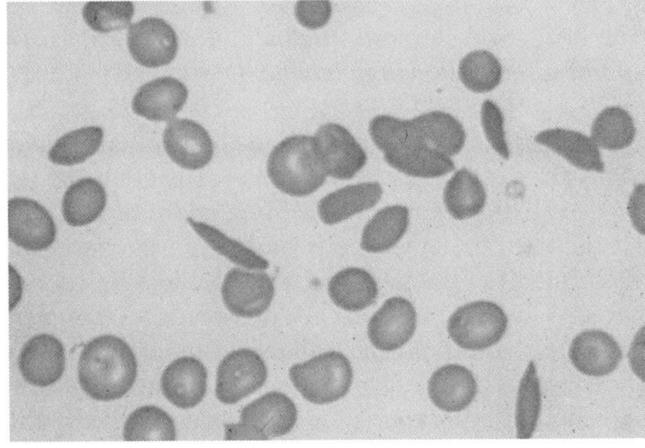

Figure 1-168 • Image Courtesy of Dr. Brenda Shinar, Banner Good Samaritan Medical Center, Phoenix, Arizona.

A. Cerebral infarction
B. Distal type 1 RTA
C. Splenomegaly in adults
D. *Streptococcus pneumoniae* osteomyelitis
E. Nephrogenic diabetes insipidus

169. A 28-year-old man with no significant medical history presents with shortness of breath and pleuritic chest pain acute in onset 4 hours ago. He arrived in Phoenix from Boston 1 day ago by plane. The patient's father has a history of recurrent DVT. On physical examination he is tachypneic, tachycardic, and oxygen saturation is 88% on room air. Pulmonary examination reveals no focal crackles, wheezes, or other abnormalities. ABG analysis shows a respiratory alkalosis with hypoxemia. The patient is admitted and an evaluation for hypercoagulable state is begun. The most likely underlying disorder in this patient would be:

A. Factor V Leiden defect
B. Antithrombin deficiency
C. Antiphospholipid syndrome
D. Malignancy
E. Protein C deficiency

170. A 25-year-old man presents to the ER complaining of a right testicular mass that has been enlarging over the past 6 weeks. He has no other significant past medical history. On physical examination, there is a 4-cm palpable mass in the right testis that does not change in size or consistency with position. It does not transilluminate with light. You are worried about possible testicular cancer and order ultrasonography of the testicle, which reveals a 4-cm heterogenous testicular mass in the right testicle with cystic areas and indistinct margins. Laboratory studies reveal the following: serum β-hCG 10,000 mIU/mL, serum alpha-fetoprotein 4 mg/mL, and lactate dehydrogenase (LDH) 800 IU. Which of the following is a true statement regarding this patient's disease?

A. Normal tumor markers would have ruled out the diagnosis of testicular cancer.
B. This patient probably has a pure seminoma.
C. This patient probably has a choriocarcinoma.
D. This patient probably has a Sertoli cell tumor.
E. This patient probably has a Leydig cell tumor.

171. A 68-year-old woman presents with a painful rash. She states that prior to the rash occurring, she had a severe, burning pain over the area, and the skin was sensitive to touch. On examination, you note groups of small vesicles and pustules on an erythematous base (Figure 1-171). Which one of the following is true about this disease?

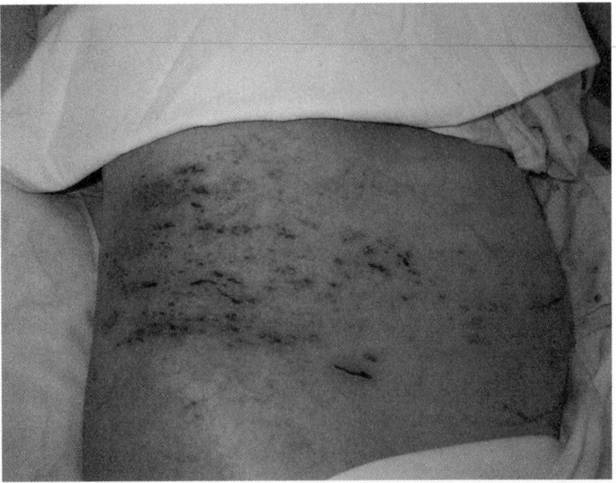

Figure 1-171 • Image Courtesy of Dr. Brenda Shinar, Banner Good Samaritan Medical Center, Phoenix, Arizona.

A. It is more common in the elderly.
B. It is not contagious.
C. It is caused by herpes simplex virus.
D. It is usually bilateral.
E. Antiviral treatment is recommended only for immunocompromised patients.

172. That same day, you see another patient in the ER with complaints of a rash on the upper right face, which began with a burning-type pain 2 days prior. You look closely and note that the rash also appears erythematous with small, grouped vesicles. There appears to be a lesion on the tip of the patient's nose as well. What is the significance of this lesion?

A. It indicates a high risk for varicella encephalitis.
B. It indicates a high risk for sinusitis.
C. It necessitates referral to a plastic surgeon.
D. It indicates a high risk for eye involvement.
E. It indicates that more than one dermatome is involved.

173. A 68-year-old woman presents to the ER with complaints of a fever and a headache for the past 3 days. This morning she noticed a weakness in her right arm, which prompted her to come in. Prior to the development of these symptoms she had been suffering from a respiratory infection with symptoms of fever and a productive cough. Her past medical history is significant for temporal arteritis for which she has been on prednisone 60 mg daily for several months. She has smoked one pack of cigarettes per day for the past 30 years. On physical examination her temperature is 101.8°C, HR 96, RR 22, and BP 103/68 mm Hg. Lung examination reveals scattered rhonchi. Neurologic examination reveals weakness of the right upper extremity. Chest radiography reveals multiple pulmonary nodules. CT of the head with contrast was performed and revealed several ring-enhancing lesions. What is the most likely etiology for her constellation of signs and symptoms?

A. *Streptococcus pneumoniae* infection
B. *Nocardia asteroides* infection
C. *Pneumocystis carinii* infection
D. Wegener granulomatosis
E. Lung cancer with brain metastases

The next two questions (items 174 and 175) correspond to the following vignette:

A 68-year-old woman presents to the emergency room after collapsing at work. She states that she felt dizzy and then passed out. After approximately 15 seconds, she regained consciousness, was alert, and was brought to the hospital by co-workers. She denies having chest pain, shortness of breath, diaphoresis, nausea, or vomiting. Her colleagues report that there were no tonic-clonic movements during that time and she did not experience incontinence. In the ER, she is afebrile with a BP of 80/48, HR of 30, and RR of 16. Results of her examination are unremarkable except for a bradycardic heart rate. You obtain an ECG (Figure 1-174).

174. The ECG demonstrates which of the following conduction abnormalities?

A. Sinus bradycardia
B. First-degree AV block
C. Type I second-degree AV block
D. Type II second-degree AV block
E. Third degree AV block

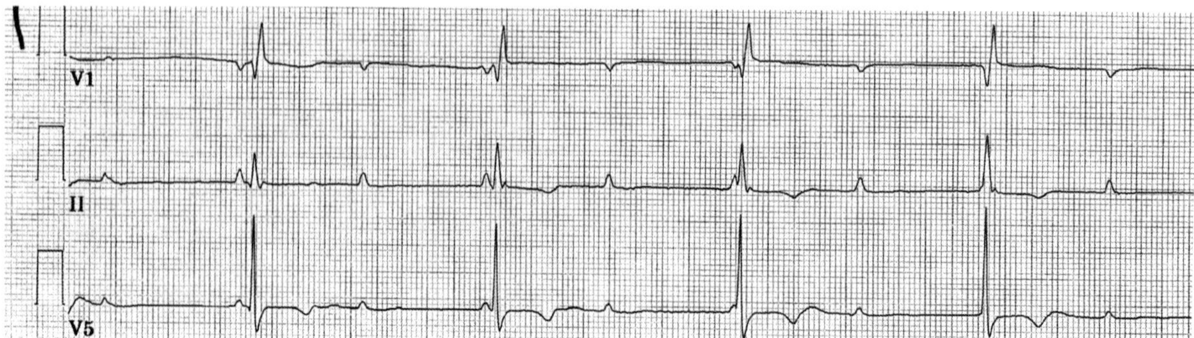

Figure 1-174 • Image Courtesy of Dr. Brenda Shinar, Banner Good Samaritan Medical Center, Phoenix, Arizona.

175. What is the most appropriate initial step in treating her condition?

A. Give her IV diltiazem
B. Give her IV metoprolol
C. Give her IV adenosine
D. Initiate transcutaneous pacing
E. Defibrillate her at 200 joules

End of Set

The next two questions (items 176 and 177) correspond to the following vignette:

A 52-year-old homeless woman is brought into the ER after friends find her passed out in a local park. It is unclear what happened to the woman or how long she has been down. No further history can be obtained. She has a BP of 118/76 mm Hg, HR of 98, and temperature of 99.4°C. She has agonal respirations and is immediately intubated and fluids are begun. Chest x-ray shows appropriate positioning of the endotracheal tube with normal lung fields. Blood is drawn, and a urinary catheter is inserted and reveals reddish brown urine, which is sent for analysis. The following laboratory results are returned: sodium 141 mEq/L, potassium 4.6 mEq/L, BUN 42 mg/dL, creatinine 2.0 mg/dL, CO_2 15 meq/L, and chloride 108 mEq/L. Urinalysis results show the urine is hazy and red in appearance, specific gravity 1.030, pH 5.5, 4+ blood, trace protein, negative for leukocyte esterase and nitrites, 0–1 WBCs/HPF, and 0–1 RBCs/HPF.

176. What is the most likely explanation for the findings on her urinalysis?

A. Urinary tract infection
B. Acute tubular necrosis from hypotension
C. Rhabdomyolysis
D. Traumatic insertion of catheter
E. Transitional cell carcinoma of the bladder

177. After beginning aggressive IV fluids, what is the next most important step in the treatment of this patient?

A. Cystoscopy
B. Alkalinization of the urine
C. IV antibiotics
D. Removal of catheter
E. Emergent hemodialysis

End of Set

The following two questions (items 178 and 179) relate to the same clinical scenario:

You are working in the ER when a 49-year-old woman is brought in unresponsive. The paramedics were notified after witnesses saw her collapse while standing at a bus stop. No other history is available. On examination, she has a BP of 65/35 mm Hg, with an HR of 130. Her temperature is 99.8°C and she has agonal respirations. Her physical examination is remarkable for rales throughout both lung fields. She is tachycardic but there are no murmurs appreciated on examination. The results of the remainder of her examination are unremarkable. She is intubated for airway protection. You give her a bolus of 2 L of normal saline IV and her BP does not change significantly. An infusion of dopamine is started and you insert a pulmonary artery catheter (Swan-Ganz) and obtain the following parameters: pulmonary artery pressure 30/20 mm Hg, pulmonary capillary wedge pressure 25 mm Hg, cardiac output 2.1 L/min, and systemic vascular resistance 1500 dynes $\times$ sec/cm^5.

178. How would you best classify the type of shock present in this patient?

A. Septic shock
B. Hypovolemic shock
C. Anaphylactic shock
D. Cardiogenic shock
E. Toxic shock

179. After the dopamine infusion is started, her BP improves to 110/76 mm Hg but her cardiac output remains relatively unchanged. What is the best choice for the next step in the treatment of this patient's shock?

A. IV broad-spectrum antibiotics
B. IV solumedrol and diphenhydramine
C. Additional boluses of normal saline
D. IV dobutamine

End of Set

180. A 21-year-old white man is brought into the trauma bay after a rollover accident on his all-terrain vehicle. He opens his eyes to painful stimuli, but otherwise they remain closed. He pulls away his arm as the nurse tries to start an IV line, but otherwise has no spontaneous movement. The patient's responses to questions are incomprehensible and he is clearly not oriented or appropriate. Which of the following best estimates this patient's Glasgow Coma Scale score?

A. 3
B. 6
C. 9
D. 12
E. 15

The next two questions (items 181 and 182) correspond to the following vignette:

A 21-year-old white woman presents to the emergency room with the complaint of a headache for the past 3 hours. The headache is located over the left frontal and temporal areas and she describes it as throbbing in nature. Bright light worsens the headache, so the patient has been lying in a dark room for the past 2 hours. She reports some nausea, but no emesis. She reports seeing some "bright and sparkling lights" in her vision prior to onset of the headache. Family history is remarkable for a mother with headaches similar to this. Neurologic examination results are normal.

181. Which of the following is a true statement regarding migraine headaches?

A. They are usually bilateral, throbbing, and last only for an hour or two.
B. Common migraines occur with an aura.
C. Classic migraines may have preceding visual symptoms, including "seeing stars and light flashes" or other abnormal visual field defects.
D. Dark rooms and sleep usually do not appreciably improve symptoms.
E. Patients usually present later in life with symptoms and very few report a family history.

182. Which of the following is a true statement regarding treatment of migraines?

A. Sumatriptan can be used as a prophylactic treatment for migraine headaches.
B. Prophylactic treatment should be started if the patient has more than four headaches per month.
C. NSAIDs are ineffective in this population and should not be used as an acute treatment.
D. Acute treatment medications are given once the headache has reached maximal intensity.
E. Sumatriptan and other triptans should not be used in patients with peripheral vascular disease or CAD because they cause sustained coronary artery constriction.

End of Set

183. A 40-year-old African-American man with a known seizure disorder is brought by ambulance to the emergency department. He is having a generalized tonic-clonic seizure that has lasted at least 30 minutes. On your arrival, his arms and legs are moving in a rhythmic tonic-clonic pattern. He is unresponsive to any stimuli, but has spontaneous respirations, a good pulse, and normal vital signs. He has an IV line placed by the paramedics, but has been given no medications. Blood glucose as checked by paramedics was normal. What is the next most appropriate step in management of this patient?

A. Paralyze and intubate
B. Lorazepam 0.1 mg/kg IV
C. Phenytoin 20 mg/kg IV
D. CT of the head
E. EEG

184. A 34-year-old Asian woman with no prior medical history presents with abrupt-onset right arm stiffness followed by jerking and twitching of the right arm for 3 to 5 minutes. The patient is conscious throughout the event, but cannot control the symptoms. She denies having any symptoms of weakness, numbness, visual changes, headache, fever, or other associated symptoms. The symptoms have occurred three times over the past 2 weeks. What is the most likely diagnosis?

A. Pseudoseizures
B. Generalized tonic-clonic seizure
C. Simple partial seizure
D. Complex partial seizure
E. Absence seizure

185. A 45-year-old man comes to the ER with complaints of a severe headache, nausea and vomiting, and fever that started the day before. He denies any recent travel or ingestion of unpasteurized dairy products. He is in otherwise good health, and has no HIV risk factors. He says that he has 10-year-old twin daughters at home who have had colds recently. On physical examination, he has a BP of 110/75 mm Hg, HR of 100, temperature of 102°C, and RR of 14. His neck is stiff, and he is unable to touch his chin to his chest. His examination is otherwise unremarkable except for some purulent sinus drainage. Laboratory studies reveal a WBC count of 18,000 with 10% bands. The rest of his CBC and laboratory results are normal. You obtain two sets of blood cultures. Choose the appropriate treatment of the patient in the correct sequence from the following choices:

A. CT of the head; lumbar puncture (LP); IV ceftriaxone, vancomycin, and dexamethasone
B. IV ceftriaxone and vancomycin; CT of the head; LP
C. IV ceftriaxone, vancomycin, and acyclovir; CT of the head; LP
D. LP; IV ceftriaxone, ampicillin, acyclovir, and steroids; no CT scan is needed
E. IV ceftriaxone, vancomycin, and dexamethasone; CT scan of the head; LP

186. A 68-year-old man with a history of coronary artery disease and tobacco abuse comes to the ER with complaints of right arm weakness and numbness that has persisted for the past 2 hours. On physical examination, his BP is 150/85 mm Hg, HR is 100, and he is afebrile. He is awake and alert and answering questions appropriately. His heart examination reveals a regular rhythm without murmurs or gallops. His lungs are clear and his abdomen is benign. His extremities are warm and without edema. He has slightly diminished pulses in the lower extremities with some loss of hair growth on the toes and feet. His neurologic examination reveals normal cranial nerves. He has 4/5 motor function of the right arm deltoid, biceps, triceps, and hand grip. His sensation is also diminished to light touch and pinprick. Reflexes of the right upper extremity are slightly brisk. Results of the rest of the neurologic examination are normal. A CT scan of the head shows no evidence of bleeding or mass in the brain. What should be done next in the management of this patient?

A. Recombinant tissue plasminogen activator (rt-PA)
B. Aspirin
C. Heparin therapy, full dose
D. MRI of the brain with diffusion weighted images
E. Lower the BP with sublingual nifedipine

187. A 40-year-old woman comes to the ER with complaints of left leg swelling and pain. You go to examine and interview the patient with a medical student; afterward, you discuss the possibility that this patient may have a DVT. You ask your medical student the following question: In which of the following scenarios would a negative D-dimer test effectively rule out thromboembolic disease?

A. A 70-year-old man with metastatic prostate cancer presents to the ER with 3 days of right lower extremity swelling and pain that involves the entire extremity.
B. A 60-year-old man on a ventilator in the ICU for the past 7 days for hypercarbic respiratory failure develops sudden worsening hypoxemia and tachycardia.
C. A 30-year-old woman who is 38 weeks pregnant comes to the ER with unilateral lower extremity swelling and pain after a 5-hour plane trip.
D. A 20-year-old woman with a history of asthma since childhood presents to the ER with increasing cough and wheezing for the past 2 days associated with the onset of a sore throat and clear rhinorrhea.
E. A 60-year-old woman with metastatic ovarian cancer who has sudden onset of dyspnea and pleuritic chest pain 2 days after undergoing a debulking surgery.

188. A 72-year-old Asian woman comes in to the ER for evaluation of shortness of breath. She has a past medical history of osteoporosis. The shortness of breath has been gradual in onset and she denies having any other respiratory symptoms. On examination she is in no respiratory distress. Her temperature is 98.8°C, HR 90, RR 20, and BP 118/72 mm Hg. Her oxygen saturation is 98% on room air. Heart and lung examinations reveal no adventitious sounds. She has severe kyphosis. Extremity examination reveals no clubbing or cyanosis. You send her for PFTs with flow volume loops. What do you expect her results to show?

A. Decreased total lung capacity (TLC), decreased vital capacity (VC), decreased residual volume (RV), normal FEV_1, normal FEV_1/FVC ratio, normal DLCO
B. Increased TLC, increased VC, increased RV, decreased FEV_1, decreased FEV_1/FVC ratio, decreased DLCO
C. Increased TLC, increased VC, increased RV, decreased FEV_1, decreased FEV_1/FVC ratio, normal DLCO
D. Decreased TLC, decreased VC, decreased RV, normal FEV_1, increased FEV_1/FVC, decreased DLCO
E. Normal TLC, normal VC, normal RV, normal FEV_1, normal FEV_1/FVC, normal DLCO

189. A 45-year-old man presents to you for evaluation of a visual disturbance. He states that for the past several weeks he has noted dark spots in his vision in the left eye. He occasionally sees a flash of light. The symptoms have remained static. He denies having any past medical history. He is homosexual and doesn't smoke or drink alcohol. Review of symptoms reveals a 20-pound, unintentional weight loss over the past several months and persistent diarrhea. On examination he is thin. His vital signs are normal. His physical examination results are within normal limits, with the exception of funduscopic examination of the left eye (Figure 1-189). What is the most likely cause of this abnormality?

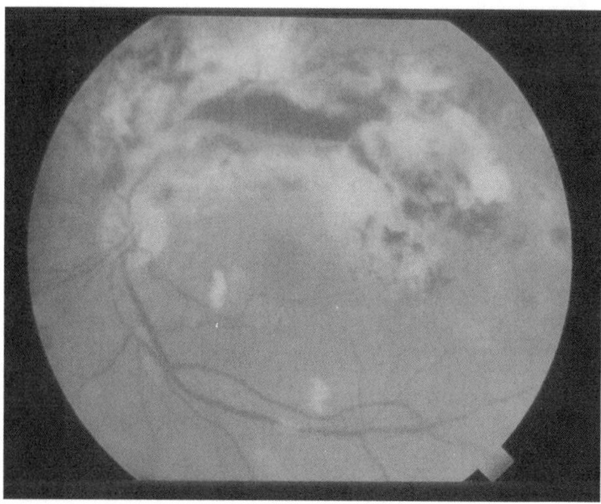

Figure 1-189 • Image Courtesy of Dr. Brenda Shinar, Banner Good Samaritan Medical Center, Phoenix, Arizona.

A. Retinal detachment
B. Central retinal vein occlusion
C. Central retinal artery occlusion
D. CMV retinitis
E. Angioid streaks

190. A 30-year-old man comes to the ER with complaints of fever, myalgias, and a diffuse maculopapular skin rash that started approximately 4 days ago. He reports being in good health prior to this episode. He works as a waiter, and is living with a roommate. He is sexually active and has sex with both men and women, telling you that he is bisexual. His last sexual experience was 2 weeks ago with a new male partner. On physical examination, he is febrile to 101°C, BP is 115/80 mm Hg, RR is 14, and HR is 90. His examination is significant for diffuse cervical and axillary lymphadenopathy and no hepatosplenomegaly. He has a fine maculopapular rash over his abdomen and back. Which of the following symptoms, if present, is most specific for acute HIV infection?

A. Fever
B. Lymphadenopathy
C. Diarrhea
D. Oral ulcers
E. Rash

191. A 42-year-old African-American man with a history of gallstones and hypertension presents to the ER with severe abdominal pain, nausea, and vomiting. He does not drink alcohol or use illicit drugs. In the ER, his temperature is 102°C, HR 100, RR 20, and BP 100/80 mm Hg. Abdominal examination reveals significant tenderness in the epigastric area and right upper quadrant. Laboratory evaluation reveals a WBC count of 14,000, amylase 4000 U/L, and lipase 3500 U/L. He is admitted to the ICU with a diagnosis of severe pancreatitis. His recovery is prolonged, and he is eventually started on total parenteral nutrition. During his hospitalization, as he is beginning to improve, he suddenly becomes tachycardic and hypotensive again. He develops a diffuse rash consisting of pustular skin. Funduscopic examination is performed (Figure 1-191). What should be the next step in the care of this patient?

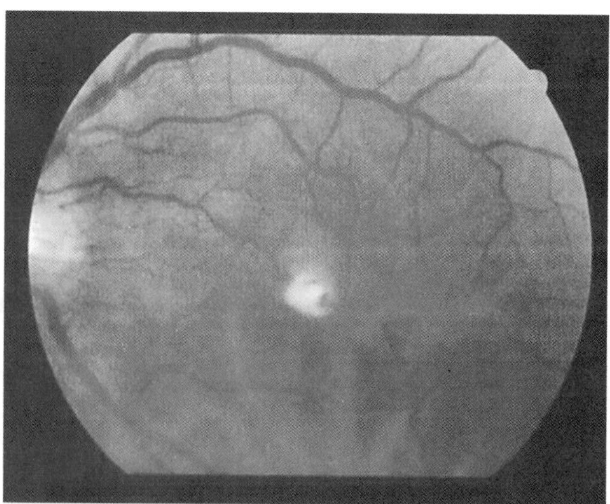

Figure 1-191 • Image Courtesy of Dr. Brenda Shinar, Banner Good Samaritan Medical Center, Phoenix, Arizona.

A. LP to rule out *Neisseria* meningitis
B. Removal of the triple-lumen catheter, initiation of IV vancomycin
C. Removal of the triple-lumen catheter, initiation of IV amphotericin B
D. CT of the abdomen to rule out necrotizing pancreatitis
E. Initiation of IV fluconazole

192. A 38-year-old man with a history of HIV on HAART comes to the ER with complaints of right flank pain and hematuria that have been present for the past 24 hours. He is miserable with the pain and is unable to lie still on the bed because of his discomfort. He has had some nausea and vomiting, but no fevers. He is unsure which medicines he is taking, but states that they are all related to his HIV. You begin the workup for the evaluation of a possible kidney stone. Which of the following antiretroviral medications is associated with nephrolithiasis?

A. Indinavir
B. Efavirenz
C. Abacavir
D. Ritonavir
E. Didanosine

193. A 58-year-old man is evaluated in the ER for a productive cough. His past medical history is significant for alcohol abuse and he continues to drink heavily. He states that for several weeks he has had a cough productive of dark, blood-streaked sputum. He has had subjective fevers and night sweats. He does not smoke and has never used any IV drugs. He is not aware of any exposure to persons with TB. He had a negative PPD skin test approximately 2 months prior while incarcerated for drunk driving. On examination he is disheveled. Temperature is 101.3°C, HR 98, RR 20, and BP 142/88 mm Hg. He has poor dentition. Lung examination reveals a few rhonchi in the right lower lung field. Chest radiography reveals an air fluid level in the right lower lobe. Sputum culture reveals usual oropharyngeal flora. Stain for AFB is negative. Results of PPD skin testing are negative. What is the most likely etiology for this patient's cavitary lesion?

A. TB
B. Pneumococcal pneumonia
C. Lung abscess
D. Squamous cell cancer
E. *Mycoplasma* pneumonia

194. A 40-year-old man with a 28-year heavy smoking history presents with complaints of a sudden onset of left chest pain and shortness of breath approximately 2 hours prior to coming to the ER. On physical examination, his BP is 120/75 mm Hg, HR 96, RR 22, and oxygen saturation 90% on room air. He is afebrile. His lung examination is significant for decreased breath sounds on the left with hyperresonance to percussion. His chest x-ray reveals a 50% pneumothorax on the left as well as diffuse micronodular shadows and cystic spaces, which spare the costophrenic angles. There is a noted lytic lesion in the lower thoracic vertebrae. Which of the following is the most likely unifying diagnosis?

A. Eosinophilic granulomatosis
B. Lymphangioleiomyomatosis
C. Eosinophilic pneumonia
D. Pulmonary alveolar proteinosis
E. Idiopathic pulmonary hemosiderosis

195. A 21-year-old woman and her college roommate both present to the ER with the complaint of nausea, vomiting, and abdominal pain. The symptoms started approximately 3 hours after the girls ate at a Chinese restaurant. What is the most likely organism responsible for their symptoms?

A. *Staphylococcus aureus*
B. *Salmonella enteriditis*
C. *Campylobacter jejuni*
D. *Bacillus cereus*
E. *Clostridium botulinum*

The next two questions (items 196 and 197) correspond to the following vignette:

A 62-year-old man is brought the ER by his wife because his right hand and leg are shaking. He first noticed the repetitive motion in his right hand a few weeks ago and was not too worried about it. Now he has developed a similar tremor in his right leg. He notices the tremor most when his hand and leg are resting. The tremor waxes and wanes in severity and seems to diminish with activity. He has no other neurologic complaints and denies any family history of neurologic problems. His only medical problem is COPD that resulted from many years of tobacco abuse. He uses albuterol and ipratropium bromide inhalers on a daily basis. On examination, his vital signs are normal and he is afebrile. Results of his HEENT, lung, and heart examinations are all unremarkable. He has a noticeable supination-pronation tremor in his right hand and forearm that has a frequency of approximately 4 Hz. The tremor decreases when you have the patient reach out to pick something up off the table in front of him. The tremor in his leg is not as noticeable. He has normal deep tendon reflexes bilaterally and has preserved and symmetric muscle strength. There is mild rigidity noted when you try to passively extend his elbow with a ratchetlike motion.

196. Which of the following classifications best describes this patient's tremor?

 A. Intention tremor
 B. Resting tremor
 C. Essential tremor
 D. Familial tremor
 E. Physiologic tremor

197. What is the most likely cause of this patient's tremor?

 A. MS
 B. Midbrain stroke
 C. Guillain-Barré syndrome
 D. Parkinson disease (PD)
 E. Medication induced

End of Set

The next two questions (items 198 and 199) correspond to the following vignette:

A 48-year-old woman presents to the ER with complaints of recurrent dizzy spells associated with nausea. Upon further questioning, you find that she has had numerous episodes over the past 4 months where she feels like the room is spinning around her and she has nausea. These episodes are short lived (<1 minute) and resolve spontaneously. She has no loss of consciousness when they occur. She has no focal neurologic changes, including weakness, numbness, or seizure-like activity. She denies any hearing loss or tinnitus. She has noticed that looking up while standing and rolling over in bed will sometimes precipitate her symptoms. She has no past medical history and takes no regular medications. On examination, she is afebrile and has normal vital signs. Her physical examination results are normal. You have her stand and look upward to try to provoke her symptoms. She states that she feels like the room is starting to spin and you notice a few beats of nystagmus.

198. What is the diagnosis?

 A. Benign positional vertigo (BPV)
 B. Vestibular neuritis
 C. Acute labyrinthitis
 D. Ménière disease
 E. Vertebrobasilar TIAs

199. Which of the following is appropriate first-line therapy?

 A. Meclizine
 B. Aspirin
 C. Salt restriction and diuretics
 D. Antibiotics
 E. No therapy

End of Set

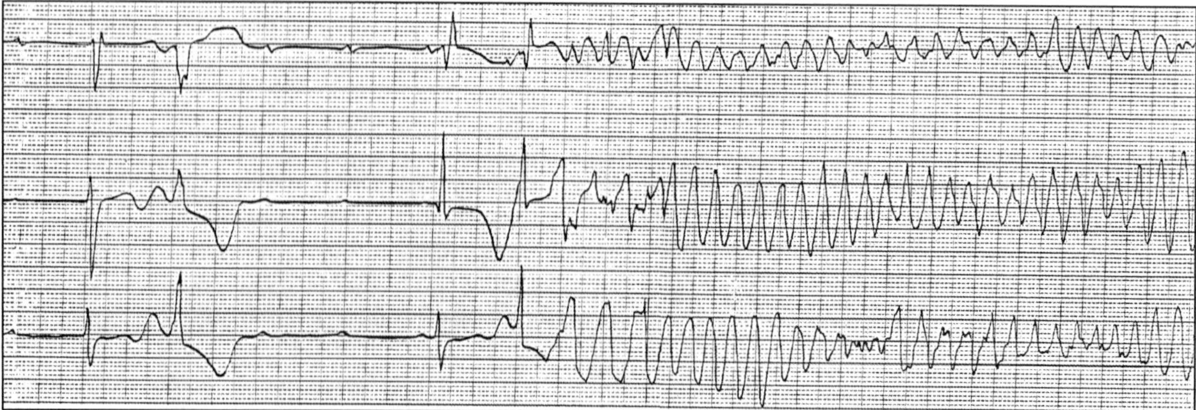

Figure 3-200 • Image Courtesy of Dr. Robert Raschke, Banner Good Samaritan Medical Center, Phoenix, Arizona.

200. A 65-year-old man with a history of CHF and CAD is brought to the ER after a syncopal event on the golf course. He had no aura or chest pain prior to the event, and he revives spontaneously before the paramedics come to get him. He is diaphoretic and nauseated with a BP of 90/45 mm Hg and an HR of 65. RR is 18, and his oxygen saturation is 94% on room air. An IV is placed in the field. He is brought to the ER and you go to examine him. As you introduce yourself, the patient becomes stuporous and you call for immediate vital signs and an ECG. His BP is 60/palpable mm Hg and his rhythm strip is seen in Figure 1-200. Which of the following is the most appropriate intervention to do first?

A. Prepare to intubate the patient
B. Open the IV fluid wide open
C. Start chest compressions and bag the patient
D. Defibrillate at 200 joules, unsyncronized
E. Give the patient a precordial thump followed by 1 mg IV epinephrine

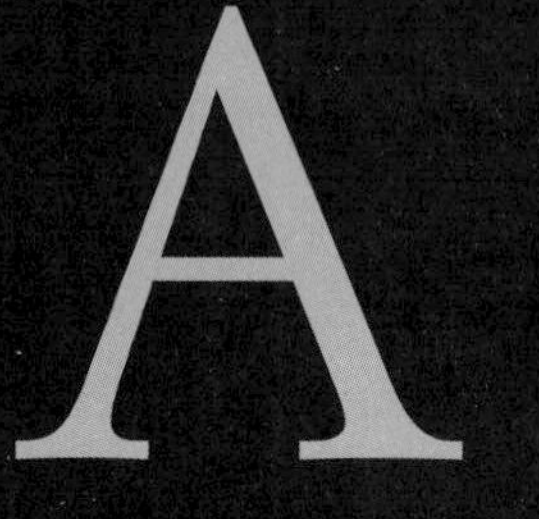

Answers and Explanations

151. A
152. A
153. D
154. D
155. E
156. B
157. D
158. A
159. A
160. B
161. C
162. B
163. D
164. A
165. B
166. C
167. B
168. A
169. A
170. C
171. A
172. D
173. B
174. E
175. D
176. C
177. B
178. D
179. D
180. C
181. C
182. B
183. B
184. C
185. E
186. A
187. D
188. A
189. D
190. D
191. C
192. A
193. C
194. A
195. D
196. B
197. D
198. A
199. A
200. D

151. A. This patient most likely has a radiopaque stone in the right ureter based on the clinical presentation and the finding of blood on urinalysis as well as a possible stone on KUB x-rays. However, KUB radiography does not evaluate the exact location of a stone, its size, and the possibility of hydronephrosis like ultrasonography or CT. Furthermore, it is often hard to distinguish a phlebolith (calcification of a vein) from nephrolithiasis on a KUB x-ray. Therefore, a more sensitive imaging test is warranted to evaluate for the exact placement of the stone, its size (to determine its likelihood of passing on its own vs. the need for urologic intervention), and any resulting hydronephrosis or hydroureter. A stone that is 5 mm or less in diameter should pass on its own with hydration.

B. Calcium oxalate and calcium phosphate stones are the most common stones, seen in 75% of stone producers. Uric acid stones make up a much smaller percentage of stones, and there are two reasons why this is not likely to be a uric acid stone. First, it is radiopaque, and uric acid stones are radiolucent. Second, uric acid stones form in patients who have very low urine pH as well as hyperuricosuria. Our patient's urine has a relatively high pH.

C. Urine culture and sensitivity should be ordered, especially if there is a possibility of struvite stones, which are formed secondary to the presence of chronic urinary infections with urease-producing bacteria, such as *Proteus* species. The high urine pH should make you concerned for the possibility of infection with urease-producing bacteria; however, this patient did not give a history of urinary tract infections, and his urinalysis was only significant for blood without WBCs, which makes infection less likely.

D, E. Twenty-four-hour urine collections for electrolyte concentrations and stone analysis are not usually performed in patients who pass kidney stones for the first time. This is reserved for patients who pass multiple stones.

152. A. This patient likely has type 1 distal RTA characterized by a hyperchloremic (nongap) metabolic acidosis, hypokalemia, and a high urine pH, seemingly inappropriate for the metabolic acidosis in the serum. (Type 1 distal RTA is the only RTA with an alkaline urine pH at a baseline.) Furthermore, type 1 distal RTA is associated with low urine citrate concentrations, and patients may present with calcium-containing kidney stones.

B. Type 4 distal RTA is characterized by a hyperchloremic (nongap) metabolic acidosis and hyperkalemia with a normal urine pH.

C. There is no such thing as type 3 proximal RTA.

D. Patients with type 2 proximal RTA have a hyperchloremic (nongap) metabolic acidosis with a normal serum potassium and a normal urine pH, unless they are bicarbonate "loaded." When bicarbonate loading is done, the bicarbonate is spilled into the urine, making the pH rise. Once the serum bicarbonate is back down to 15 mEq/L or so, the urine pH remains appropriately acidic.

E. There is enough information to determine the type of renal tubular acidosis that this patient likely has.

153. D. Chronic active hepatitis is a cause of type 1 distal RTA. Other causes include medications like amphotericin B and lithium. This patient has elevation of his transaminases and a history of IVDA, which puts him at high risk for chronic hepatitis. Therefore, the complete picture of this patient is that he has chronic active viral hepatitis with associated type 1 distal RTA and associated calcium-stone nephrolithiasis.

A, B. Heavy metal poisoning and multiple myeloma are causes of proximal type 2 RTA. Fanconi disease is also a cause of this RTA in children.

C, E. Diabetic nephropathy is probably the most common cause of type 4 distal RTA because of its prevalence. Other causes of type 4 RTA include sickle cell anemia and the medication spironolactone.

154. D. The patient has an elevated potassium on initial laboratory study results. This is due to the transcellular shift of potassium via the hydrogen/potassium pump on the cell's surface. The acidosis is driving the hydrogen ions into the cells and the potassium out of the cell. Once the acidosis starts to correct, potassium will decrease.

A. This patient is not truly hyponatremic. For each 100 mg/dL increase in glucose, measured sodium decreases by 1.6 mEq/L secondary to the transcellular shift of fluid. This patient's corrected sodium is 140 mEq/L, which is in the normal range.
B. Initial treatment of DKA should be fluid resuscitation followed by an insulin drip. Bicarbonate is not indicated in this patient.
C. The sodium would be expected to correct to normal when glucose returns to normal. Hyperglycemia causes measured sodium to decrease, so with correction of glucose to normal, measured sodium would rise back to normal. (See also answer A).
E. This patient has an anion gap metabolic acidosis. Anion gap is calculated by the following equation: Na − (bicarbonate + chloride). This patient's anion gap is 34. In order to evaluate for respiratory compensation, Winter's formula is used: Expected pCO_2 = (1.5 × serum bicarbonate) + 8 (±2). This patient's expected pCO_2 would be 26, which is within 2 of the measured value of 25, indicating adequate compensation.

155. E. This patient has ECG findings consistent with hyperkalemia. Calcium gluconate should be given first to stabilize the cardiac cell membrane. Onset of action is within minutes, making it the fastest acting medication in the regimen of medications given for hyperkalemia.

A. The patient has ECG findings of hyperkalemia and must first have the cardiac membrane stabilized by the treatment with calcium gluconate. The furosemide can be given next to help eliminate potassium from the kidneys, but it will take too long to correct the hyperkalemia, and the patient is in immediate danger because of cardiac cell membrane instability.
B. Sodium bicarbonate has a transient effect in hyperkalemia by driving potassium into the cells. Onset of action is 15–30 minutes. This can be given as a temporary therapy to lower potassium after calcium gluconate is given.
C. Insulin and glucose have a transient effect in hyperkalemia by driving potassium into the cells. Onset of action is 15–30 minutes. This can be given as a temporary therapy to lower potassium after calcium gluconate is given.
D. Sodium polystyrene sulfonate acts to decrease total body potassium by increasing intestinal excretion of potassium. Onset of action is 1–2 hours, so this would not provide the immediate therapy necessary in a patient with ECG changes.

156. B. Red man syndrome secondary to vancomycin. This side effect of vancomycin is an anaphylactoid reaction, which results in erythema and pruritis, particularly of the head and torso. It characteristically follows the first dose and may be avoided if the infusion time is slowed. The reaction is due to a release of histamine. Vancomycin is used in the empiric treatment of bacterial meningitis if penicillin-resistant *Streptococcus* pneumonia is suspected or if it is likely based on the susceptibility patterns in the area.

A. Infection with *Neisseria meningitidis* may result in meningitis as well as an associated rash. However, the rash associated with meningococcal infection is usually purpuric and not diffuse erythema.
C. Toxic shock syndrome can cause a diffuse, erythematous rash. This syndrome is usually secondary to staphylococcal or streptococcal species. It is most commonly seen in very young and very old patients. A soft tissue infection is the most common etiology for the syndrome, but it may also be due to tampon use in menstruating women. Patients present with hypotension, which is often severe and which our patient did not have. In addition, the neurologic symptoms seen in our patient are not usually part of the toxic shock syndrome.
D. Patients with psoriasis may develop a diffuse erythroderma that can be triggered by infection. However, our patient has no prior history of psoriasis.
E. Staphylococcal scalded skin syndrome is rare in adults unless they are immunocompromised. The disease is usually seen in infants. It is usually preceded by a skin infection, and large bullae often develop and rupture, leaving denuded skin. The neurologic signs seen in our patient are not a part of this syndrome.

157. D. This patient has the classical physical examination findings associated with AS. The systolic murmur noted on her examination is the

result of turbulent blood flow across the stenotic valve during systole. It takes longer for the left ventricle to eject its volume of blood through the stenotic valve, which results in a slower carotid upstroke (called parvus et tardus) and sustained apical impulse.

A. The murmur of aortic insufficiency, which is located best in the third and fourth intercostal spaces to the left of the sternum, results from retrograde blood flow across the valve (back into the left ventricle) during diastole. It is a diastolic murmur heard best with the patient leaning forward at end expiration.

B. Pulmonary stenosis is a systolic murmur that is best heard in the left upper sternal border area. Severe pulmonary stenosis more often presents with evidence of right-sided ventricular failure, not left-sided.

C. The regurgitation, or retrograde blood flow, across the mitral valve that occurs throughout systole results in a holosystolic murmur that is best heard in the apical area. This murmur often radiates into the axillary region.

E. Mitral stenosis results in a murmur caused by turbulence of blood flow across the stenotic valve that occurs during diastole. Severe mitral stenosis results in elevated left atrial pressures, atrial dilatation, and ultimately an increased pressure in the pulmonary vasculature (i.e., pulmonary hypertension). As a result, these patients classically present with atrial arrhythmias and hemoptysis.

158. **A. Echocardiography is the optimal test to assess the severity of her disease. It is a relatively rapid, noninvasive way of estimating the degree of stenosis, as well as showing the degree of LVH and the EF.**

B. Cardiac catheterization can also give you the above information, but it is much more invasive, is more expensive, and takes longer to obtain. Therefore, it is not the best choice to initially assess the severity of her AS.

C. Results of the exercise treadmill stress test will suggest if she has underlying coronary artery disease and may induce her exercise-associated syncope; however, it does not give you an objective assessment of the severity of her disease. More importantly, strenuous exercise, including stress tests, are contraindicated in patients with severe AS.

D. ECG can suggest the presence of LVH, but it does not provide an assessment of the ejection fraction or valvular area.

E. Vasodilator therapy will not provide any insight into the severity of the AS, and actually should be avoided in patients with severe AS.

159. **A. Patients with severe AS who become symptomatic have an extremely high risk for mortality over the next 5 years. If they have chest pain with exertion that is relieved by rest (angina), it portends a 5-year survival. This angina may occur despite normal coronary arteries because of the tremendous hypertrophy that the ventricle undergoes to overcome the fixed obstruction at the aortic valve. The hypertrophied muscle may have a hard time relaxing during diastole (which is the time of coronary perfusion). Patients who have exertional syncope have an approximate 3-year survival without valve replacement. The valve has become so stenotic that when the patient exerts himself, the left ventricle cannot increase to cardiac output appropriately in response to the vasodilation of the skeletal muscle enough to perfuse the brain. This results in presyncope or syncope. Finally, if the ventricle can no longer work hard enough to push the blood out of the stenotic aortic valve, heart failure ensues. Once left ventricular failure develops, patients will survive approximately 1 year without valve replacement.**

B, C, D, E. See explanation for A.

160. **B. The most important initial treatment for this patient is to control her HR. Although she is symptomatic, she is stable, so emergent cardioversion is not indicated. The choice of medication used to obtain rate control in atrial fibrillation should be chosen based on your patient. Digoxin can be considered when a patient has a history of a low EF because of its positive inotropic effect, but it is not appropriate to use alone for long-term rate control because it will not slow the HR when the patient is active. (It works by augmenting parasympathetic tone, but doesn't inhibit sympathetic tone.) Given that she leads an active lifestyle and has no evidence of CHF on examination, digoxin would not be the first-line therapy for rate control in this case. Other medications that slow AV nodal conduction such as calcium channel blockers or beta blockers are a better choice for initial treatment in this patient.**

A. See explanation for B.
C, D. Although amiodarone is an acceptable way of attempting medical cardioversion, this is not indicated in this patient at this time. Given that her symptoms have been present for >48 hours and she is currently stable, she should not be cardioverted until she is either fully anticoagulated for 3 weeks or until TEE can be performed to exclude the presence of a thrombus in her left atrium.
E. Although the prevention of thromboembolic disease in patients with atrial fibrillation is important, it is not the first step in the treatment of this disease.

161. **C. If atrial fibrillation has been present <48 hours, a patient can be anticoagulated with IV heparin, cardioverted and discharged home on warfarin for 4 weeks or longer. There are two ways to approach cardioversion if the patient has been in atrial fibrillation longer than 48 hours, or for an unknown period of time. First, if a TEE can be performed and shows no evidence of thrombus in the left atrium (TTE is not sufficient to rule out thrombus in the left atrium), the patient can be cardioverted and discharged home on warfarin therapy. If there is thrombus present, the patient should be fully anticoagulated for 3 weeks or longer prior to attempting cardioversion. The patient should then be continued on warfarin therapy for a minimum of 4 weeks afterward. (The AFFIRM trial suggested that patients should be anticoagulated for life, regardless of whether the physician thinks that they have remained in sinus rhythm, because their risk for stroke was the same as for people who remained in atrial fibrillation who were not anticoagulated or were subtherapeutic on their INR.) If a TEE cannot be completed, the patient should be treated with warfarin for 3 or more weeks, electively cardioverted, and continued on warfarin for an additional 4 weeks or longer. Given that the duration of her atrial fibrillation was >48 hours and our only choice was to use TTE, the correct answer is C.**

A. See explanation for C.
B. This answer is incorrect for two reasons. First, a TTE is not sufficient, as discussed above. Second, a patient should not be discharged after cardioversion without being started on full anticoagulation. Once the atria are converted back into sinus rhythm, it takes several weeks before they begin to contract normally again. During this time, there is still risk for stasis of blood in the atria and subsequently for development of thrombus.
D. This patient is not a low-risk patient for thromboembolism. Clinical risk factors include history of TIA/CVA, hypertension, DM, CHF, and age >65 years. She has three identified risk factors, making her a high-risk patient for thromboembolism. Therefore, she should be anticoagulated for prophylaxis against CVA.
E. She is not unstable and does not require emergent cardioversion. In addition, the reason for using TEE in the management of atrial fibrillation is to assess for the presence of a thrombus in the left atrium before cardioversion, not after.

162. **B. Based on the information given, the most likely diagnosis in this patient is acute cholecystitis, although each of the choices is in the differential diagnosis for this patient's complaints. Patients with acute cholecystitis often have epigastric and right upper quadrant abdominal pain with nausea and vomiting and fever. This patient is obese, female, and in her forties, which puts her at risk for gallstone disease. Her laboratory results are significant for an elevated alkaline phosphatase and total bilirubin compared with the normal levels of hepatocellular enzymes. This suggests an obstructive picture, and you must ascertain whether there is extrahepatic obstruction or intrahepatic obstruction via abdominal ultrasonography.**

A. The amylase is mildly elevated, but this is not specific for pancreatitis. An elevated amylase may be seen in many disorders of the GI tract, such as salivary gland abnormalities, pancreatitis, cholecystitis, and intestinal ischemia. In addition, the lipase is normal, and this is both sensitive and specific for pancreas inflammation. Therefore, at this point in time, our diagnosis of cholecystitis is more appropriate.
C. Mesenteric ischemia classically presents with complaints of abdominal pain that is sudden in onset and out of proportion to the amount of tenderness on physical examination.

Patients may have an anion gap acidosis from an increase in lactate. They also may have an increase in amylase, which is released from the injured small bowel. Usually patients are older and have risks for atherosclerotic vascular disease, atrial fibrillation (a source for embolism), or vasculitis signs and symptoms.

D. A perforated peptic ulcer may cause an increase in amylase along with abdominal pain, nausea, and vomiting. Patients may have melena or hematemesis. Patients with this diagnosis usually have peritoneal signs on examination and at least guaiac-positive stool if not frank blood.

E. DKA can cause abdominal pain and elevated amylase levels secondary to the acidosis. This patient had a history of type 2 diabetes, and her blood sugar was high, but not at the point that we usually see with DKA. Her urine was negative for ketones, which makes this diagnosis unlikely. It is more likely that something (like the patient's gallbladder) is making her sick and causing a release of cortisol that is increasing her blood sugar. She should have frequent monitoring of her blood sugars while you are trying to make the diagnosis.

163. D. The most concerning issue with this patient at this time is his hypotension. Two large-bore IVs should be placed, and crystalloid should be administered wide open.

A. A gastroenterologist should be called so that endoscopy can be scheduled, but the patient needs to be stabilized first.

B. It is more than likely that this patient will require a blood transfusion. The blood should be ordered, but it will unlikely be available immediately. Crystalloid replacement is the best first choice.

C. A nasogastric tube should eventually be placed in this patient, but again, his hypotension is more of a concern at this point. Varices are not a contraindication to placing a nasogastric tube.

E. A continuous octreotide infusion can be started once the patient has been resuscitated.

164. A. The patient has evidence of an inferior MI, and on physical examination he has elevated jugular venous pressure, mild hepatomegaly, mild pedal edema and clear lungs, which may represent some degree of right-sided heart failure. A right-sided ECG should be ordered to look for possible posterior wall involvement, which is seen best in V_4R. Patients with inferior infarcts usually have involvement of the right coronary artery, which also supplies the AV node. Thus, these patients are at risk for AV node ischemia with resulting AV block. Keeping some atropine at the bedside is a good idea. If he developed a significant heart block, beta blockers would be contraindicated, and they should therefore be used with caution. Also, patients with inferior infarcts may develop poor right ventricular compliance due to ischemia. Therefore, they may require large volumes of fluid to keep their pressures up. Anything that reduces preload, such as IV nitroglycerin, may precipitate severe hypotension and should also be used with caution.

B, C, D, E. See explanation for A.

165. B. A young woman with abdominal pain or pelvic pain needs to have a pregnancy test. If her pregnancy test result is positive, the next test would be a serum quantitative hCG and transvaginal ultrasonography. Transvaginal ultrasonography is performed to evaluate for an intrauterine pregnancy, any ovarian pathology, or evidence of an ectopic pregnancy. The patient may be presenting with an ectopic pregnancy or she may be miscarrying an intrauterine pregnancy that was undetected. If her pregnancy test result is negative, she may be experiencing an ovarian torsion or ruptured ovarian cyst.

A. Patients with PID usually present with pelvic pain, vaginal discharge, fever, and an elevated WBC count. On physical examination, they may have a purulent discharge from the cervix and cervical motion tenderness. (This test is nonspecific, however, and patients with inflammation or blood in the cul de sac from ruptured ectopic pregnancy or ovarian cyst rupture may also have cervical motion tenderness.) Because the patient did not have fever, discharge, or an elevated WBC count, I would not pursue PID first as a diagnosis in this patient. Also, cultures may be negative up to 50% of the time when searching for evidence of PID, so it is a diagnosis often made on clinical grounds.

C. Pelvic ultrasonography should be performed in this patient, but a urine pregnancy test needs to be done first to know whether or not you are dealing with pregnancy-related pathology, such as described above.
D. Urinalysis should be evaluated in a patient who complains of abdominal or pelvic pain, but the priority test in this patient is a urine pregnancy test.
E. CT scan of the abdomen and pelvis is often done to help diagnose appendicitis, although the diagnosis is really made clinically. Appendicitis should be thought of as a possible diagnosis in this patient, but she does not have fever, elevated WBC count, or anorexia, making the diagnosis of appendicitis less likely.

166. C. This patient has hemochromatosis. Hemochromatosis is a disease that is inherited in an autosomal-recessive fashion that results in too much absorption of iron from the GI tract and systemic iron overload. The treatment of this disease includes defuroximine, which combines with ferric ions to form ferrioxamine. These combined products can then be excreted by the kidneys. Additionally, phlebotomy is performed to keep the patient chronically iron deficient as determined by ferritin levels.

A. Transferrin saturation will be extremely elevated in hemochromatosis. Transferrin is the carrier protein for iron in the serum. Normal iron saturation levels of transferrin are less than 50% in women and less than 60% in men. This test is a useful screening tool for iron overload. Patients with hemochromatosis often have saturations of 95% or higher, but patients with alcoholic liver disease also may have high transferrin saturations, which can make the diagnosis confusing. This is when a liver biopsy can be helpful.
B. Liver biopsy is the gold standard for the diagnosis of hemochromatosis, and the hepatic iron index can be measured from the sample. This index is useful to determine whether or not a patient has increased transferrin saturation from hemochromatosis or from alcoholic liver disease. In hemochromatosis, the hepatic iron index is elevated, whereas in alcoholic liver disease, the hepatic iron index is normal.
D. Hemochromatosis is a disease of iron overload. As a result, iron is deposited in various tissues and organs in the body. The skin, liver, pancreas, heart, and testes are the most commonly effected. Deposition of iron leads to a "bronzing" of the skin, cirrhosis, diabetes, CHF, and primary hypogonadism.
E. The inheritance of hereditary hemochromatosis is autosomal recessive.

167. B. This patient has G6PD deficiency. In patients with this enzyme defect, hemolysis of RBCs is triggered by oxidative drugs. There is a long list of offending drugs that includes primaquine, sulfa, dapsone, and nitrofurantion.

A. G6PD deficiency is an X-linked inherited disorder.
C. Splenectomy is not indicated in patients with G6PD deficiency. Patients should avoid oxidative drugs to prevent episodes of hemolysis.
D. The enzyme defect described in this answer is pyruvate kinase deficiency. G6PD works in the glutathione production pathway and is the enzyme that reduces NADP to NADPH.
E. The reticulocyte count would be elevated. In a hemolytic anemia, the bone marrow would increase production of RBCs.

168. A. Sickle cell anemia is caused by a substitution of a valine for a glutamic acid as the sixth amino acid in the beta-globin chain, resulting from a DNA substitution of thymine for adenine. Sickle cells obstruct small blood vessels because of their shape and abnormal adherence to endothelium, resulting in many different complications. Cerebral infarction affects children and young adults more commonly and results from occlusion of major cerebral vessels.

B, E. There are several renal manifestations of sickle cell anemia. Tubular complications include distal type 4 RTA, resulting in hyperkalemia (not type 1 RTA). The concentrating ability of the kidney is often diminished because of destruction of the vasa recta in the medulla, resulting in maximum urine osmolality of around 400 mosm/kg as compared with 900–1200 mosm/kg in normal patients. Other renal complications include renal papillary necrosis and renal infarction.

C. Patients with sickle cell anemia have enlarged spleens in infancy and throughout childhood. However, by the time patients are adults, they have had recurrent perivascular hemorrhage and infarction that reduces the organ to a small vestige.

D. Osteomyelitis occurs with increased frequency in all age groups, and over half of the cases are related to *Salmonella* infection, unlike the normal population, in which 80% of cases are due to staphylococcal organisms. Patients with sickle cell disease are at increased risk for infection with encapsulated organisms due to the functional asplenia.

169. **A. Factor V Leiden is the most common inherited hypercoagulable state, accounting for nearly 50% of inherited thrombophilic disorders. Estimated prevalence of the defect is 2%–5%, with whites having the highest prevalence. The risk for venous thrombosis in patients who are heterozygous for this defect is approximately seven times that of persons without the defect. Several factors should alert the clinician to an underlying defect, including family history of thrombosis, age of first thrombotic event at age less than 50, and recurrent thrombotic events.**

B. Antithrombin serves to inactivate procoagulant factors, including factors II, IX, and X. Initial presentation with thrombosis typically occurs before age 50. This defect also has a prevalence of less than 1%.

C. Antiphospholipid antibodies occur in 2%–5% of otherwise healthy people, but are most frequent in patients with autoimmune disorders such as lupus. Patients with this syndrome are at risk for both venous and arterial thrombosis.

D. Malignancy is a risk factor for a hypercoagulable state, but this patient has nothing in the history to suggest this as an underlying diagnosis. It is not usually recommended to go searching for an underlying malignancy in a patient who presents with a new clot, but it is important to make sure that the normal cancer screening examinations are performed appropriate to the patient's age.

E. Protein C deficiency is less common, with a prevalence of <1%. Protein C, once activated, serves to break down factors V and VIII. There is a high incidence of thrombosis, even among patients who are heterozygous for the deficiency. Most present in their twenties or thirties with a venous thromboembolism.

170. **C. This patient has a 4-cm mass in the testicle, which is cancer until proven otherwise. Ninety-five percent of cancers of the testes are GCTs. The remaining 5% are stromal tumors (Leydig or Sertoli cell origin.) The GCTs are divided into seminomas (60%) and nonseminomas (40%). The nonseminomas are divided into three types: embryonal, teratoma, and choriocarcinoma. This patient's ultrasound shows a heterogeneous mass with cystic areas and indistinct margins, which is more concerning for a nonseminomatous type of tumor such as an embryonal tumor, teratoma, or choriocarcinoma. His β-hCG is significantly elevated, which suggests choriocarcinoma as a diagnosis.**

A. Tumor markers are useful for diagnosis, staging, and monitoring for recurrence, but they are not sensitive or specific enough to make the diagnosis of testicular cancer without a tissue diagnosis. Therefore, normal tumor markers do not rule out a diagnosis of testicular cancer.

B. Seminomas do not produce alpha-fetoprotein. Therefore, if the alpha-fetoprotein is elevated, there is no possibility of a pure seminoma as the diagnosis. Seminomas also are more homogeneous, well marginated, and usually do not have cystic components on ultrasonography.

D, E. Leydig cell tumors and Sertoli tumors are of stromal origin and statistically less common than GCTs. They are often seen in children, although Leydig tumors may be seen in adults and are likely to be malignant in adults. Children with stromal tumors may present with precocious puberty or gynecomastia with a testicular mass.

171. **A. It is more common in the elderly. Older age is one of the most significant risk factors for the development of herpes zoster, which is depicted in the figure.**

B. Herpes zoster is less contagious than varicella (chicken pox). However, it may result in varicella in household contacts not previously exposed to varicella zoster virus.

C. Herpes zoster is caused by varicella zoster virus, a herpesvirus related to herpes simplex. Herpes zoster is due to reactivation along a dermatome of latent varicella virus present from a prior exposure to varicella.
D. Herpes zoster is usually unilateral, as it usually respects a single dermatome.
E. Antiviral treatment in immunocompetent patients can decrease the duration of the rash, can prevent spread of the rash to other areas, and can prevent postherpetic neuralgia. Therefore, oral antiviral treatment is recommended for all patients with herpes zoster. The best results are obtained if the treatment is initiated within 72 hours of the onset of the rash.

172. **D. It indicates a high risk for eye involvement. When a patient has an episode of herpes zoster affecting the trigeminal nerve dermatome, a lesion on the tip of the nose reflects involvement of the ophthalmic division of the trigeminal nerve. This involvement places patients at risk for herpes zoster keratitis, corneal involvement of the herpes zoster. These patients should be referred to an ophthalmologist for evaluation.**

A. Herpes zoster in any branch of the trigeminal nerve may result in the complication of varicella zoster virus encephalitis. The complication is not specific to the ophthalmic division.
B. Sinusitis is not a complication of herpes zoster.
C. Consultation with a plastic surgeon is usually not necessary in caring for a patient with herpes zoster. Severe lesions or superinfected lesions may heal with some scarring, but plastic surgery is not usually necessary.
E. A lesion on the tip of the nose indicates that the ophthalmic division of the trigeminal nerve is involved; it does not indicate involvement of more than one dermatome.

173. **B. Nocardiosis is an infection caused by *Nocardia* organisms, which are usually found in soil. Most commonly, immunocompromised patients, particularly those on chronic corticosteroids, are at risk for this disease which may cause pulmonary, CNS, and skin infections. Pulmonary manifestations include most commonly pulmonary nodules, but consolidation, interstitial infiltrates, cavitary lesions, and pleural effusions are possible as well. CNS manifestations include brain abscesses, which present as ring-enhancing lesions on CT of the brain. Skin involvement usually consists of a pustule or nodule with regional lymphadenopathy.**

A. *Streptococcus pneumoniae* may present with pneumonia and CNS involvement, but usually, meningitis rather than brain abscesses is the complication seen with this infection.
C. *Pneumocystis carinii* causes pneumonia in immunocompromised patients, particularly those with HIV infection. It does not cause brain abscesses.
D. Wegener granulomatosis usually causes sinusitis and may cause pulmonary symptoms, but it does not cause brain abscesses.
E. Lung cancer may present similarly to pneumonia with a productive cough and even fever. However, the appearance on CT of brain metastases is usually not a ring-enhancing lesion, which is more classic for an abscess.

174. **E. Third-degree AV block occurs when all atrial depolarizations fail to conduct through to the ventricles. This results in the atria and the ventricles having their own independent rates and rhythms. The P waves, which indicate atrial depolarization, march to their own regular rate and do not correlate with any of the QRS complexes. On the ECG, the PR interval is constantly changing from one beat to the next. The QRS is also regular, but usually slower than the atrial rate and independent of the atrial rhythm. If the QRS complex is narrow in third-degree AV block, then the focus of origin of the ventricular depolarization is coming from the AV junction or the bundle of His. If the QRS is wide, then the focus of ventricular depolarization is coming from the distal conduction fibers within the ventricle.**

A. Sinus bradycardia is defined as a sinus rhythm with a rate of <60 beats/min. Characteristics of a sinus rhythm include a constant PR interval, each P wave is followed by a QRS complex, each QRS complex is preceded by a P wave, and the P waves are upright in lead II and inverted in lead aVR. As a rule of thumb, for an HR of 60, there should be at least five large boxes between each QRS complex.

B. First-degree AV block is present when there is a prolonged PR interval of >200 msec (one large square). The block is occurring between the atria and the ventricles, but all atrial impulses are conducted to the ventricles. The PR interval, although prolonged, remains constant in first-degree AV block. If there is variation in the PR interval from one beat to the next, then you should be thinking of other types of heart block, not first-degree.

C. There are two types (referred to as Mobitz types) of second-degree AV block. Mobitz type I, also known as Wenckebach, is present when the PR interval becomes progressively longer between beats until a beat (QRS) is completely dropped. After the dropped beat, the PR interval usually shortens again and repeats the cycle. The QRS complex is usually narrow in Mobitz I block. This is because the block is occurring within the AV node.

D. The second type of second degree AV block is Mobitz type II. In Mobitz type II, the PR interval remains constant and the QRS complex is dropped periodically. The QRS complex in Mobitz type II is usually wide, showing a preexisting bundle branch pattern. This is because the block is usually occurring distal to the bundle of His, in the bundle branches.

175. D. The use of a transcutaneous pacemaker is the best initial treatment in the patient described above with third-degree heart block. Because the atrial depolarizations are unable to make it through the AV node, the ventricles are left to function on their own. The inherent rate of ventricular depolarization is much slower than the atrial rate of depolarization. Therefore, in third-degree AV block, the ventricular rate is usually much slower than the rate that would be present in normal sinus rhythm, which leads to clinical symptoms (syncope, dyspnea, etc.). As a result, a transcutaneous pacemaker is the best option to use to increase this patient's ventricular rate until a more permanent pacemaker can be placed. A trial of atropine may also be useful in increasing the ventricular rate, but its effects may be short lived, requiring frequent repeated doses. In general, atropine and other autonomic maneuvers are more successful in more proximal blocks such as first degree or Mobitz type I, and less successful as the blocks move distally.

A. Synchronized cardioversion is indicated in the treatment of various arrhythmias such as supraventricular tachycardia and unstable atrial fibrillation and flutter. Using synchronized cardioversion attempts to "reset" the rhythm to sinus rhythm by delivering a set amount of energy across the myocardium at a precise time. In the synchronized mode, the instrument detects the QRS complexes and delivers the energy (shock) at a precise time so as not to induce ventricular arrhythmias.

B. IV metoprolol actually slows conduction through the AV node and in high enough doses can cause third-degree AV block. Therefore, it is not the treatment of choice for third-degree AV block (and is actually contraindicated).

C. Diltiazem also slows conduction through the AV node. So, similar to IV metoprolol, diltiazem should not be used in the treatment of third-degree AV block.

E. Defibrillation is also used to deliver a set amount of energy across the myocardium in an attempt to "reset" the underlying abnormal rhythm. However, unlike with synchronized cardioversion, there is no coordination between the timing of the QRS complexes and when the shock is delivered.

176. C. Rhabdomyolysis is a syndrome defined by muscle necrosis and the release of the muscle cell contents into the circulation. Etiologies of rhabdomyolysis include crush injuries, severe strenuous exertion, certain drugs, prolonged comatose states (due to compression injury,) postictal states, and inflammatory myopathies to name a few. When large amounts of muscle cells necrose, several serious complications can occur. The most worrisome complication is renal failure due to the nephrotoxicity of the heme pigment in the myoglobin. Hyperkalemia can be severe and refractory due to the renal failure and the release of potassium from the destroyed myocytes. This patient was "found down," a presentation that should make you think of rhabdomyolysis. Her urinalysis has characteristic features of rhabdomyolysis. First, the myoglobin (i.e., heme pigment) that is excreted in the urine gives it the reddish brown appearance. Secondly, the urine dip was strongly positive for "blood," but the urinalysis showed a paucity of RBCs. This is a strong clue to alert you toward the diagnosis of rhabdomyolysis. An elevated serum CPK level would help to confirm the diagnosis.

A. Urinary tract infections can cause hematuria, but there is usually also other evidence of infection on microscopy such as white blood cells and bacteria. Other evidence for infection is a urine dip that is positive for leukocyte esterase. Nitrates on urine dip may be positive or negative in infection.
B. Changes typically seen on urinalysis in the presence of ATN include "muddy brown granular casts" as well as epithelial casts. It usually does not cause a gross color change of the urine and it should not cause the degree of "blood" detected on our patient's urine dip.
D. Traumatic insertion of a urinary catheter is a relatively common cause of blood being detected on urinalysis. However, in this setting you should also see numerous RBCs present on the microscopic examination.
E. Transitional cell carcinoma of the bladder is another cause of hematuria, but you should also see RBCs on your urinary examination.

177. **B. Fluid resuscitation and hydration are the cornerstone of the treatment of rhabdomyolysis. This allows for an increase in renal perfusion and urinary flow, which will help remove any obstructing casts that have developed. After IV fluids have been started, alkalinization of the urine and forced diuresis is the next most important therapeutic maneuver. This is especially true in patients who demonstrate acute renal insufficiency and metabolic acidosis from the rhabdomyolysis. By raising the urine pH above 6.5 with an alkalinizing agent, the solubility of the heme pigments increases and their excretion is facilitated. It is important to remember that alkalinization of the urine does carry potential risks, such as hypocalcemia by precipitation of calcium phosphate.**

A. Cystoscopy would be indicated for the evaluation of a possible bladder mass, but this patient does not have evidence of this.
C. IV antibiotics would be used in the treatment of a urinary tract infection in a patient who appears septic or is unable to take oral antibiotics (such as our patient). However, it has no role in the treatment of rhabdomyolysis.
D. If there is significant hematuria present after a urinary catheter is placed, then it should be removed and reassessed. In the situation above, there is no clear indication to remove the catheter. Actually, one could argue to leave the catheter in so that urinary output could be followed more accurately given her increased creatinine.
E. Emergent hemodialysis is indicated in patients with rhabdomyolysis if they have refractory hyperkalemia or have respiratory compromise from fluid overload as a result of their acute renal failure, neither of which our patient has.

178. **D. There are three basic types of shock: hypovolemic, cardiogenic, and distributive. Each type of shock is characterized by its usual values for wedge pressure, cardiac output, and SVR in Table 1-178. Our patient has an elevated PCWP of 25. The wedge pressure is measured with the Swan-Ganz catheter and gives us a pressure that reflects the pressure in the left ventricle at the end of diastole (left ventricle end-diastolic pressure or LVEDP, also sometimes called the "filling pressure"). Normal wedge pressure is around 11. The elevated wedge pressure implies that the preload is high, or that the volume filling the ventricle is high. (But remember that wedge pressure is not synonymous with volume.) It can also**

TABLE 1-178 Shock Classifications

Type of Shock	Pulmonary Capillary Wedge Pressure (i.e., Preload)	Cardiac Output (Heart Rate × Stroke Volume)	Systemic Vascular Resistance (i.e., Afterload)
Hypovolemic	↓	↓	↑
Cardiogenic	↑	↓	↑
Distributive	↓	↑	↓

mean that the compliance of the ventricle is poor, requiring a high pressure to fill the ventricle. It is a number that is very useful in clinical medicine, but it must be used in combination with the other numbers and the clinical judgment of the clinician. The cardiac output is calculated by the following formula: Heart Rate × Stroke Volume = Cardiac Output. Our patient's cardiac output is low, at 2.1 L/min. Normal cardiac output is 4–8 L/min. The cardiac output may be low because of pump failure, in which case the wedge pressure would be high because of "backed up" volume. The cardiac output also may be low because of inadequate filling in the case of hypovolemia, but in that case you would expect the wedge pressure to also be low. Lastly, the SVR is a measure of the resistance of the arterial bed vasculature throughout the body, or the "squeeze" of the arterial circulation. Normal SVR is 800–1200 dynes × sec/cm^5. In cases of poor perfusion due to hypovolemia or pump failure, the adrenergic stimulus causes a "clamping down" of the systemic blood vessels in an effort to improve perfusion. Therefore, in our patient, a high wedge, a low cardiac output, and a high SVR are indicative of cardiogenic shock. The pump failure caused a "back up" of fluid, resulting in a high wedge pressure, and the SVR increased in an attempt to improve perfusion. In distributive causes of shock, due to sepsis, anaphylaxis, or neurogenic causes, the SVR decreases. The heart compensates with increased stroke volume and HR in an effort to improve cardiac output. There is usually a low wedge pressure because of inadequate preload due to vasodilation and third spacing.

A, B, C, E. See explanation for D.

179. D. This patient is in cardiogenic shock, and the cardiac output has not responded optimally to your management thus far. Given that the PCWP ("wedge") is not low and the SVR is not low, further boluses of fluid are unlikely to be helpful. Her shock is the result of pump failure. Dobutamine is an inotropic agent that will help increase contractility and, ultimately, cardiac output, and it should be started now. Because dobutamine works predominantly by agonist action of beta-1 and beta-2 adrenergic receptors, it can cause arterial vasodilation (beta-2) in addition to its inotropic (beta-1) increase in cardiac contractility. Therefore, it is usually advised to use it in conjunction with another pressor that will help support the blood pressure. (In this case, dopamine is already "on board.")

A. IV broad-spectrum antibiotics are indicated for the treatment of septic shock. A patient with septic shock would be expected to have increased cardiac output with significantly decreased SVR.

B. IV solumedrol and diphenhydramine can be used as part of the treatment for anaphylactic shock. Like septic shock, anaphylactic shock should show a very low SVR with increased cardiac output.

C. Additional boluses of normal saline are not indicated at this time. The elevated PCWP indicates that the patient's preload is already high. Additional fluid poses the risk for causing pulmonary edema.

180. C. The Glasgow Coma Scale is divided into three categories for scoring: eye opening, verbal response, and motor response. This tool can be used in the initial evaluation of a patient's level of consciousness. The lowest score that can be attained is 3 and the highest is 15. Eye opening is scored as follows: 4 points if spontaneous, 3 if to speech, 2 if to pain, and 1 if none. This patient opened his eyes to pain, giving him 2 points in this category. Motor response is scored as follows: 6 points if following command, 5 points if localizing, 4 points for withdrawal, 3 points for flexing, 2 points if extending, and 1 point if no movement. This patient appeared to localize the pain of his IV line placement by pulling away the appropriate arm, giving him 5 points. Finally, verbal response is scored as follows: 5 points if oriented, 4 points if confused, 3 points if inappropriate, 2 points if incomprehensible, and 1 point if no verbal response is made. This patient receives 2 points because he is incomprehensible. The total score is 9.

A, B, D, E. These scores are incorrect. See explanation for C.

181. **C. Classic migraines typically have an aura of visual changes prior to onset of the headache. The visual disturbances can vary widely, but many patients report seeing flashing lights, sparkles, or having blurred vision.**

A. Migraines can have some variance in presentation, but are mostly reported as unilateral and throbbing in nature. Most last for several hours or more.

B. Common migraines do not present with a preceding aura of any kind. Classic migraines present with an aura, most often visual changes including lights, sparkles, or blurred vision.

D. Most patients report that dark rooms, sleep, and quiet all improve their symptoms.

E. Most patients with migraines present initially in adolescence or early adulthood. Many of them report a family history of migraine.

182. **B. Prophylactic treatment is indicated in patients with four or more migraines per month. Medications are taken on a daily basis and migraine incidence should decrease after 2–4 weeks of taking prophylactic medications. Beta blockers, tricyclic antidepressants, calcium channel blockers, and anticonvulsants are all used for prophylaxis. It is also helpful for the patient to identify any triggers, such as caffeine, stress, or lack of sleep, which may bring on the headache.**

A. Sumatriptan is a serotonin agonist used in the acute treatment of migraines. The entire family of triptans cause vasoconstriction and inhibit pain mechanisms in the brain. Preparations include oral, nasal, and injection. This is important in the acute setting of migraine, when patients may be nauseated or vomiting.

C. NSAIDs are still first-line treatment for migraine abortive therapy. Many patients respond to acetaminophen, ibuprofen, or other NSAIDs. If these medications fail, then the triptan family of medications should be tried next.

D. Treatment of migraine in the acute setting should be initiated at first sign of the migraine. Patients should not wait until the migraine has reached maximal intensity prior to taking medications.

E. Ergotamine, not the triptans, causes prolonged coronary artery constriction, making it absolutely contraindicated in patients with CAD. Although this is a medication that can be used in the abortive treatment of migraine, the medication's many side effects have made it a less desirable treatment. In addition the coronary artery constriction side effects include rebound headaches. This medication should not be used in patients with hypertension, hepatic disease, renal disease, or peripheral vascular disease.

183. **B. This patient has been seizing for at least 30 minutes and is in status epilepticus. The seizure should be stopped in order to prevent brain hypoxia and damage. Benzodiazepines are the first choice of medication to be given in this situation and doses can be repeated. Phenytoin should be given at a loading dose of 20 mg/kg. If the patient is still seizing following these medications, phenobarbital should be loaded at 20 mg/kg. If the patient is still seizing, anesthesia should be called for to place the patient in a pentobarbital coma.**

A. This patient is spontaneously breathing. Although the "A,B,C's" (airway, breathing, circulation) should be the first priority in any patient, this patient's airway is intact. By paralyzing the patient, any seizure activity will be masked. This should be avoided unless absolutely necessary to secure an airway. If paralytics are indicated to obtain an airway, a continuous EEG monitor should be used to monitor for further seizure activity.

C. Phenytoin should be given after benzodiazepines if the patient is still seizing or if scheduled antiepileptic drugs will be indicated. A loading dose of 20 mg/kg is appropriate. This should be given with continuous monitoring of the BP, because it can precipitate hypotension.

D. This patient may need a CT of the head to evaluate for an intracranial process. However, it should not be the next step in management. The seizure should be under control prior to imaging.

E. The patient is visibly seizing. An EEG may be indicated for further workup in determining the cause of the seizure, but is not the next step in management.

184. C. This patient is having focal tonic-clonic motor activity without loss of consciousness or a simple partial seizure. When the motor cortex is involved, as in this patient, it is called a jacksonian seizure. The motor activity is usually a reflection of the region of cortex that is involved in the abnormal activity. Further investigations of new-onset seizure should be pursued, including imaging, EEG, electrolytes, liver function tests, renal function, and glucose.

A. Pseudoseizures are seizures that are not physiologic, but psychological in etiology. Diagnosis is one of exclusion, and video EEG is often helpful in making the diagnosis.

B. Generalized tonic-clonic seizures are nonfocal tonic-clonic movements with loss of consciousness. The patient will initially stiffen, lose consciousness, and then have jerking movements of the muscles. The seizure is followed by a postictal phase of sleepiness. Patients are often incontinent of bowel and bladder during the seizure.

D. Complex partial seizures are similar to simple partial seizures with focal neurologic involvement, but the patient will have impaired consciousness.

E. Absence seizures are usually seen in children. The child will typically have a sudden staring spell with impaired consciousness that lasts only a few seconds. There is no postictal phase. EEG will show a distinct three-per-second spike-and-wave pattern. Most children outgrow this type of seizure.

185. E. Bacterial meningitis is a medical emergency, and this man has a very high pretest probability for bacterial meningitis because of his fever, headache, and nuchal rigidity. Antibiotics should be given without delay in this patient to cover such organisms as *Streptococcus pneumoniae, Haemophilus influenzae,* and *Neisseria meningitidis.* The antibiotics that are recommended are ceftriaxone 2 g IV every 12 hours (note the high dose) and vancomycin 15 mg/kg IV every 6–12 hours to cover for penicillin-resistant *S. pneumoniae* strains. This patient is not at risk for *Listeria* meningitis, which is more commonly seen in children and the elderly or in patients with impaired cellular immunity. If *Listeria* infection is suspected, coverage with ampicillin in meningeal doses (2 g IV every 4–6 hours in adults) is recommended along with gentamicin for synergy. He is also not likely to need coverage for herpes meningitis/encephalitis because his presentation is more likely to be bacterial. For this reason, acyclovir should not be given empirically at this point. Steroids are recommended at the time of IV antibiotic treatment in adults with bacterial meningitis. This is because of a randomized controlled trial published in *The New England Journal of Medicine* in November 2002 (vol. 347, pp. 1549–1556). The trial showed that early treatment with dexamethasone in addition to IV antibiotics reduced the risk for both unfavorable outcome and death. Often, a CT scan is ordered prior to an LP being performed in the unlikely event that something will be seen on CT that will contraindicate an LP. If there will be any significant delay in doing the LP, the antibiotics and steroids must be given first, and then the CT scan and the LP can be done.

A, B, C, D. These management sequences are incorrect. See explanation for E.

186. A. rt-PA has been shown to benefit patients with acute onset of ischemic stroke within 3 hours of onset of symptoms. This is according to the National Institute of Neurologic Disorders and Stroke trial, which randomized patients presenting within 3 hours of onset of stroke symptoms to rt-PA versus placebo. Complete or very nearly complete recovery was seen at 3 months in 38% of those treated with rt-PA versus 21% of the placebo-treated group. There was no difference in mortality in 3 months despite a 10-fold increase in cerebral hemorrhage in the thrombolytic group. Patients who present later than 3 hours after symptom onset should not get lytic therapy, because studies have shown much less benefit to these patients and, potentially, much more harm.

B. Aspirin has been shown to improve mortality when it is given to a patient with an acute thrombotic stroke within 48 hours of the onset of symptoms. The combined data of two randomized, controlled trials (the International Stroke Trial and the Chinese Acute Stroke Trial) demonstrated that aspirin therapy reduced the risk for stroke with residual impairment and death in 13 per 1000 patients. Aspirin should not be given to patients who are undergoing thrombolytic therapy.

C. Full-dose unfractionated heparin and low-molecular-weight heparin are not recommended for the treatment of acute ischemic stroke. Many trials have confirmed that full-dose heparin is not efficacious in preventing death or a dependent state following a stroke, and that it increases the risk for significant bleeding complications. Therefore, full-dose anticoagulation is not recommended for patients who present with ischemic stroke. This does not preclude the use of low-dose heparin therapies for deep venous thromboembolus prophylaxis, and DVT prophylaxis should be used in the appropriate patient.

D. MRI of the brain with diffusion-weighted images is a useful tool in the diagnosis of stroke. The stroke can be identified within minutes of its occurrence. A CT scan will not show evidence of the acute stroke for approximately 12–24 hours. A CT scan is immediately sensitive, however, for acute bleeding, and it should be obtained prior to giving the patient lytics to ascertain that the stroke is thrombotic and not hemorrhagic. An MRI with diffusion-weighted images can be ordered to make the diagnosis, but the patient should be given lytics first, because time is of the essence.

E. Patients with stroke often have elevated blood pressure. This may be for two reasons: the patient may have high BP at baseline, which is his risk factor for stroke; or, the patient may have transient hypertension related to the stroke event. The elevated BP will help to perfuse brain tissue, which has lost the ability to autoregulate its perfusion. For this second reason, it is important not to lower the BP acutely in a patient who presents with a stroke, and it may even be important to let the BP run "a little high" to avoid extending the infarct. Generally, a week or so after the stroke is sufficient time to allow before restarting the BP medicines to obtain optimal control.

187. D. The D-dimer is a noninvasive test that can be used to help in the diagnostic workup of VTE. It is important to realize that there are many different assays used for measuring D-dimer levels, and the assays are not equal in their sensitivity or specificity. The traditional enzyme-linked immunosorbent assays produce the most accurate results, with a sensitivity of 95%–99%. In general, the specificity of the test is not as high as the sensitivity. Therefore, a positive result is not as helpful to rule in VTE as a negative result is to rule out

TABLE 1-187 Scoring System for Clinical Prediction of Deep Venous Thrombosis

Finding	Point*
Paralysis, paresis, or recent immobilization of legs	1
Bed-bound for >3 days recently or major surgery in the past month	1
Calf of symptomatic leg is 3 cm larger than calf of asymptomatic leg†	1
Edema of entire lower extremity	1
Pitting edema in symptomatic leg	1
Tenderness along course of deep vein	1
Nonvaricose collateral superficial veins	1
Active cancer	1
Alternative diagnosis as likely or greater than deep venous thrombosis	−2

*A composite score of 3 points indicates a high probability of deep venous thrombosis; 1 or 2 points, a moderate probability; and 0 or fewer points, a low probability. Data from Wells et al.

†Measured 10 cm below the tibial tuberosity

Reprinted with permission from Mayo Clinic Proceedings. S.D. Frost, D.J. Brotman, and F.A. Michota. November 2003; Vol. 78., No. 11, p. 1385.

VTE in the appropriate setting. (There are many comorbid conditions, including advanced age, which may produce elevated D-dimers in the absence of thromboembolic disease.) So, how should the D-dimer be used to evaluate a patient for the presence of VTE? Eleven prospective clinical management trials have studied approximately 7000 patients by evaluating the role of D-dimer testing to rule out VTE. The first thing to realize is that D-dimers alone should not be used to exclude DVT or pulmonary embolism, but they should be used in combination with either noninvasive testing (such as Doppler ultrasonography) or a structured assessment of clinical probability. A patient with low or moderate pretest probability by structured clinical probability rules (Table 1-187) and a negative D-dimer can be safely ruled out for VTE, but not a patient with high pretest probability. Each of the patients described in the scenarios except the patient described in answer D are considered high risk for VTE, and therefore the diagnosis cannot be excluded based on a negative D-dimer test result alone.

A, B, C, E. See explanation for D.

188. **A. This pattern is consistent with a restrictive lung disease. It is likely extraparenchymal given the normal flow volumes and DLCO. Restrictive patterns have as their hallmark decreased lung volumes, including TLC, VC, and RV. Flow rates are preserved. Restrictive lung disease may be parenchymal or extra-parenchymal. Extra-parenchymal causes are characterized by either inspiratory dysfunction or both inspiratory and expiratory dysfunction. The PFT results are similar in both conditions, although in the inspiratory/expiratory type the residual volume may be elevated due to inability to expire all the inspired gas. The pattern described in A is consistent with an extra-parenchymal disorder affecting primarily inspiration. This pattern may be seen in diseases of the chest wall such as kyphosis or obesity.**

B. This pattern is an obstructive pattern consisting primarily of decreased flow rates. Because of the airway obstruction of expiration, the lung volumes are elevated. The DLCO is decreased, indicating the airway obstruction is more likely due to emphysema.

C. This pattern is also obstructive and is very similar to the pattern seen in choice B. The difference is that the DLCO is normal, making these results more likely due to asthma because asthma is not an alveolar disease.

D. This pattern is a restrictive pattern similar to that seen in A, but the decreased DLCO is indicative of a parenchymal etiology for the restriction such as pulmonary fibrosis.

E. These are normal PFT values. With such severe kyphosis we would expect to see some degree of restriction on pulmonary function tests.

189. **D. This picture is consistent with CMV retinitis. CMV retinitis is usually segmental, involving only portions of the retina. The vessels often have a "frosted branch" appearance. With his history of homosexual behavior, he is at risk for contracting HIV. His history of weight loss and diarrhea is concerning for this infection as well as possible AIDS.**

A. A retinal detachment may result in the patient seeing floaters and flashes of light. It also will usually involve only a portion of the retina. However, rather than a frosted branch appearance, a retinal detachment may appear as a tear or flap appearance on funduscopic examination. Complaints from patients also involve seeing a "curtain" come down over their vision, which did not occur in this patient.

B. A central retinal vein occlusion will usually result in sudden visual loss. The funduscopic appearance of a central retinal vein occlusion consists of multiple hemorrhages and edema as well as congestion of the vessels, particularly near the optic nerve. Central retinal vein occlusion is not consistent with the history or physical examination in this patient.

C. A central retinal artery occlusion will usually also result in a sudden loss of vision. The appearance on funduscopic examination of a central retinal artery occlusion is that of a pale fundus, often with a cherry red spot, which is the choroidal vasculature visible beneath the macula. Again, the symptoms and examination findings in this patient are not consistent with a central retinal artery occlusion.

E. Angioid streaks are breaks in the retina that have the appearance and distribution of blood vessels. They are due to collagen diseases such as pseudoxanthoma elasticum or Ehlers-Danlos syndrome. They are usually asymptomatic.

190. D. The syndrome of primary HIV infection is so nonspecific that it is generally underdiagnosed. It usually consists of a mononucleosis-like syndrome that includes malaise, fever, rash, lymphadenopathy, and sore throat. Without a high index of suspicion by inquiring into the patient's social history, it is easy to see how the diagnosis can be overlooked. If suspected, the diagnosis of acute HIV infection may be confirmed with a high viral load or positive p24 antigen. If the patient is found to have HIV disease, immediate treatment should be started. The symptoms of acute HIV infection include fever, lymphadenopathy, sore throat, oral ulcers, rash, myalgias, arthralgias, headache, nausea, vomiting, diarrhea, and weight loss. The symptoms usually last 1–2 weeks. The characteristics that are most specific for acute HIV infection are oral ulcers, as well as the duration of symptoms.

A. Fever is nonspecific but is seen in almost all patients with acute HIV infection. The temperature usually ranges from 38° to 40°C.
B. Also nonspecific, lymphadenopathy occurs in the majority of patients with acute HIV infection. The adenopathy is nontender and located mainly in the axiallary, cervical, and occipital nodes.
C. Diarrhea is nonspecific and just one of the many gastrointestinal symptoms that may occur in acute HIV infection. Others include nausea, vomiting, and anorexia.
E. The rash seen in acute HIV infection usually consists of a macular or maculopapular rash that is pink to red in color. It involves the chest and face. The palms and soles may also be affected. Like many of the other symptoms of acute HIV infection, the rash is nonspecific.

191. C. This patient has disseminated candidemia, which is evidenced by the fluffy white lesions seen on the funduscopic examination (*Candida* retinitis) as well as the diffuse pustular skin rash. (If the rash were examined via biopsy, it would reveal fungal elements.) Risk factors for systemic candidemia include broad-spectrum antibiotic treatment, a history of recent surgery (especially abdominal procedures), central venous catheters, and parenteral nutrition. Blood cultures are helpful only if the results are positive. (Negative blood culture results for fungus do not rule out candidemia, because they are not very sensitive.) The treatment of disseminated candidiasis is IV antifungal medications, including fluconazole or amphotericin B. In addition, all central catheters must be removed.

A. Although *Neisseria* meningitis may cause a rash, it is usually a purpuric rash and not pustular. Also, this patient does not have any other symptoms of meningitis, and *Neisseria* meningitis is not a nosocomially acquired illness.
B. Although the triple-lumen catheter should be removed, initiation of IV vancomycin should be started only if an infection with a gram-positive organism is suspected, particularly a resistant strain of *Staphylococcus aureus.* The clinical scenario on this patient is much more suggestive of infection with *Candida albicans* than *S. aureus* because of the pustular rash and funduscopic findings.
D. Although necrotizing pancreatitis is a concern in a patient with known pancreatitis who worsens clinically, the rash and eye findings point to a new problem because they are not manifestations of pancreatitis.
E. IV fluconazole or amphotericin B may be used in patients with disseminated candidiasis. However, removal of the triple-lumen catheter in addition to initiation of antifungal medications is essential, making C a better choice.

192. A. Indinavir is a protease inhibitor. It is known to cause nephrolithiasis. This side effect more commonly occurs in children than adults. Because of this side effect, it is recommended that patients drink at least 48 ounces of water per day. If signs or symptoms of nephrolithiasis develop, the drug should be discontinued and the patient should be evaluated.

B. Efavirenz is a non-nucleoside reverse transcriptase inhibitor. It may cause a rash and vivid dreams. Another side effect, one that is common to the nonnucleoside reverse transcriptase inhibitors, is elevation of the aminotransferase levels.
C. Abacavir may cause a hypersensitivity reaction in about 5% of patients, which may be lethal. Symptoms of this hypersensitivity reaction include, but are not limited to, anaphylaxis, fever, rash, and diarrhea. If a patient develops a hypersensitivity reaction while taking abacavir, the drug should be stopped immediately. If the patient survives the reaction, repeat challenge with the drug should never be performed because a recurrent reaction could be fatal.

D. Ritonavir is another protease inhibitor. Side effects common to the protease inhibitors include hyperglycemia and dyslipidemia as well as a redistribution of fat. Nausea is a common side effect of ritonavir but can be minimized by starting at a low dose and escalating the dose over a period of several days. Another side effect of ritonavir is perioral numbness.

E. Didanosine is a nucleoside reverse transcriptase inhibitor, most of which have the possible side effect of pancreatitis. Didanosine also may cause peripheral neuropathy. Retinal changes and optic neuritis may also occur; therefore, patients should have a dilated retinal examination every 6–12 months while taking didanosine.

193. C. Lung abscesses are usually caused by anaerobic bacteria and result from aspiration of oral bacteria. They are common in alcoholics and people with poor dentition. When due to aspiration, the most common location for a lung abscess is the upper segment of the right lower lobe. Lung abscesses usually appear as an infiltrate on chest radiography. Air-fluid levels indicate rupture into a bronchial tree. Sputum examination is usually not helpful and most often results in growth of usual oral flora. The diagnosis can often be made clinically. Definitive diagnosis requires invasive testing such as bronchoscopy. Treatment is directed at the causative organism if one is found. Otherwise, the patient is given penicillin. In addition to antibiotics, postural drainage and chest physiotherapy are crucial to treatment of lung abscesses. Surgery is reserved for complications. Given our patient's alcoholism and poor dentition, lung abscess is the most likely etiology for the fluid-filled cavitary lesion seen on chest radiography.

A. TB may result in cavitary lesions and may occur in alcoholic patients. It also may result in symptoms similar to those about which the patient is complaining. Arguing against TB in this patient is the negative PPD skin test results on two occasions as well as the lower lobe location of the lesion. Primary TB usually affects the upper lobes of the lungs.

B. Pneumococcal pneumonia may result in a lung abscess. However, this patient's history of alcohol abuse and poor dentition make an anaerobic abscess secondary to aspiration more likely. In addition, the location of the lesion is typical for aspiration. Sputum Gram stain and culture, although not very sensitive, would be expected to show gram-positive diplococci in pneumococcal pneumonia, whereas in this patient these studies only showed oral flora.

D. Squamous cell cancer may result in cavitary lesions on chest radiograph up to 20% of the time. However, this cancer is highly associated with smoking, and our patient does not smoke. It is more likely that he has a lung abscess than lung cancer.

E. *Mycoplasma* pneumonia only rarely causes lung abscesses. It would be much more likely for this alcoholic man to have a lung abscess related to aspiration.

194. A. Eosinophilic granuloma (also known as Langerhans cell granuloma or histiocytosis X) is a proliferation of the dendritic cell that affects the lung, bones, and viscera. In the lung, it causes an interstitial lung disease with small cystic spaces. These may result in a spontaneous pneumothorax. The pulmonary disease is seen virtually exclusively in smokers. The disease may also affect the bone, causing lytic bone lesions. It also may affect the posterior pituitary, causing diabetes insipidus. It is one of the few diseases that cause a combined restrictive and obstructive picture on PFT. It is treated by smoking cessation. Steroids are usually not helpful.

B. Lymphangioleiomyomatosis is a disease that is usually seen in women of childbearing years. Patients present with dyspnea, cough, and hemoptysis, but they also may present with spontaneous pneumothorax. Chest x-ray findings, like eosinophilic granulomatosis, also include cystic lesions. Lymphangioleiomyomatosis is caused by a proliferation of immature smooth muscle cells in lung tissue throughout bronchial, vascular, and lymphatic structures. Chylous effusions may be seen in this disease. There are no associated bone changes.

C. Eosinophilic pneumonias can be associated with chronic asthma and fungal hypersensitivity such as that seen in allergic bronchopulmonary aspergillosis or with chronic pneumonias and an eosinophilia. They may need to be diagnosed by lung biopsy. Eosinophilic pneumonias and eosinophilic granulomatosis are not related.

D. Pulmonary alveolar proteinosis is a disease that is categorized in the "interstitial lung disease" category. Chest x-rays show diffuse alveolar consolidation or nodular shadows that radiate from the hilar regions. On biopsy, the aveoli are filled with a granular material that stains with periodic acid-Schiff reagent. Treatment may include whole-lung lavage. There is no associated increased risk for pneumothorax or bone involvement.

E. Diffuse alveolar hemorrhage can result in idiopathic pulmonary hemosiderosis. The diagnosis is made when all other causes of alveolar bleeding (such as connective tissue disease and vasculitis) are ruled out. There is no associated pneumothorax or bone involvement.

195. **D. *Bacillus cereus* infection causes two different food poisoning syndromes. The first is an emetic form caused by an emetic toxin that is most often found in fried rice, particularly rice that has been reheated. It results in a food poisoning syndrome identical to that caused by *Staphylococcus aureus* and usually begins 1–6 hours after ingestion of the contaminated food. The diarrheal form is caused by a diarrheal toxin and results in watery diarrhea, abdominal pain, and tenesmus. It is caused by ingestion of contaminated meat or vegetables. The patients in question have a syndrome very similar to *S. aureus* food poisoning, but their history of eating at a Chinese restaurant makes *B. cereus* food poisoning more likely. Treatment is supportive.**

A. *S. aureus* causes a food poisoning syndrome similar to that of *B. cereus*. It is also due to a toxin. Symptoms begin 2–6 hours after ingestion, and the syndrome begins abruptly with nausea, vomiting, abdominal pain, and diarrhea.

B. *Salmonella enteriditis* causes a food poisoning syndrome after ingestion of contaminated food, usually eggs or chicken that is undercooked. A distinguishing characteristic of *Salmonella* infection is the large inoculum needed to produce illness. The disease then has a 6- to 24-hour incubation period followed by nausea, vomiting, fever, nonbloody diarrhea, and abdominal cramps. Symptoms are self-limited and generally last 3–7 days. Treatment is supportive because antibiotics may prolong the carrier state. However, patients over 50 who are immunosuppressed or have heart valve abnormalities or vascular grafts should be treated with antibiotics. Acceptable antibiotics include quinolones and trimethoprim-sulfamethoxazole.

C. *Campylobacter jenuni* is the most common cause of bacterial gastroenteritis in the United States. It is caused by ingestion of contaminated food, but because the incubation period can last 2–4 days, the etiology may not always be obvious. Symptoms begin with crampy abdominal pain and fevers, and then profuse watery diarrhea develops. Stool may contain blood. Symptoms are usually self-limited, but erythromycin may be used in patients with severe disease. Interesting complications of *Campylobacter* infection include Guillain-Barré syndrome and postinfectious arthritis.

E. *Clostridium botulinum* may result in a foodborne illness that is caused by a toxin. The symptoms varies widely, from mild illness for which no medical attention is sought, to a severe, life-threatening disease. The incubation period is 18–36 hours followed by a symmetric descending paralysis. This paralysis may lead to respiratory failure and death. Nausea and vomiting and abdominal pain may be seen just prior to the development of the paralysis. Treatment is supportive and may also include administration of equine antitoxin.

196. **B. The are several types of tremors that can be simplified into two categories: tremors that occur with movement and tremors that occur at rest. Everyone has some degree of repetitive motion in their extremities, a physiologic tremor, but most people's extremities move at such slow rhythms or with such tiny amplitudes that the tremor is not visible. Certain conditions such as fatigue, stress, medications, and others can exaggerate this underlying tremor and make it more noticeable. It's a normal tremor that becomes visible at times, so it is referred to as a physiologic tremor. The most common cause of a resting tremor is Parkinson disease. The tremor occurs at rest, hence the name, and initially decreases in intensity with voluntary motion. The speed at which the tremor occurs is about 4–6 Hz. The tremor is typically a**

supination-pronation type of tremor and not a flexion-extension type of tremor. Postural tremors occur when patients have a tremor while they are holding their extremities in a fixed position (out to their side, holding an object, etc.). Of the postural tremors, essential tremor is the most common. This is referred to as familial tremor when there is a family history or sporadic when there is not. Essential tremor should be fairly easy to distinguish from a resting tremor. Last of the major groups of tremors are the intention tremors. These do not usually occur at rest, but become quite obvious as patients move closer to the object they are trying to reach. There are a couple of other less common types of tremors, which include cerebellar tremors and neuropathic tremors. Cerebellar tremors can either be resting, essential, or intention in their appearance. The distinguishing feature is usually the presence of other cerebellar signs. Neuropathic tremors are associated with the recovery phase of demyelinating diseases such as Guillain-Barré. The patient described above has classic findings of a resting tremor (present at rest, low frequency/Hertz, improves with initial voluntary movement).

A, C, D, E. See explanation for B.

197. **D. As discussed above, the most common cause of resting tremor is PD. The tremor associated with PD usually starts in one extremity and is then followed by involvement of the ipsilateral extremity (e.g., the right arm is followed by the right leg). The contralateral side is then affected next. The patient has other signs on his examination that are suggestive of PD as well. For example, the "ratchet" motion described above is called cogwheeling and is suggestive of the diagnosis when it is seen on examination.**

A. MS is a demyelinating disease that can produce tremor, but it is not usually of the resting type (it's usually an intention tremor).
B. Midbrain stroke can also cause tremor, but similar to MS, it is usually an intention tremor.
C. Guillain-Barré syndrome, as discussed above, can cause a neuropathic tremor during the recovery phase of the disease as the myelin is being repleted.
E. Medications can cause a physiologic tremor to be present by unmasking the underlying normal tremor. When this occurs, the tremor may occur at rest, but the frequency of motion is usually much faster (10–12 Hertz, not 4–6 Hertz).

198. **A. The patient in this scenario has characteristic findings of BPV. The complaint of dizziness can often be a challenge to sort out because many patients have difficulty putting their feelings or sensations into words. The timing of events, associated symptoms, and precipitating causes can sometimes be more helpful than the description of the actual event. Patients who have BPV experience recurrent episodes of vertigo that are usually brief. These episodes are often triggered by changes in position and usually do not have other associated symptoms such as hearing loss, tinnitus, or focal neurologic changes. The presence of nystagmus while you are doing a provocative test helps confirm the diagnosis. BPV is often associated with prior head trauma, but not always. BPV frequently recurs but it is rarely refractory to therapy.**

B. Vestibular neuritis can cause an abrupt episode of vertigo, but it is not positional. Vestibular neuritis is often self-limiting and there is not normally hearing loss associated with it.
C. Acute labyrinthitis can appear similar to vestibular neuritis except that there is an associated hearing loss with acute labyrinthitis.
D. Ménière disease usually affects people in their thirties and forties and presents with vertigo, tinnitus, and hearing loss. It usually only involves one ear early in the course and then both.
E. Vertebrobasilar TIAs can cause intermittent and abrupt vertigo, but these are much easier to diagnose because of associated symptoms such as vision loss, dysarthria, diplopia, ataxia, and weakness.

199. **A. There are several maneuvers that may be used to help abate the symptoms of BPV. Meclizine is used in patients with BPV, not necessarily during one of their brief episodes, but if they are having increased frequency of the episodes.**

B. Aspirin may be beneficial in a patient with recurrent TIAs but its use in BPV is not indicated.
C. Salt restriction and diuretics is indicated for the treatment of Ménière disease, but not BPV.
D. Antibiotics are rarely indicated, even in the face of acute labyrinthitis.
E. See A above.

200. **D. This patient is in ventricular tachycardia, is hypotensive and stuporous, and is in immediate need of defibrillation, before any other resuscitative efforts are done. Always assess the patients rhythm when you are called to evaluate a patient at a code situation. Others may have started CPR in the meantime, while they are waiting for you to arrive with defibrillator paddles, and that is appropriate. However, the first thing that should be done in evaluation of the patient is to place the defibrillator paddles to his chest to assess the rhythm. If he is in ventricular tachycardia or fibrillation, you must shock him with 200 joules of unsynchronized electricity and immediately assess the rhythm. If he is still in ventricular tachycardia or ventricular fibrillation, go up on the joules to 300, and reshock, immediately reassessing the rhythm again. If he is still in ventricular tachycardia or ventricular fibrillation, then go up to 360 joules and shock again. These initial shocks are most likely to convert the patient into a more stable rhythm, and you may continue resuscitative efforts with intubation and drugs at that point. Each of the other measures mentioned take less priority than the electrical therapy in this scenario.**

A, B, C, and E, see D above.

Section

2 Obstetrics & Gynecology

SETTING 1: COMMUNITY-BASED HEALTH CENTER

You work at a community-based health facility where patients seeking both routine and urgent care are encountered. Many patients are members of low-income groups; many are ethnic minorities. Several industrial parks and local businesses send their employees to the health center for treatment of on-the-job injuries and employee health screening. There is a facility that provides x-ray films, but CT and MRI scans must be arranged at other facilities. Laboratory services are available.

The next two questions (items 1 and 2) correspond to the following vignette.

A 33-year-old G_1P_0 is seen in clinic at 39 weeks GA. Her fundal height measures 36 cm. You send her for US, which shows an estimated fetal weight of 3500 g, an amniotic fluid index (AFI) of 3.0, and normal uterine artery Dopplers. An US done earlier in the pregnancy showed normal amniotic fluid volume.

1. What is the most appropriate next step?

    A. Induction of labor
    B. Cesarean delivery
    C. Bed rest
    D. Maternal hydration
    E. Repeat US in 1 week

2. Which of the following is a possible etiology of oligohydramnios?

    A. Tracheoesophageal fistula
    B. Rh alloimmunization
    C. Gestational diabetes
    D. Renal agenesis
    E. Fetal hydrops

End of Set

3. A 20-year-old presents 3 weeks past her missed period. She had unprotected intercourse once with someone not well known to her. Her office urine pregnancy test is positive. The patient wishes to terminate her pregnancy. Which of the following statements is true regarding pregnancy termination?

    A. In 1972, maternal mortality from illegal abortions was 52%; in 1974 it was 6%.
    B. General anesthesia is now the major cause of mortality from pregnancy termination.
    C. A single induced abortion does not cause future pregnancy complications or sterility.
    D. Cervical dilation in the second trimester cannot safely be achieved by using laminaria.
    E. Surgical termination is associated with a greater blood loss than is medical termination.

4. A 31-year-old G_1P_0 presents to clinic at 26 weeks GA complaining of decreased fetal movement for 3 days. She has no medical problems and her pregnancy has been uncomplicated. She had a normal Level I US at 20 weeks GA. The patient's BP is normal, and her fundal height measures 26 cm. You are unable to auscultate fetal heart tones with a Doptone. Office US confirms fetal demise. Your partner comes in to confirm your finding, which you then explain to the patient. Which of the following do you recommend to the patient?

    A. Induction of labor
    B. Formal US to confirm findings
    C. Expectant management and await spontaneous labor
    D. Cesarean delivery
    E. Amniocentesis

The next two questions (items 5 and 6) correspond to the following vignette.

A 35-year-old G_4P_3 presents to clinic at 33 weeks GA after being involved in a minor motor vehicle accident. While pulling into your parking lot, another car collided with her front passenger door. The patient was wearing a seat belt, which had been placed low and across her lap, under her pregnant abdomen. She estimates that the other car was driving 5 to 10 miles per hour and reports minor damage to her car. She is unsure whether she hit her abdomen, and complains of mild left abdominal and shoulder pain. Your exam is unremarkable.

5. What is the most appropriate next step?
   A. 4 hours of fetal monitoring
   B. Draw a hematocrit
   C. Discharge home with follow-up in 1 week
   D. Rupture membranes to check for abruption
   E. Instruct the patient to follow fetal kick counts

6. Which of the following is true regarding management of a patient with major trauma during pregnancy?
   A. US can identify the majority of abruptions.
   B. Pregnant patients generally show signs of shock later than nonpregnant patients.
   C. Any pregnant patient with loss of consciousness should undergo emergent cesarean delivery.
   D. If CPR is necessary, it can be performed similar to nonpregnant patients regardless of the trimester of pregnancy.
   E. Fetal injury from trauma is common.

End of Set

7. An 18-year-old G_1P_0 presents to clinic at 36 weeks GA complaining of copious watery vaginal discharge that has run down her legs for the past 24 hours. Which of the following is the initial step in her evaluation?
   A. Culture for chlamydia
   B. Urine stream assessment for chlamydia
   C. Speculum exam and nitrazine test
   D. Cultures for herpes
   E. Office US

8. A 26-year-old woman presents complaining of a painful swollen mass near her vagina. She noticed a small lump approximately 2 weeks ago. During the last 2 days, the lump has become exquisitely tender and has grown significantly larger. The patient also reports subjective fevers. She has noticed no drainage, is not sexually active, and denies chills, myalgias, or vaginal discharge. On exam, you find a 4-cm, erythematous, nondraining vulvar mass to the right side of the posterior fourchette (Figure 2-8). What is the next step in management?

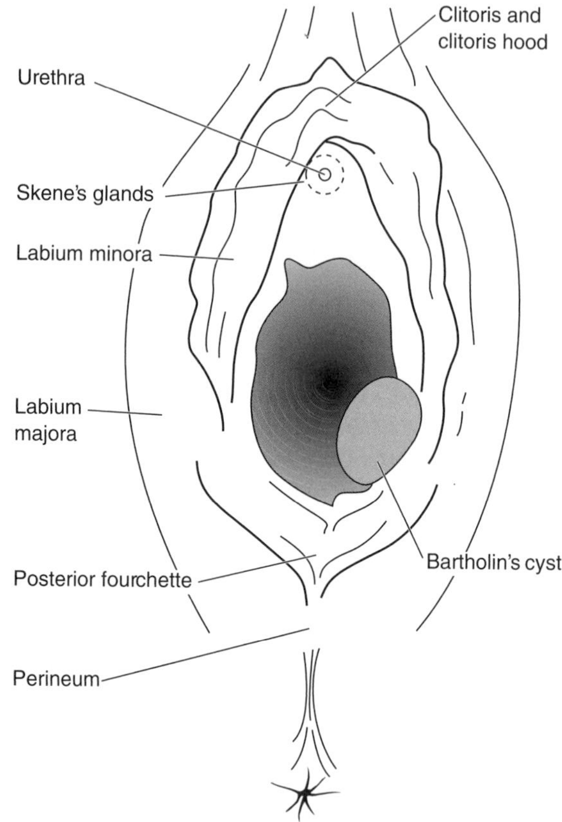

Figure 2-8 • Reproduced from Callahan T. Blueprints Obstetrics & Gynecology. 3rd ed. Blackwell, 2004: Fig 13-4, p. 126.

   A. Oral antibiotics and follow-up in 1 week
   B. Hospitalization and intravenous antibiotics
   C. Full screen for sexually transmitted infections
   D. Warm compresses
   E. Incision and drainage

9. A 27-year-old G_0 presents with intermittent post-coital spotting for the past week. Her friend was recently diagnosed with cervical cancer, and the patient is extremely concerned that her bleeding is related to a similar diagnosis. She is

sexually active with her husband only and has never had a sexually transmitted disease. She has had normal annual Pap smears for the past 5 to 6 years, with the most recent being 4 months ago. What is the most important initial diagnostic test?

A. Pap smear
B. Urine pregnancy test
C. Chlamydia and gonorrhea culture
D. Pelvic US
E. Urine culture

10. A 47-year-old G_0 complains of moderate vaginal bleeding 3 weeks after her period, which lasted several hours, moderately stained two pads, and then stopped. She otherwise feels well, is non-obese, and is in good general health. Her menses are usually regular, occurring every 28 days and lasting for 3 to 4 days. Which of the following is the most important next step?

A. Endometrial biopsy
B. Pap smear
C. Cervical cultures
D. Pelvic US
E. Hysteroscopy

11. A 39-year-old G_2P_0 presents after trying to become pregnant for 2 years. She is monogamous and sexually active with her husband twice a week. Her infertility evaluation has been normal, revealing normal cycles, normal thyroid and prolactin levels, and patent fallopian tubes. Her husband's semen analysis is normal. For the past one-and-a-half years she has experienced increasingly heavy menstrual periods, and she has had two miscarriages. A pelvic US with injected saline is obtained (Figure 2-11). What is the most appropriate next step in management?

A. Adoption
B. Recommend a gestational carrier
C. Myomectomy
D. Intra-cytoplasmic sperm injection (ICSI)
E. In vitro fertilization (IVF)

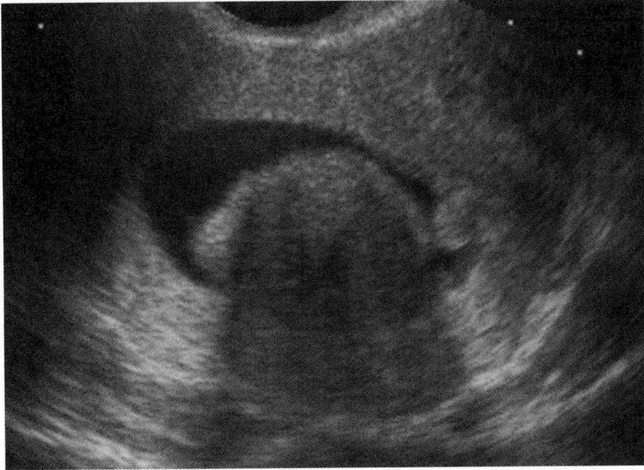

Figure 2-11 • Image Provided by Departments of Radiology and Obstetrics & Gynecology, University of California, San Francisco.

12. A 27-year-old woman presents to the clinic reporting, "I have a skin rash down there." She believes the rash has been present for approximately 2 weeks. Other than a prior history of chlamydial infection at age 21, she denies any significant gynecologic or medical history. Which of the following is the most common noninfectious vulvar disease in members of this age group?

A. Eczema
B. Lichen simplex chronicus (LSC)
C. Lichen sclerosis
D. Melanoma
E. Basal cell carcinoma

13. A 36-year-old woman visits your clinic complaining of lesions on her labia. She denies any pain associated with the lesions, which appeared 3 days ago. She denies vaginal discharge, dysuria, or pruritis. On exam, you observe three 1 cm round, painless ulcers on her labia majora, and you note inguinal adenopathy. You suspect primary syphilis. Which of the following statements is true regarding this STD?

A. Early syphilis is treated with metronidazole for 14 days.
B. Primary syphilis is characterized by a painless chancre that develops approximately 3 weeks after inoculation.
C. The causative agent is a gram-positive rod.
D. Secondary syphilis occurs when the lesions become painful and a rash appears on the backs of the hands and feet.
E. Tertiary syphilis is characterized by notched teeth and saber shins.

14. A 17-year-old G_1 student presents to the clinic for her second prenatal visit with uncertain GA. She was first seen 10 weeks ago, when she was unable to provide the date of her LMP, and was dated at 30 weeks by US (normal anatomy and amniotic fluid). Prenatal labs were drawn and were unremarkable except for an elevated 50-g glucose load

test (GLT) of 163. The patient did not return for follow-up despite multiple messages being left by the clinic staff. She has never been counseled or treated for diabetes. This morning, she returns because she is extremely uncomfortable; however, she reports no symptoms of labor. She explains that she has not returned to clinic for fear of needing insulin injections like her mother and aunt, both of whom have diabetes. Her BP is 110/65. Urine dipstick shows 2+ glucose and trace protein. Her fingerstick blood glucose is 160, and the patient is certain that she has not eaten yet today. US estimates fetal weight at 5100 g, and fetal anatomy and amniotic fluid are normal. Fetal heart tracing is reactive. Which of the following diagnostic tests will be most useful in planning the obstetrical management of this patient?

A. Amniotic fluid lecithin:sphingomyelin ratio
B. 3-hour oral glucose tolerance test (OGTT)
C. Serum hemoglobin A_{1c} level
D. Cervical exam to assess Bishop score
E. Quantitative β-hCG

The following two questions (items 15 and 16) relate to the same clinical scenario.

A 28-year-old G_2P_1 woman at 32 weeks GA presents for a routine prenatal visit. Her previous pregnancy was uncomplicated, and she has had no problems in this pregnancy. Her BP in the office is noted to be elevated at 155/110, and her urine dips trace protein. She denies a prior history of hypertension. Her pressures have been normal earlier in this pregnancy. The patient does not complain of visual disturbances, headache, or epigastric discomfort. Her BPs are carefully monitored, and remain in the range 135–155/95–110. She is admitted to the hospital to rule out preeclampsia and to monitor her BPs. A 24-hour urine collection yields 160 mg of protein. The patient remains asymptomatic, and her pressures improve but remain elevated. The decision is made to discharge her to home with oral antihypertensive medication. She will monitor her BPs and urine protein at home.

15. Which of the following medications is the most appropriate choice in this setting?

    A. Labetolol
    B. Captopril
    C. Magnesium sulfate
    D. Losartan
    E. Furosemide

16. Over the next 4 weeks, the patient's BPs improve, and are generally in the range 110–125/80–95 with the use of her medication. Her urine occasionally dips trace proteinuria, but never higher. At 36 weeks GA, her membranes spontaneously rupture, and she delivers a healthy boy several hours later without complication. She now returns for her 6-week postpartum visit and brings a log of BPs, which are in the range 100–115/65–80. The patient explains that she is unsure what to tell friends and family about the reasons for her hospitalization during pregnancy. What is the most appropriate diagnosis of this patient's hypertension?

    A. Mild preeclampsia
    B. Severe preeclampsia
    C. Chronic hypertension
    D. Chronic hypertension with superimposed preeclampsia
    E. Gestational hypertension

End of Set

17. A 38-year-old G_0 African American premenopausal woman presents to clinic for an annual exam. Her last exam was 3 years ago. She is 5 ft 7 in. tall and weighs 129 lb. Her physical exam is within normal limits except for the pelvic exam. On bimanual exam, you note a left adnexal mass, distinct from her uterus, which is retroverted and retroflexed. The mass is nontender and palpates approximately 6 to 7 cm in diameter. You order a pelvic US, which reveals an 8 cm × 7 cm × 5 cm complex left ovarian mass. No ascites or omental thickening is seen. The other ovary appears entirely normal. When considering how to counsel this patient about her differential diagnosis, which of the following statements is true regarding the major types of ovarian tumors?

    A. Epithelial cell tumors are the most common.
    B. Epithelial cell tumors are more frequent among girls and young women.
    C. Germ cell tumors include granulosa-theca and Sertoli-Leydig tumors.
    D. Germ cell tumors are more frequent among women in their late fifties.
    E. Sex-cord stromal tumors include mucinous and endometrioid tumors.

The next two questions (items 18 and 19) correspond to the following vignette.

A mother brings her 15-year-old daughter to clinic, concerned because of the girl's abdominal pain. The pain began 2 months ago and has become constant. The patient is virginal and in good health. She has normal monthly menses and denies fevers, chills, nausea, vomiting, and weight loss. Pelvic US reveals a complex 8 × 6 cm left ovarian mass (Figure 2-18). The patient is taken to the operating room 2 days later for exploratory laparotomy and left salpingo-oophorectomy. The mass is removed without complication and sent to pathology for intraoperative frozen section analysis of tumor histology.

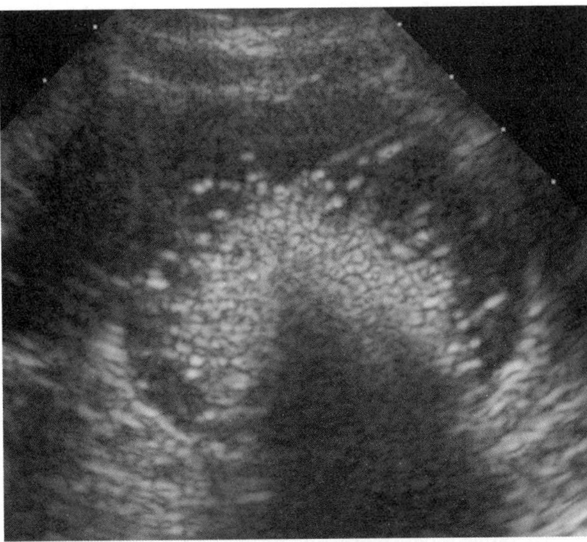

Figure 2-18 • Image Provided by Departments of Radiology and Obstetrics & Gynecology, University of California, San Francisco.

18. Which of the following associations is most accurate?
    A. Dysgerminoma arises from trophoblastic (placental) tissue.
    B. Embryonal carcinoma arises from undifferentiated germ cells.
    C. Endodermal sinus tumor arises from undifferentiated germ cells.
    D. Choriocarcinoma arises from embryonic (fetal) tissue.
    E. Immature teratoma arises from extraembryonic (yolk sac) tissue.

19. Postoperative management of patients with ovarian tumors can include monitoring serum markers for evidence of persistent disease. Which of the following germ cell tumors is correctly matched to its associated serum tumor marker?
    A. Dysgerminoma and lactate dehydrogenase (LDH)
    B. Embryonal carcinoma and LDH
    C. Endodermal sinus tumor and CA-125
    D. Choriocarcinoma and alpha-fetoprotein (AFP)
    E. Immature teratoma and hCG

End of Set

The next three questions (items 20, 21, and 22) correspond to the following vignette.

A 29-year-old G_0 woman presents to the clinic with a nontender mass found on routine breast self-exam. Her family history is notable for breast cancer in an aunt at age 37. On physical exam, a firm, immobile mass is palpated in the upper outer quadrant of the left breast. No other masses are palpable, but axillary lymph nodes on the left side are firm and fixed. There is no discharge from the nipple. A bilateral mammogram is nondiagnostic (due to dense breast parenchyma). US identifies a 4 cm solid mass. MRI with contrast is consistent with infiltrating carcinoma. No involvement is seen on the right side, but several clinically occult lesions are apparent on the left side. Core biopsy of the 4 cm mass demonstrates histology consistent with medullary carcinoma, infiltrating the basement membrane. Tumor cells are found to be negative for estrogen receptors, progesterone receptors, and c-erbB-2 overexpression. Significant aneuploidy and a high S-phase fraction are seen. Axillary lymph node biopsy is positive for metastasis, but no other evidence of metastatic disease is noted on additional imaging or lab testing. The patient is determined to do everything possible to maximize her chances of curative therapy.

20. The planned surgical procedure will include resection of the breast tissue, nipple-areolar complex, overlying skin, and axillary lymph nodes. The pectoralis major muscle will be spared. What is the most accurate description of this procedure?
    A. Modified radical mastectomy
    B. Total (simple) mastectomy
    C. Subcutaneous mastectomy
    D. Radical mastectomy
    E. Wide local excision

21. Which of the following medical therapies would be most appropriate to start for this patient postoperatively?

A. Hormonal therapy (e.g., tamoxifen)
B. Combination chemotherapy (e.g., cyclophosphamide/methotrexate/5-fluorouracil, also known as CMF)
C. Strontium-89
D. Herceptin (trastuzumab)
E. No therapy

22. Which of the following features of this patient's history and presentation has the most favorable impact on her prognosis?

A. The tumor is negative for estrogen receptors.
B. The tumor is negative for progesterone receptors.
C. A high percentage of tumor cells is seen in the S phase.
D. The tumor is classified as medullary.
E. The patient is premenopausal.

End of Set

23. A 52-year-old G_0 waitress presents to the clinic after a screening mammogram identified a 3-cm lesion in the upper inner quadrant of her right breast. Physical exam is unremarkable, with no palpable breast masses. US-guided biopsy of the mass is positive for infiltrating intraductal carcinoma. A radionucleotide bone scan is negative for evidence of metastasis; chest and abdominal CT are unremarkable. A complete blood count and liver function tests are within normal limits. During surgery, the right axillary lymph nodes are noted to be firm, fixed, and positive for metastasis by intraoperative biopsy. No other evidence of metastasis is seen. Which of the following is the most accurate staging of this patient's disease?

A. Tis N0 M0 (Stage 0)
B. T1 N1 M0 (Stage IIa)
C. T3 N0 M0 (Stage IIb)
D. T2 N2 M0 (Stage IIIa)
E. T2 N2 M1 (Stage IV)

24. A 16-year-old African American woman presents to the clinic after 5 days of worsening low abdominal pain. She reports nausea and vomiting, fever, and vaginal discharge. She is sexually active, currently has three partners, and is unsure of her LMP. She was seen in the ED 3 days ago and given "some pills," which she admits she did not take. On exam, she has uterine tenderness and pain with cervical motion. You note bilateral adnexal tenderness but cannot palpate her adnexa definitively. Her urine pregnancy test is negative. You diagnose PID. Which of the following is the best next step in management?

A. Transvaginal US to rule out tubo-ovarian abscess
B. Serum β-hCG since she is unsure of her LMP
C. Oral antibiotics with another clinic appointment within 24 hours
D. Admission for laparoscopy
E. Admission with intravenous antibiotics

25. A 36-year-old G_3P_3 presents to your clinic 8 days after an uncomplicated IUD insertion. She noted increasing pain and vaginal spotting. Her recent cervical cultures for gonorrhea and chlamydia were negative at the time of the IUD insertion, and she reports no intercourse with her husband in the last 5 weeks. She is afebrile but has uterine tenderness on bimanual exam. Which of the following is the best option for management?

A. Admission with intravenous antibiotics
B. Outpatient oral antibiotics
C. Removal of IUD and oral antibiotics
D. Repeat cultures and prescribe NSAIDs
E. Check a urine pregnancy test

26. A 27-year-old woman and her boyfriend of 8 months regularly engage in sexual relations using condoms as their sole form of birth control. They are careful and have never had a problem with breakage or slippage in the past. Two days after their last sexual encounter, however, the woman receives a call from her boyfriend, who states that the condom may have broken during sex. He had refrained from saying something sooner because he wasn't sure and did not want to worry her, but after giving the matter more thought now feels that the breakage did indeed occur. Fearing the worst, the woman considers using emergency contraception, or "the morning after pill," to prevent pregnancy. Which of the following statements is most accurate regarding the benefit of emergency contraception for this woman?

A. She will not benefit because the event occurred more than 24 hours prior to taking the pill.
B. She may not benefit because the failure rate with emergency contraception approaches 25%.
C. She may benefit depending on her ability to obtain a prescription from her gynecologist promptly.
D. She may benefit as long as she is willing to accept the risk of teratogenicity to the fetus should the regimen fail.
E. She may benefit because she has never used an IUD.

27. A 32-year-old woman had a low-grade squamous intraepithelial lesion (LSIL) on her annual Pap smear. She underwent colposcopic evaluation. At the time of colposcopy, the transformation zone (TZ) was visible clockwise from 1 o'clock to 10 o'clock. Two areas of concern were biopsied. An endocervical curettage (ECC) was also done. The pathology from one biopsy was "Normal exocervix," and that from the other biopsy was "High-grade squamous intraepithelial lesion (HSIL). No evidence of invasion." The ECC pathology was negative. Which of the following options should this woman be offered?

   A. Hysterectomy
   B. Repeat colposcopy in 3 months
   C. Loop electrosurgical excision procedure (LEEP)
   D. Localized radiation therapy
   E. Cryotherapy

28. A 32-year-old G_4P_3 woman presents at 19 weeks GA for a routine prenatal appointment immediately prior to her scheduled US. She has had an uncomplicated antenatal course with normal first-trimester labs. In addition, her triple screen returned negative for neural tube defects or aneuploidy. The patient and her husband are looking forward to the US because they have three daughters and are hoping for a son. You discuss the indications for a Level I obstetric US. Which of the following is a routine component of this US?

   A. Fetal extremities
   B. Fetal gender
   C. Fetal kidneys
   D. Umbilical cord insertion into the placenta
   E. Fetal face

29. A 20-year-old G_1P_0 woman at 16 weeks GA by LMP has decided she wants to terminate the pregnancy. She is healthy and denies prior medical or surgical history. What is the safest and most appropriate method to induce an abortion in this patient?

   A. Suction curettage
   B. Vaginal prostaglandin administration
   C. Menstrual regulation
   D. Hysterectomy
   E. D&E

30. A 37-year-old G_3P_3 woman asks you to discuss birth control options. She does not want to risk becoming pregnant again at her age, but feels that sterilization is "a bit drastic." She has a history of postpartum depression, no other past medical history, smokes one-half pack of cigarettes a day, and has no allergies to medications. What is the safest, most efficacious method of contraception for this patient?

   A. Depo-Provera
   B. Combined OCPs
   C. Progestin-only OCPs
   D. Diaphragm
   E. Copper-T IUD

31. A 16-year-old woman has just recently become sexually active and comes to your clinic for her first annual exam. At the end of the exam, she expresses interest in starting OCPs to prevent pregnancy while she finishes school. Her health counselor once told her, however, that some women should not take birth control pills because it could be hazardous to their health. She is concerned that she may be one of those women. To allay her concerns, you decide to take a more thorough history and highlight for her the factors that would be considered dangerous. Of the following, what additional history would be considered an absolute contraindication to combined OCPs?

   A. History of diabetes mellitus type I
   B. Concurrent hypertension (HTN)
   C. Uterine leiomyoma (fibroid)
   D. Family history of breast cancer
   E. Concurrent symptomatic hepatitis C infection

32. A 35-year-old G_2P_1 woman presents to your clinic 4 weeks after spontaneous abortion of a highly desired pregnancy at 10 weeks GA. She reports 1 week of persistent, intermittent vaginal bleeding and 2 days of hemoptysis. Physical exam is notable for tachycardia and an enlarged uterus. Speculum exam reveals only a small amount of blood in the vaginal vault. A β-hCG level is drawn and is found to be elevated at 25,000 mIU/mL. Suction curettage is performed, and after pathology confirms the diagnosis, imaging is ordered. Multiple pulmonary nodules are identified on chest X-ray; chest CT confirms the nodules seen on plain film. CT of the abdomen and brain are within normal limits, with no focal lesions identified. What is the most appropriate medical treatment to initiate for this patient?

A. Single-agent chemotherapy (e.g., methotrexate)
B. Multiple-agent chemotherapy (e.g., etoposide/methotrexate/dactinomycin)
C. Hysterectomy
D. Exploratory laparotomy and local excision of uterine lesion
E. Radiation therapy to pelvis

33. A 24-year-old G_1P_0 woman—a patient of another physician in your practice who is currently on vacation—presents to your office 6 weeks after suction evacuation of an incomplete molar pregnancy. She was started on OCPs at that time, and has been compliant with her medication. Her β-hCG level today is 3000 mIU/mL, slightly lower than the value of 5000 mIU/mL measured last week. Today, the patient expresses her desire to conceive, and says that she does not understand why she needs to continue with contraceptives. What is the most compelling reason for her to continue taking the OCPs?

A. She is at increased risk for GTD in future pregnancies, and the risk is significant enough to discourage future pregnancy.
B. She is at increased risk of spontaneous abortions, complications, and congenital malformations in future pregnancies, and these risks are significant enough to discourage future pregnancy.
C. OCPs reduce the risk of persistent locally invasive moles.
D. OCPs reduce the risk of malignant choriocarcinoma.
E. Reliable prevention of pregnancy is necessary to allow accurate measurement of β-hCG levels to rule out persistent or malignant trophoblastic disease.

34. A 39-year-old G_2P_0 presents for a routine office visit at 30 weeks GA. Her pregnancy has been unremarkable, and she has no history of medical problems or UTIs. Today in the clinic, her BP is 90/60. A routine urine dipstick reveals trace protein, trace blood, trace leukocyte esterase, and 1+ WBCs. She denies dysuria, fevers, chills, contractions, vaginal bleeding, and leakage of fluid, and reports good fetal movement. What is the most appropriate next step?

A. Send a urine culture
B. Counsel her to follow up if she becomes symptomatic
C. Treat with antibiotics
D. Do nothing
E. Renal biopsy

35. A 15-year-old G_1P_0 woman presents at 33 weeks GA complaining of constant abdominal pain for 2 days. She has been leaking fluid for approximately 1 week. She feels otherwise well and denies symptoms of an upper respiratory tract infection, nausea, vomiting, diarrhea, or dysuria. Her appetite is normal. On exam, she is febrile to 101.1°C, her pulse is 120, her abdomen is tender to palpation, and she has a foul-smelling, purulent vaginal discharge. There is no pool of fluid in her vagina, but a fern pattern is seen on a slide, and nitrazine paper turns dark blue when touched with the swab. The patient's cervix appears long and closed. Office US reveals a fetus in cephalic presentation and an amniotic fluid index of 2. What is the most appropriate next step?

A. Cesarean section
B. Antibiotics and observation
C. Amniocentesis for culture
D. Tampon dye test
E. Induction of labor

36. A 27-year-old G_3P_0 presents to clinic at 26 weeks GA complaining of constant vaginal wetness that began 3 weeks ago. She now wears a pad in her underwear because of her symptoms. She experiences occasional vaginal itching and mild pain. The patient has no medical problems, and her pregnancy has been uncomplicated. She denies contractions, vaginal bleeding, and abnormal discharge, and reports active fetal movement. What is the most important and appropriate next step in this patient's management?

A. Observation at home with further evaluation if the symptoms worsen
B. Sterile speculum exam with tests for a pool of fluid with a fern pattern and a basic pH
C. Sterile speculum exam with a KOH and wet prep
D. Vaginal and rectal swab for Group B *Streptococcus*
E. US

37. A 34-year-old G_3P_2 at 32 weeks GA calls your clinic concerned because her son's friend, who just slept overnight at their home, awoke with a vesicular rash, which has been confirmed to be

chickenpox. The patient is unsure whether she has had chickenpox. She is feeling well and has no medical problems. Her pregnancy has been uncomplicated. You recommend that she do which of the following?

A. Go to the clinic for an exam
B. Go to the ED designated area for varicella zoster immunoglobulin (VZIG)
C. Go to the pharmacy and fill a prescription for oral acyclovir
D. Alert the pediatrician so that the infant may be prophylaxed after delivery
E. Go to the ED designated area and have a varicella zoster virus (VZV) titer drawn

38. A 20-year-old G_3P_0 presents at 16 weeks GA for her first prenatal visit. Her prenatal labs are normal except her RPR, which is reactive. She has no medical problems and takes no medications. She has had three sexual partners during the last year, has had sexual contact with two of the partners in the last 3 months, and has used condoms only occasionally. She had a full STD-screen 1 year ago, including an RPR, which was negative. She feels well in general, but during the last 6 months has experienced three episodes of arthritis of her hands, lasting approximately 2 weeks before resolving spontaneously. She reports intermittent fatigue during the last 2 years, which was not significant enough to prevent her from exercising but has worsened since she became pregnant. She denies fever, rash, and photosensitivity. What is the most appropriate next step?

A. Send an ANA
B. Arrange a consult with rheumatology
C. Send an MHA-TP
D. Treat with benzathine penicillin G
E. Repeat the RPR

39. A 37-year-old G_2P_1 Caucasian woman presents to you at 33 weeks GA with her third complaint of decreased fetal movement in the last 3 weeks. You send her for a nonstress test, which is reactive. She appears tremendously relieved. An amniocentesis at 16 weeks was normal, and US revealed an appropriately grown fetus without identifiable anomalies and a posterior placenta. Her fundal height measures appropriately. She is 5 ft 5 in. tall, weighs 140 lb, and has gained 12 lb during this pregnancy. She reports that poor appetite has been a problem, and she has been trying to increase her caloric intake. She is married, and describes her husband as somewhat ambivalent about the pregnancy because of financial concerns. During this pregnancy, she has come in nearly weekly complaining of any variety of mild symptoms, including headaches, abdominal pain, decreased fetal movement, joint pains, and heartburn, each time wanting reassurance that the baby is okay. She is well known to you because you delivered her first child, and she did not have multiple somatic complaints during that pregnancy. What is the most appropriate next step in this patient's management?

A. Biophysical profile
B. Screen for domestic violence
C. Evaluate for anorexia nervosa
D. US for fetal weight
E. Weekly nonstress tests

40. A mother brings her 16-year-old G_0 daughter to the clinic because she has not yet begun to menstruate. On exam, the girl is 5 ft 9 in. tall and weighs 100 lb. Her breasts are enlarged, and the areolae project to form secondary mounds. She shaves her axilla and has a mid-escutcheon on her mons. Her vagina appears well estrogenized, there is no septum, and her cervix appears normal. On palpation, a uterus is present, and her ovaries feel normal. Which Tanner stage of development (Figure2- 40a) best describes this patient?

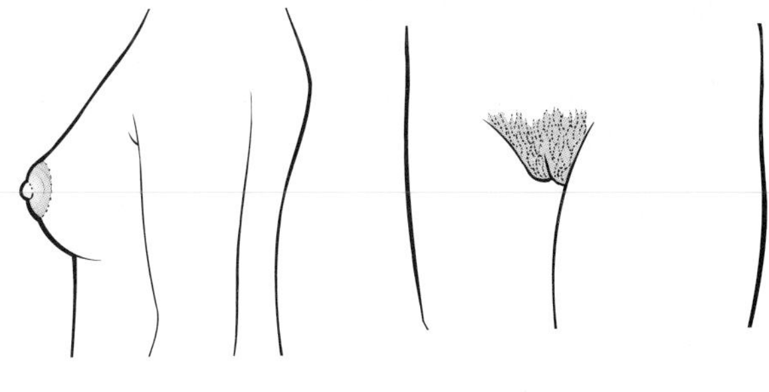

A

Figure 2-40A • Reproduced from Callahan T, Caughey AB. Blueprints Obstetrics & Gynecology, 4e. Baltimore: Lippincott Williams & Wilkins, 2007. Figs. 20-2 and 20-3.

A. Stage 1
B. Stage 2
C. Stage 3
D. Stage 4
E. Stage 5

41. A 16-year-old adolescent female is brought in by her mother for what appears to be primary amenorrhea. Upon further questioning, she admits that she had her first period at age 14, had four periods every 1 to 2 months after that, and has not a period for more than 1 year. You ask her mother to leave the room. The patient reports that she has lost 20 lb during the last year and a half as a result of dieting and exercising 1 hour a day. Reluctantly, she admits that she feels fat, and she describes her friends as serial dieters. The patient does not like to discuss her weight with her mother, who has encouraged her to gain weight. She is 5 ft 9 in. tall and weighs 100 lb. Her exam is normal, and development is otherwise appropriate for her age. She has no medical problems, is virginal, and has never had surgery. A urine pregnancy test is negative. Which of the following is the most likely cause of this patient's secondary amenorrhea?

   A. Cervical stenosis
   B. Asherman's syndrome
   C. Premature ovarian failure (POF)
   D. Hypothalamic amenorrhea
   E. Polycystic ovarian syndrome (PCOS)

42. A 21-year-old G_0 woman presents complaining of profuse, foul-smelling, greenish vaginal discharge, which worsened 2 days after the end of her LMP. She complains of itching and irritation. She is sexually active, has had two partners during the last 3 months, and does not use condoms. On sterile speculum, she has a frothy gray-green discharge. You perform a wet prep in clinic and see actively moving, flagellated organisms. Figure 2-42 shows a scanning electron micrograph of the organism. Which of the following statements is true regarding this patient?

   A. She can be treated immediately with 2 g of oral metronidazole (Flagyl).
   B. Her partners do not need treatment, as men do not manifest symptoms of this infection.
   C. She can be treated with 250 mg of oral azithromycin (Zithromax).
   D. There is no need to be screen for STDs such as *Neisseria gonorrhea*, *Chlamydia trachomatis*, and HIV.
   E. Diagnosis cannot be made on wet prep alone; prior to treatment, a culture should be sent to confirm the diagnosis.

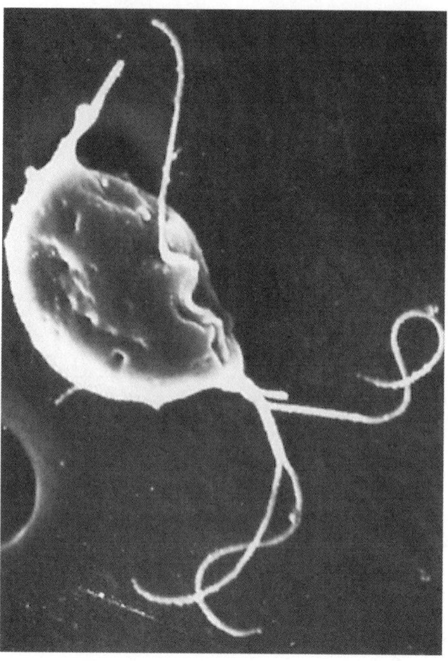

Figure 2-42 • Reproduced with Permission from Cox FEB, ed. Modern Parasitology: A Textbook of Parasitology, 2nd ed. Blackwell Science, 1993: Fig. 9.

43. A 22-year-old G_1P_1 woman complains of a foul-smelling vaginal discharge and dyspareunia for 3 days. She has been sexually active with her new partner for 1 month and uses oral contraception, but not condoms. She has had one other sexual partner during the last year and did not use condoms. Her LMP was 8 days ago. The patient is compliant and well known to you. On exam, she is afebrile. Her abdomen is nontender. Her pelvic exam is pertinent for mucopurulent discharge coming from her cervical os, cervical-motion tenderness, and a nontender uterus and adnexae. Which of the following is the most appropriate initial treatment?

   A. Ceftriaxone 250 mg IM once
   B. Ceftriaxone 250 mg IM once and azithromycin 1g PO once
   C. Doxycycline 100 mg PO BID (× 7 days)
   D. Azithromycin 1 g PO once
   E. Cefoxitin 2 g IV q6 hours and doxycycline 100 mg IV q12 hours

44. A 48-year-old G_2P_2 woman presents with menorrhagia, bloating, and pelvic pressure. During the past 2 years, her menses have lasted longer and are heavier. She has also begun to experience dyspareunia and constipation. Rectovaginal exam is remarkable for fullness. Pelvic US reveals an 8 cm × 8 cm × 6 cm homogenous fibroid in the posterior uterine wall. Which of the following statements is true about fibroids?

A. Most women with fibroids eventually become symptomatic.
B. Fibroids should be removed because of their malignant potential.
C. Fibroids tend to regress during pregnancy.
D. Fibroids are associated with infertility.
E. Fibroids are most common among Hispanic women.

45. A 31-year-old G_0 woman is found to have moderate cervical intraepithelial neoplasia (CIN II) on her Pap smear. Colposcopically directed biopsies are consistent with CIN II at two small sites on the exocervix. The endocervical curettage (ECC) is normal. The patient has always had normal annual Pap smears, with the most recent occurring 1 year ago. She has had a new sexual partner for the last 6 months and uses oral contraception. What is the most appropriate next step in this patient's treatment?

A. Serotype for HPV
B. Cryotherapy or laser therapy
C. Loop electrosurgical excision procedure (LEEP)
D. Cold knife cone (CKC)
E. Repeat colposcopy and biopsies in 3 months

46. A 62-year-old G_2P_2 woman, postmenopausal for 12 years, presents to the clinic complaining of abdominal bloating for 6 months. During the past 2 months she has been unable to button her pants, despite a 10-lb weight loss achieved without dieting. A pelvic US reveals massive ascites and a 9 cm × 10 cm complex right ovarian mass as shown in Figure 2-46. In addition to obtaining lab work, what is the next step in this patient's management?

A. Observation with repeat US in 4 weeks
B. Exploratory laparotomy
C. Diuretic treatment for relief of her ascites
D. A second opinion
E. Chemotherapy

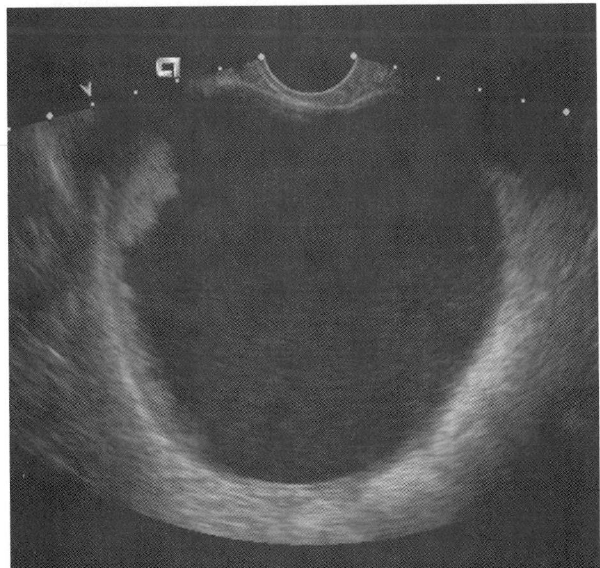

Figure 2-46 • Image Provided by Departments of Radiology and Obstetrics & Gynecology, University of California, San Francisco.

47. A 24-year-old G_1P_0 woman at 18 4/7 weeks GA presents to the clinic after her scheduled US. The radiologist calls you to report an abnormality, which is shown in Figure 47. The patient had an expanded AFP (XAFP) serum screening test sent off 3 days ago as well, but the results are not back yet. Based on the findings in the US in Figure 2-47, what are the likely results of her XAFP?

A. Decreased MSAFP, decreased estriol, elevated hCG
B. Decreased MSAFP, decreased estriol, decreased hCG
C. Elevated MSAFP, normal estriol, normal hCG
D. Elevated MSAFP, elevated estriol, elevated hCG
E. Normal MSAFP, decreased estriol, elevated hCG

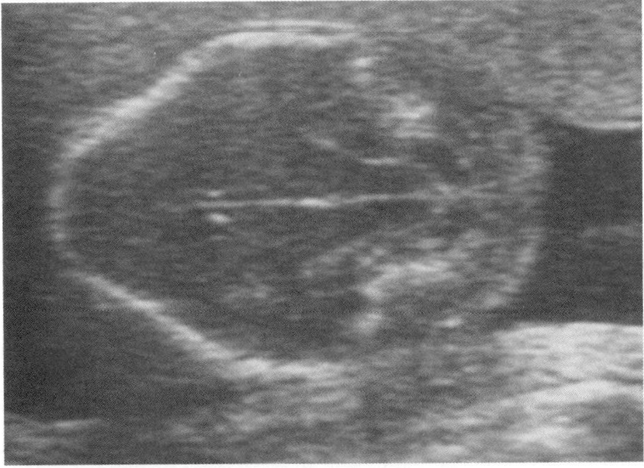

Figure 2-47 • Image Provided by Departments of Radiology and Obstetrics & Gynecology, University of California, San Francisco.

48. A 23-year-old G_0 woman presents with intermittent left lower quadrant pain. The pain began 2 months ago, a couple of weeks before her monthly menses. She describes the pain as mild, sharp, focal, nonradiating, and never severe. The patient is virginal and takes no medications. She is afebrile and well appearing. Pelvic exam reveals fullness is the left adnexa. A pelvic US demonstrates a 2-cm simple left adnexal cyst. What is the most appropriate next step?

   A. Oral progestin-only pills
   B. Laparoscopic cystectomy
   C. Fine-needle aspiration
   D. Hospitalization and observation
   E. Outpatient observation

49. A 55-year-old woman comes to the clinic with complaints of a vulvar lesion for at least the past 6 months. The mass appears suspicious for malignancy, and you perform a vulvar biopsy, which returns as Paget's disease. Which of the following statements is true about Paget's disease of the vulva?

   A. Treatment is wide local excision or vulvectomy without radiation or chemotherapy.
   B. It is caused by HPV.
   C. It is associated with a lower incidence of an underlying internal carcinoma than other forms of Paget's disease.
   D. It is most common in premenarchal females.
   E. It is commonly associated with HSV-1.

50. A 18-year-old African American woman presents to the clinic after 5 days of worsening lower abdominal pain. She reports nausea and vomiting, fever, and vaginal discharge. She is sexually active with three partners and is unsure of her LMP. She was seen in the ED 3 days ago and given "some pills," which she admits she did not take. On exam, she is afebrile and has uterine and cervical motion tenderness. You also note bilateral adnexal tenderness and no vaginal discharge. Her urine pregnancy test is negative. You diagnose pelvic inflammatory disease and emphasize the importance of taking the prescribed antibiotics. However, the patient returns 4 days later still complaining of pain. She now has a fever. An US reveals bilateral tubo-ovarian abscesses (TOAs). Which of the following statements is true regarding TOA?

   A. TOA results from a mixed polymicrobial infection with a high proportion of anaerobes.
   B. Management should begin with drainage of the complex.
   C. TOA is most commonly caused by appendicitis, pelvic surgery, or diverticulitis.
   D. Fever and elevated WBC count are the most common features of TOA.
   E. TOA is not associated with future infertility as compared to PID.

A Answers and Explanations

1. A
2. D
3. C
4. A
5. A
6. B
7. C
8. E
9. B
10. A
11. C
12. B
13. B
14. A
15. A
16. E
17. A
18. E
19. A
20. A
21. B
22. D
23. D
24. E
25. C
26. B
27. C
28. C
29. E
30. E
31. E
32. A
33. E
34. A
35. E
36. B
37. E
38. C
39. B
40. D
41. D
42. A
43. B
44. D
45. B
46. B
47. C
48. E
49. A
50. A

1. **A. An AFI of less than 5 cm is diagnostic of oligohydramnios. Late in pregnancy, unexplained oligohydramnios should prompt concern for placental insufficiency and nonreassuring fetal status. A stressed fetus shunts blood away from the kidneys and toward the brain, resulting in decreased renal perfusion, decreased urine production, and eventually oligohydramnios. A fetus with oligohydramnios at term should be delivered. Induction of labor is reasonable, although the fetus may not tolerate labor well.**

   B. Cesarean delivery is not necessary based on the finding of oligohydramnios alone. A positive contraction stress test, or fetal intolerance of labor, would prompt a recommendation for cesarean delivery.

   C, D. Bed rest and maternal hydration are thought to improve uterine perfusion, which in turn may improve fetal perfusion and amniotic fluid volume. Oligohydramnios may indicate nonreassuring fetal status and should indicate prompt delivery at term. These options might be employed if the fetus is premature.

   E. Waiting 1 week is not appropriate. Antepartum fetal testing is performed to identify the fetus at risk for intrauterine fetal demise or abnormal outcome.

2. **D. Amniotic fluid is produced primarily by the fetal kidneys and less by the fetal lungs. Thus renal agenesis leads to oligohydramnios or anhydramnios. Amniotic fluid provides an acoustic window for US, which is quite limited in the setting of anhydramnios or severe oligohydramnios. US with Doppler can be used to identify the renal arteries, which suggest the presence of kidneys. Absence of the renal arteries suggests absence of kidneys.**

   A. From the second trimester onward, fetal swallowing and urination result in continuous circulation of amniotic fluid. Disorders of the gastrointestinal tract, such as tracheoesophageal fistula, generally result in polyhydramnios, not oligohydramnios.

   B, E. Rh alloimmunization (known also as isoimmunization) leads to fetal hemolysis, anemia, and eventually fetal hydrops. This results in polyhydramnios rather than oligohydramnios.

   C. Uncontrolled gestational diabetes can be associated with fetal macrosomia and polyhydramnios similar to pregestational diabetes.

3. **C. Having one or more prior abortions is unlikely to be associated with an increased risk of adverse outcomes in subsequent pregnancies. A history of three or more induced abortions appears to be associated with pregnancy complications such as placental abruption, premature rupture of the membranes, low birth weight, preterm delivery, and bleeding in the first and third trimesters as compared to women with a history of two or fewer induced abortions.**

   A. Illegal abortions resulted in significant maternal mortality (some studies reported rates as high as 39% prior to legalization of abortion), but the rate was not as high as 52%. A mere 2 years after the *Roe v. Wade* decision in 1972, maternal mortality fell dramatically to 6%, largely due to increased access to procedures performed sterilely in adequate medical facilities by trained, accountable practitioners. Today, maternal mortality is close to zero in the United States in patients with no medical complications who undergo routine procedures.

   B. General anesthesia is rarely needed in pregnancy termination, except in cases of extreme anxiety, mental retardation, or psychotic disorders. While general anesthesia poses the greatest risk to a woman undergoing pregnancy termination, most such procedures are performed with the use of a paracervical block, often in combination with a sedative. Thus general anesthesia is not a major cause of mortality due to pregnancy termination.

   D. Laminaria, often composed of hygroscopic seaweed, are placed into the cervix to facilitate cervical dilation prior to the procedure. The laminaria take on liquid, which results in their expansion and gentle dilation of the cervix. Gradual dilation reduces the risk of cervical trauma and is safe for usage in both first- and second-trimester terminations.

   E. Medical termination is associated with more bleeding than surgical termination. However, overall blood loss from both procedures is low.

4. **A. Upon the diagnosis of intrauterine fetal demise (IUFD), immediate delivery is offered. Case reports do cite maternal coagulopathy developing in association with IUFD, but this complication has been shown to occur only when the IUFD took place 3 weeks or more beforehand. Many patients with IUFD may want to delay delivery for a few days to grieve prior to**

undergoing the stress of labor. As long as the risk of coagulopathy is explained to the patient and screened for, this is reasonable management. Occasionally, patients will not want to go through labor with an IUFD and will request a cesarean delivery. Because of the risks to the patient from cesarean delivery as well as its effects on all future pregnancies, this is not a reasonable course of action. Patients and their partners should be encouraged to name, hold, and view the demised fetus. At the time of delivery, a nurse or assistant may take the stillborn to another room to examine it and describe it to the family, especially if the stillborn is macerated or anomalous. He or she should then swaddle and place a hat on the stillborn, like a newborn, and, if the parents have agreed, bring it to them. Viewing, holding, and naming the baby have been shown to facilitate the grieving process. In the case of anomalous or macerated fetuses, studies have shown that the actual experience of viewing the baby is better than the nightmarish fantasies that people may otherwise have.

B. Fetal demise should be confirmed by a second person skilled in US. Both examiners should observe absence of fetal cardiac activity for at least 3 minutes. You appropriately asked your partner to confirm the diagnosis. A third US is not necessary. Note that if the patient had not had an US performed for anatomy, it would not be unreasonable to obtain an US to look for an anatomic cause for fetal demise (e.g., congenital abnormality or syndrome). However, the best way to identify such an etiology is with post-delivery exam by pathology.

C, D. See the explanation for A.

E. Amniocentesis may be performed most commonly in the second trimester for prenatal diagnosis to obtain fetal cells to perform a karyotype or other genetic tests. It is also performed later in pregnancy to assess fetal lung maturity. There would be no reason to obtain these tests at this point. However, a karyotype would be one aspect of the postpartum work-up of the IUFD.

5. **A. The incidence of perinatal mortality following minor trauma is 0.5%. Thus all seemingly minor traumas must be evaluated. The standard of care is to assess the fetal heart rate and tocometer for 4 to 6 hours following trauma, looking for contractions that may not be apparent to the patient, and performing fetal evaluation. Monitoring should be extended, with consideration for delivery, if the fetal testing is nonreassuring, there are signs of placental abruption, or the trauma is significant.**

B. A hematocrit will not be helpful in guiding management after this minor trauma. A Kleihauer-Betke test may be used to screen for fetal–maternal hemorrhage due to placental abruption. Pregnant women generally have a physiologic anemia, and a single hematocrit is not useful. In cases of severe trauma, serial hematocrits may be appropriate.

C. Placental abruption may develop over hours or even a couple of days. Thus, if the patient is discharged home after 4 hours of fetal monitoring, she should be advised to follow up for any symptoms of uterine contractions, abdominal pain, or decreased fetal movement. Before discharge home, however, the patient should be monitored as in the explanation for A.

D. If the patient was full term and her cervix was favorable, one could consider induction of labor after minor trauma, particularly if monitoring was nonreassuring. Rupture of membranes, when appropriate during induction, might reveal blood-tinged amniotic fluid following trauma. In the absence of concerning findings, however, rupture of membranes is inappropriate and the pregnancy should be continued and monitored as in the explanation for A.

E. The patient should be instructed to follow fetal kick counts if she is discharged home after at least 4 hours of monitoring. However, this is not the most appropriate initial step in management.

6. **B. Pregnant women are volume expanded and often manifest signs of shock after greater loss of volume as compared to nonpregnant women. Any trauma patient presenting with seizures should be treated with magnesium sulfate and assessed rapidly for preeclampsia. Women with eclampsia, especially if they are driving, may sustain significant trauma.**

A. US of the placenta identifies only 25% of abruptions, which must be quite large to be seen. Thus a normal US cannot be too reassuring. Abruptions are commonly identified retrospectively, after delivery of the placenta. Often, clinical decisions are guided by a suspicion for abruption based on symptoms and signs such as decreased fetal movement, nonreassuring fetal testing, and uterine contractions.

C. While a small subset of patients who suffer loss of consciousness (LOC) may need emergent cesarean delivery to enhance resuscitation, the best resuscitation for the fetus typically is to resuscitate the mother. Thus LOC alone is not an indication for emergent delivery.

D. The large gravid uterus impedes effective administration of CPR. Thus, if a pregnant patient in the third trimester requires CPR, generally an emergent cesarean delivery is required to improve the results of CPR.

E. The uterus and amniotic fluid protect the fetus during most blunt abdominal traumas. Thus injury to the fetus is rare.

7. C. One should have a low threshold to rule out rupture of membranes in any patient complaining of increased vaginal discharge. If missed, this condition may lead to significantly increased rates of infection and preterm delivery, in addition to potential loss of treatment options such as antibiotics and, if indicated, steroids for fetal lung maturity. The description of fluid "running down her legs" in this particular patient makes rupture of membranes the most likely etiology. A sterile speculum exam should be performed to examine the vagina for a "pool" of amnionic fluid, check the fluid's pH with nitrazine paper, and collect a small amount of fluid on a slide that should exhibit a ferning pattern when dried. If this patient does have rupture of membranes, the management would be immediate induction of labor to reduce the probability of maternal and neonatal infection.

A. Chlamydia should be screened for in a patient with the complaint of vaginal discharge. This is not the best answer to this question for two reasons: (1) The patient's complaint of watery discharge is less consistent with chlamydial infection and more consistent with rupture of membranes, bacterial vaginosis, trichomoniasis, or physiologic discharge. Generally, a chlamydial infection will lead to a more purulent discharge. (2) If this patient did rule out for rupture of membranes, a chlamydia DNA test has far higher sensitivity than a culture.

B. While the urine chlamydia test is a DNA test, it can be done after determining whether the patient has ruptured membranes, which is the more likely diagnosis.

D. Herpes infection generally presents with pain, burning or itching, and blistering lesions. It is not typically associated with increased vaginal discharge. If the patient has a history of herpes, one should have a low threshold for evaluation and culture, but this patient's symptoms do not suggest herpes.

E. In patients in whom the diagnosis of rupture of membranes is questionable, but the patient gives a very good history (as this patient does), it is reasonable to perform an US to look for amniotic fluid volume. In this patient, this step would be secondary to the primary diagnostic techniques for amnionic fluid leakage (i.e., sterile speculum exam).

8. E. The patient's symptoms and exam are consistent with an infected Bartholin's cyst, also called a Bartholin's abscess. The Bartholin's glands are found in the vulva, on both sides of the vaginal fourchette. They normally secrete mucin, which drains into the vagina. Obstruction of the duct leads to formation of a cyst. Infection of the cyst, or abscess formation, may occur rapidly. The infection tends to be polymicrobial, involving mixed bacterial organisms and sometimes *Neisseria gonorrhea.* A Bartholin's abscess must be drained. Drainage is accomplished with local anesthesia, a small incision, and drainage of the infected material. The abscess must be allowed to continue to drain. A Word catheter, with a balloon tip, may be placed to maintain patency of the abscess cavity.

A. A Bartholin's abscess is extremely uncomfortable, and the pain is immediately reduced significantly with drainage. Management with antibiotics alone is inappropriate. If the abscess is unrelated to *Neisseria gonorrhea*, the patient may not need antibiotics at all.

B. Hospitalization and treatment with IV antibiotics is unnecessary. Incision and drainage are most important, and likely curative.

C. A screen for STDs may be performed, but incision and drainage are the most important order of management. Bartholin's abscess was initially thought to be highly associated with *Neisseria gonorrhea*, but further data suggest that the association is not so strong.

D. Warm compresses will not help if the duct is blocked. In the days and weeks after the cyst has been incised, they may help to facilitate further drainage.

9. **B. Any woman of reproductive age with abnormal bleeding or spotting should be evaluated for pregnancy. Spotting can occur with implantation or—more concerning—can be a sign of ectopic pregnancy. If the patient is pregnant, she should be evaluated further with a pelvic US to confirm that the pregnancy is intrauterine and not ectopic.**

   A. Post-coital spotting can be a sign of cervical cancer, although cervical polyps or infections are more common. Patients should have Pap smears performed if they have not had one within the past year.
   C. Cervical cultures should also be sent, after the urine pregnancy test is performed.
   D. Pelvic US is not indicated, unless the patient is pregnant.
   E. A urinary tract infection may cause pink spotting, although this is rare.

10. **A. Midcycle spotting may be hormonal in origin, or may be caused by a lesion such as endometrial cancer, cervical or uterine polyps, or fibroids. Uterine cancer is often detected early because 90% of patients present with abnormal bleeding and can, therefore, be treated successfully. Women older than age 35 with unexplained, irregular bleeding should be evaluated by endometrial biopsy, with endocervical curettage.**

   B. While some patients with endometrial cancer will have abnormal Pap smears, most will have normal Pap smears. Regardless, the patient should be up-to-date on her Pap smears to ensure that she does not have cervical cancer.
   C. Cervicitis and STDs can cause abnormal cervical bleeding. However, the patient must first be evaluated for endometrial cancer.
   D. Pelvic US may add data on the thickness and contour of the endometrial stripe, suggesting a polyp or, especially among postmenopausal women, abnormal thickening. However, US is never diagnostic. In this case, tissue is important for diagnosis.
   E. Hysteroscopy, looking for polyps, fibroids, or locations for directed biopsies, should be considered if the endometrial biopsy is normal.

11. **C. Uterine fibroids may distort the uterine cavity, impairing implantation or causing infertility. This patient has achieved pregnancy twice. Fibroids may be associated with spontaneous abortion, preterm labor, and infertility. The patient is 39 years old and her fertility will likely decline rapidly. Given her history, myomectomy is a reasonable option.**

   A. Consideration of adoption is a personal issue and one that is often discussed with patients undergoing infertility treatments. While adoption should be considered, myomectomy is a reasonable option that should be offered to the patient.
   B. A gestational carrier is a woman who carries a pregnancy for another couple (a "surrogate mother"). The couple's own sperm and egg often create the pregnancy. This option is relevant to a woman who cannot carry a pregnancy, often because of anatomic problems such as cervical incompetence. Such an approach is controversial and often expensive. This patient's history does not suggest the need for a gestational carrier.
   D. ICSI is reserved for situations in which the sperm is qualitatively or quantitatively unlikely to enter the egg on its own. This couple has a normal semen analysis and, more importantly, has achieved two pregnancies without ICSI. Thus they do not need this technology.
   E. The patient has already been able to conceive, so IVF is unnecessary.

12. **B. LSC is the result of an irritant causing pruritis and subsequent mechanical irritation (scratching) that leads to epidermal hyperplasia. On exam, the area appears diffusely red with hyperplastic or hyperpigmented plaques. Treatment includes topical steroids and antipruritics.**

   A. Eczema does not commonly occur on the vulva; common locations include the antecubital fossa and hands.
   C. Lichen sclerosis is also characterized by vulvar pruritis and diffusely involves the vulva. In contrast to LSC, lesions are thin and whitish, commonly termed "onion skin" lesions. Furthermore, lichen sclerosis tends to occur in postmenopausal women, and occasionally in premenarchal girls, but rarely in women in their twenties. Treatment is topical steroids. This disorder poses no increased risk for vulvar carcinoma.
   D, E. Melanoma, squamous cell carcinoma, and basal cell carcinoma are the three most common vulvar cancers, but are certainly much less common than LSC, particularly in this age group.

13. **B. The incubation period for syphilis is 14 to 21 days. This patient has an early infection of syphilis with painless ulcerations on her labia. An ulcer or *chancre,* may occur on any mucosal surface, including the vulva, vagina, penis, cervix, anus, nipples, and lips.**

A. The treatment for early (less than 1 year) syphilis is a single intramuscular injection of benzathine penicillin. If syphilis has gone undetected for more than a year, three doses should be administered. Treatment for neurosyphilis includes aqueous crystalline penicillin G, 2–4 million units IV every 4 hours for nearly 2 weeks, followed by three weekly doses of benzathine penicillin.

C. Syphilis is caused by the spirochete *Treponema pallidum*.

D, E. Early syphilis can progress to secondary syphilis 1 to 3 months after initial infection as the chancres disappear and a characteristic maculopapular rash appears on the palms of the hands and soles of the feet. Syphilis, which is known as the "great imitator," may have a multitude of manifestations, including hepatitis, meningitis, and nephritis. If left untreated, the disease enters a latent phase, which is highly variable and may last for several years. The disease culminates in tertiary syphilis, which is characterized by skin gummas (granulomas), infection of the aorta (aortitis), and neurosyphilis with meningovascular disease, tabes dorsalis, and paresis. Notched teeth and saber shins are characteristics of neonatal syphilis rather than tertiary syphilis.

14. **A. In this patient with very uncertain dates, obtaining evidence of fetal lung maturity is essential before actively initiating delivery. Because of the increased risks of traumatic birth due to macrosomia, and higher rates of intrauterine fetal demise, patients with gestational diabetes treated with insulin are regularly induced at 39 to 40 weeks. If dating is certain, assessment of fetal lung maturity is not necessary so close to term. Importantly, organ development, including lung maturity, in fetuses of diabetic mothers is actually delayed. Biochemical evidence of fetal lung maturity (e.g., amniotic fluid lecithin:sphingomyelin ratio) is needed, as the risk of respiratory distress syndrome may outweigh the risk of continued gestation.**

B, C. An OGTT could formally establish a diagnosis of diabetes, which is hardly in question given the patient's extremely elevated fasting blood sugar. The HbA_{1c} level would allow assessment of blood glucose control over the last 1 to 2 months, and is almost certain to be elevated in this patient with untreated disease. Both measurements provide valuable information for the management of this patient, but neither will substantially alter obstetrical decisions made at this point. Blood sugars can be controlled with insulin, and the fetus should be delivered if fetal lung maturity is documented. Of note, although this patient does not give a history of overt diabetes, today's fasting glucose is highly suggestive of pregestational disease; the American Diabetes Association considers a fasting glucose level higher than 126 to be diagnostic of overt diabetes.

D. This patient's fetus is markedly macrosomic (more than 4500 g). Cervical exam would be critical if induction of labor for vaginal delivery was planned, but an estimated fetal weight exceeding 4500 g is an indication for cesarean delivery to avoid the incidence of shoulder dystocia and its sequelae.

E. Quantitative β-hCG would not be useful in managing this patient (although it should be noted for screening purposes that β-hCG is decreased in pregnancies complicated by diabetes).

15. **A. Without significant proteinuria, this patient does not have evidence of preeclampsia. Thus, if no other etiology for her hypertension is identified, discharge home with oral hypertensives may be appropriate. Labetolol and Aldomet are generally considered first-line therapy in this situation. Aldomet (methyldopa) enjoys the benefit of the most clinical experience and is thought to be very safe, but is not a very effective antihypertensive. Labetolol is the beta blocker of choice in pregnancy, is more effective than Aldomet, and is also considered safe (there is some suggestion of intrauterine growth restriction with atenolol). Another agent that is increasingly used but is not an answer choice here is nifedipine, a calcium-channel blocker.**

B, D. ACE inhibitors are contraindicated in pregnancy because of evidence for fetal renal toxicity when given in the second and third trimesters. Similarly, angiotensin receptor blockers are contraindicated in pregnancy.

C. Magnesium sulfate is used in preeclampsia for seizure prophylaxis; it does *not* treat hypertension.

E. Diuretics are generally avoided in pregnancy due to concerns about intravascular volume depletion. They are not absolutely contraindicated, but better options for control of hypertension exist.

16. **E. Gestational hypertension is a retrospective diagnosis, in which hypertension in pregnancy is not preceded by pregestational (chronic) hypertension and does not result in significant proteinuria (and thus is not a form of preeclampsia). As long as BPs normalize by 12 weeks postpartum, the patient can be reassured that she does not have chronic hypertension.**

A, B. The diagnosis of preeclampsia requires proteinuria (300 mg on 24-hour collection) or repeated spot urine protein (more than 30 mg/dL, equivalent to 1+). Although urine protein can fluctuate, this patient was never observed to have significant proteinuria.

C, D. Chronic hypertension is defined as hypertension preceding pregnancy, or hypertension measured at less than 20 weeks GA. Chronic hypertension puts patients at increased risk for preeclampsia. This patient has evidence of neither chronic hypertension nor preeclampsia.

17. **A. Classification of ovarian neoplasms is based on the cell of origin: surface epithelial, germ, or sex-cord stromal cells. Epithelial cell tumors are the most common (90% of malignant ovarian tumors and 65% to 70% of all ovarian tumors). Major categories of epithelial tumors include serous and mucinous tumors, endometrioid clear cell, undifferentiated carcinoma, and Brenner tumor.**

B. While epithelial cell tumors can affect women age 20 and older, they are most frequently observed among women in their late fifties.

C, D. Germ cell tumors include teratomas, dysgerminomas, endodermal sinus tumors, and choriocarcinoma. They generally affect girls and women of 0 to 25 years of age. Like all tumors, however, they may be seen at any age.

E. The major types of sex-cord stromal tumors include granulosa-theca and Sertoli-Leydig cell tumors as well as gonadoblastomas.

18. **E. Immature teratoma, a germ cell tumor, is derived from embryonic (fetal) tissue. In both types of teratomas, fat, hair, and bone can be seen. In Figure 2-18, hair can be seen consistent with a teratoma (most likely a mature teratoma).**

A. Dysgerminomas arise from the undifferentiated germ cells.

B. Embryonal carcinoma includes the embryonic, yolk sac, and placental cell lines.

C. Endodermal sinus tumor arises from extraembryonic (yolk sac) tissue.

D. Choriocarcinoma arises from trophoblastic (placental) tissue.

19. **A. Dysgerminoma, a germ cell tumor of the ovary predominantly affecting girls and young women, is remarkable for its secretion of LDH as a tumor marker. Patients commonly present with a rapidly enlarging adnexal mass and abdominal pain.**

B. Embryonal carcinomas may produce AFP, as well as hCG and CA-125.

C. Endodermal sinus tumors may produce AFP.

D. Choriocarcinoma is a germ cell tumor and also a form of gestational trophoblastic disease that secretes hCG.

E. Immature teratoma or immature dermoid cysts may produce CA-125.

20. **A. A "radical" mastectomy entails en bloc resection of the anterior chest, including resection of breast tissue, nipple-areolar complex, overlying skin, axillary lymph nodes, and pectoralis muscles; it is termed "modified" when the pectoralis major is spared. The modified radical mastectomy is often the procedure chosen for node-positive disease, as it offers cosmetic advantages with equivalent disease-free and overall survival rates.**

B. Total (simple) mastectomy includes resection of breast tissue, nipple-areolar complex, and overlying skin, but spares lymph nodes. It is often used for ductal carcinoma in situ (DCIS) or lobular carcinoma in situ (LCIS). When combined with radiation therapy, results are comparable to those achieved with radical procedures for these localized malignancies. Total mastectomy is not appropriate for node-positive disease.

C. Subcutaneous mastectomy includes resection of breast tissue only, sparing the nipple-areolar complex, skin, and lymph nodes. It is not indicated for treatment of breast cancer.

D. See the explanation for A.

E. Wide local excision entails breast-conserving removal of the tumor ("local") with tumor-free margins ("wide"). Appropriate candidates for this procedure are patients who have tumors smaller than 4 cm, no fixation to muscle or the chest wall, no involvement of the overlying skin, no multicentric lesions, and no fixed lymph nodes. This patient is not an appropriate candidate.

21. **B. Younger women with more aggressive tumors generally respond best to chemotherapy, especially if the tumor is hormone receptor negative (as in this patient). The standard adjuvant treatment for node-positive premenopausal women includes 6 months of CMF combination therapy, regardless of hormone-receptor status.**

A. Hormonal therapy is less effective in hormone-receptor–negative tumors, but some response is seen. Hormonal therapy may, in fact, be the preferred choice for an older patient prioritizing quality of life in the short term, as these agents are better tolerated than chemotherapeutic agents and are often better for palliative therapy.

C. Strontium is sometimes used as a bone-targeting isotope for multifocal bone metastases. This patient shows no evidence of bone metastases.

D. Herceptin is a monoclonal antibody directed against the c-erbB-2 signal transduction protein. This patient does not overexpress this protein and is unlikely to benefit from this therapy.

E. See the explanation for B.

22. **D. Medullary carcinoma is more frequent in younger patients and, despite being rather aggressive, carries a relatively favorable prognosis. Tubular carcinoma and mucinous (colloid) carcinoma are other, less common subtypes that carry better prognoses than intraductal carcinoma.**

A, B. Tumors that are positive for hormone receptors carry more favorable prognoses.

C. Aneuploid tumors with a high S-phase fraction tend to be more aggressive and carry poorer prognoses than diploid tumors with a low S-phase fraction. It should be noted that tumor stage is more predictive than histology in determining prognosis.

E. Premenopausal women tend to have more aggressive disease and higher associated mortality.

23. **D. The TNM system stages breast malignancies by the size of the primary tumor (T), regional nodal involvement (N), and distant metastases (M). This patient has a tumor larger than 2 cm but smaller than 5 cm (T2), metastases to the axillary lymph nodes that are fixed (N2), and no evidence of distant metastasis (M0). This corresponds to stage grouping IIIa.**

A, B, C, E. See the explanation for D and Table 2-23.

24. **E. This young woman has PID. She should be admitted to the hospital and receive intravenous antibiotics as she is *unable to tolerate oral medications* and has failed outpatient management. She has many risk factors for PID, including some of the following: age (15- to 19-year-old age group), early onset of sexual activity, and multiple partners. Other risk factors may include partner infection with gonorrhea or chlamydia, personal history of recurrent STDs, personal history of PID, douching, and even cigarette smoking, all of which have all been shown to increase the risk of contracting PID. Barrier contraception appears to be protective against PID.**

A. If this patient does not improve within 24 to 48 hours with IV antibiotics, a pelvic US may be obtained to diagnose tubo-ovarian abscess(es), but is unnecessary at this point.

B. A urine pregnancy test routinely can detect an elevated serum β-hCG of 20 or more, so obtaining a serum β-hCG is not necessary in this case. In the future, secondary to this episode of PID, the patient is at risk for ectopic pregnancy (as well as infertility and pelvic pain).

C. This patient is not a candidate for outpatient management of her infection. She has failed an outpatient regimen due to noncompliance and is ***unable to tolerate oral medications.*** Other contraindications to outpatient management would include pregnancy, an immunocompromised state, a pelvic abscess, or a patient with a surgical abdomen.

D. Laparoscopy has been used as the "gold standard" to make the diagnosis of PID in small clinical studies. However, it is rarely used in this way because of the risks of surgery. Laparoscopy would be reasonable in a patient with a tubo-ovarian abscess that is resistant to intravenous antibiotics or that has ruptured.

TABLE 2-23 TNM Classification of Breast Cancer

T: Primary Tumor	
T_x	Primary tumor unassessable
T_0	No evidence of primary tumor
T_{is}	Carcinoma in situ
T_1	<2 cm
T_2	>2 cm, <5 cm
T_3	>5 cm
T_4	Any tumor extending to the chest wall or skin
N: Regional Lymph Nodes	
N_x	Regional lymph nodes cannot be assessed
N_0	No regional lymph node metastases
N_1	Metastasis to mobile ipsilateral axillary node
N_2	Metastasis to ipsilateral axillary node, fixed
N_3	Metastasis to ipsilateral internal mammary node
M: Distant Metastases	
M_x	Presence of distant metastasis cannot be assessed
M_0	No evidence of distant metastasis
M_1	Distant metastasis

25. **C. The patient has post-IUD insertion endometritis or an infection of the endometrium. When the infection spreads into the myometrium, it is called endomyometritis. There is considerable overlap with the diagnosis of PID—only the clinical situation differentiates them. Risk factors include instrumentation of some type such as IUD insertion, D&C or D&E, normal spontaneous vaginal delivery, or cesarean section. In addition to pain and tenderness, affected patients often have a fever and leukocytosis. The best course of management is removal of the IUD and antibiotics. The antibiotics of choice are identical to those used to treat PID.**

    A. This patient does not have any contraindications for outpatient management of endometritis, and it is safe to treat her with an outpatient regimen. The CDC currently recommends the following: oral ofloxacin (400 mg PO BID) or levofloxacin (500 mg PO QD) with or without metronidazole (500 mg PO BID); another regimen involves ceftriaxone (250 mg IM once) or cefoxitin (2 g IM once) plus probenecid (1 g PO once) followed by doxycycline (100 mg PO BID) with or without metronidazole (500 mg PO BID). This treatment should last 14 days.

    B. Oral antibiotics are appropriate only after the foreign body is removed.

    D. Repeat cultures are unlikely to be positive and would not change the management. Additionally, the treatment you provide would eradicate any gonorrhea and chlamydia present. This infection likely resulted from contamination of the IUD with bacteria from the vagina or cervix. NSAIDs would be helpful for pain management.

    E. The patient is not likely to be pregnant. A pregnancy test is usually obtained at insertion time. Additionally, she reports no intercourse in more than 4 weeks. It is important to remember that if she does get pregnant, she is at increased risk for an ectopic pregnancy.

26. **B. Emergency contraception formulations have a relative failure rate of approximately 25%. Therefore, these pills decrease a woman's absolute pregnancy risk from 8% to 2%. Progestin-only pills fare slightly better, having a relative failure rate of 11%. The most common side effect of either regimen is nausea, although the side-effect rate is much higher with preparations including estrogen.**

    A. Any of the emergency contraception types can be used up to 72 hours after the time of unprotected sexual intercourse.
    C. Emergency contraception can be obtained from a variety of sources, including primary care doctors, pharmacists, local community clinics, and Internet Web sites.
    D. Numerous studies have shown that OCPs taken inadvertently during pregnancy pose no threat to the developing embryo. This is generally believed to be true regarding emergency contraception as well.
    E. Prior use of an IUD has no bearing on the effectiveness of emergency contraception.

27. **C. The patient has a tissue diagnosis and needs treatment for her disease. The appropriate treatment is a LEEP. This patient is not a candidate for cryotherapy (see the explanation for E).**

    A. A hysterectomy is too aggressive and not warranted given the pathology report.
    B. A colposcopy is generally considered a diagnostic tool as opposed to a treatment for dysplasia and is not the standard of care after a tissue diagnosis of HSIL.
    D. This patient does not need radiation therapy. Radiation therapy is the mainstay treatment for bulky advanced disease, not disease that is confined to the cervix.
    E. This patient is not a candidate for cryotherapy because the transformation zone was not visualized in its entirety at the time of colposcopy; thus the patient needs a LEEP. A colposcopy is termed "satisfactory" only if the entire TZ is visualized. An "unsatisfactory" colposcopy is one of the three indications for a LEEP as opposed to cryotherapy; the other two are a positive ECC and a two-step discrepancy between the Pap smear and biopsy results.

28. **C. Fetal kidneys are examined on a routine obstetric US. Of note, renal pelvis dilation has been associated with aneuploidy and urinary obstruction. A Level I US usually includes location of pregnancy (i.e., intrauterine versus ectopic), location of placenta, amniotic fluid assessment, fetal lie, fetal biometric data for dating, and basic fetal anatomy. The anatomy scan routinely identifies cerebral landmarks such as the ventricles, thalamus, cerebellar hemispheres and posterior fossa, four-chamber view of the heart, stomach, spine, kidneys, bladder, and umbilical cord insertion.**

    A. Examining fetal extremities is not a part of the routine Level I US.
    B. Despite the fact that many patients hope to find out fetal gender at the 18- to 22-week Level I US, it may be easily disclosed in only 80% to 90% of cases, and is not a component of the routine obstetric US.
    D. While an image of the umbilical cord insertion into the fetal abdomen is important to rule out omphalocele, its insertion into the placenta is not a routine component of the obstetric US.
    E. The fetal face is not a routine component of the Level I obstetric US.

29. **E. D&E is most appropriate for this patient. It involves serial dilation of the cervix, followed by manual removal of fetal parts and placenta using specialized forceps and suction, as well as sharp curettage of the uterus. D&E is very effective for mid-trimester pregnancies up to 18 weeks GA, and can be done on an outpatient basis with less invasive anesthesia. While risks for adverse events including hemorrhage, perforation, and infection exist, this method has proven to be safest among the mid-trimester abortion methods such as vaginal prostaglandins or hypertonic saline instillation.**

    A. Suction curettage involves the use of a cannula attached to pump suction that is placed in the uterine cavity to suction out intrauterine contents. It usually requires a small amount of cervical dilation and is the most widely used method of induced abortion in the world. It has a very low risk of adverse events. However, sole use of this method is generally effective only in pregnancies up to approximately 12 weeks GA, after which time D&E is usually necessary.

B. Placement of prostaglandins such as prostaglandin E_2 in the vagina causes abortion via labor induction. The agent is administered every 3 to 4 hours until delivery has occurred. This procedure is appropriate for mid-trimester abortions, but is more time-consuming and associated with higher maternal morbidity than D&E.
C. Menstrual regulation involves the aspiration of endometrium within 14 days of a missed period or by 42 days after the beginning of the LMP. This safe and quick procedure can be done in the doctor's office, usually without anesthesia. It is a reliable and relatively inexpensive means of abortion. However, it must be done almost immediately after pregnancy is suspected to be effective, and is therefore not applicable to this patient.
D. Hysterectomy is not a method of pregnancy termination, particularly in this young patient who will likely desire preservation of fertility. Also, hysterectomy is generally not indicated in any patient unless other attempts at mid-trimester abortion have failed or the patient suffers from comorbid conditions, such as cervical stenosis, that would be satisfactorily addressed with hysterectomy.

30. **E. The copper-T IUD is the safest form of contraception for this patient. Given her need for long-term contraception, she would benefit most from a method that does not involve daily interventions. Of the two listed (Depo-Provera and the copper-T IUD), the IUD has not been associated with mood disturbances, likely because it is a physical device as opposed to a hormonal barrier. Depo-Provera, by contrast, utilizes hormonal agents and has been associated with depressive symptoms. This association is especially prominent among women with a history of postpartum depression, although any history of mood disorders warrants avoidance of Depo-Provera as a contraceptive method.**

A. See the explanation for E.
B. Given her smoking history and age greater than 35 years, combination OCPs are contraindicated in this patient, as they significantly raise the risk of DVT, pulmonary embolism, and stroke. Daily regimens increase the chance of missed doses, and because this patient will presumably not want a quick reversal of contraception in the future, there is no need to keep that as an option. With proper use, however, combination OCPs offer the best protection overall, with a theoretical failure rate of 0.1%.
C. Progestin-only OCPs are even more restrictive than combination OCPs, needing to be taken within a very specific time window every day to work. Also, their failure rate is higher—0.5%.
D. The diaphragm is similarly a *daily affair,* and the failure rate is quite high at 6%.

31. **E. Impaired hepatic function is considered an absolute contraindication to combination OCPs. Other absolute contraindications include thrombophlebitis, cerebral/coronary vascular disease, hyperlipidemia, undiagnosed vaginal bleeding, smoking if greater than 35 years old, pregnancy, known or suspected breast cancer, and hepatic neoplasm.**

A. Vascular disease mediated by diabetes mellitus (DM) can be exacerbated by combination OCPs; in patients younger than 35, however, the risks of pregnancy outweigh the risks of this potential vascular pathology. Thus DM is only a relative contraindication in this case.
B. HTN is only a relative contraindication. If the patient is younger than 35 and her BP is well controlled, the benefits of contraception outweigh risks.
C. In the past, fibroids were considered a contraindication; however, modern combination OCPs have sufficiently low doses of estrogen to render fibroid growth unaffected.
D. Only a personal history of breast cancer is a contraindication. Family history is not considered to be a contraindication.

32. **A. This patient presents with metastatic choriocarcinoma. Appropriate treatment for patients without "poor prognosis" risk factors is single-agent chemotherapy. Choriocarcinoma is a malignant, necrotizing tumor arising from trophoblastic tissue. It is often rapidly metastatic, spreading hematogenously to the lungs (most commonly) and also to the vagina, pelvis, brain, liver, and kidneys. Left untreated, this rapid metastasis can result in death within months. Fortunately, like other forms of gestational trophoblastic disease (GTD), choriocarcinoma is exquisitely sensitive to chemotherapy. Single-agent therapy is indicated for patients with nonmetastatic disease and**

patients with metastatic disease with no "poor prognosis" risk factors. Choriocarcinoma is one of the few malignancies where single-agent therapy remains the standard of care in modern medicine. It is important to note that only 50% of choriocarcinomas develop after a preceding molar pregnancy; 25% follow normal term pregnancy, and 25% follow ectopic pregnancy or abortion.

B. Multiple-agent chemotherapy is indicated for patients with metastatic choriocarcinoma and "poor prognosis" risk factors—namely, duration of disease greater than 4 months, serum β-hCG greater than 40,000, metastasis to the brain or liver, choriocarcinoma following term pregnancy, or unsuccessful single-agent chemotherapy. This patient does not have any of these risk factors.

C. Hysterectomy has a very limited role in choriocarcinoma, as the tumor is highly sensitive to chemotherapy and is often metastatic. Hysterectomy is an option only for patients who do not desire future fertility and who show no evidence of metastatic disease, but it results in a higher complication rate. This procedure is the treatment of choice for placental-site trophoblastic tumors, which are extremely rare tumors arising from the placental implantation site. Surgery is indicated for these patients because the tumor is poorly responsive to chemotherapy and rarely metastatic.

D, E. Because GTD is sensitive to chemotherapy and often metastatic, surgical intervention and radiation do not generally play a role in its treatment.

33. **E. Treatment of molar pregnancy consists of immediate evacuation of the uterus, followed by monitoring for persistent trophoblastic proliferation by serial β-hCG levels. This follow-up period should last at least one year, during which time reliable contraception is required to allow accurate measurement. The method of contraception is not critical, but OCPs offer the advantages of high efficacy and low incidence of irregular bleeding (which could be confused with persistent disease).**

A. While it is true that the risk of GTD in future pregnancies is higher for this patient than for members of the general population (about 1% versus 0.1%), prompt diagnosis has reduced the mortality from molar pregnancies to near zero and morbidity to an acceptable level. The risk is not considered sufficiently high to discourage future pregnancy beyond the period required for monitoring of β-hCG levels.

B. Patients who are cured of molar pregnancy have no increase in the rate of spontaneous abortions, complications, or congenital malformations in future (nonmolar) pregnancies.

C, D. The risk of persistent and/or malignant trophoblastic disease is estimated at about 5% for a partial (incomplete) mole and 20% for a complete mole. OCPs do not reduce this risk (in fact, a weak association may exist between OCP use and persistent disease).

34. **A. Roughly 5% of all pregnancies are complicated by asymptomatic bacteriuria of more than 100,000 colonies on culture. The incidence of asymptomatic bacteriuria during pregnancy is similar to that for the nonpregnant population. During pregnancy, however, urinary stasis increases due to progesterone-induced relaxation of the ureters and bladder, and direct obstruction by the uterus. Consequently, pregnant women with untreated asymptomatic bacteriuria are more likely to develop UTIs, cystitis, and, most seriously, pyelonephritis. In 15% of pregnant patients with pyelonephritis, severe complications occur such as bacteremia, sepsis, and adult respiratory distress syndrome (ARDS). Because asymptomatic bacteriuria can progress to severe infection in the pregnant patient, it should be evaluated further—in this case, with a urine culture.**

B. Symptoms of UTI during pregnancy may be somewhat nonspecific. Increased blood flow to the bladder and pressure from the uterus cause most pregnant women to experience frequency and sometimes urgency. Pregnant women may develop pyelonephritis without any preceding symptoms of UTI.

C. Vaginal flora and discharge may explain the urine dip results. Treating all patients presumptively with antibiotics will lead to increased microbial resistance, allergic reactions, and maternal side effects. Patients with a history of pyelonephritis, urologic surgery, or frequent UTIs may require suppressive therapy during pregnancy.

D. To ignore a urine dip suggestive of a UTI might result in progression of asymptomatic bacteriuria to pyelonephritis.
E. There is no indication for renal biopsy in this situation.

35. **E. The patient has clear signs of chorioamnionitis, or infection of the chorion and amnion. Chorioamnionitis is the most common cause of neonatal sepsis, which poses a significant risk for neonatal death or cerebral palsy. Given the signs and the risks, and despite the early GA, the patient should be delivered. The patient should also be treated with intravenous fluids, Tylenol, and broad-spectrum antibiotics that include coverage for group B *Streptococcus.***

A. Cesarean section in this setting should be reserved for a persistently nonreassuring fetal heart tracing, malpresentation, or failed induction. A cesarean section in the setting of chorioamnionitis is associated with increased postpartum complications such as wound infection, abscess, and fistula formation.
B. The patient should receive antibiotics, but observation in the setting of diagnosed chorioamnionitis is inappropriate.
C. Amniocentesis for culture is sometimes performed when the diagnosis is unclear. In this case, the patient clearly has chorioamnionitis. Amniocentesis for culture would merely waste critical time.
D. The tampon dye test involves the placement of a tampon in the vagina with injection of indigo carmine into the amniotic cavity; the tampon is removed 1 hour later. Blue dye on the tampon confirms rupture of membranes. In this patient's case, the diagnosis of ruptured membranes has already been made by history, the ferning pattern caused by the high sodium concentration in the amniotic fluid, the nitrazine test, and the oligohydramnios, making the tampon dye test unnecessary.

36. **B. The patient's symptoms are concerning for ruptured membranes, the most ominous of the possibilities suggested by the tests. Some patients leak fluid slowly after membrane rupture; as such, any patient complaining of vaginal wetness should be evaluated for membrane rupture. A sterile speculum must be used to reduce the risk of infection if the membranes have indeed ruptured. A pool of fluid may not be seen if the patient has a high leak or oligohydramnios. Fluid loss may be provoked by asking the patient to cough during the exam. Amniotic fluid contains a high concentration of sodium, which crystallizes on a slide when it dries, creating a fern-like pattern. Amniotic fluid is basic and should turn pH paper blue. If all tests are negative, and the suspicion for ruptured membranes is high, an US should be performed to check the amniotic fluid index. A tampon dye test may be performed if the suspicion for rupture is high but the above-mentioned tests are negative.**

A. Observation at home when rupture of membranes is suggested by history is inappropriate following initial evaluation, and inappropriate management if rupture is confirmed and the fetus is viable.
C. In addition to evaluation for ruptured membranes, the patient should be checked with a wet prep to rule out bacterial vaginosis or a candidal infection. Either could explain her symptoms.
D. A Group B *Streptococcus* culture is appropriate for any patient at risk for preterm delivery. In this case, however, one must first assess membrane status.
E. US may be performed to assess fluid as part of the evaluation for ruptured membranes. First, however, one must perform a sterile speculum exam to assess for leakage of fluid.

37. **E. This patient has been exposed to VZV, or chickenpox, and is at risk because she may not have had the disease before. Chickenpox during pregnancy can be severe, carrying as high as a 25% risk of maternal mortality should varicella pneumonia develop. If the patient contracts varicella infection 5 days before or after delivery, the neonate is at risk for life-threatening neonatal varicella infection. This patient is within 72 hours of the time of exposure, so she may benefit from VZIG if she has never had varicella. Fortunately, 70% to 90% of patients who think they have never had chickenpox show detectable antibodies, and thus do not need VZIG. Rapid VZV screening for prior exposure is available. The patient should go to an area of the ED designated for patients with exposures to potentially infectious diseases and have a VZV titer drawn. If the titer is negative, she should return later in the day for VZIG. You should call the ED and alert them that she is coming.**

A. The patient must be advised to avoid the clinic, where she could potentially infect other pregnant women.
B. While the patient qualifies for VZIG because she is within the 72-hour window, she may not need passive immunity if she has previously had the disease. A rapid VZV titer should be drawn prior to VZIG administration.
C. Oral acyclovir, when administered within 24 hours of the appearance of the rash, may reduce the duration of new lesion formation and the total number of lesions. Oral acyclovir is safe in pregnancy and may provide symptomatic relief. It does not reduce the risk of vertical transmission. This patient is not clearly infected with varicella and prescription of acyclovir is premature.
D. VZIG should be given to infants born to women who develop a varicella infection between 5 days prior to and 2 days after delivery. If this patient develops varicella infection and delivers within 5 days, the pediatrician needs to be alerted and the infant prophylaxed.

38. **C. The RPR and the VDRL are both nonspecific antibody screening tests for *T. pallidum*, or syphilis. Diagnosis is confirmed with either the more specific microhemagglutination assay for antibodies to *T. pallidum* (MHA-TP) or the fluorescent treponemal antibody-absorption (FTA-ABS) technique. Nonspecific screening tests such as the RPR or the VDRL yield many false-positives and must be followed with confirmatory testing before action is taken. In this case, sending an MHA-TP is appropriate. Because congenital syphilis can be quite severe and treatment for syphilis is available, this infection is screened for universally in pregnancy.**

A, B. Patients with rheumatologic disease may falsely screen positive for syphilis and are sometimes identified this way. This patient's intermittent arthritis and fatigue are somewhat nonspecific, and she may merit further evaluation for rheumatologic disease. However, evaluation for syphilis is the most appropriate next step.
D. Confirmatory testing is needed prior to treatment, with the possible exception of a case involving a highly noncompliant patient at high risk for syphilis (e.g., with a known positive partner).
E. Rather than repeat a nonspecific test, one should send the more specific confirmatory test. Repeating the RPR merely wastes time. A negative result would not erase the fact that the first test was positive and would simply raise concerns for a false-negative or a lab error.

39. **B. Domestic violence increases during pregnancy, and occurs in 4% to 8% of pregnancies. The perpetrator is usually a current or prior intimate partner. A controlling partner and multiple somatic complaints may be present. Domestic violence often goes unrecognized, and universal screening must be undertaken. This patient's frequent, nonspecific complaints suggest that she is reaching out for help. She needs to be asked about domestic violence in a supportive manner. Studies have shown that most women support and appreciate universal inquiry about domestic violence. Examples of screening questions include the following:**

- **Has anyone close to you ever threatened to hurt you?**
- **Have you ever been afraid of your partner?**
- **Do you feel safe at home?**
- **Has anyone ever hit, kicked, choked, or hurt you physically?**
- **Has anyone, including your partner, ever forced you to have sex?**

A. The biophysical profile is typically used to follow up a nonreactive NST.
C. The patient should be asked about her weight gain in a supportive manner. The Institute of Medicine recommends that normal-weight women gain between 25 and 35 lb during pregnancy. Maternal weight gain often occurs most rapidly during the third trimester.
D, E. There is no indication for US or weekly nonstress tests at this point.

40. **D. In addition to breast enlargement, the patient has a secondary mound caused by projection of the areola and papilla. This is characteristic of Tanner stage 4 (see Figure 2-40a). In addition, her pubic hair appears mid-escutcheon, characteristic of Tanner stage 4. The patient's exam suggests the presence of circulating estrogens, as well as normal anatomy, both of which are important in the evaluation of primary amenorrhea.**

A, B, C, E. Preadolescent breasts, with elevation of the papilla only, characterize Tanner stage 1. Pubic hair is absent. Breast buds characterize Tanner stage 2. The breast and papilla are elevated, and the areola is engorged. Presexual axillary and pubic hair may be present. Tanner stage 3 is characterized by further development of breast size, without separation in contour from the breast and the areola. Axillary and sexual pubic hair may be present. Tanner stage 5 is the mature stage. The breasts have an adult contour, with recession of the areola. Axillary hair and a female escutcheon are present (Figure 2-40b).

41. D. The most common cause of secondary amenorrhea is pregnancy. This patient reports that she's never been sexually active, and her urine pregnancy test is negative. The patient is extremely thin, and she must be evaluated for anorexia nervosa. Weight loss, anorexia nervosa, stress, and exercise can all cause hypothalamic dysfunction and disruption in the pulsatile secretion of GnRH, resulting in hypogonadotropic hypogonadism. Most adolescents experience some degree of hypothalamic amenorrhea during the first few years after menarche.

A. Cervical stenosis can lead to secondary amenorrhea and is usually caused by scarring of the cervical os as a result of obstetric trauma or surgery; this patient has had neither.

B. Asherman's syndrome is the presence of intrauterine synechiae or adhesions and is usually caused by infection or surgery. D&C, cesarean section, myomectomy, and endometritis, which are not part of this patient's history, may lead to Asherman's syndrome.

C. POF is defined by menopause that occurs before age 40. Chromosomal analysis is sent before the age of 35 to rule out a genetic basis for POF. It may result from radiation, chemotherapy, infection, or ovarian surgery, but is most often idiopathic. While it is a possible diagnosis in this case, the patient has no other symptoms of menopause, and POF is not the most likely diagnosis.

E. PCOS, originally described as Stein-Leventhal syndrome, represents a spectrum of disease characterized by oligomenorrhea and some degree of chemical or clinical androgenization. While it is a possible diagnosis in this case, the patient has no evidence of androgenization, and it is not the most likely diagnosis.

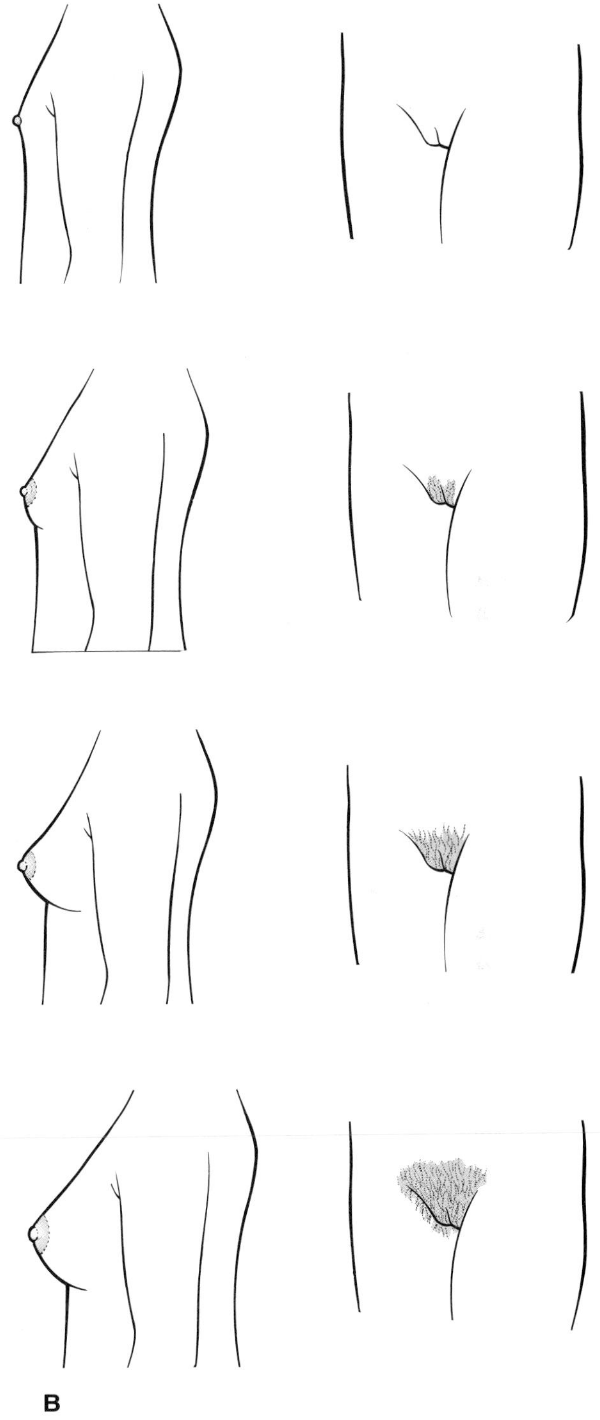

Figure 2-40B • Reproduced from Callahan T, Caughey AB. Blueprints Obstetrics & Gynecology, 4e. Baltimore: Lippincott Williams & Wilkins, 2007. Figs. 20-2 and 20-3.

42. A. Metronidazole (Flagyl), dosed orally at 2 g once, is often sufficient treatment for *Trichomonas vaginalis,* the infection from which this patient suffers. The presence of actively moving, flagellated organisms seen on wet prep is diagnostic of *Trichomonas* infection.

B. Partners must always be treated or they will continue to pass the infection back and forth to each other.
C. Alternative treatment for *Trichomonas* infection includes azithromycin (Zithromax) at 1 g orally given once.
D. Any patient diagnosed with an STD is at risk for all STDs and needs full screening.
E. Diagnosis of *Trichomonas vaginalis* infection can be made based on wet prep alone. A culture is unnecessary when the wet prep is positive, and may result in delayed treatment or lost treatment opportunity.

43. B. This patient's presentation strongly suggests cervicitis, and not PID, likely caused by infection with *Neisseria gonorrhoeae* (GC) or *Chlamydia trachomatis* (CT). GC can be treated by a single dose of ceftriaxone; CT can be treated with either a single dose of azithromycin (1 g) or a 7-day course of doxycycline. Some small studies support a 2 g dose to treat GC as well as CT. If left untreated, cervicitis may progress to PID. The three major criteria used to diagnose PID are abdominal pain, adnexal pain, and cervical motion tenderness; this patient has only cervical motion tenderness. Hospitalization and treatment with IV antibiotics would constitute overtreatment and are not indicated in the setting of uncomplicated cervicitis. Cervical cultures should be performed prior to presumptive treatment. The patient's partner also needs treatment. In addition, this patient should be counseled to use condoms because of their relative protection against STDs, and she should be offered full STD screening, including an HIV test. Among sexually active women, 20- to 24-year-olds have the highest prevalence of gonococcal and chlamydial infections.

A. While ceftriaxone covers GC, it does not cover CT adequately, and these infections can often occur together.
C. Doxycycline does not adequately cover GC.
D. As noted in the explanation for B, a 2g regimen has some coverage for GC, but a 1 g dose is not the standard recommended regimen to cover GC.
E. IV cefoxitin and doxycycline are appropriate for inpatient treatment of PID.

44. D. Uterine fibroids are the sole cause of infertility in 2% to 10% of cases. Fibroid-related infertility may be due to distortion of the endocervical canal, endometrial cavity, or fallopian tubes, which interferes with conception or implantation and may cause spontaneous abortion.

A. An estimated 20% to 30% of American women develop fibroids by age 40, and 50% to 65% have no clinical symptoms. The most common symptom is abnormal vaginal bleeding, as seen in this patient. Pressure-related symptoms are relatively common as well. Symptoms generally depend on the location of the fibroids. In this patient, the posterior location of her fairly large fibroid has also caused dyspareunia and constipation.
B. Studies suggest that the degeneration of a fibroid to a leiomyosarcoma occurs rarely, on the order of 1 in 1000 cases. Rapidly enlarging fibroids in women who are postmenopausal or who have uncertain diagnoses are causes for concern. The decision to perform myomectomy, however, is often not based on a concern for malignant potential.
C. Estrogen stimulates fibroid growth, causing some fibroids to increase significantly during pregnancy and to regress after menopause. Fibroid growth during pregnancy may cause infarction and severe pain as a fibroid outgrows its blood supply. Fibroids may also cause intrauterine growth restriction (IUGR), uterine distortion causing fetal malpresentation, preterm labor, and dystocia, or blockage of the presenting part necessitating a cesarean section.
E. African American women have three to nine times the incidence of uterine fibroids as compared to Hispanic, Asian, and Caucasian women.

45. B. CIN II, or moderate dysplasia, also described as high-grade squamous intraepithelial lesion (HSIL), may progress to cervical cancer if left untreated. Destruction or excision of the lesion is needed. The endocervical curettage was performed to assess the endocervical canal, which cannot be viewed during colposcopy. This patient has no abnormal tissue identified by endocervical curettage. Her lesions are small, non-invasive, and confined to the exocervix, making her a candidate for cryotherapy or laser therapy. She will still require follow-up. See Table 2-45.

TABLE 2-45 Management of Abnormal Pap Smears

Abnormality		Treatment
ASC-US		HPV serotype testing • If (+) for high-risk HPV: colposcopy • If (−) for high-risk HPV: repeat Pap smear in 1 year
ASC-H		Colposcopy
LSIL	CIN I (mild dysplasia)	Colposcopy • If confirmed LSIL on colposcopic biopsy: colposcopy every 4 to 6 months • If persistent LSIL (more than 1 to 2 years) on colposcopy: o Confined to exocervix: cryotherapy, laser therapy, or LEEP o Involving endocervical canal: cervical conization via LEEP or CKC
HSIL	CIN II (moderate dysplasia) CIN III (severe dysplasia)	Colposcopy • If confirmed HSIL on colposcopic biopsy: o Confined to exocervix: cryotherapy, laser therapy, or LEEP o Involving endocervical canal: cervical conization via LEEP or CKC

ASC-US: Atypical squamous cells of undetermined significance.
HPV: Human papillomavirus.
ASC-H: Atypical squamous cells, cannot exclude high-grade squamous intraepithelial lesion.
LSIL: Low-grade squamous intraepithelial lesion.
CIN: Cervical intraepithelial neoplasia.
LEEP: Loop electrosurgical excision procedure (removing a cone-shaped piece of cervix with a cauterized wire loop).
CKC: Cold knife cone biopsy (removal of a wedge-shaped portion of the cervical stroma and endocervical canal).
HSIL: High-grade squamous intraepithelial lesion.

A. HPV infection is the primary cause of cervical cancer and premalignant lesions. Virus serotypes 16, 18, and 31 are especially closely correlated with cervical cancer. HPV serotype testing is currently used at some institutions to direct management of Pap smears read out as atypical squamous cells of undetermined significance (ASC-US). However, because CIN II already represents precancerous changes (i.e., HSIL), further testing for HPV serotype would not alter the patient's management.

C, D. LEEP and CKC are generally performed when CIN II or III involves the endocervix, or when there is a discrepancy between the Pap smear and colposcopy.

E. Patients with ASC-US and CIN I may be followed with colposcopy every 3 to 4 months. If left untreated, approximately 30% of CIN I lesions will resolve. It takes about 7 years for CIN I lesions to progress to cervical cancer.

46. B. A complex ovarian mass in a postmenopausal woman is highly suspicious for cancer and requires a diagnostic and staging laparotomy. The patient's signs and symptoms—in particular, a complex mass in the setting of ascites—are particularly concerning for ovarian cancer. The US image shows a large ovarian mass that is both cystic and solid. The worrisome finding on the image suggestive of malignancy is the appearance of the internal excrescences. Exploratory laparotomy is performed for diagnosis and, if cancer is found, for staging and debulking of the tumor.

A. The postmenopausal ovary does not cycle. A complex ovarian cyst in a postmenopausal woman is highly suspicious for carcinoma and is not expected to resolve. A delay in diagnosis is potentially harmful.
C. Diuretic treatment of ascites has little efficacy, as fluid reaccumulates. When fluid returns to the third space, the patient may become intravascularly depleted and dehydrated. Thus diuretic treatment of ascites can be harmful.
D. A second opinion is reserved for cases in which management is unclear or controversial, which is not applicable here. A patient may always seek a second opinion herself, a move that should be supported.
E. If ovarian carcinoma is found, the patient will undergo a surgical debulking of her tumor followed by chemotherapy. Until an accurate tissue diagnosis is made, chemotherapy should not be given. Debulking the tumor is also thought to increase the percentage of tumor in the S phase, making the tumor relatively more responsive to chemotherapy than the patient's normal tissue.

47. **C. The image shown in the US depicts the fetal head in a case of a neural tube defect known as spina bifida. The two anomalies seen in the image are the "lemon" sign, which is exhibited by the concavities of the frontal bones, and the "banana" sign, evidenced by the abnormal shape of the cerebellum. While the defect in spina bifida is usually one of the lower spinal cord, it can be difficult to diagnose on US directly. Rather, the findings in the fetal brain tend to make the US diagnosis. Spina bifida was the first fetal anomaly to be screened for with maternal serum screening. Mothers with fetuses who have neural tube defects have an elevated MSAFP, but the other analytes (estriol and hCG) should be normal.**

A. Decreased MSAFP, decreased estriol, and an elevated hCG are seen in fetuses with Down syndrome. US findings in cases of Down syndrome include a short humerus and femur, the "double bubble" sign of pyloric stenosis, endocardial cushion defects, nuchal thickening, and soft findings of echogenic intracardiac focus and pyelectasis. Notably, nearly 50% of Down syndrome fetuses will have a normal US.
B. Fetuses with trisomy 18 may have a decrease in all three analytes in the XAFP.
D, E. These two patterns of XAFP analytes are not associated with any particular syndrome.

48. **E. The patient has a small, functional cyst, which will most likely resolve spontaneously. Cysts that are larger than 5 cm pose a significantly increased risk of ovarian torsion, of which this patient has no symptoms.**

A. Combination OCPs reduce the likelihood of formation of new cysts through suppression of ovulation, but will not cause the regression of existing cysts. If the patient wishes prophylaxis for the future, combination OCPs are a reasonable choice. Progestin-only pills are less effective in the suppression of ovulation, so they would be less effective in this patient.
B. Laparoscopic cystectomy is reserved for patients who are symptomatic for ovarian torsion. Such symptoms may include severe pain, fever, nausea, vomiting, and absent arterial and venous Doppler flow to the ovary on US.
C. Fine-needle aspiration of an ovarian cyst is often unsuccessful and is not indicated here.
D. Hospitalization and observation are indicated if a patient shows signs of intermittent torsion. This patient's symptoms are extremely mild, and torsion of a 2 cm cyst is unlikely. She should, however, be given precautionary information about returning for any signs or symptoms of ovarian torsion.

49. **A. Treatment of Paget's disease consists of excision of all involved tissue with wide margins. Recurrence is more common than in vulvar intraepithelial lesions.**

B. HPV infection has not been associated with Paget's disease of the vulva.
C. Paget's disease of the vulva is associated with a higher incidence of internal carcinoma, most commonly of the breast or colon.
D. Paget's disease is seen most commonly in postmenopausal women.
E. HSV-1 infection is most commonly associated with oral/labial lesions, but can also cause vulvar and vaginal lesions. HSV-2 infection is more commonly associated with genital tract lesions but can also cause oral lesions. Neither HSV type is associated with Paget's disease.

50. A. TOA or TOC most commonly results from PID; therefore, the same organisms are involved. Pathogenic organisms such as gonorrhea or chlamydia may be present and cultured from the cervix or the TOA at the time of surgical therapy. The most commonly found bacteria in TOAs are species of skin flora, gram-negative rods, and anaerobes such as *Streptococcus* spp., *Staphylococcus* spp., *Klebsiella* spp., *E. coli*, *Proteus* spp., *Bacteroides* spp., *Gardnerella vaginalis*, *Prevotella* spp., and *Peptostreptococcus*, among others. After 24 to 48 hours of IV antibiotics without improvement or if the patient develops signs of sepsis, drainage of the abscess should be performed. There are several modalities (e.g., laparotomy, laparoscopy, or imaging-guided needle drainage) to accomplish this to limit morbidity and mortality. Although TOA is most often associated with PID, it has been linked to other sources of pelvic infection, including diverticulitis, appendicitis, and pelvic surgeries and procedures.

B. As in the explanation for A, management is begun conservatively with antibiotics. Only if these measures fail to improve symptoms is drainage or surgery utilized.

C. TOA is most commonly a sequela of untreated PID, but it is also associated with ruptured appendicitis, pelvic surgery, hysterosalpingogram, and diverticulitis.

D. The most common feature in TOA is pain. In fact, more than 90% of patients report persistent low abdominal pain. Only 60% to 80% of patients have fever or leukocytosis. The patient invariably will have uterine tenderness, adnexal tenderness, and cervical motion tenderness. She may or may not have a palpable pelvic mass.

E. TOA is really a more severe subset of PID and carries with it all of the same risks of future infertility.

SETTING 2: OFFICE

Your office is in a primary care generalist group practice located in a physician office suite adjoining a suburban community hospital. Patients are usually seen by appointment. Most of the patients you see are from your own practice and are appearing for regular scheduled return visits, with some new patients as well. As in most group practices, you will often encounter a patient whose primary care is managed by one of your associates; reference may be made to the patient's medical records. You may do some telephone management, and you may have to respond to questions about articles in magazines and on television that will require interpretation. Complete laboratory and radiology services are available.

51. A 22-year-old sexually active woman comes into your office for a follow-up gynecological exam after her annual Pap smear 1 month ago showed morphology suggestive of cervical intraepithelial neoplasia type I (CIN I). On this visit, you perform a colposcopy with directed biopsies of small lesions seen in the transformation zone, as well as an endocervical curettage (ECC). Which of the following test results or historical information is an indication for further diagnosis and treatment via conization?

    A. White epithelium is visible on colposcopy
    B. Directed biopsies show changes consistent with CIN type III
    C. The patient douches once per month
    D. Punctation and mosaicism are seen on colposcopy
    E. The patient is pregnant

52. A 52-year-old G_2P_2 woman presents with complaints of vaginal spotting, especially after intercourse, and a 15-pound weight loss in the last four months. On speculum exam, she is found to have a friable-appearing, cauliflower-shaped lesion in the transformation zone of her cervix. Subsequent biopsy of the lesion identifies it as squamous cell carcinoma. Which of the following would be considered a risk factor for cervical carcinoma in this patient?

    A. She had her first child at age 31
    B. She used a cervical cap as her primary mode of contraception for 30 years
    C. She has a history of infection with HPV type 11
    D. She has a 25 pack/year smoking history
    E. She achieved menarche at the age of 15

53. A 29-year-old G_2P_1 woman presents at 27 weeks GA for a routine prenatal visit and third trimester labs. She has had an uncomplicated antenatal course up to this point. She weighs 82 kg now and her 3-year-old son's birthweight was 4500 g. The patient had a long labor with that delivery, which resulted in a cesarean section when she failed to dilate beyond 7 cm. She had an elevated glucose load test (GLT) in her last pregnancy of 147, but a normal 3-hour glucose tolerance test (GTT) of 80, 177, 151, and 122. She has a maternal aunt who developed diabetes at age 57, but no other relatives with diabetes. In her history, which of the following is the biggest risk for her to have gestational diabetes (GD) in this pregnancy?

    A. Previous elevated GLT
    B. Prior macrosomic fetus
    C. Aunt with type 2 diabetes
    D. Prior gestational diabetes
    E. Prior cesarean delivery

54. A 56-year-old postmenopausal woman is experiencing occasional vaginal bleeding and has had malodorous discharge, oliguria, and weight loss over several months. Vaginal exam reveals a cervical tumor involving much of the lower third of the vagina. On rectal exam, it is found that the tumor has obliterated the pouch of Douglas and extended all the way to the pelvic wall (Figure 2-54). A pelvic CT is remarkable for hydronephrosis of the left kidney; however, cytoscopy and proctoscopy are normal. The patient is diagnosed with cervical carcinoma. Based on these findings, what is her likely 5-year survival rate?

    A. 4%
    B. 40%
    C. 72%
    D. 88%
    E. 95%

55. A 20-year-old woman presents to you with new onset of hair growth on her lower back, chest, and face. She reports no menstrual changes and no changes in her body shape or voice. She is not currently on any medications. Her FSH, LH, testosterone, and androgen precursor levels are

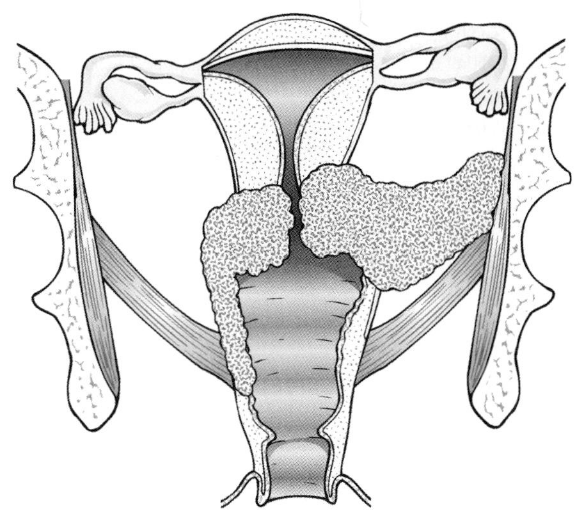

Figure 2-54 • Reproduced from Callahan T. Blueprints Obstetrics & Gynecology, 2nd ed. Blackwell Science, 2001: Fig. 26-2, p. 212.

all within the normal range. Exam reveals no pelvic mass, no changes in fat distribution, and no anatomical changes other than increased hair growth throughout her body. In the absence of a clear etiology, you diagnose this patient with constitutional (idiopathic) hirsutism. What is the best treatment option for her?

A. Danazol
B. Dehydroepiandrosterone (DHEA)
C. Cyclosporine
D. Spironolactone
E. Minocycline

56. A 28-year-old G_0 woman presents with a 7-month history of acne, deepening of her voice, and amenorrhea. She has never had menstrual irregularity in the past, and her past medical history is otherwise negative. Her exam is remarkable for a palpable pelvic mass and an enlarged clitoris. Labs show a negative pregnancy test; marked suppression of LH, FSH, and plasma androstenedione; and increased free testosterone levels. A pelvic US is obtained (Figure 2-56). You suspect a Sertoli-Leydig cell tumor, and promptly arrange for surgical removal. Which of the following statements is true regarding these tumors?

A. In the normal progression of disease, breast atrophy and amenorrhea precede clitoral hypertrophy.
B. With successful treatment of disease, there are no lasting sequelae.

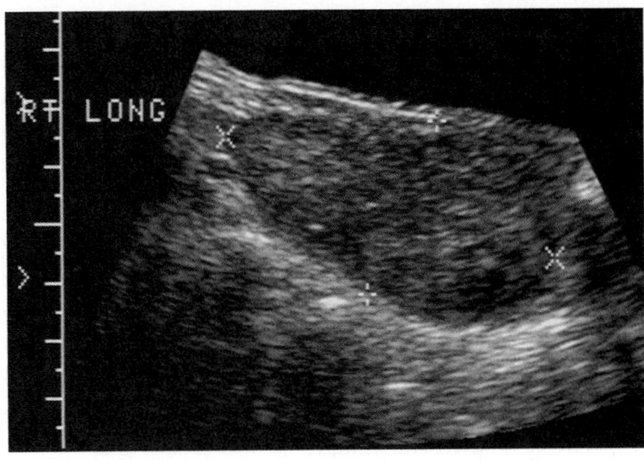

Figure 2-56 • Image Provided by Departments of Radiology and Obstetrics & Gynecology, University of California, San Francisco.

C. Hirsutism is not a part of this syndrome.
D. The mortality rate for this tumor approaches 60%.
E. In the majority of cases, both ovaries are affected.

57. A 19-year-old woman in a stable, monogamous relationship wishes to begin hormonal contraception. She has done some research and decided that she would prefer hormones over barrier methods because the latter are cumbersome and "ruin the mood." She does want to know more about specific hormone-based contraceptive methods, however, to help make her decision. Which of the following statements is most accurate regarding hormonal contraception?

A. Combination OCPs exert their effect predominantly by use of estrogen to stimulate LH secretion.
B. Progestin-only pills allow more flexibility in dosing as compared to combination OCPs.
C. Progestin-only pills are contraindicated in lactating women.
D. The transdermal patch system has been shown to be twice as effective as combination OCPs.
E. Depo-Provera can safely be used in patients with epilepsy.

58. A 19-year-old G_0 Caucasian woman presents to your office with complaints of lower abdominal and pelvic pain. She has experienced cyclic pain with her menses since the age of 14, but notes that over the past 12 to 15 months this pain has

been increasing, leaving her unable to go to work for 2 to 3 days each month. For the past 2 months, she has had pain that occurs several times between her periods and lasts for several days. The patient has been sexually active since age 15, has used only condoms for contraception, and has never had any pelvic infections to her knowledge. She is currently in a monogamous sexual relationship, but has not been sexually active for the past month secondary to dyspareunia. She does note some relief of symptoms with 400 mg of ibuprofen. What is the next step in her diagnosis and treatment?

A. Laparoscopic resection of adhesions
B. Monophasic or continuous OCPs
C. Gonadotropin-releasing hormone (GnRH) analog therapy (Lupron)
D. Pain consult/psychiatry consult
E. Antibiotics

59. You are asked to see a couple regarding reversal of a sterilization procedure performed 4 years prior to their current visit. At that time, the couple had discussed a vasectomy, but the husband could not allay the many concerns he had regarding his ability to function sexually after the procedure. As a consequence, his wife decided to undergo a sterilization procedure, although she cannot recall which type. Now, however, the couple want another child. They cannot afford IVF, and feel that adoption would not be fulfilling because they believe that "one of the greatest joys of life is seeing each other in our children." Which of the following sterilization procedures, if done 4 years ago, would now offer the best chance of a successful reversal?

A. Falope ring
B. Pomeroy tubal ligation
C. Hulka clip
D. Electrocautery
E. Colpotomy

60. A 32-year-old G_1P_1 woman gave birth to a Down syndrome baby nearly 7 years ago. She now wants another child, but has concerns regarding this next pregnancy and her chances of having another child with Down syndrome. She therefore makes an appointment with a genetic counselor, who decides to screen her and her husband for a possible genetic predisposition to Down syndrome. The results of the karyotypes are as follows: Father: 46,XY; Mother: 45,XX, –21,–21, + t(21q;21q). What is the theoretical risk of their second-born child having Down syndrome?

A. 25%
B. 33%
C. 50%
D. 100%
E. Unable to determine from the information given

The next two questions (items 61 and 62) correspond to the following vignette.

A 34-year-old G_1P_0 woman at 17 weeks GA by LMP presents to your clinic for a follow-up appointment. At her last visit, she had an expanded AFP/maternal serum triple screen test. The results of the test came back with a low maternal serum alpha-fetoprotein (MSAFP), a low estriol level, and a high β-hCG. You are concerned, so you perform an US, which confirms that fetal size equals dates. Figure 2-61 is an image of the fetal abdomen.

61. These screening test results are most consistent with which of the following disorders/defects?

A. Edward's syndrome (trisomy 18)
B. Neural tube defects
C. Patau's syndrome (trisomy 13)
D. Down syndrome (trisomy 21)
E. Turner's syndrome (monosomy X)

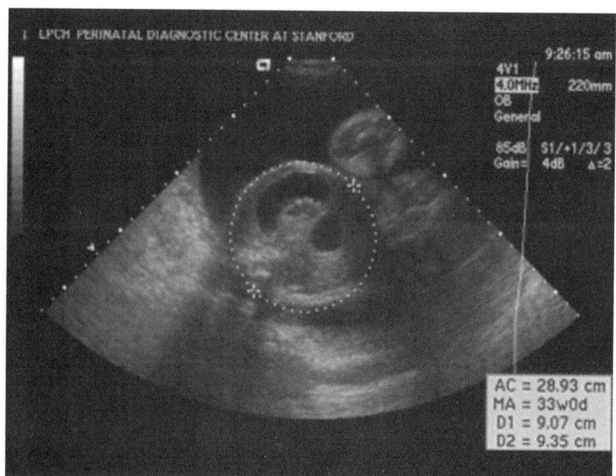

Figure 2-61 • Image Courtesy of Susan H. Tran, Kaiser San Francisco Hospital, San Francisco, California.

62. What is the recommended next step in this patient's management?
    A. Amniocentesis
    B. Cordocentesis
    C. CT scan of the abdomen
    D. Chorionic villi sampling (CVS)
    E. Nothing is indicated at this time; the fetus is not far enough along for accurate testing

End of Set

63. A 23-year-old woman presents to your office with complaints of vulvar and vaginal pruritis. She became sexually active 2 weeks ago with a new partner and is concerned that these signs may be symptomatic of a STD. She complains of an increase in a white, clumpy discharge without odor. She notes no abdominal pain or fever. On physical exam, you note some erythematous punctate macular lesions bilaterally near the perineum, but no papular or vesicular lesions. On speculum exam, you observe a white discharge that has a negative whiff test; a KOH prepared slide reveals the image in Figure 2-63. What is the treatment of choice?
    A. Oral acyclovir
    B. Topical acyclovir applied to the lesions
    C. Oral metronidazole (Flagyl)
    D. Vaginal metronidazole (Metro-gel)
    E. Oral fluconazole (Diflucan)

64. A 26-year-old woman presents for her first prenatal visit after having a positive home pregnancy test 2 weeks ago. Her LMP began 7 weeks and 1 day ago. After taking a medical history, you perform a physical exam, perform a Pap smear, and take cultures for gonorrhea and chlamydia. In addition to these tests, which of the following would also be done at this visit?
    A. Triple screen of maternal serum alpha-fetoprotein, estriol, and β-hCG
    B. Diabetes mellitus screen
    C. Rh factor and antibody screen
    D. Group B *Streptococcus* culture
    E. Pelvic US

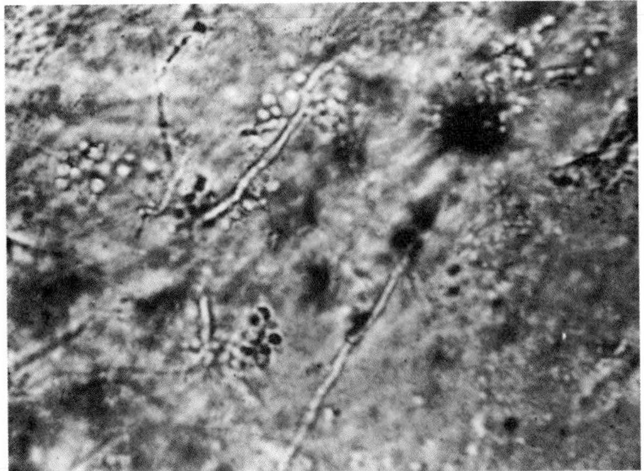

Figure 2-63 • Reproduced with Permission from Crissey JT. Manual of Medical Mycology. Blackwell Science, 1995: 90.

The next two questions (items 65 and 66) correspond to the following vignette.

A 32-year-old G_4P_2 woman sees you for her second prenatal visit at 17 weeks GA. She has two healthy children at home, both full-term vaginal deliveries following uncomplicated pregnancies. She agreed to an HIV test at her first visit, which is part of the universal screening that your clinic offers. Both the Western blot and ELISA are positive for HIV. The patient had never received a blood transfusion or used intravenous drugs. She is monogamous with her husband and believes their relationship to be mutually monogamous. He has no known exposures. She feels well in general and has no symptoms of opportunistic infections. Her viral load is undetectable. She is very concerned about passing the virus on to her baby, and has spent the last several days doing research on the Internet. Her understanding is that she will be started on antiretroviral therapy immediately and that she will need to have a cesarean delivery (although she desires vaginal delivery).

65. Which of the following corrections to her understanding best reflects the current standard of care for prevention of vertical transmission of HIV in the United States?
    A. If her viral load remains low, she will benefit from neither antiretroviral therapy nor cesarean section.
    B. Antiretroviral therapy does not need to be initiated until she is in labor, but cesarean section is indeed indicated.
    C. Antiretroviral therapy should never be given to pregnant women because of concerns about teratogenicity; cesarean section is indeed indicated.

D. Antiretroviral therapy should be initiated now; if her viral count remains undetectable, a cesarean section is not necessarily indicated.
E. Antiretroviral therapy should be initiated now; the fetus should be closely monitored with a scalp electrode as soon as the patient begins to labor, and cesarean section performed only for signs of distress.

66. This patient breastfed her previous two children, and is hoping to breastfeed this child as well. What is the most appropriate recommendation?

A. Her HIV status should have no bearing on breastfeeding choices, as the virus is not expressed in breast milk.
B. She should not breastfeed, because she is HIV positive.
C. She should not breastfeed, because the baby will require optimal nutrition to maximize immune system function, and this is best achieved with formula feeding.
D. Breastfeeding should be encouraged, as maternal immunoglobulins may protect the baby from infection.
E. Breastfeeding should be encouraged, as antiretroviral drugs given to the mother have been shown to be expressed in breast milk and provide a protective effect on the baby.

End of Set

67. A 37-year-old G_1 actress presents at 26 weeks GA for a routine prenatal visit and review of her third-trimester labs. She is dated by LMP, which was consistent with a normal 10-week US. Her antenatal course has been uncomplicated, although fatigue has forced her to limit her rehearsal schedule. Amniocentesis at 16 weeks GA (for advanced maternal age) showed a normal karyotype (46,XX). Last week her 50g GLT was found to be elevated at 157. This morning she completed her 3-hour OGTT, which has just been reported to you as 86, 193, 173, and 128. The patient denies personal or family history of diabetes. She is not obese and has no history of spontaneous abortions. As you begin to discuss the results of the OGTT, the patient becomes very tearful, explaining that she recently read in a magazine article that the risk of birth defects is increased in diabetic mothers. Which of the following is the most accurate way to counsel this patient regarding her concern?

A. The article is wrong; there is no connection between maternal diabetes and congenital anomalies
B. This patient probably has gestational diabetes (GD), which, unlike overt (pregestational) diabetes, is not believed to carry an increased risk of fetal congenital anomalies
C. There is an increased risk of congenital anomalies in children of diabetic mothers, but her normal US at 10 weeks makes the risk of malformation very remote
D. There is an increased risk of congenital anomalies in children of diabetic mothers, but these are usually chromosomal in origin, so her normal amniocentesis result is very reassuring
E. The risk of birth defects is indeed increased, and oral hypoglycemic agents should be started to minimize this risk

68. A 13-year-old African American adolescent female presents to your office with complaints of lower abdominal pain that began 6 months ago. The pain lasts for 4 to 6 days and then decreases. For the last 2 months, the pain has lasted longer, and the patient now notes a fullness in her lower abdomen. She is not sexually active and has not begun menstruating yet. On physical exam, she is Tanner stage III. On abdominal exam, you note mild lower abdominal tenderness and a palpable fullness in her lower abdomen. On pelvic exam, you note that she has an intact hymeneal ring and a foreshortened vaginal vault of only 2 cm above the hymenal ring. Figure 2-68 depicts her internal genitalia. What is the most likely diagnosis?

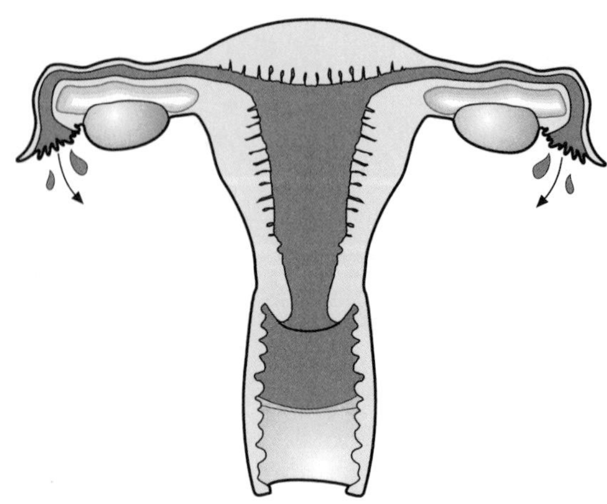

Figure 2-68 •

A. Testicular feminization
B. Imperforate hymen
C. Transverse vaginal septum
D. Labial fusion
E. Rudimentary uterine horn

69. A 32-year-old nonpregnant woman presents with complaints of minor changes to her body hair growth and changing voice beginning 2 months ago. She denies changes to her menses, and she is not currently taking any medications. Exam reveals mild increases in facial hair and low back hair growth, a slight deepening of her voice, and a blood pressure of 135/85. You suspect an endocrine disorder and begin a work-up. You find that her 24-hour free cortisol level is normal, but her free testosterone level is elevated at 220 ng/dL. A CT scan of her abdomen and pelvis is negative for masses. You decide to perform an ACTH stimulation test, which shows extremely elevated plasma levels of 11-deoxycorticosterone, but otherwise normal hormonal levels. Which of the following enzyme deficiencies could result in this finding?

A. 21-Hydroxylase
B. 11b-Hydroxylase
C. Aromatase
D. 3β-hydroxysteroid dehydrogenase
E. 5α-reductase

The next two questions (items 70 and 71) correspond to the following vignette.

A 61-year-old G_0 woman presents for routine gynecologic exam. Her LMP was 7 years ago, and her last office visit was 2 years ago. She reports that she is in generally good health, but has felt vague abdominal discomfort for the last couple of months, which she attributes to stress resulting from adapting to a new format for the evening news. On bimanual exam, you note a unilateral, mobile adnexal mass on the left. The mass feels regular in shape.

70. Which one of the following is most concerning for malignancy, independently requiring further work-up?

A. The mass is unilateral
B. The mass is mobile
C. The mass feels regular
D. The cul-de-sac is smooth
E. The patient is postmenopausal

71. A pelvic US is performed, which confirms a cystic mass measuring 4 cm on the left (Figure 2-71). Smooth internal and external contours are noted, as are multiple septations within the mass. No ascites are observed. Which of the following radiological findings is most suggestive of malignancy?

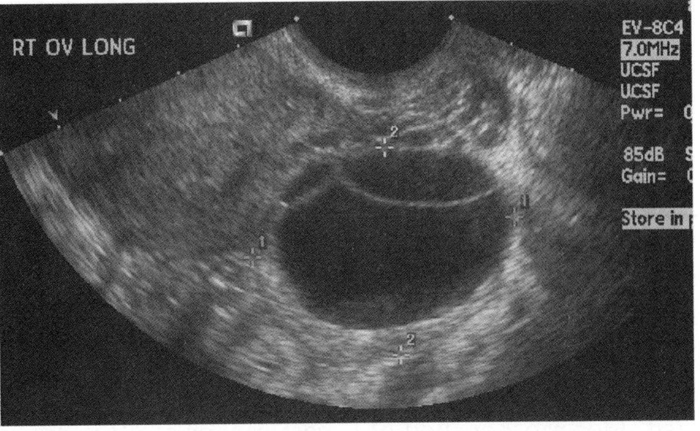

Figure 2-71 • Image Provided by Departments of Radiology and Obstetrics & Gynecology, University of California, San Francisco.

A. The mass is cystic
B. The mass is smaller than 5 cm
C. The mass has smooth contours
D. The mass is septated
E. No ascites are observed

End of Set

72. A 49-year-old G_0 woman presents for routine annual exam. Her LMP was 3 years ago. She used OCPs for 7 years in her early twenties. At age 31, she had a 6-month course of clomiphene citrate for unexplained infertility, but later discovered that the basis of her inability to conceive was male factor. At age 33, no longer desiring pregnancy, she underwent bilateral tubal ligation. During today's visit, she expresses her concern about ovarian cancer because a friend was recently diagnosed with it. The patient has no family history of ovarian or breast cancer. Which of the following elements of this patient's history is most likely to increase her risk for ovarian cancer?

A. Her age at menopause
B. Her history of OCP use
C. Her nulliparity
D. Her tubal ligation
E. Her history of clomiphene treatment

The next two questions (items 73 and 74) correspond to the following vignette.

A 35-year-old G_3P_3 who is 4 weeks postpartum presented 2 days ago with fever, chills, and left breast pain and erythema. She was diagnosed with mastitis and given outpatient oral antibiotics. Her systemic symptoms have greatly improved, but she continues to have mildly elevated temperatures to 100.08F and persistent left breast pain. On physical exam, her left breast is not engorged but there is a deep, firm, 2 cm mass at the 3 o'clock position. It is difficult to assess fluctuance given the depth of the mass. The patient has continued to breastfeed from both breasts and has taken her antibiotics as prescribed since her prior visit. Her mother died of breast cancer at 49 years of age, and her sister is currently undergoing a work-up for a breast mass.

73. What should be the next step in evaluation?
    A. A core biopsy
    B. A breast US
    C. Incision and drainage in the OR
    D. A CT scan to evaluate for an abscess
    E. Reevaluation in 1 week

74. What is the most common pathogen in mastitis?
    A. *Staphylococcus aureus*
    B. *Staphylococcus epidermidis*
    C. *Pseudomonas aeruginosa*
    D. *Proprionobacterium acnes*
    E. *Lactococcal ductalis*

End of Set

The next two questions (items 75 and 76) correspond to the following vignette.

A 26-year-old G_1P_1 had an uncomplicated normal, spontaneous vaginal delivery of a highly desired and healthy baby girl 4 days ago. Her husband calls the office stating that he is worried about his wife. Since coming home 2 days ago, she has experienced periods of crying for 1 to 2 hours at a time, followed by normal behavior, extreme irritability with him, and insomnia. He reports with concern that she forgot pots on the stove twice and burned the contents, which is very unusual for her because she is a professional chef. She has no known psychiatric history.

75. What is the most likely diagnosis?
    A. Postpartum depression
    B. Bipolar disorder
    C. Postpartum blues
    D. Malingering in the husband
    E. Postpartum psychosis

76. A woman who had postpartum depression after the birth of her first child has what statistical risk for recurrence after her next birth?
    A. 10%
    B. 25%
    C. 50%
    D. 75%
    E. 90%

End of Set

77. A 26-year-old G_0 female had a routine Pap smear done at the time of a sexually transmitted infection screening visit. She was diagnosed with bacterial vaginosis and given a prescription for metronidazole vaginal gel at the appointment. Her Pap smear results are reported as HSIL. Her gonorrhea, chlamydia, syphilis, and HIV tests were all negative. What should be the next step in evaluating this patient?
    A. Cold knife conization (CKC)
    B. Repeat Pap smear every 4 months for 2 years until three consecutive smears are negative; do a colposcopy if and when a second smear is abnormal
    C. Colposcopy and ECC
    D. Cryotherapy
    E. Treat her again for bacterial vaginosis and then repeat the Pap smear

78. A 37-year-old African American G_1P_0 woman at 41 weeks GA presents for her routine prenatal visit. Her pregnancy is complicated by a history of severe hyperemesis gravidarum until 16 weeks gestation that required two brief hospital stays for aggressive hydration. She has felt fine during the second half of her pregnancy. All of her routine prenatal labs have been within

normal limits, and she had an amniocentesis performed at 15 weeks, which revealed a 46,XX fetus. She now presents 1 week after her due date wanting to know when she will deliver. On exam, her cervix is closed, but soft, and 50% effaced. She has a nonstress test (Figure 2-78). Given its appearance, you will reassure her that she is at lower risk for what condition over the ensuing week?

A. Gestational diabetes (GD)
B. Intrauterine fetal demise (IUFD)
C. Meconium in the amniotic fluid
D. Macrosomia
E. Preeclampsia

79. A 27-year-old attorney presents to your gynecologic clinic for an annual exam. She has not had an exam for 3 years, but has not experienced any problems prior to her current visit. She presents because she is interested in birth control, as she is now in a monogamous sexual relationship. As part of this routine exam, you perform a Pap smear, test for gonorrhea and chlamydia, and start the patient on a monophasic oral contraceptive pill. The Pap smear returns with a result of LSIL/CIN I. You meet with the patient 2 weeks later to discuss the ramifications of this finding. You tell her the following in your discussion:

A. With CIN I, the average length of time to the development of cervical cancer is 3 to 4 years
B. 10% of CIN I lesions resolve spontaneously
C. The next step in management is cryotherapy
D. Cervical dysplasia is highly associated with HPV subtypes 16 and 18
E. The next step in management is laser therapy

80. A 66-year-old African American woman presents to the office complaining of external vaginal dryness and itching for the last 3 months. She suspected a yeast infection and tried two over-the-counter antifungal creams with no relief. She has also tried vinegar douches with no relief. She is not sexually active, and her LMP was 12 years ago. She does not take HRT. On exam, you find moderate vaginal mucosal atrophy and a small (less than 1 cm), white-based, nontender ulcer on the inferior left labia majus. No exophytic lesions are noted. Which of the following steps should you take?

A. Prescribe a topical estrogen cream and reevaluate in 3 weeks
B. Prescribe a topical steroid cream and reevaluate in 3 weeks
C. Perform a wide local excision in the office
D. Perform a punch biopsy
E. Reassure her that vulvar pruritis is normal in postmenopausal women and offer her HRT

81. A 67-year-old female patient of yours notes an abnormal vaginal discharge on and off for longer than 6 months. Each time she thought it was a yeast infection like those she experienced as a young woman and used an over-the-counter antifungal vaginal cream with minimal relief. She came to your office on this occasion because she noticed a bloody tinge to the discharge. On exam, you note a foul-smelling discharge and a large mucosal abnormality on the upper-left vaginal wall. You take a biopsy and have a high suspicion for vaginal carcinoma. Where does squamous cell carcinoma of the vagina most commonly occur?

A. At the introitus
B. In the upper one-third of the vagina
C. In the lower two-thirds of the vagina
D. On the labia majora
E. Equally in all vaginal areas

The next two questions (items 82 and 83) correspond to the following vignette.

A non–sexually active 42-year-old woman was found to have a large mass in the mucosa of the posterior fornix on pelvic exam as part of a work-up for recurrent UTIs. On bimanual exam, the mass was felt to extend to the left pelvic sidewall. A biopsy was done and returned as "invasive squamous cell carcinoma with lymphatic invasion."

82. Which of the following lymph nodes would you first expect to be positive?

A. None; vaginal cancer spreads hematogenously
B. Femoral triangle nodes
C. Internal and common iliac nodes
D. Supraclavicular
E. Posterior cervical

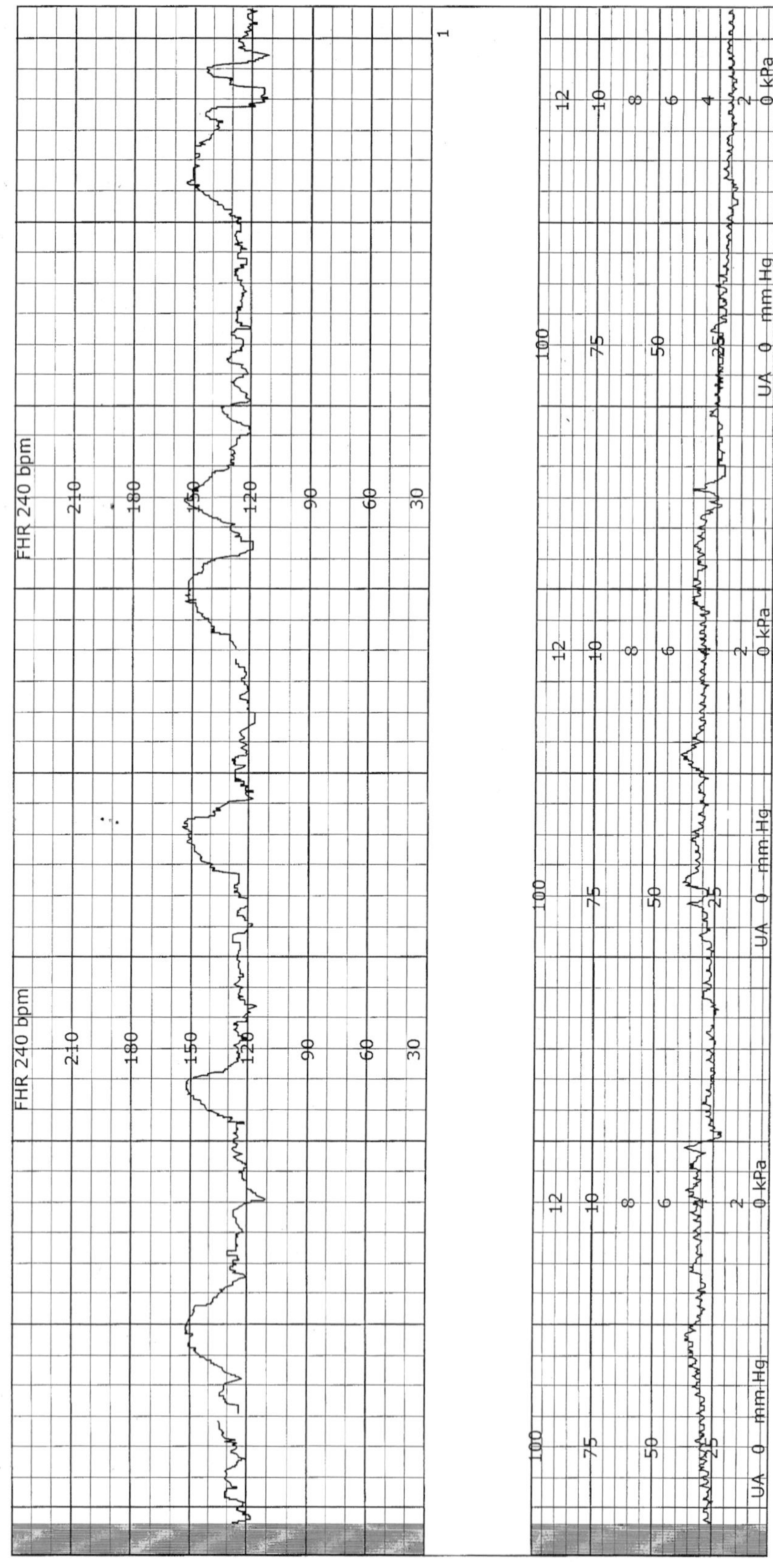

Figure 2-78 • Image Provided by Departments of Radiology and Obstetrics & Gynecology, University of California, San Francisco.

83. Given the above information, what stage is this woman's disease?

A. Stage I
B. Stage II
C. Stage III or IV
D. Stage V
E. Unable to assign until tissue borders are evaluated on the pathologic specimen

End of Set

84. A 27-year-old G_1P_1 presents to your office for preconception counseling. Her prior delivery was significant for a primary low transverse cesarean section for fetal intolerance of labor. She desires a trial of labor for her subsequent pregnancy. You counsel her that:

A. Her risk of uterine rupture is 5% to 10%
B. Management of uterine rupture includes expectant management and laparoscopy
C. Risk of uterine rupture is increased by induction of labor
D. Fetal mortality rate is greater than 50% should uterine rupture occur
E. Use of oxytocin during labor may decrease her risk for uterine rupture

85. A 36-year-old G_1P_0 at 42 0/7 weeks GA presents for a routine prenatal appointment followed by antenatal testing (nonstress test and amniotic fluid index). Her NST is reactive and her amniotic fluid index is 6. On exam, her cervix is found to be favorable with a Bishop's score of 6. She declines your recommendation to proceed with post-term labor induction. In counseling the patient, you tell her that post-term pregnancy (more than 42 weeks GA) includes an increased risk of:

A. Polyhydramnios
B. Meconium aspiration
C. Rh sensitization
D. Low birthweight
E. Respiratory distress syndrome

86. A 32-year-old G_2P_1 with a twin pregnancy at 26 4/7 weeks GA presents for her prenatal visit. She is noted to have size greater than dates on physical exam and is sent for a formal US for further evaluation. The US is notable for polyhydramnios of one twin and oligohydramnios and growth restriction of the other twin. In addition, the image in Figure 2-86 is obtained of the twin with polyhydramnios. What is the most likely diagnosis?

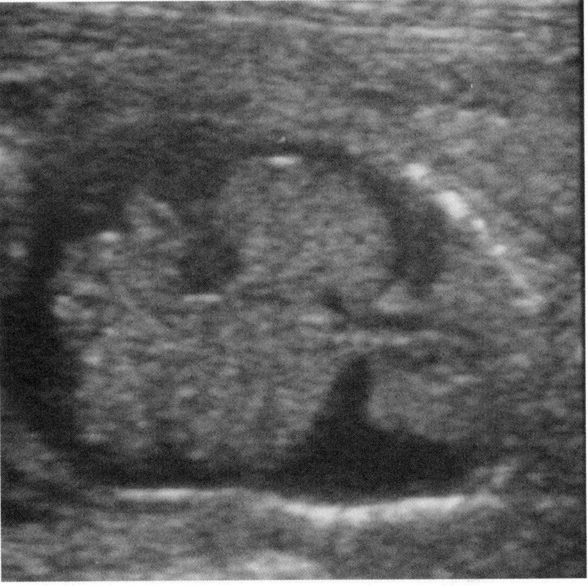

Figure 2-86 • Image Provided by Departments of Radiology and Obstetrics & Gynecology, University of California, San Francisco.

A. Twin–twin transfusion syndrome
B. Rh incompatibility
C. "Siamese" twinning
D. Normal variant of monozygotic twinning
E. Congenital rubella syndrome

87. An 18-year-old woman presents for her annual exam requesting OCPs and complaining of 3 months of amenorrhea. She experienced menarche at age 12 and had regular menses every 28 days until the last 3 months. She became sexually active at age 16 and is currently monogamous with her boyfriend of 4 months. She is completing her freshman year as a premedical student and is a member of the freshman track team. Despite her rigorous exercise regimen, she notes a 5 lb weight gain over the past 4 months. What is the most likely cause of secondary amenorrhea in this patient?

A. Kallman's syndrome
B. Hypothyroidism
C. Pregnancy
D. Exercise
E. Stress

88. A 36-year-old G_2P_1 Asian woman presents for her fourth prenatal visit at 17 weeks GA. She had some nausea and vomiting in the first trimester that resolved by 14 weeks gestation; otherwise, she has had an entirely uncomplicated pregnancy. At her last appointment at 15 weeks gestation, she underwent screening for maternal serum alpha-fetoprotein (MSAFP). The result returned 2 days ago with a value that is 4.5 multiples of the median (MoMs). Which of the following is the most likely etiology of this abnormal result?

A. Anencephaly
B. Twin gestation
C. Gastroschisis
D. Trisomy 18
E. She is actually 19 weeks GA

89. A 26-year-old woman with no significant past medical history presents to you for evaluation after having two miscarriages in the past 2 years. During an office US, you note a bicornuate uterus (Figure 2-89). To evaluate further, you order a hysterosalpingogram. Which of the following is associated with a bicornuate uterus?

A. Endometriosis
B. Uterine cancer
C. Premature labor
D. Urinary tract infections
E. Fetal anomalies

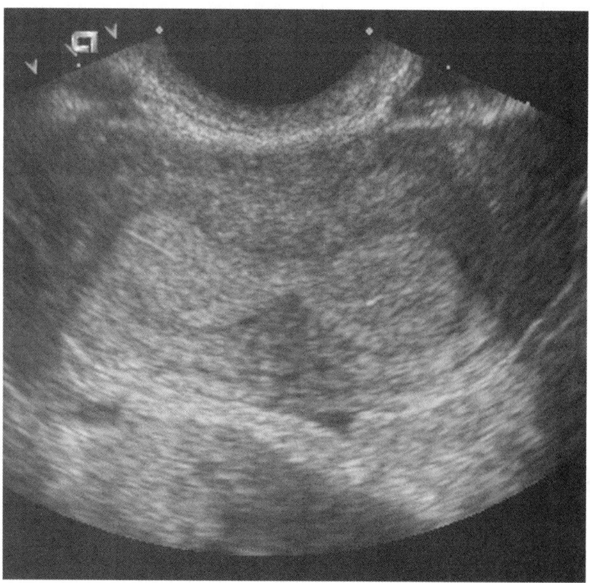

Figure 2-89 • Image Provided by Departments of Radiology and Obstetrics & Gynecology, University of California, San Francisco.

90. A 33-year-old G_3P_0 visits your office for consultation regarding her pregnancy history of three consecutive pregnancy losses at 10, 13, and 11 weeks of gestation. She and her partner are interested in an evaluation for the etiology of the losses. You explain that possible causes may include thrombophilia, genetic abnormalities in one or both of the partners, uterine cavity abnormalities, and endocrine or immune system dysfunction. Which of the following choices correctly matches a cause with the best treatment for the losses?

A. Septate uterus–surgery
B. Balanced translocation–Clomid with intrauterine insemination
C. Antiphospholipid antibody syndrome–corticosteroids
D. Hyperprolactinemia–corticosteroids
E. Group B *Streptococcus*–antibiotics

91. You are seeing a 26-year-old woman in her second trimester of pregnancy who has a history of a prior cesarean delivery. She inquires about a trial of labor (TOL) to achieve a vaginal birth after cesarean section (VBAC). Which of the following is a contraindication to TOL in this setting?

A. History of prior cesarean section being 7 months ago
B. History of cesarean section for breech
C. History of Kerr (low transverse) incision with a "T" extension into the active segment
D. History of Kronig (low vertical) incision
E. History of successful VBAC complicated by postpartum hemorrhage

92. A 33-year-old G_3P_2 Caucasian woman at 14 weeks GA presents for her second prenatal visit. She has had two prior uncomplicated births: a daughter, age 7, and a son, age 3. Her first-trimester prenatal labs done at 11 weeks of gestation revealed that she is Rh-negative and has an anti-D antibody titer of 1:4. She found out that she was Rh-negative in her first pregnancy; at birth, her daughter was also Rh-negative. The patient's last pregnancy was uncomplicated, and she had a negative antibody titer throughout. Her son was Rh-positive. The patient received RhoGAM (anti-D immune globulin) in her last two pregnancies at 28 weeks, but not after delivery in either one. Her Caucasian husband is

the father of all of her pregnancies. Given that the rate of Rh-negative individuals is 16% among Caucasians, which of the following statements is true regarding this patient?

A. Her husband has a 48% chance of being heterozygous.
B. There is a possibility that her husband is Rh-negative.
C. The probability that this fetus is Rh-negative is 0.5.
D. A dose of RhoGAM in this pregnancy will be protective.
E. This patient will need serial amniocentesis in this pregnancy if the fetus is Rh-positive.

93. An obese 78-year-old G_0 female presents to your office with complaints of heavy vaginal spotting for the last 2 weeks. She is concerned because her periods stopped 22 years ago. She reports an uneventful transition to menopause after a long history of irregular periods. She tells you that she has never liked taking pills and did not use OCPs or HRT. What is the best way to care for this patient?

A. US
B. Reassurance and a follow-up appointment in 2 weeks
C. Endometrial biopsy
D. Pap smear
E. D&C

94. You are a urogynecologist evaluating a 67-year-old female for urinary stress incontinence. Your patient reports that she wears a large panty shield at all times because of her fear of leaking urine. She tells you she has been wearing the pads for 1 year and now is concerned that the pads are causing an allergic reaction because she has been suffering from severe vulvar itching over the last 2 months. Upon exam, you note a raised white lesion. Your clinical suspicion is that this lesion is most likely which of the following?

A. Contact dermatitis
B. Yeast infection
C. Lichen simplex chronicus
D. Lichen sclerosus et atrophicus
E. Vulvar cancer

95. A 27-year-old G_3P_2 woman presents to your office at 19 weeks GA after just having had her obstetric US. You call the ultrasonologist for the results and find that the fetus had a normal US except for bilateral choroid plexus cysts (Figure 2-95). The patient's pregnancy has been uncomplicated to this point, and her second-trimester serum screening results returned with lower than age-related risks of both trisomies 21 and 18. You prepare to tell her that this finding has been associated with which of the following?

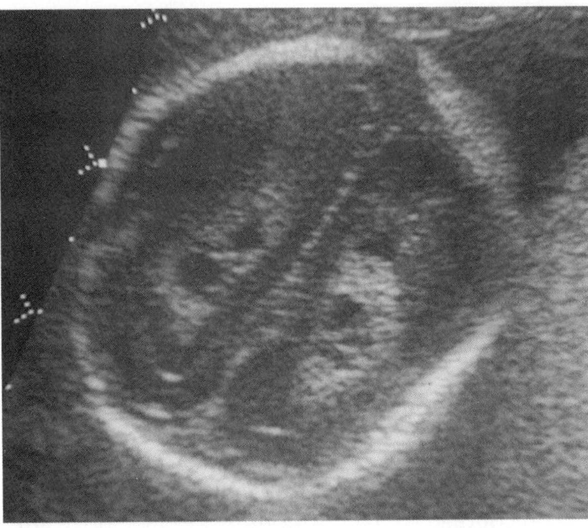

Figure 2-95 • Image Provided by Departments of Radiology and Obstetrics & Gynecology, University of California, San Francisco.

A. Trisomy 18
B. Anencephaly
C. Neural tube defects (NTDs)
D. Developmental delay
E. Turner's syndrome

96. A 22-year-old G_0 Korean woman presents with complaints of increased body and facial hair. She has noticed increased hair growth on her upper lip, chin, upper back, and lower abdomen for about 5 years. She denies deepening of her voice, balding, or enlargement of her clitoris. None of the other women in her family have any of these symptoms, and she feels quite self-conscious as a result. The patient underwent menarche at age 13, has irregular menses every 25 to 45 days, and has never been sexually active. On physical exam, she is 5 ft 4 in. tall and weighs 154 lb. She has some generalized acne on her face and back in addition to acanthosis nigricans. There are a few terminal hairs on her back as well as some stubble on her cheeks and upper lip. Her escutcheon is diamond-shaped. Lab tests show

the following results: normal 17-α-hydroxyprogesterone, normal testosterone, a luteinizing hormone to follicle-stimulating hormone ratio (LH:FSH) of 4, normal DHEA-S, and normal function of 5-α-reductase. What is the most likely diagnosis?

A. Sertoli-Leydig cell tumor
B. Congenital adrenal hyperplasia (CAH)
C. Testicular feminization
D. Germ cell tumor
E. Polycystic ovarian syndrome (PCOS)

97. A 32-year-old G_2P_2 woman presents complaining of vaginal fullness and occasional vaginal pain and urinary urgency. She denies urinary or fecal incontinence. Her symptoms began shortly after the birth of her second child 3 months ago and worsen when she exercises. Her delivery was vaginal and uncomplicated, and the baby weighed 7 lb 4 oz. The patient is not breastfeeding. A pelvic exam reveals a first-degree cystocele (Figure 2-97), but the remainder of the exam is unremarkable. Urinary and cervical cultures are negative, and her postpartum Pap smear was negative. What is the most appropriate next step?

A. Estrogen therapy
B. Anterior repair
C. Kegel exercises
D. Colpocleisis
E. Pessary

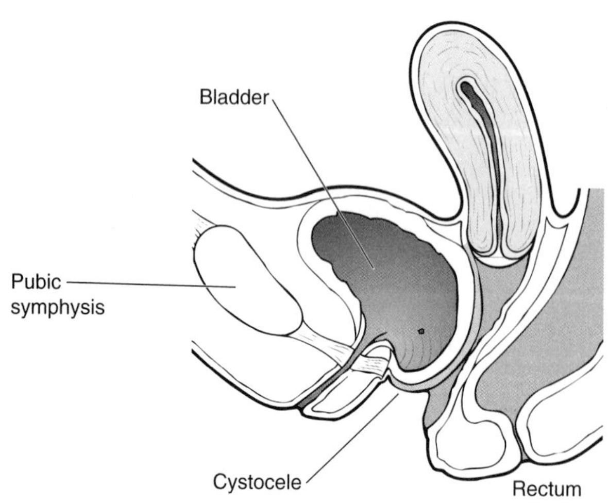

Figure 2-97 •

98. A 63-year-old woman presents with complaints of leaking urine. She started noticing occasional leakage about 6 months ago, occurring approximately once or twice a week during physical activity (hiking or yoga). Over the past month, however, she has noted an increase in frequency, leaking small amounts of urine several times a day. The patient developed an upper respiratory infection 2 weeks ago and noticed that she leaked urine whenever she coughed. She does not notice any leakage while she sleeps or while she is seated, but will have a small leak when she rises from sitting. She denies dysuria or inability to control micturition if she feels a urinary urge. Other past medical history reveals that she is a G_5P_4 with four vaginal deliveries. She went through menopause at age 51 and is not currently taking HRT. On physical exam, you note mild uterine descensus and a grade I cystocele. A Q-tip test (Figure 2-98) is positive with an angle change from 10° to approximately 45°. You tell her she most likely has:

A. Stress incontinence
B. Urge incontinence
C. Detrusor instability
D. Total incontinence
E. Overflow incontinence

99. A 24-year-old G_2P_0 woman presents at 18 weeks GA for her routine obstetric US. She notes no fevers, chills, changes in bowel or urinary function, or abdominal pain. She has had an uncomplicated pregnancy up to this point and had an elective termination of her last pregnancy at 12 weeks. The US is performed, and the resulting image of the cervix and vagina is shown in (Figure 2-99). A sterile speculum exam is performed and reveals no evidence of ruptured membranes, trichomoniasis, or bacterial vaginosis. At this point, her management could include which of the following?

A. Oral metronidazole (Flagyl)
B. Termination of pregnancy
C. Vaginal clindamycin (Cleocin)
D. Tocolysis with magnesium sulfate
E. Betamethasone for fetal lung maturity

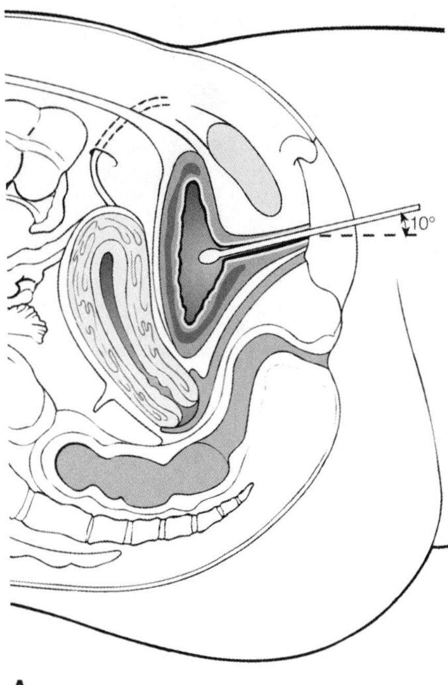

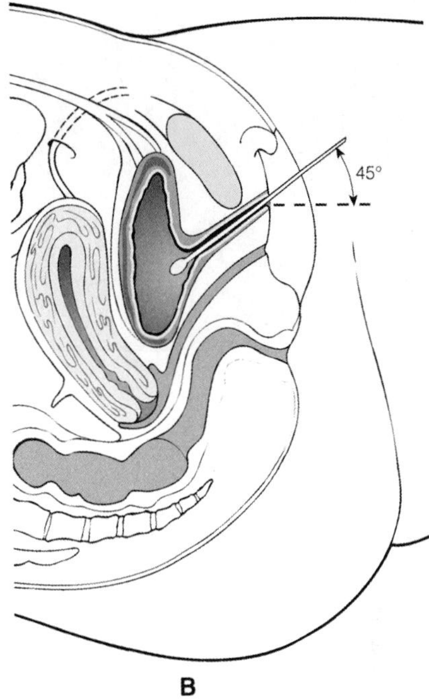

Figure 2-98 • Reproduced from Callahan TL, Caughey AB. Blueprints Obstetrics & Gynecology, 4th ed. Baltimore: Lippincott Williams & Wilkins, 2007. Fig. 19-4, p. 202.

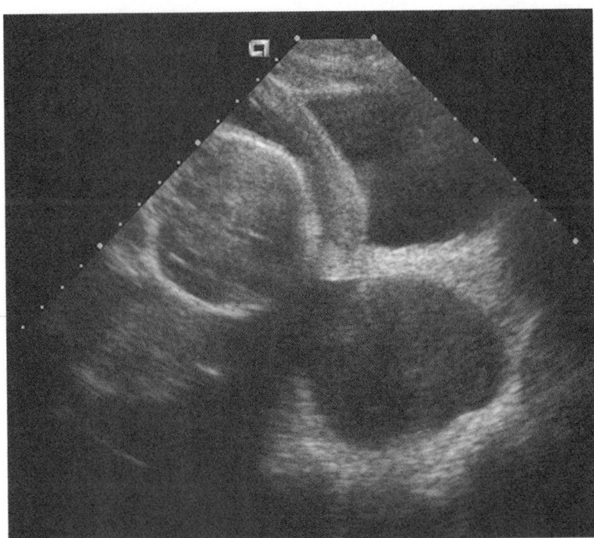

Figure 2-99 • Image Provided by Departments of Radiology and Obstetrics & Gynecology, University of California, San Francisco.

100. A 19-year-old G_1P_0 woman at 28 weeks GA by LMP is Rh-negative, while her husband is Rh-positive. When you perform an antibody screen of the mother for Rh sensitivity, you find that she is unsensitized (i.e., she does not possess antibodies to Rh factor). What is the appropriate next step in the management of this patient?

   A. Schedule an amniocentesis
   B. Recheck the father's Rh status, as this result is incompatible with the mother's current antibody status
   C. Counsel the couple about the high likelihood that this baby will be born with a hemolytic anemia
   D. Administer 300 μg of RhoGAM immediately
   E. No intervention other than close monitoring is indicated at this time

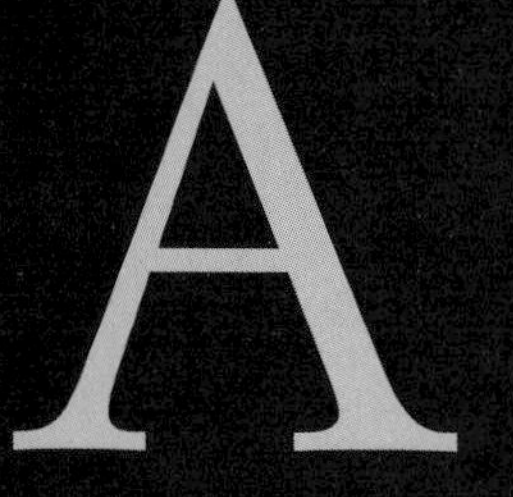

Answers and Explanations

51. B
52. D
53. B
54. B
55. D
56. A
57. E
58. B
59. C
60. D
61. D
62. A
63. E
64. C
65. D
66. B
67. B
68. C
69. B
70. E
71. D
72. C
73. B
74. A
75. C
76. B
77. C
78. B
79. D
80. D
81. B
82. C
83. C
84. C
85. B
86. A
87. C
88. D
89. C
90. A
91. C
92. C
93. C
94. C
95. A
96. E
97. C
98. A
99. B
100. D

51. **B. Conization (also called cone biopsy) is a procedure in which a cone-shaped piece of cervical tissue is removed for analysis. It can be performed using either a scalpel, known as a cold knife cone, or an electrocautery device. The specimen taken includes the entire squamocolumnar junction (SCJ), any visible ectocervical lesions, and a portion of the endocervical canal. One indication for this procedure is a two-step discrepancy between Pap smear and subsequent guided biopsies, as seen in this case where the Pap smear shows CIN I and the biopsies show CIN III. Such a large difference warrants further testing, and a cone biopsy aids in resolving this discrepancy. A second indication for conization is an unsatisfactory colposcopy, where either the SCJ or margins of abnormal areas cannot be visualized in their entirety. In this situation, conization allows for better visualization of both areas. A positive ECC showing signs of dysplasia is a third indication for conization. ECC provides cytologic information for areas located farther inside the cervical canal. Because ECC does not provide any information on tissue orientation, however, it is impossible to determine the degree of dysplasia present in these samples. Conization provides the means for further analysis. Of note, conization can also be used as a therapeutic measure, usually to remove portions of the cervix that contain high-grade dysplastic changes or frank cervical carcinoma in situ.**

A. Colposcopy helps to better visualize the TZ, where 95% of cervical cellular changes are found. The cervix is first prepped with acetic acid to dehydrate cells and precipitate proteins in the nucleus. Because neoplastic cells contain higher nuclear:cytoplasm ratios, they appear whiter than the surrounding epithelium. This white epithelium helps to guide biopsies but does not indicate the need for further work-up or treatment. Other signs of neoplasia on colposcopy include abnormal vasculature and visible punctate lesions.

C. While douching is known to predispose a woman to bacterial vaginosis and trichomoniasis by raising the pH in the vagina, it is not linked to cervical dysplasia or cancer.

D. Punctation and mosaicism are visual signs of dysplastic cells and deserve colposcopic-directed biopsy. Only if those biopsy results are consistent with more aggressive disease does the patient need to progress to conization.

E. Pregnancy is an absolute contraindication to conization because there is significant risk for the development of cervical incompetence and premature delivery.

52. **D. Smoking is believed to increase the risk for cervical cancer by decreasing the body's ability to clear cancer-causing HPV (see the explanation for C) from the body. Other major risk factors for cervical cancer include early age at first coitus (especially within 1 year of menarche), multiple sexual partners, young age at first pregnancy, high parity, low SES, and *divorce.***

A. See the explanation for D.

B. While cervical caps have been linked to cervicitis, inflammation, and toxic shock syndrome, they play no role in the pathogenesis of cervical cancer.

C. HPV is the principal causative agent of cervical cancer. Leading theories link HPV with dysplasia, with evidence suggesting that it may induce epithelial cells to undergo abnormal maturation processes and unchecked mitosis. However, only certain types of HPV are linked to cancer and/or dysplasia—namely, 16, 18, 31, 33, 35, 39, 45, 51, 52, 56, and 58. HPV type 11, as well as type 6, is a proven cause of condyloma acuminata (venereal warts), but not cervical cancer.

E. Menarche, regardless of age, is not correlated with cervical cancer.

53. **B. GD is a phenomenon seen in pregnancy related to diminished ability to metabolize and utilize carbohydrates efficiently. It is likely a product of a combination of factors, including a baseline mild carbohydrate intolerance combined with anti-insulin agents synthesized by the placenta (e.g., human placental lactogen, HPL) that increase throughout the second and third trimesters of pregnancy. GD is classified into two types: A1 (diet controlled) and A2 (medication dependent). GD has been associated with increased birthweight and birth injury, but not with fetal anomalies as has pregestational diabetes. It is also associated with increased likelihood of maternal type 2 diabetes in the future. This patient's biggest risk factor for developing GD is history of a**

prior macrosomic fetus. Other risk factors include prior GD, first-degree relative with diabetes, and Latina, South Pacific Islander, or Native American ethnicity.

A. Because the GLT is a screening test and has many false-positive results, an elevated GLT in a prior pregnancy has not been shown to increase risk of diabetes in a subsequent pregnancy.
C. While a history of affected second-degree relatives has not been well studied as a risk factor, it seems likely that there is a mild association with the development of GD. However, this correlation is not as strong as that noted with the other risk factors listed in the explanation for B.
D. The patient did not have GD in her last pregnancy. Otherwise, that would be the major risk factor.
E. Prior cesarean section has not been associated with GD in epidemiologic studies.

54. **B. This patient presents with Stage IIIB cervical cancer. Hallmarks include involvement of the lower one-third of the vagina, extension to the pelvic wall, and renal dysfunction that is not otherwise explained. The 5-year survival rate in general for Stage III cancer ranges from 36% to 44%. Stage I cancer is preclinical. It is confined to the cervix with minimal stromal invasion and microscopic lesions not larger than 7 mm across and 5 mm deep. The 5-year survival rate for Stage I cancer ranges from 85% to 100%. Stage II cancer extends beyond the cervix, but has not reached the pelvic wall. It may involve the vagina, but has not yet extended to the lower one-third. The 5-year survival rate for Stage II cancer ranges from 68% to 80%. Stage IV cancer has extended beyond the true pelvis to adjacent organs (bladder/rectum) or distant sites. Most commonly affected organs include lung, liver, and bone. Overall 5-year survival rates are dismal—only 2% to 15%.**

A, C, D, E. See the explanation for B.

55. **D. Spironolactone is traditionally used as a diuretic agent due to its effect on aldosterone receptors. However, this drug also decreases production of testosterone and works in hair follicles to decrease local binding of dihydrotestosterone (DHT, a potent stimulator of hair growth) to androgen receptors via competitive inhibition, leading to resolution of abnormal hair growth.**

A. Danazol is a weak androgenic drug used for treatment of endometriosis. It can actually cause hirsutism and other virilizing changes in some women. It is not an appropriate therapy for constitutional hirsutism.
B. DHEA is an important precursor of androstenedione and testosterone. It is not appropriate therapy for hirsutism.
C. Cyclosporine is an immunosuppressive agent used to treat inflammatory bowel disease, aplastic anemia, psoriasis, and various types of cancer. It is not known to decrease androgenic concentrations in hair follicles but has been shown to cause hirsutism in some patients.
E. Minocycline is a tetracycline-class antibiotic used primarily for the treatment of acne vulgaris. Common side effects include staining of teeth; hyperpigmentation of skin, nails, conjunctiva, tongue, and internal organs; and other rare autoimmune disorders. However, this agent does not affect hair growth.

56. **A. Sertoli-Leydig cell tumor is a rare ovarian neoplasm that accounts for less than 0.5% of all ovarian tumors. Peak incidence is between 20 and 40 years of age. Generally, a characteristic clinical course is observed, in which defeminizing changes such as amenorrhea, breast atrophy, and loss of subcutaneous fat precede the masculinizing changes of clitoral hypertrophy, hirsutism, and deepening voice. Progression is rapid, however, with most of these changes occurring within 6 months. Treatment is prompt surgical removal of the tumor; the 10-year survival rate for this type of cancer exceeds 90%.**

B. Some of the masculinizing changes such as clitoral enlargement and terminal hair growth do not regress after the tumor has been removed. However, temporal balding, menstrual changes, female body habitus, and future hair growth patterns do return to normal.
C. See the explanation for A. Hirsutism is a major symptom of this disorder.
D. See the explanation for A. This is generally a low-grade, highly curable disease.
E. Bilateral ovarian involvement is relatively rare, though when this diagnosis is made it is imperative that the contralateral ovary be inspected for gross changes.

57. **E. Depo-Provera does not interfere with the metabolism or action of antiseizure medications, and thus is safe for use in patients with epilepsy. Furthermore, progesterone has been associated with diminished seizure activity. Combination OCPs, on the other hand, are relatively contraindicated due to interference by most antiseizure medications on combination OCP metabolism and efficacy.**

A. Combination OCPs exert their effect mostly by use of progestins to block LH secretion, thereby preventing ovulation. Progestins also serve to thicken cervical mucus, thereby inhibiting sperm passage and decreasing fallopian tube peristalsis, which interferes with zygote transport and implantation. The estrogenic component is important in blocking FSH secretion, which prevents the development of a dominant ovarian follicle. When used in combination, these hormones effect atrophic changes in the uterine lining, thereby hindering implantation.

B. Progestin-only OCPs exert essentially the same effects as do the progestin components of combination OCPs. However, the low doses of progestin are not as effective in preventing ovulation, which can happen as much as 40% of the time. In addition, the low doses of progestin necessitate taking progestin-only OCPs at almost the same time every day to reduce the risk of failure, making them inherently less flexible.

C. Progestin-only OCPs have no effect on the contents or production of breast milk, and there is no evidence of nursing infants being adversely affected by progestin-only OCPs. Lactating women actually have a lower failure rate with progestin-only OCPs compared to the general population, however, because high circulating prolactin levels further suppress ovulation.

D. Numerous studies have confirmed the equal efficacy of the transdermal patch with traditional combination OCPs.

58. **B. This patient gives an excellent history for endometriosis. It is likely she has endometrial implants in her pelvis that undergo the same cycle as her endometrium and become inflamed each month with her menses. Over time, these implants can become scarred, cause adhesions, and lead to pain that is intermenstrual and eventually continuous. This pain can become quite debilitating, leading to change in work, school, and social habits. The first step in the treatment of endometriosis involves the administration of OCPs and NSAIDs. If the patient notes relief from pain except during menses, the OCPs can be given continuously with just one or two withdrawal bleeds per year.**

A. Laparoscopy in the setting of endometriosis and pelvic pain in general should be used after the patient has failed medical treatment. Laparoscopy is the gold standard for diagnosis of endometriosis, allowing biopsy for pathological confirmation and resection of endometrial implants. Resection of the implants and lysis of adhesions have also been shown to give symptomatic relief. This relief, however, is rarely permanent.

C. The GnRH analog Lupron (leuprolide) is used in severe cases of endometriosis. It causes ovarian suppression and effectively produces a menopausal-like state. While this can give symptomatic relief, it can also lead to other problems due to the prolonged hypoestrogenic state, such as osteoporosis. Any patient undergoing GnRH therapy should have a bone density scan at baseline and be followed during treatment.

D. Consultation with the pain and psychiatry services can be an important aspect of management. However, this can often lead to alienation of the patient, who may infer that you think her pain is "in her head." Thus it is better to provide medical therapy first and form a therapeutic bond with the patient. If the medical therapy fails, then you should consider these consults prior to surgery.

E. Although both chronic PID and endometritis are causes of chronic pain treatable with antibiotics, this patient's story is not consistent with either diagnosis. Cultures should be taken at the initial exam to rule out PID.

59. **C. This procedure involves placing a plastic clip (Figure 2-59a) similar to a staple on the isthmus of the tube to occlude passage of ova. It is the most easily reversed procedure (success rates are as high as 50% to 75%), because only a very small portion of the tubes is damaged during the procedure. It also carries the highest failure rate for this reason—as high as 1%.**

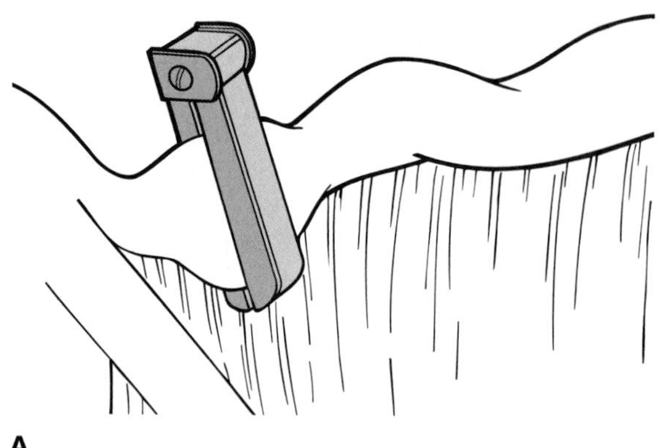

Figure 2-59A • Reproduced from Callahan TL, Caughey AB. Blueprints Obstetrics & Gynecology, 4th ed. Baltimore: Lippincott Williams & Wilkins, 2007.

A. The Falope ring (Figure 2-59b) is similar to the Hulka clip, except that it involves placement of a single ring around two adjacent portions of the tube. It has a slightly lower failure rate, and a lower rate of successful reversal, than the clip.

B. This is the most commonly used of the ligation techniques, whereby the proximal and distal borders of the middle third of the tube are ligated and the section of tube in between is removed (Figure 2-59c). The ends then

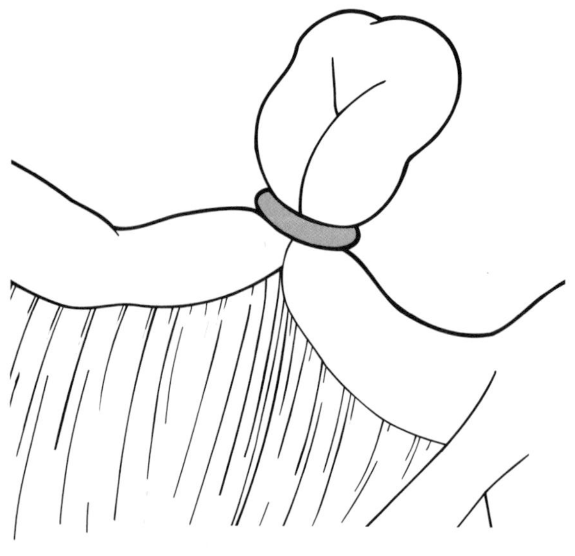

Figure 2-59B • Reproduced from Callahan TL, Caughey AB. Blueprints Obstetrics & Gynecology, 4th ed. Baltimore: Lippincott Williams & Wilkins, 2007.

seal closed over time. This procedure presents a much more difficult reversal task, and success rates hover near 25% to 50%.

D. Electrocautery involves electrical ligation of portions of the tube using coagulation forceps. It is fast and very reliable, and the most difficult procedure to reverse because of the extensive damage done to the tube. There is also a higher risk of damage to adjacent organs during the procedure.

E. Colpotomy describes the surgical approach through the vagina taken to sterilize a patient, and is not a procedure in itself. Any of the laparoscopic or laparotomy procedures can be performed via this approach.

60. **D. The mother's karyotype represents a balanced Robertsonian translocation, in which her two copies of chromosome 21 (which are acrocentric) have lost their very short p sections and subsequently joined their q sections into one chromosome. Because karyotypes are done on cultured lymphocytes from peripheral blood, this represents the karyotype of all her cells, including germ cells. Therefore, when her germ cells undergo meiosis, 50% of them will have two copies of chromosome 21 (joined as a single chromosome), while the other 50% will have no copies of chromosome 21. When these gametes subsequently join with a normal paternal gamete containing one copy of chromosome 21, half of the resulting embryos will be trisomic for 21, and the other half will be monosomic for 21. One would conclude, then, that this couple's chance of having a Down syndrome baby is 50%. However, because monosomy 21 is incompatible with life and all such embryos are spontaneously aborted, all live births will be trisomy 21 births, leaving this couple with a 100% chance that their next baby will have Down syndrome.**

    A, B, C, E. See the explanation for D.

61. **D. The combined pattern of elevated β-hCG, low MSAFP, and low estriol is concerning for Down syndrome. However, many factors contribute to the interpretation of these results, including maternal age, weight, ethnicity, mother's diabetic status, and multiple gestations. A likelihood of Down syndrome is then determined based on these factors. Note that**

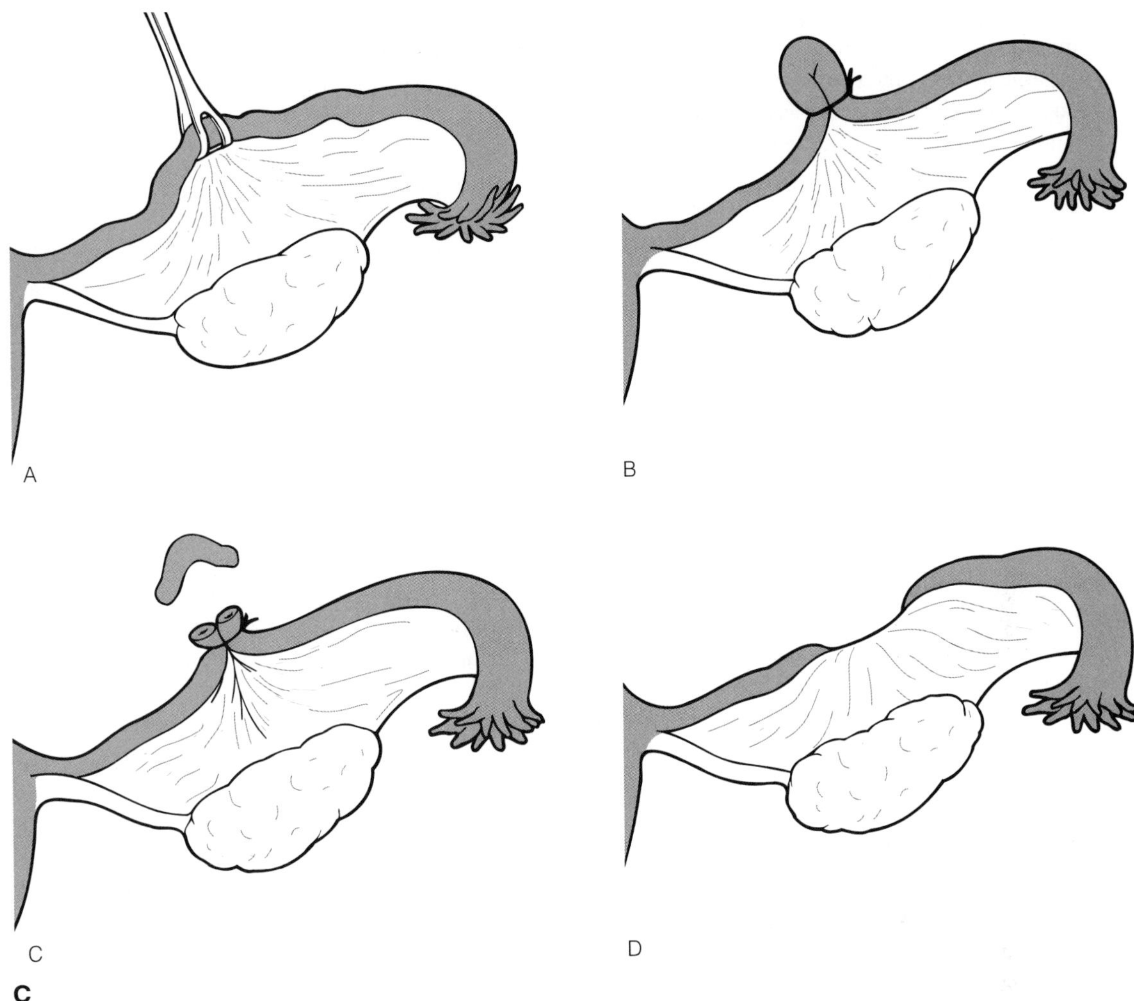

Figure 2-59C • Reproduced from Callahan TL, Caughey AB. Blueprints Obstetrics & Gynecology, 4th ed. Baltimore: Lippincott Williams & Wilkins, 2007.

the vast majority of mothers with a positive triple screen will deliver normal, healthy infants. In addition to the triple screen abnormalities, the finding on US of a likely pyloric stenosis or duodenal atresia as indicated by the "double-bubble" sign increases the likelihood of Down syndrome.

A. Edward's syndrome (trisomy 18) is similar to Down syndrome, except that symptoms are much more severe. Edward's syndrome infants usually do not survive more than a few days after birth, and only 10% will live 1 year. They present with severe mental retardation and defects in many organ systems. This is usually represented by low estriol (similar to Down syndrome) and low β-hCG (opposite of Down syndrome) levels.

B. Neural tube defects include such disorders as spina bifida, meningocele, and anencephaly. Generally, these abnormalities are indicated by an elevated MSAFP (opposite of Down syndrome), elevated amniotic AFP, and, in the case of anencephaly, a low β-hCG (also opposite of Down syndrome). Depending on severity, some types of neural tube defects can be corrected surgically.

C. Trisomy 13 (Patau's syndrome) is the least common and most severe of the autosomal trisomies. It is characterized by severe mental retardation, neurologic abnormalities including holoprosencephaly (the brain does not divide into distinct hemispheres), cardiac and other organic structural defects, and death within 3 days. This disorder is not associated with any findings on the triple screen.

E. Turner's syndrome presents as a girl with short stature, webbed neck, amenorrhea, and absence of secondary sex characteristics. Generally, this disorder is not diagnosed until puberty, when these findings become much more noticeable. As with trisomy 13, there is no association between Turner's syndrome and the triple screen.

62. **A. The combination of results is associated with a higher risk of a fetus with Down syndrome. An abnormal result can also be seen with a pregnancy that is earlier than predicted by LMP. However, this outcome is less likely in this case because the US confirmed that the fetus's GA is the same as its calculated age by LMP. To evaluate for Down syndrome, a formal karyotype of the fetus is needed. This can be accomplished by using either amniocentesis (a process by which amniotic fluid is drawn via a needle using US guidance), cordocentesis, or chorionic villi sampling. Amniocentesis is generally performed at or around 15 weeks, making it the most appropriate choice in this case.**

B. Cordocentesis is done by inserting a spinal needle, via US guidance, into an umbilical cord vessel to draw blood for analysis. It has a much higher complication rate than amniocentesis and is reserved for situations where rapid diagnosis is important.

C. A CT scan would not provide any additional information.

D. CVS involves sampling of chorionic villi taken either through the cervix or through the abdomen. This procedure is generally done at 9 to 12 weeks GA.

E. See the explanation for A.

63. **E. The patient has vulvovaginal candidiasis, which presents with pruritis and a white discharge, and which may have an instigator such as a change in sexual habits, undergarments, or a course of antibiotics. Treatments include over-the-counter antifungal preparations (Monistat), prescription topical agents (Terazole cream), and oral fluconazole (Diflucan). The oral treatment is more than 85% effective from a one-time dose and is much more convenient than the topical agents.**

A. Oral acyclovir would be used to treat or prophylax against herpes simplex virus (HSV) lesions.

B. Topical acyclovir is more often used for herpes labialis or herpetic lesions on the upper lip than for herpes vaginalis or vulvar lesions.

C. Metronidazole can be used to treat bacterial vaginosis. Common dosing regimens include 500 mg PO BID and 250 mg PO TID.

D. Metronidazole can also be given in a vaginal preparation (Metro-gel).

64. **C. Rh incompatibility is a serious problem that can present in pregnancy. It occurs in the setting of an Rh-negative mother and an Rh-positive fetus. At some point during the pregnancy, but particularly at delivery, a feto-maternal hemorrhage typically occurs that leads to maternal production of IgG antibodies to Rh-positive erythrocytes. Because these antibodies can freely cross the placenta, they attack fetal blood, leading to a hemolytic anemia and erythroblastosis fetalis. The first child is usually safer from this fate than subsequent children, because blood mixing does not occur until late in pregnancy or at birth, which does not allow enough time for maternal generation of antibodies to affect the fetus. Prevention of Rh sensitization is accomplished by giving all Rh-negative pregnant women IM injections of IgG (RhoGAM) at 26 to 28 weeks of pregnancy and postpartum if the fetus is Rh-positive. Rh factor is screened for at the first prenatal visit; also at this visit, a broad antibody screen to all of the erythrocyte antigens is performed, as some of these antigens more rarely cause hemolysis in the fetus.**

A. The triple screen is calibrated to screen between 15 and 20 weeks of gestation.

B. Screening for gestational diabetes is usually done at 26 to 28 weeks GA, as it is dependent upon the increasing production of the human chorionic somatomammotropin by the placenta.

D. GBS culture is usually performed at 36 weeks of gestation.

E. Pelvic US is typically not performed until 18 to 20 weeks GA, unless it is required for dating in the setting of unknown LMP.

65. **D. Antepartum antiretroviral therapy is the central treatment modality for reducing the risk of vertical transmission in HIV-positive women. The recommended regimen consists of zidovudine (ZDV; for women with low viral loads) or a combination of zidovudine, another nucleoside analog, and either a non-nucleoside analog or a protease inhibitor (for women with viral loads exceeding 1000 or those who desire combination therapy despite low viral loads). Patients who are compliant with antiretroviral therapy decrease the risk of transmission (which is 25% if untreated) by more than 60%. Delivery by cesarean section was once recommended for all HIV-positive women, as it reduces fetal exposure to maternal HIV and has been shown to clearly reduce the risk of vertical transmission in women who have not taken antiretroviral therapy. Currently, for women who have received appropriate antiretroviral therapy and achieve undetectable viral loads, cesarean delivery is thought to be of very marginal value, if any, and is usually reserved for obstetrical indications.**

    A. Treatment should be initiated regardless of viral load, as vertical transmission is possible even when viral mRNA is undetectable.
    B. Intrapartum ZDV and short courses of antepartum ZDV (e.g., beginning at 36 weeks) have been shown to reduce transmission rates, but these strategies are not as effective as prolonged combination therapy. These short-course antepartum regimens play an important role in countries where antiretroviral medications are prohibitively expensive, but they are not the standard of care in the United States. Although the majority of vertical transmission is believed to be intrapartum, the virus is also passed transplacentally, and any intervention limited to the perinatal period will not address this additional risk.
    C. Some concerns have been raised about the effects of antiretroviral medications on the fetus, but these are thought to be outweighed by the risk of transmitting the virus if they are withheld. In general, optimal therapy should not be altered because a patient is pregnant. For patients who are known to be HIV infected before pregnancy, some controversy exists regarding whether these drugs can be held during the critical period for organogenesis. Depending on the clinical situation, treatment may be delayed until 12 weeks gestation. At 17 weeks GA, this patient should clearly begin therapy.
    E. Invasive monitoring is a risk factor for vertical transmission and should be avoided whenever possible. Other peripartum risk factors for increased rates of transmission include prolonged rupture of membranes and genital ulceration.

66. **B. Vertical transmission of HIV occurs not only transplacentally and during birth, but also via breast milk. In the United States, where alternative sources of infant nutrition are readily available, breastfeeding by HIV-positive mothers is absolutely contraindicated. The patient needs to be made aware of the risk that breastfeeding poses to her newborn. In developing countries, where alternative infant nutrition is often not available, most infants are breastfed, which leads to high rates of vertical transmission.**

    A. HIV is known to be expressed in breast milk, and breastfeeding carries an increased risk of transmitting the virus.
    C. Breast milk offers multiple advantages for the neonate over formula feeding, including provision of passive immunity, but the risk of transmitting the virus clearly outweighs these benefits.
    D. A protective effect of maternal immunoglobulins has not been demonstrated, and the risk of transmitting the virus outweighs any theoretical benefit.
    E. While several antiretroviral drugs (e.g., ZDV, 3TC, and nevirapine) have been shown to be present in breast milk, a protective effect has not been demonstrated, and the risk of transmitting the virus outweighs any theoretical benefit. ZDV can be given directly to high-risk neonates.

67. **B. There is a threefold increase in congenital anomalies in patients with overt (pregestational) diabetes, but this increase is not seen in true gestational diabetes. This patient's elevated 3-hour OGTT could, of course, represent the unmasking of pregestational diabetes, but this patient has no pertinent positive features in her history. Statistically, the majority of diabetes diagnosed for the first time in pregnancy is true pregnancy-induced diabetes, depending on the patient population and their prepregnancy risk.**

A. Pregestational maternal diabetes is clearly associated with an increase in congenital anomalies. Cardiac abnormalities and neural tube defects are the most common anomalies; sacral agenesis, while less common, is an anomaly highly specific to diabetes.

C. Early sonography can detect some malformations associated with diabetes (e.g., anencephaly), but many other congenital anomalies (e.g., cardiac defects) may not be apparent until later in gestation (18 to 20 weeks).

D. Diabetes—whether gestational or overt—is not independently associated with an increased risk of chromosomal abnormalities.

E. While oral hypoglycemic agents are a recent addition to the armamentarium to treat patients with GD, they would not decrease the risk of fetal anomalies at this GA. Although some concerns had been voiced over the use of these agents, and a weak and theoretical association with fetal nephrotoxicity and hypoglycemia had been hypothesized, recent studies do not suggest that either of these outcomes is of concern. Now that this patient has been diagnosed with GD, she should be counseled regarding diet and exercise, and she should check her blood sugars four times per day. If they remain persistently elevated despite these measures, oral hypoglycemic agents or insulin can be initiated.

68. **C. This patient's history is a classic presentation of one of the uterine outflow obstruction syndromes. These syndromes include imperforate hymen, transverse vaginal septum, and vaginal agenesis with either a rudimentary uterine horn or entire uterus. When these patients go through menarche, the lack of vaginal egress of menses leads to retrograde menstrual flow into the peritoneal cavity and subsequent cyclic pain. In addition, patients with imperforate hymen and transverse vaginal septum can experience a buildup of menses that collects in the upper vagina; this buildup can stretch over time and contain a large volume of old menstrual discharge. In this case, the diagnosis is either imperforate hymen or transverse vaginal septum because of the fullness noted by the patient and the clinician. The latter is the more likely diagnosis because a normal, patent hymeneal ring is noted.**

A. Testicular feminization also may present with a foreshortened vagina. Because affected patients do not have a uterus, however, the history regarding cyclical pain is inconsistent with testicular feminization.

B. Imperforate hymen is the second most likely diagnosis; it is often indistinguishable from transverse vaginal septum. However, the presence of a clear hymeneal ring near the introitus with the vagina beyond confirms the diagnosis of transverse vaginal septum.

D. Labial fusion is seen more commonly in newborns, young children, or postmenopausal women secondary to a hypoestrogenic state and/or excessive androgenic state.

E. Patients with transverse vaginal septum are most likely to have a normal uterus, tubes, and ovaries.

69. **B. 11β-hydroxylase deficiency is found in one form of congenital adrenal hyperplasia (CAH). This enzyme catalyzes the conversion of 11-deoxycorticosterone to 11-deoxycortisol (compound S), which is one step involved in the production of cortisol. Due to the redundant pathways in which cortisol is made, cortisol deficiency is not generally observed. Buildup of the 11-deoxycorticosterone precursor due to enzyme deficiency, however, does lead to excess androgen production via shunt pathways. Hallmarks of this form of CAH include mild hirsutism, mild hypertension, and virilization.**

A. 21-Hydroxylase is another enzyme involved in cortisol and aldosterone synthesis. Deficiency of this enzyme is the most common form of CAH, affecting approximately 2% of the population. Buildup of progesterone and 17α-hydroxyprogesterone due to this enzyme deficiency leads to excess production of DHEA, which is a precursor protein for androstenedione and testosterone synthesis. Virilization tends to be more severe in this disorder than in 11β-hydroxylase deficiency.

C. Aromatase converts androgens to estrogens in adipose tissue, muscle, and hepatocytes. While a deficiency in this enzyme could theoretically lead to virilization, it would not cause the large elevation in 11-deoxycorticosterone levels observed in this patient.

D. 3β-hydroxysteroid dehydrogenase is another enzyme implicated in some forms of CAH. A deficiency of this enzyme would lead to increased levels of 17-hydroxypregnenolone. 11-Deoxycorticosterone levels would not be markedly elevated.

E. 5α-reductase converts testosterone to dihydrotestosterone (DHT) in peripheral sites such as hair follicles. DHT is a more potent form of testosterone involved in hair growth and, during embryonic development, in the formation of various external genital structures. A deficiency in 5α-reductase would not affect 11-deoxycorticosterone levels.

70. **E. The characteristics on physical exam are more consistent with a benign mass, but any adnexal mass in a postmenopausal woman is considered cancer until proven otherwise. While the large majority of women of reproductive age with this presentation will be found to have functional cysts or other benign processes, an ovarian mass in a woman older than age 50 is more likely to be malignant than benign. If this patient were younger and premenopausal, the chances of malignancy would be sufficiently small that (after appropriate imaging) she could be simply observed for probable resolution of the mass (with no further action required at this time). In contrast, a postmenopausal patient with a mass larger than 3 cm should be scheduled for exploratory surgery.**

A. Although malignant tumors are more commonly unilateral than bilateral, the finding of a bilateral mass carries a greater risk of malignancy than does the finding a unilateral mass.
B. A fixed mass is suggestive of malignancy.
C. An irregular mass is suggestive of malignancy.
D. A nodular cul-de-sac is suggestive of malignancy that has spread to the pelvic cavity.

71. **D. A septated mass is concerning for malignancy.**

A. A solid mass is more suggestive of malignancy.
B. Masses larger than 5 cm are more likely to be malignant than are smaller masses.
C. Irregular contours are suggestive of malignancy.
E. Ascites are suggestive of malignancy.

72. **C. Many of the major risk factors for ovarian cancer, other than family history, are thought to be secondary to an increased period of "chronic uninterrupted ovulation." Nulliparity is a very strong risk factor, as it contributes to this effect. Similar risk factors include early menarche and late menopause.**

A. The average age of menopause in the United States is 50 to 51 years, so this patient's menopause would not be considered late onset.
B. OCPs have been found to be significantly protective against ovarian cancer, presumably through suppression of ovulation. Five years' use of OCPs has been shown to reduce the risk of ovarian cancer in a nulliparous woman by about half.
D. Tubal ligation is associated with a decreased risk of ovarian cancer. One hypothesis is that disruption of communication between the ovary and the external environment may limit exposure to carcinogens ascending the reproductive tract.
E. Infertility treatment, including clomiphene citrate, has not been shown to be an independent risk factor for ovarian cancer. Infertility itself is a risk factor (presumably ovarian dysfunction leads to both infertility and a greater risk of malignancy), and as a result there is a noncausal association between women who have received infertility treatment and the risk of ovarian cancer. This patient is presumably not infertile (with the diagnosis of male factor) and does not have this increased risk.

73. **B. The history is consistent with development of a breast abscess in the setting of mastitis. Approximately 10% of women with mastitis develop a breast abscess despite antibiosis. The next appropriate step in evaluation is to get a breast US not only to confirm a breast abscess, but also to evaluate the location and extent of the abscess. Abscesses that undermine the nipple may jeopardize the vascular supply of the nipple and require consultation with the general or plastic surgery service.**

A. Despite the patient's concerning family history, her clinical course is more consistent with an abscess than breast cancer. Core biopsies are done in evaluation of solid breast masses that are concerning for a neoplasm.
C. In this patient with a difficult exam, it is not entirely clear whether she has an abscess. However, if there is an abscess on US, the patient will subsequently need incision and

drainage of the abscess. Cultures and sensitivity of the purulent fluid from the abscess should be sent because many babies (and thus organisms of mastitis and subsequent abscesses) are colonized with methicillin-resistant staphylococcal strains while in the nursery during their newborn hospitalization.

D. US is the standard imaging for breast abscesses; a CT scan is not warranted.

E. Given the progressive nature of the breast process and outpatient-regimen failure, reevaluation in 1 week would be inappropriate.

74. **A. *Staphylococcus aureus* is the most common pathogen in mastitis and breast abscesses. The organism usually arises from the infant's mouth and nose and enters via a crack or fissure in the nipple. Thus, it is safe, and recommended, that the mother continue to feed her infant from the infected breast. Good breast care and routine use of emollient creams, such as lanolin, help prevent nipple fissures. Proper breast care should be a routine part of postpartum teaching.**

B. *Staphylococcus epidermidis* is part of normal skin flora, but is not a common cause of mastitis.

C. *Pseudomonas* is a more common pathogen of the respiratory or urinary tract.

D. *Propionobacterium acnes* is the bacteria most commonly associated with acne.

E. *Lactococcal ductalis* is not a real organism.

75. **C. This woman's symptoms are most consistent with postpartum blues, which typically has an onset on postpartum days 2–6 and subsides by 2 weeks after parturition. Postpartum blues occur in approximately 50% of new mothers.**

A. Postpartum depression occurs in approximately 10% of new mothers and usually has an onset at 3 to 6 months after delivery. Postpartum depression is diagnosed by the presence of at least five of the following symptoms that have at least a 2-week duration: depressed mood most of the day, diminished pleasure and interest in activities, weight changes without intentional effort to cause such, insomnia or hypersomnia, psychomotor agitation or retardation, fatigue, feelings of worthlessness or excessive guilt, difficulty concentrating or recurrent thoughts of death or suicide without a specific plan or attempt.

B. Bipolar disorder is characterized by alternating periods of depression and mania. The short nature of this patient's mood swings are inconsistent with bipolar disorder. Bipolar disorder cannot be diagnosed based on 4 days of behavior.

D. Malingering is the intentional faking of physical or psychological illness or symptoms to gain something—often medication, disability, or money. Neither the patient nor her husband is malingering nor is there evidence that any of the reported symptoms are not legitimate.

E. Postpartum psychosis is rare. Women who have an underlying depressive, manic, schizophrenic, or schizoaffective disorder, or who have a history of a severe life event in the prior year are predisposed to its development.

76. **B. Approximately one-fourth of women who have had a postpartum mental disorder will suffer from a recurrent event with a future pregnancy. Therefore, patients with prior episodes of postpartum depression should have a number of prophylactic measures taken, including an intact support environment of family and friends, appointments with professional counseling postpartum, and antidepressant medications.**

A, C, D, E. All of these are incorrect.

77. **C. A Pap smear is a screening test and does not give a pathological tissue diagnosis. According to the Bethesda System, the appropriate next step in evaluation after a Pap smear is reported as HSIL is to perform a colposcopy and ECC with biopsies as indicated.**

A. A CKC is a treatment procedure that is done only after a tissue diagnosis is obtained. Although they were very popular in the past, cold knife cones have since been largely replaced by LEEPs. The advantage of a CKC over a LEEP is easier evaluation of the tissue borders by the pathologist. If the patient's colposcopy evaluation reveals a high-grade lesion, conization would be indicated at that point.

B. This is one standard-of-care option for LSIL (the other being to go directly to colposcopy and ECC), but not for HSIL.

D. Cryotherapy is a treatment procedure once a tissue diagnosis is obtained. To be a candidate for cryotherapy, a patient must have had a "satisfactory" colposcopy (the entire

TZ was visualized) and show no evidence of advanced disease.

E. Bacterial vaginosis does not lead to HSIL. Thus, it would not be appropriate to retreat the patient and then to repeat the Pap smear. Vaginal infections such as *Gardnerella* vaginitis, chlamydia, candidiasis, gonorrhea, and trichomoniasis can lead to a Pap smear being read as "reactive" or "inflammatory." With either of these Pap smear reports, it would be appropriate to treat the infection and repeat the Pap smear.

78. **B. Antepartum testing that is performed beyond 41 or 42 weeks gestation in pregnancy is called post-dates testing. The nonstress test shown has two fetal heart rate accelerations that are at least 15 beats per minute higher than the baseline and is deemed reactive and thus reassuring. Patients with reassuring testing have been shown to have lower rates of IUFD as compared to high-risk patients without testing. Options for testing include the following: nonstress test (NST), contraction stress test (CST), modified biophysical profile (BPP, consisting of an NST and amniotic fluid assessment), and a complete BPP (evaluation of five diagnostic criteria including fetal tone, movement, and breathing motion, along with amniotic fluid assessment and an NST). In many high-risk pregnancies, this testing is begun between 32 and 34 weeks of gestation.**

A. GD is diagnosed early in the third trimester (if not earlier). It is never tested for in the post-dates period.

C. The likelihood of meconium in the amniotic fluid increases with GA. Its most dangerous complication is the risk of meconium aspiration syndrome, which carries a high rate of morbidity for the fetus. This syndrome cannot be identified by a nonstress test.

D. Macrosomia (fetal weight greater than 4000 to 4500 g by varying definitions) is seen at higher rates in post-dates pregnancies. It is also associated with increased rates of cesarean delivery and shoulder dystocia at birth. This condition cannot be identified by a nonstress test.

E. Patients with preeclampsia should undergo early antepartum testing starting at 32 to 34 weeks of gestation. There is no association between an abnormal nonstress test and development of preeclampsia.

79. **D. There is a strong association between cervical dysplasia and cervical cancer with HPV. In particular, the subtypes that put one at risk include 16, 18, and 31; in contrast, subtypes 6 and 11 predispose to condyloma formation.**

A. The average length of time to the development of cervical cancer with CIN I is 7 to 10 years, whereas CIN II can develop into carcinoma in 3 to 4 years. However, some lesions progress much faster, so most patients are managed aggressively.

B. Approximately 60% of CIN I lesions resolve spontaneously.

C, E. The next step in the management of a CIN I lesion would be scheduled colposcopy and directed biopsy. Colposcopy allows a better view of the cervix and uses acetic acid to bring out the possible lesions by turning them white. Once a formal diagnosis is made, CIN I lesions are usually followed every 3 to 6 months with colposcopy until the lesions either regress or progress. If a diagnosis is made at that time, cryotherapy or laser can be used. However, an excisional procedure that can demonstrate clear margins is often the procedure of choice with either LEEP or a CKC biopsy.

80. **D. Vulvar carcinoma accounts for 4% of gynecologic malignancies, with 90% of cases involving the squamous cell variety. It typically arises in postmenopausal women 65 to 70 years of age, and the most common presenting complaint is vulvar pruritis. Lesions most commonly arise in the inferior two-thirds of either labium majus. A punch biopsy should be performed.**

A. Topical estrogen is often prescribed to relieve symptoms of postmenopausal vaginal atrophy. However, the presence of an ulcer is not consistent with routine atrophy.

B. Topical steroids are used to treat lichen sclerosis, lichen simplex chronicus, psoriasis, and lichen planus. The described lesion is not typical for any of these diagnoses, and delay of further evaluation would be inappropriate.

C. One needs a tissue diagnosis prior to performing a therapeutic excisional procedure, and wide local vulvar excisions are not done in the office.

E. Atrophy with pruritis is quite common in postmenopausal women and prescription of HRT can alleviate these symptoms in appropriate patients. However, this patient has a discrete ulcerated lesion that is suspicious for vulvar carcinoma and should be biopsied.

81. **B. The upper vagina is the most common place for vaginal carcinoma to arise. The most common complaint with vaginal cancer is a vaginal discharge that is often bloody. However, urinary symptoms can arise with bulky disease given the close proximity of the upper vagina to the bladder neck.**

A, C, D. These are not the most common locations for vaginal carcinoma to arise. The labia majora is not part of the vagina.

E. Vaginal cancer has a predilection for the upper vagina.

82. **C. The upper vagina is drained by the internal and common iliac nodes.**

A. Vaginal cancer does not spread hematogenously.

B. The lower vagina is drained by the regional nodes in the femoral triangle.

D. The supraclavicular nodes are not in the immediate chain of nodes that drain the genitourinary system. The presence of a palpable supraclavicular node should alert the clinician to the possibility of other malignancies—specifically, lung, breast, GI, and hematogenous.

E. The posterior cervical chain of nodes is in the neck, not the pelvis. These nodes are commonly enlarged with viral and oropharyngeal infections (strep pharyngitis).

83. **C. Stage III extends to the pelvic sidewall. Stage IV extends beyond the true pelvis or involves the mucosa of the bladder or rectum. This patient has at least Stage III disease but may well have Stage IV disease. Her urinary symptoms could be secondary either to mucosal invasion or mass compression. Five-year survival rates are 40% for Stage III disease and 0% for Stage IV disease.**

A. Stage I is limited to the vaginal mucosa.

B. Stage II involves the submucosa but does not extend to the sidewall.

D. There is no Stage V.

E. Vaginal cancer is clinically staged, not pathologically staged.

84. **C. Induction of labor has been associated with a two- to fivefold increase in the rate of uterine rupture. This rate of uterine rupture is further increased by the use of prostaglandins for induction by three- to fourfold. Thus, in most patients undergoing indicated induction of labor who had a prior cesarean delivery, mechanical means with a Foley bulb are typically utilized.**

A. The risk of uterine rupture in women with one prior low transverse cesarean scar is 0.5% to 1%. This risk would be increased if the patient underwent induction of labor, but would still be below the 5% to 10% range.

B. Management of uterine rupture requires immediate laparotomy, delivery of the fetus, and repair of the rupture site or hysterectomy if bleeding cannot be controlled.

D. In some early studies, fetal mortality in the event of uterine rupture was as high as 30% to 40%. However, with the ready availability of obstetricians and anesthesiologists, as well as earlier recognition of uterine rupture, mortality rates in one recent large study were closer to 5%.

E. Injudicious use of oxytocin during labor increases the risk of uterine rupture in patients with prior uterine scars.

85. **B. Post-term pregnancies are at increased risk for fetal demise, macrosomia, meconium aspiration, and oligohydramnios. The management of post-term pregnancy includes more frequent office visits, increased fetal testing, and plans for eventual labor induction. This patient has a favorable cervix for induction. Beyond 42 weeks, however, most patients will be counseled toward labor induction regardless of the cervical exam.**

A. The opposite is true, with amniotic fluid volume decreasing toward the end of pregnancy.

C. The risk of Rh sensitization does not increase with postdates pregnancy.

D. The opposite is true, with the rate of macrosomia increasing among post-term pregnancies. The risk of low birthweight (less than 2500 g) would be quite low among post-term infants.

E. The rate of respiratory distress syndrome falls with increasing GA until 39 weeks, at which point it remains stable.

86. **A. Twin–twin transfusion syndrome can occur in monochorionic/diamnionic twin gestations. Vascular communication between twins can result in one fetus with hypervolemia, cardiomegaly, glomerulotubal hypertrophy, edema, ascites, and polyhydramnios, while the other twin has hypovolemia, growth restriction, and oligohydramnios. The US image shows fetal ascites and large pleural effusions.**

B. Rh sensitization may occur when an Rh-negative woman is exposed to fetal blood that is Rh-positive, resulting in maternal production of antibodies (i.e., sensitization). In sensitized patients with Rh-positive fetuses, these antibodies can cross the placenta and cause hemolysis of fetal blood cells, leading to varying degrees of fetal anemia and possibly erythroblastosis fetalis.

C. In "Siamese" twinning, or conjoined twinning, the fetuses are monochorionic/monoamniotic (i.e., they share one placenta and an amniotic sac).

D. This is not a normal variant of twinning.

E. Congenital rubella syndrome, like any teratogenic infection, would be likely to affect both twins.

87. **C. In reproductive-age women, pregnancy is the most common cause of secondary amenorrhea. In this patient who has a history of being sexually active, a urine pregnancy test should be performed in the office to obtain a diagnosis. The other clue in her history is the weight gain despite her athletic training.**

A. Kallman's syndrome involves a congenital absence of GnRH (commonly associated with anosmia) and is a hypothalamic cause of primary amenorrhea. Primary amenorrhea is the absence of menses in women who have not undergone menarche by age 16 or who have not begun menstruating by 4 years after thelarche.

B. Secondary amenorrhea is the absence of menses for three menstrual cycles or a total of 6 months in a woman who has had previously normal menses. Common causes of secondary amenorrhea include pregnancy, anatomic abnormalities (e.g., Asherman's syndrome), ovarian dysfunction, hypothyroidism, prolactinomas and hyperprolactinemia, and CNS or hypothalamic disorders.

D, E. Exercise and stress can both lead to hypothalamic dysfunction, producing amenorrhea. Certainly in this patient who is a competitive athlete, as well as likely to have a stressful academic life, these issues would be the next in line as likely etiologies for her secondary amenorrhea.

88. **D. Screening for trisomy 18 is via serum screening, of which MSAFP is a part. Both trisomy 18 and trisomy 21 (Down syndrome) are increased with an MSAFP value that is lower than normal. The triple screen (MSAFP, estriol, and β-hCG) differ between trisomy 18 and Down syndrome in that all three values are diminished in trisomy 18, whereas β-hCG is actually increased in the setting of Down syndrome.**

A. In cases of anencephaly, AFP is released from the neural tissue into the amniotic fluid, and subsequently crosses into maternal circulation leading to higher MSAFP levels.

B. Because of the increased number of fetuses, more AFP crosses into the maternal circulation.

C. AFP is primarily produced in the fetal neural tissue and liver. Thus any break in the fetal abdominal integument can allow increased levels to be released into the amniotic fluid and subsequently into the maternal circulation.

E. Use of MSAFP as a screening test is dependent upon accurate dating of the pregnancy. Because MSAFP increases during the second trimester, elevated values can occur if a patient is actually several weeks further along in pregnancy than indicated by her dating.

89. **C. Premature labor, second-trimester abortions, and fetal malpresentation (i.e., breech or transverse lie) are likely due the size limitations of a bicornuate uterus.**

A. Endometriosis is not associated with a bicornuate uterus. It has been found in association with blind uterine horns.

B. In the case of uterine anomalies associated with DES use by a patient's mother, there is an increase in vaginal cancer. However, increased rates of uterine cancer have not been documented.

D. While uterine anomalies are associated with urinary tract anomalies, they are not particularly associated with increased rates of UTIs.

Embryologically, the superior vagina, cervix, uterus, and fallopian tubes all originate from fusion of the paramesonephric (Mullerian) ducts. The urinary tract develops from the neighboring urogenital sinus. If the paramesonephric ducts fail to fuse during embryogenesis, urinary tract anomalies can also result given the proximity of these two developing areas. Further investigation is warranted, often in the form of an intravenous pyelogram.

E. There does not appear to be a genetic component to uterine anomalies, and they are not commonly found in familial case series. Similarly, no other fetal anomalies are associated with uterine anomalies.

90. **A. Surgery is the correct treatment for a correctable uterine anomaly including septate uterus. After successful surgical intervention, 70% to 80% of patients successfully deliver a viable fetus. A simple uterine septum can be excised hysteroscopically. Metroplasty procedures, in which a segment of the uterine wall is resected, have been utilized in cases of thicker uterine septums.**

B. If one or both partners have a genetic anomaly such as a balanced translocation, Clomid and intrauterine insemination will not increase their likelihood of having a normal pregnancy. In addition to genetic counseling, this couple might consider using a donor egg or sperm.

C. Antiphospholipid antibody syndrome is typically treated with low-dose aspirin (81 mg) with or without low-dose heparin (5000 to 10,000 units SQ q12 hours). Corticosteroids have been described as an alternative treatment, but benefits from this treatment have not been supported in clinical trials.

D. Patients with recurrent pregnancy loss (RPL) and hyperprolactinemia receive bromocriptine therapy.

E. Group B *Streptococcus* is not known to cause recurrent pregnancy loss.

91. **C. Several criteria must be met for a safe attempt at a VBAC. An obstetrician must be immediately available 24 hours a day, and an anesthesiologist must be on call. A prior classical hysterotomy (a vertical incision that extends to the fundus of the uterus) is a contraindication to TOL after prior cesarean section. Knowledge of the previous incision and no history of extension into the cervix or active portion of the uterus are also usually regarded as requirements for TOL to be allowed. In addition, patients must have signed an informed consent form for a TOL to be attempted.**

A. A number of obstetric history risk factors lead to an increased risk for uterine rupture—namely, interpregnancy interval of less than 18 months, infection at the time of a prior cesarean section, single-layer closure of the prior cesarean section, and more than one prior cesarean section. While all of these increased risks should be mentioned in the counseling, none of them is considered an absolute contraindication to a subsequent trial of labor after cesarean.

B. The specific reason for previous cesarean section does not affect the safety of the cesarean delivery but affects the likelihood of successful VBAC.

D. Kerr and Kronig incisions are both associated with a low rate of uterine rupture during a subsequent trial of labor (0.5% to 1%). Classical cesarean section, which extends above the insertion of the round ligaments, has been associated with a 6% to 12 % rate of uterine rupture and is a contraindication to TOL.

E. A postpartum hemorrhage after VBAC does not affect a safe attempt at vaginal delivery. At the same time, preparations must be made to ensure that morbidity is limited if the patient were to experience a repeat hemorrhage (e.g., confirm availability of blood products).

92. **C. An Rh-negative mother who is sensitized against anti-D creates IgG antibodies that cross the placenta and can attack fetal erythrocytes, leading to fetal hemolytic anemia and eventually high output failure, known as fetal hydrops. In this case, the father is known to be Rh-positive because he previously fathered an Rh-positive child with an Rh-negative woman; he is heterozygous because he also fathered an Rh-negative child. Given the Hardy-Weinberg equation ($p^2 + 2pq + q^2 = 1$, where p = probability of dominant allele and q = probability of recessive allele), we can calculate several probabilities. The numerator is half of the probability of the**

heterozygotes ($\frac{1}{2} * 2pq = pq$). The denominator is equal to the probability of having at least one D allele ($2pq$). Thus the overall probability is $pq / (2pq) = \frac{1}{2}$. It can also be seen that because the father is heterozygous, there is a 50% chance that he will pass on the D allele and a 50% chance that he will pass on the "–" allele. In this case, "–" is used instead of "d" because there is no recessive allele.

A. With no other information, there is a $2pq$ probability of being heterozygous. This equals $2 \times 0.4 \times 0.6 = 0.48$ in Caucasians. However, this patient's husband previously fathered an Rh-negative child and an Rh-positive child, so he must be heterozygous.
B. The husband is Rh-positive.
D. RhoGAM has no use in patients who are already sensitized.
E. As long as the antibody titer remains at 1:8 or lower, there is no reason to perform any amniocenteses. Serial amniocenteses for hemoglobin breakdown products are only necessary at titers of 1:16 or beyond.

93. **C. Bleeding in a postmenopausal woman is assumed to be endometrial cancer until proven otherwise. This patient also has several risk factors for endometrial hyperplasia or carcinoma—namely, obesity, nulliparity, late menopause (more than 55 years old at menopause), and likely chronic anovulation given her history of irregular menses. The most important evaluation of bleeding in a postmenopausal woman is an office endometrial biopsy (EMB). Bleeding is suspicious for endometrial hyperplasia or carcinoma, and a tissue sample is necessary for a pathologic diagnosis. Hyperplasia is the proliferation or overgrowth of the glands and stroma of the endometrium. It can result in histologic changes (simple or complex) of the cellular architecture with or without cellular atypia. There is a spectrum of hyperplasia ranging from simple hyperplasia without atypia (fairly benign) to atypical complex hyperplasia that progresses to carcinoma in approximately 29% of untreated cases.**

A. US can offer some reassurance if the endometrial strip is smaller than 5 mm and homogeneous. However, a tissue diagnosis is still warranted.
B. Although patient reassurance is always an important part of patient care, investigating the source of her bleeding is most important.
D. A Pap smear is helpful in screening for cervical cancer.
E. If the patient is unable to tolerate an office EMB, a D&C would be the next best means of evaluation.

94. **C. This patient's lesion is caused by chronic irritation of the vulva by her routine pad use leading to a hypertrophic area, called lichen simplex chronicus. It most likely started as a moist, erythematous lesion and, with continued abrasion from the pads and the patient's scratching, transformed into a white raised lesion. The best treatment is hydrocortisone cream.**

A. Contact dermatitis can be caused by an irritant in the pads that the patient uses for her incontinence, but the time course is inconsistent, typically lasting hours rather than weeks. The most common cause of contact dermatitis is oleoresin found in poison ivy and oak.
B. Vaginitis due to yeast infection is a common diagnosis. Affected patients complain of vaginal pruritis, burning, and vaginal discharge. Exam reveals vulvar edema and a discharge that exhibits hyphae and spores on microscopic evaluation.
D. Lichen sclerosis et atrophicus is a similar condition often diagnosed in postmenopausal women secondary to atrophy due to decreased estrogenization of the vulvar tissue. It can also present with pruritis and white lesions, but usually involves tissue thinning. The treatment for lichen sclerosis et atrophicus is hydrocortisone cream to decrease pruritis and inflammation and 2% testosterone cream to support the atrophic epithelium.
E. A biopsy of any suspicious vulvar lesion should be examined by a pathologist because the above two conditions can easily be mistaken for vulvar cancer.

95. **A. Choroid plexus cysts (CPCs) have been associated with trisomy 18. CPCs can be formally diagnosed by amniocentesis. Trisomy 18 can be screened for by obstetric US, which can identify the following associated major structural defects: rocker-bottom feet, club foot, overriding digits, omphalocele, and cerebral malformations such as holoprosencephaly.**

B. The lack of a fetal skull on US exam is usually how anencephaly is diagnosed. The most severe form of neural tube defect, it is not compatible with life.

C. NTDs can be difficult to diagnose by US, but cerebral findings such as the "lemon" sign (indentation of the frontal bones) and the "banana" sign (obliteration of the posterior fossa by the cerebellar hemispheres that appear to be pulled posteriorly) can help. Most NTDs are found by elevated MSAFP on second-trimester serum screening.

D. CPCs have not been associated with any long-term poor outcomes in fetuses with normal chromosomes.

E. Turner's syndrome is a sex chromosomal abnormality (45,XO) that results in a syndrome of short stature, webbed neck, shield-shaped chest, wide-spaced nipples, and often infertility. Affected women have relatively normal intelligence. Turner's syndrome has not been associated with CPCs.

96. **E. This patient's syndrome of hirsutism and anovulation along with physical findings of acanthosis nigricans (velvety, thickened skin in the axilla and nape of the neck) is consistent with PCOS. Also known as PCOD or simply PCO, this syndromic condition was first described by Stein and Leventhal in the setting of hirsutism, virilism, anovulation, amenorrhea, and obesity. It is also associated with insulin resistance and hence type 2 diabetes. Without any other etiology for her symptoms, this diagnosis can be made. An LH:FSH ratio of greater than 3 is also used to confirm this diagnosis of exclusion, but sole reliance on this ratio can miss the diagnosis in morbidly obese anovulatory patients who have suppression of their gonadotropins and thus will not have an elevated ratio.**

A, D. Ovarian tumors that can lead to hirsutism and virilism include the sex-cord mesenchymal tumors, granulosa-theca cell tumors, germ cell tumors, and the Sertoli-Leydig cell tumors. These tumors can all secrete testosterone; hence a testosterone elevation is often observed. Furthermore, virilism due to ovarian tumors usually presents more acutely with rapid onset of symptoms.

B. CAH results from a constellation of enzyme deficiencies, with the most common being an absence of 21-α-hydroxylase, which results in excess 17-α-hydroxyprogesterone and can lead to the complete inability to synthesize cortisol or mineralocorticoids. Adult-onset CAH can be quite mild, characterized by anovulation and androgenization, but should still be notable for elevated dehydroepiandrosterone sulfate (DHEA-S) and/or testosterone.

C. Testicular feminization is most commonly related to absence or dysfunction of the testosterone receptor. These patients are genetically 46,XY but are phenotypically female. Because of the testosterone receptor dysfunction, they cannot become hirsute or virilized.

97. **C. Kegel exercises entail isometric contraction of the pubococcygeus muscles to increase their strength. Performance of regular Kegel exercises may reduce the patient's symptoms. While not always effective, Kegel exercises are noninvasive and inexpensive, and they should be used as the initial management of mild pelvic prolapse.**

A. Estrogen therapy may improve mild pelvic relaxation and should be offered if the patient's symptoms do not improve with Kegel exercises.

B. Anterior repair, or anterior colporrhaphy, is surgical treatment and should be reserved for patients with severe symptoms, after conservative measures have failed.

D. Colpocleisis involves the surgical closure of the vagina and is not indicated. The procedure is usually reserved for elderly, non-sexually active women with symptomatic vaginal prolapse, who have failed to respond to other measures.

E. A pessary is a device, often made of rubber or Lucite, that is placed into the vagina to hold pelvic organs in place. It is usually reserved for women as an alternative to surgery.

98. **A. This patient's history and physical exam are most consistent with stress incontinence, although a formal diagnosis is usually made with urodynamics testing. The fact that she leaks only with valsalva and physical activity is consistent with stress incontinence. Her risk factors include mild pelvic relaxation, childbirth, and the postmenopausal anestrogenic state. Her positive Q-tip test on physical exam further confirms the diagnosis. Stress incontinence can be**

treated medically with exercises, estrogen administration, and surgical restoration of the bladder neck to its original anatomic position.

B. Urge incontinence patients feel the urge to micturate and then urine begins to leak before they can get to the bathroom.
C. Detrusor instability is one etiology of urge incontinence. In addition, patients will occasionally have detrusor instability along with stress incontinence symptoms. Various stressors such as coughing can trigger detrusor contraction, leading to an appearance of stress incontinence that is actually detrusor instability. This can be diagnosed with urodynamics that reveal a detrusor contraction several seconds after a valsalva and leakage that occurs with the detrusor contraction rather than with the valsalva.
D. Total incontinence is rare and results from complete inability to maintain continence. It is most commonly seen in patients with fistulae from the bladder to the vagina or skin, or from the urethra or ureters to the vagina.
E. Overflow incontinence results from detrusor insufficiency or areflexia; that is, the bladder wall contracts weakly or not at all. In this case, urine collects in the bladder and dribbles out when the bladder capacity is exceeded.

99. **B. This patient presents with incompetent cervix—that is, silent, painless dilation of the cervix without contractions, usually occurring in the mid to late second trimester. Unfortunately, most diagnoses of incompetent cervix are made when it is too late to intervene to benefit the current pregnancy. Future management is to place a prophylactic cerclage between 12 and 14 weeks of gestation. In this patient with dilation that has allowed a large portion of her membranes to prolapse into the vagina as shown in the image, there are only two reasonable forms of management. The first is termination of this pregnancy with either induction of labor or D&E. The second is expectant management, which many patients will wish to attempt in the hope of achieving a viable pregnancy (24 weeks or later GA). If the patient chooses the latter option, she must be followed with serial abdominal exams, temperatures, and WBC counts. If any signs or symptoms of infection appear, the patient should be encouraged to undergo a termination of pregnancy at that point. An emergent cerclage placement in the setting of prolapsing membranes is not advised due to the increased risk of complications such as infection and ruptured membranes.**

A. Bacterial vaginosis (BV) is associated with preterm delivery and can be treated with oral metronidazole. This patient does not have BV.
C. While vaginal clindamycin is another way to treat BV, it is not indicated in this patient.
D. This patient has had no contractions, making tocolysis unnecessary at this time.
E. Betamethasone and dexamethasone have been shown to decrease rates of respiratory distress syndrome in neonates when given between 24 and 34 weeks of gestation. At this GA, the fetus is previable, so it is of little use to give antenatal corticosteroids.

100. **D. This is a classic setup for Rh incompatibility. Because the father is Rh-positive, there is a chance he passed the Rh-positive allele to the fetus, making it Rh-positive as well. Given that the mother is Rh-negative, any exposure to Rh-positive fetal blood would induce her immune system to produce antibodies, including IgG, to Rh factor. Because IgG freely crosses the placenta, production of anti-Rh IgG could produce serious consequences for the fetus, including hemolytic anemia and hyperbilirubinemia leading to kernicterus, heart failure, ascites, and many other problems collectively known as erythroblastosis fetalis. Usually the first child is relatively protected from this condition because fetal–maternal blood mixing does not occur until late in pregnancy or at birth, and the mother does not have sufficient time to mount a strong antibody response before the baby is born. However, if this response is mounted, all future Rh-positive fetuses will be in danger of being attacked by the mother's now primed immune system. Therefore, RhoGAM (anti-Rh immunoglobulin) is given to the mother during the third trimester—even during the first pregnancy—as a precaution. These antibodies bind to the Rh-positive cells before the mother can detect them, thereby preventing an immune response from being mounted and keeping this and all future pregnancies safe from attack.**

A. Amniocentesis is not indicated for an Rh-incompatibility workup. To the contrary, amniocentesis is not advisable in this patient as this procedure can lead to fetal–maternal blood mixing and subsequent sensitization, the very consequence you are trying to prevent. If amniocentesis must be performed in an Rh-negative woman, RhoGAM should be administered after the procedure.
B. See the explanation for D. Because mixing of fetal–maternal blood does not typically occur until late in pregnancy, it is entirely possible that the patient has not yet been exposed to fetal blood, and therefore has not yet mounted an immune response. There is no reason to recheck the father's Rh status.
C. Because this is their first child, it is highly unlikely that the mother will mount a sufficient immune response to cause any lasting problems in the fetus.
E. See the explanation for D. RhoGAM is certainly indicated.

SETTING 3: INPATIENT FACILITIES

You have general admitting privileges to the hospital. You may see patients in the critical care unit, the pediatrics unit, the maternity unit, or recovery room. You may also be called to see patients in the psychiatric unit. A short-stay unit serves patients who are undergoing same-day operations or who are being held for observation. There are adjacent nursing home/extended-care facilities and a detoxification unit where you may see patients.

101. A 29-year-old G_2P_1 woman at 39 2/7 weeks GA presents in active labor. She has been contracting for 4 hours and on admission is contracting painfully every 2 to 3 minutes. Her cervix is 4 cm dilated and the fetal head is at –1 station. The patient's prior labor lasted 13 hours and culminated in a spontaneous vaginal delivery of a 9 lb 4 oz boy (4200 g) after a 60-minute second stage. By US and Leopolds, this fetus, a baby girl, is approximately 3700 g. The patient progresses slowly in labor, dilating approximately 1 cm every 1 to 2 hours during the next 12 hours. At this time, she feels the urge to push; on exam, she is fully dilated, –1 station, and left occiput transverse (LOT) position. She begins the second stage. After pushing for 2 hours, station is unchanged, and the fetal position is as shown in Figure 2-101. The patient requests assistance with a forceps or vacuum delivery because of exhaustion. Which of the following might be considered a contraindication for forceps delivery?

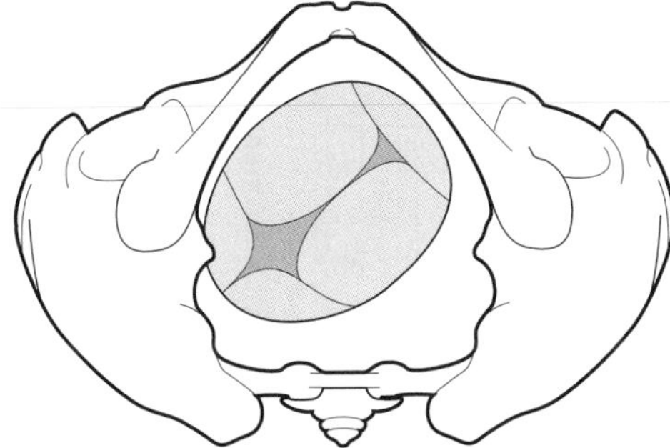

Figure 2-101 • Reproduced from Callahan TL, Caughey AB. Blueprints Obstetrics & Gynecology, 4th ed. Baltimore: Lippincott Williams & Wilkins, 2007. Fig. 4-5H, p. 40.

A. Lack of epidural anesthesia
B. Fetal station
C. Prior infant greater than 9 lb
D. Fetal position
E. Maternal exhaustion

102. A 19-year-old G_1P_0 woman at 39 5/7 GA presents with uterine contractions every 3 to 4 minutes. On exam, she is 4 cm dilated, 100% effaced, +1 station. She is admitted to labor and delivery. Over the next 2 hours, she changes her cervix to 6 cm dilation, +1 station, and left occiput anterior position (LOA). At this point, she requests an epidural. One hour after epidural placement, her exam is unchanged at 6 cm and +1 station. Artificial rupture of the membranes (AROM, or amniotomy) is performed, and Pitocin (oxytocin) is begun for augmentation of labor. Over the ensuing 2 hours, she contracts every 3 to 5 minutes, and she changes to 7 cm and +1 station. After 2 more hours, she maintains the same exam of 7 cm and +1 station, with a position of LOA. At this point, the diagnosis of failure to progress in labor is suggested. Which of the following is most important to making this diagnosis?

A. Placement of an IUPC to measure contractions
B. Cervical change of less than 1.5 cm per hour
C. At least 2 hours of Pitocin augmentation
D. No change in station over a period of 4 hours
E. An active phase of the second stage of labor greater than 5 hours

103. A 33-year-old G_4P_3 woman at term presents in active labor at 5 cm dilation. She has a reactive fetal heart tracing with a baseline in the 150s. Contractions are occurring every 2 to 3 minutes. Estimated fetal weight is 3600 g, and she had rupture of membranes approximately 3 hours prior to presentation. During the next hour, the FHR tracing begins to show decelerations (Figure 2-103). These decelerations are called _____ and are likely secondary to______.

A. Early decelerations; head compression
B. Variable decelerations; uteroplacental insufficiency
C. Late decelerations; uteroplacental insufficiency
D. Late decelerations; head compression
E. Early decelerations; a nuchal cord

104. A 19-year-old G_1P_0 woman at 41 2/7 weeks GA has just undergone a spontaneous vaginal delivery of a viable 4425 g boy. She had been diagnosed with preeclampsia and has been on magnesium sulfate for seizure prophylaxis for 26 hours. She spiked a fever to 101.8°F five hours ago and is being treated with cefotetan for presumed

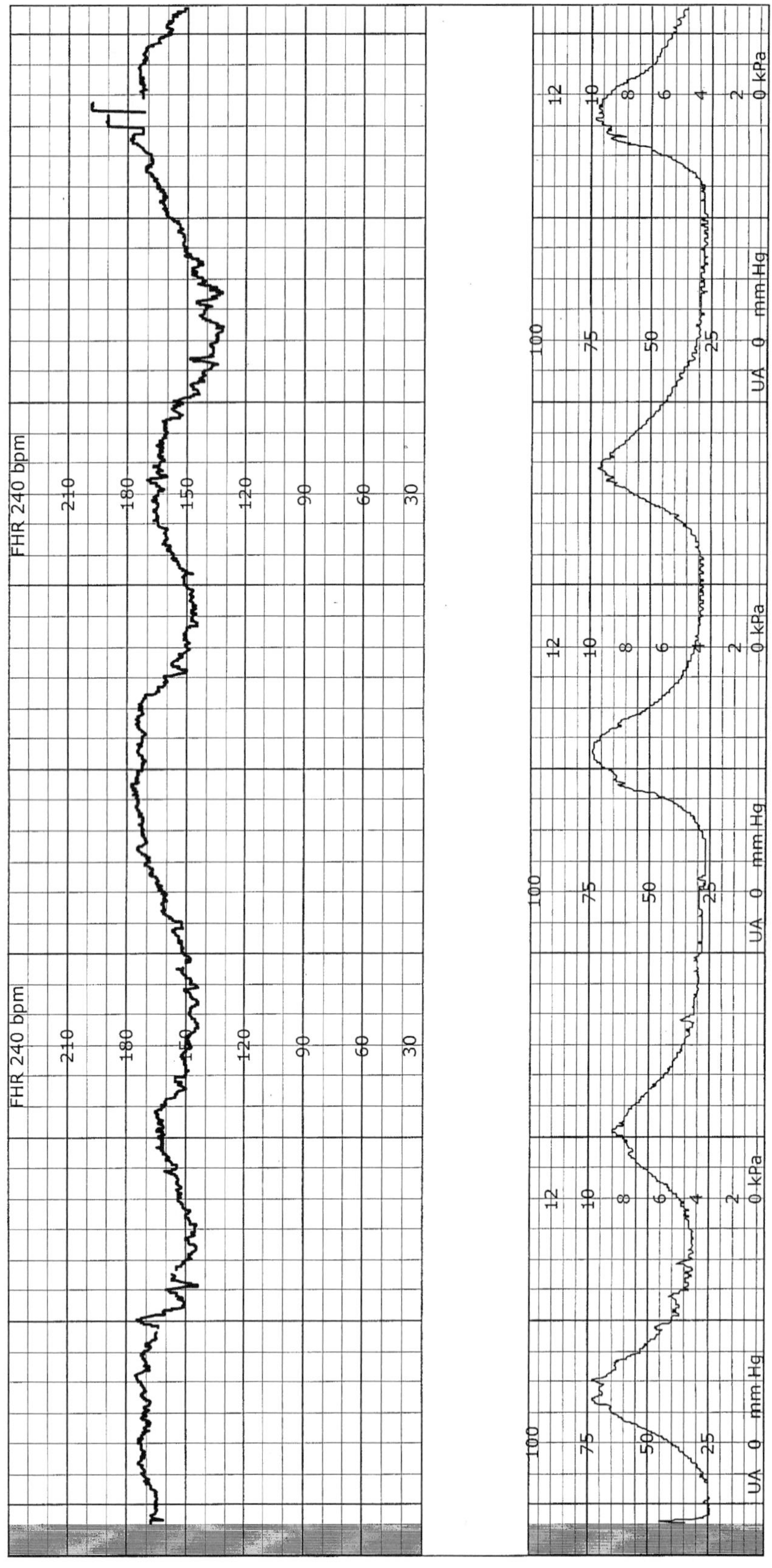

Figure 2-103 • Image Provided by Department of Obstetrics & Gynecology, University of California, San Francisco.

chorioamnionitis. After the delivery of the placenta, which appears intact and without obvious vessels traveling into the membranes, she begins to have a postpartum hemorrhage. During the next minute she loses 300 cc of blood, for a total of approximately 1 L. Which of the following is the most likely etiology in this clinical situation?

A. Cervical laceration
B. Vaginal laceration
C. Ruptured hemorrhoidal vessels
D. Uterine atony
E. Retained POCs

105. A 17-year-old G_1P_0 woman at 37 2/7 weeks GA presents with blood pressures elevated to 146–158/93–102. A urine dipstick shows 2+ proteinuria. She denies headache or visual changes, but she does note some swelling of her hands. On physical exam, you note no papilledema, no right upper quadrant tenderness, brisk 3+ deep tendon reflexes (DTRs), and 2+ pitting edema of the lower extremities. She is admitted to labor and delivery, magnesium sulfate is administered to her for seizure prophylaxis, and her labor is induced. Which of the following lab tests, if the results are elevated, would help make the diagnosis of HELLP syndrome?

A. Creatinine
B. Hematocrit
C. Aspartate transaminase (AST)
D. Uric acid
E. Platelet count

106. A 32-year-old G_2P_1 woman presents at 36 4/7 weeks GA with a dichorionic/diamnionic twin gestation. Her twin gestation was diagnosed by US at 8 weeks. An anatomic survey and amniocentesis were performed at 17 weeks, and both were normal. The fetal karyotypes are 46,XY and 46,XX. The patient had another US at 29 weeks GA, which showed concordant fetal growth with percentile weights of 46% and 57%, respectively. The patient now presents with contractions every 2 to 3 minutes and a cervical exam of 2 cm dilation, 90% effacement, and 0 station. You counsel her that which of the following is commonly accepted in the delivery of twins?

A. Trial of labor for breech-presenting twin, cephalic second twin
B. High-dose Pitocin after delivery of the first twin to remove the placenta
C. Immediate delivery of the second twin with forceps, even if the cervix is no longer fully dilated
D. Elective cesarean delivery for a cephalic-presenting first twin and cephalic-presenting second twin
E. After delivery of the first twin, immediate breech extraction of the second twin

107. A 28-year-old G_3P_2 woman at 38 2/7 weeks GA presents in active labor, 4 cm dilated, 90% effaced, and +1 station. The fetus is breech, which it had been 2 weeks earlier. A prior attempt at external cephalic version failed. CT scan for pelvimetry found the pelvis to be adequate for breech delivery. After a discussion of the risks and benefits of breech delivery with her primary obstetrician, the patient elects to attempt a trial of labor. Which of the following is generally considered necessary in the decision to allow a trial of labor for a breech-presenting fetus?

A. Estimated fetal weight less than 4500 g
B. Fetal head is flexed
C. Patient has an epidural for anesthesia
D. Prior vaginal delivery
E. No prior cesarean deliveries

108. A 22-year-old G_1P_0 woman at 29 2/7 weeks GA presents with complaints of recurrent lower back pain. She is placed on the fetal heart monitor and tocometer and is found to be contracting every 2 to 3 minutes. She has no complaints of fluid leakage, but notes that she had some spotting the last time she urinated. A sterile speculum exam is negative for pooling, nitrazine, and ferning. On sterile vaginal exam, she is 2 cm dilated, 85% effaced, at +1 station, and cephalic presenting. Which of the following management choices has been demonstrated to have the greatest effect on neonatal outcomes?

A. 6 g IV bolus of magnesium sulfate
B. 500 mg IV bolus of erythromycin
C. 12 mg IM dose of betamethasone
D. 0.25 mg SC dose of terbutaline
E. 5 million unit IV dose of penicillin

109. A 31-year-old G_2P_1 patient at 37 2/7 weeks GA presents complaining of leaking clear fluid for the last hour. One hour prior to presenting, she had a large gush of about 100 cc of fluid, and has had smaller leaks since then. She has not experienced any contractions or bleeding. On sterile speculum exam, you note a small pool of clear fluid in the vagina. A sample of this fluid is dried on a slide (Figure 2-109). On inspection, the cervix is long and closed. The FHR tracing is reactive and without decelerations. Which of the following is the most commonly accepted approach to management based on existing literature?

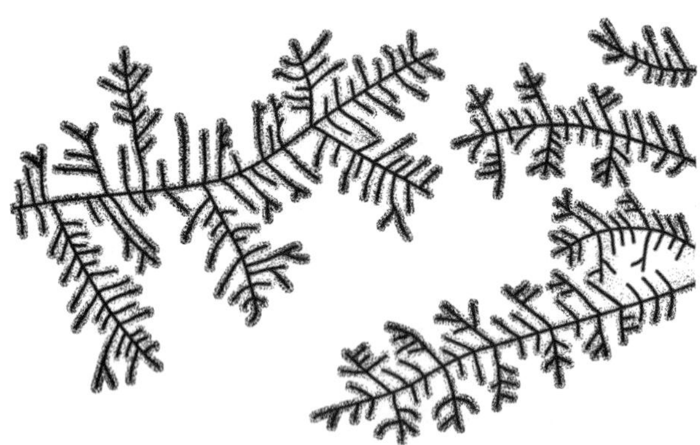

Figure 2-109 • Reproduced with Permission from Marbas L. Blueprints Clinical Procedures. Blackwell, 2004: Fig. 60-1, p. 174.

A. Discharge home
B. Immediate induction of labor with oxytocin
C. Treat with antibiotics
D. Treat with a course of betamethasone
E. Expectant management at home for the next 96 hours

110. A 23-year-old G_1P_0 woman presents in active labor. She progresses rapidly to complete dilation and undergoes a 30-minute second stage. She delivers a viable fetus with Apgar scores of 8 and 9. Upon inspection of the fetus, you note that the infant has either an enlarged clitoris or a very small penis, and partially fused labioscrotal swellings. You order a 17-hydroxyprogesterone test, which is elevated. In addition to telling the patient and her husband the likely sex of the child, you also mention that which of the following treatments will be necessary for the child?

A. Immediate surgery to correct the genitalia
B. Estradiol
C. Progesterone
D. Testosterone
E. Prednisone

111. A 26-year-old G_1P_0 woman presents in active labor at 39 2/7 weeks GA. She had an uncomplicated antepartum course and has a history of scleroderma. Her disease is currently under control with the use of prednisone. In labor, you begin stress-dose steroids. Two hours later, you are called by nursing for a prolonged deceleration. Upon pelvic exam, you note a prolapsed umbilical cord beyond the fetal head. The FHR tracing is obtained (Figure 1-111). The patient is moved to the operating room (OR) for an emergent cesarean delivery as you continue to elevate the fetal head off the umbilical cord. In the OR, the obstetric anesthesiologist asks about your preference for anesthesia. What is your response?

A. Epidural anesthesia is preferred
B. Spinal anesthesia is preferred
C. She needs to be given general anesthesia
D. You can use local anesthesia with conscious sedation
E. A pudendal block can be placed

112. A 31-year-old G_2P_1 woman presents in active labor at 39 5/7 weeks GA. She is 5 cm dilated, 90% effaced, and +1 station. The FHR tracing is reassuring with no decelerations, and the tocometer reveals contractions every 2 to 3 minutes. The patient has had an uncomplicated prenatal course. Her obstetrical history is remarkable for a cesarean delivery 4 years ago for failure to progress past 7 cm dilation. On labor and delivery, she requests an epidural, which is placed without complication. On her next exam 2 hours later, she is 7 cm dilated and +2 station, but her contractions have decreased to every 5 to 7 minutes. She is begun on oxytocin for augmentation. An hour later, the FHR tracing appears as in Figure 2-112. On exam, the cervix is now 8 cm dilated, but the fetal head cannot be easily palpated, indicating that it is at least above –3 station. What is the next step in the management of this patient?

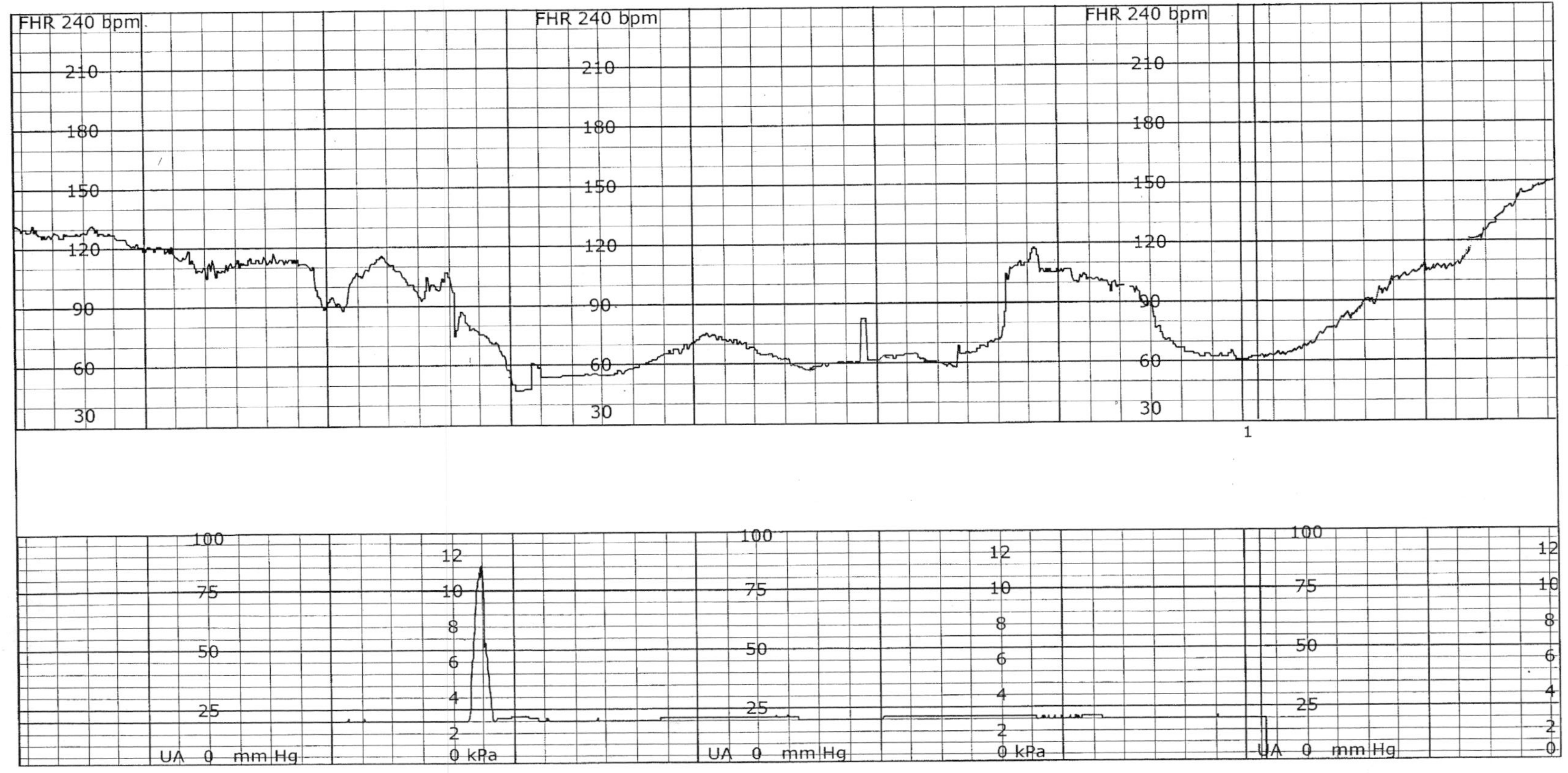

Figure 2-111 • Image Provided by Department of Obstetrics & Gynecology, University of California, San Francisco.

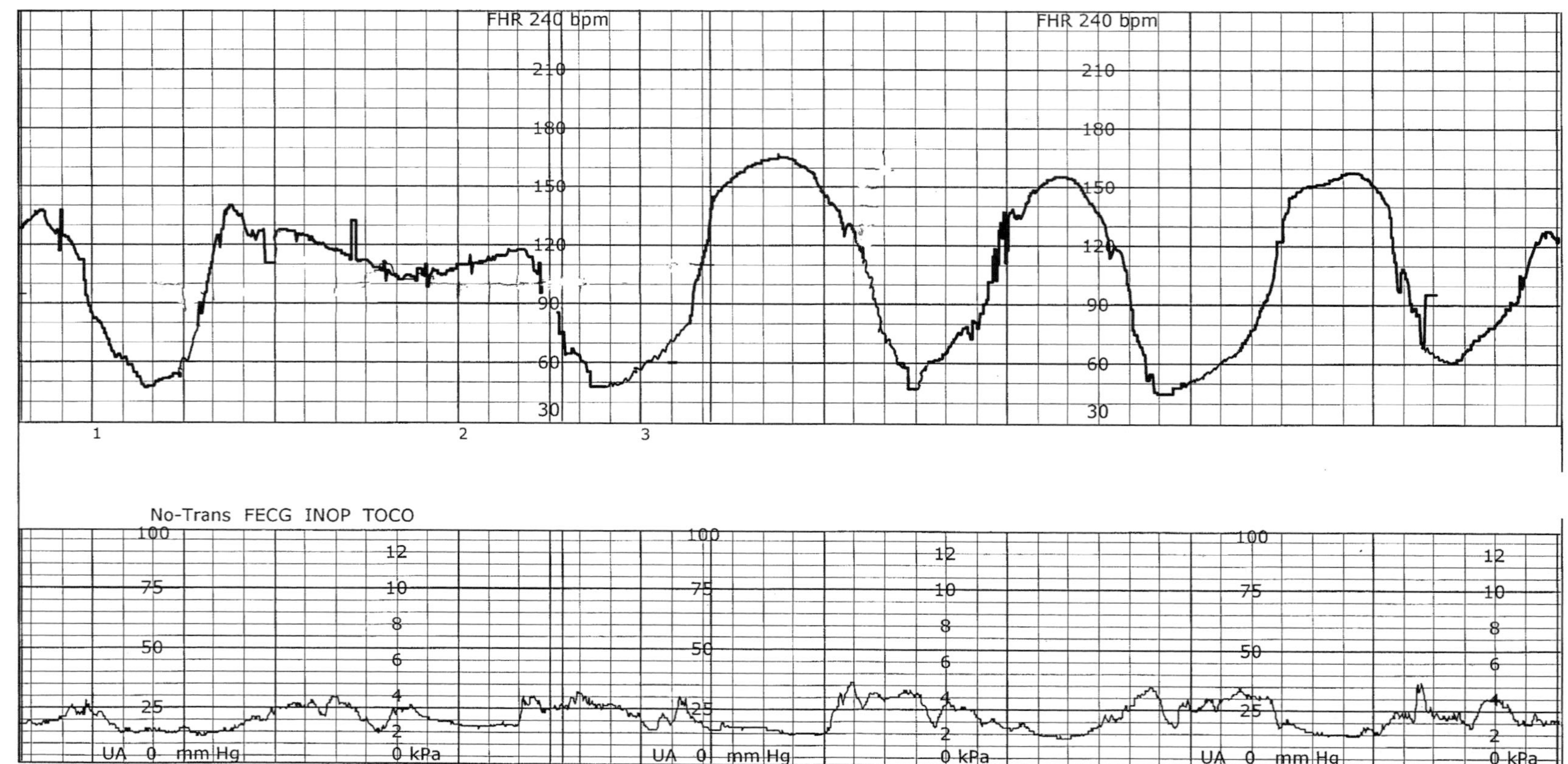

Figure 2-112 • Image Provided by Department of Obstetrics & Gynecology, University of California, San Francisco.

A. Fetal scalp pH
B. Cesarean delivery
C. Forceps delivery
D. Expectant management
E. Restart Pitocin to help bring the head back down

113. A 57-year-old woman underwent a total abdominal hysterectomy and bilateral salpingo-oophorectomy (TAH-BSO) with bilateral pelvic lymph node sampling for stage I, grade III endometrial cancer. She was discharged home on postoperative day 3 with oral cephalexin (Keflex) because of a wound cellulitis. She now returns 2 days later with complaints of leaking pus from the lateral edge of the incision. On physical exam she is obese, with a Pfannenstiel skin incision that has surrounding erythema 3 to 4 cm superiorly. The left aspect of the incision is slightly open; when you palpate the area, a small amount of thick, yellowish discharge is extruded. You attempt to probe the incision with a cotton swab, but it cannot be passed into the small opening. What is your next step?

A. Start the patient on IV antibiotics
B. Schedule the patient for an incision and drainage of the wound in the OR
C. Using local anesthesia, open the lateral edge of the incision with a scalpel for further exploration
D. Using an IV catheter, irrigate the small opening at the lateral edge of the incision
E. Order a CT scan to examine the incision

114. A 66-year-old woman is 12 hours postoperatively from an exploratory laparotomy and debulking procedure for ovarian cancer. At the time of the surgery, approximately 4 L of ascites was removed from the abdomen. You are called by nursing because the patient has made only 15 cc of urine over the last hour. Her fluid intake and output for the day are recorded in Table 2-114. Over the past 3 hours her urine output has progressively slowed from 30 cc/h to 25 cc/h and finally 15 cc/h. What is the next step in this patient's management?

A. Bolus 500 cc IV crystalloid
B. Bolus 2000 cc IV crystalloid
C. Bolus IV colloid, salt-poor albumin
D. IV furosemide (Lasix)
E. PO furosemide (Lasix)

TABLE 2-114 Fluid Balance

	In	Out
Operating room	1600 cc crystalloid	700 cc EBL, 200 cc urine
Postoperative	1200 cc crystalloid	250 cc drains, 520 cc urine

115. A 53-year-old obese woman is undergoing a TAH-BSO for stage I, grade I endometrial cancer. During the procedure, a clamp on the left uterine artery slips and the patient loses a total of 1500 cc of blood. Her preoperative hematocrit was 42. During the procedure, she received 3500 cc of crystalloid. At the end of the procedure, there was no obvious bleeding from this pedicle. Six hours postoperatively, she has a hematocrit drawn, which returns 28. At this time, her blood pressure is 108/64 and her heart rate is 88. Her urine output over the prior 3 hours has been 55 cc, 50cc, and 65 cc. What is the next step in this patient's management?

A. Follow serial hematocrits
B. This is an appropriate drop—check hematocrit in the morning
C. Return to operating room for immediate exploration
D. Transfuse 2 units of PRBCs
E. Check PT/PTT

116. A 23-year-old woman presents 3 days postoperatively with complaints of abdominal pain and fever. She had undergone a laparoscopic resection and fulguration of endometriosis with unipolar cautery. She is seen in the ED by her primary physician. On physical exam, she has a temperature of 101.4°F, tachycardia to the 120s, and an abdominal exam with rebound tenderness. Her bimanual exam shows some slight cervical motion tenderness. She is given the diagnosis of postoperative PID. She is admitted to the Gynecology floor and started on triple antibiotics. Three hours after admission, you are consulted because her abdominal pain is increasing, her temperature has increased to 102.3°F, her blood pressure is 80/40, and her heart rate is in the 130s. Her abdomen is diffusely tender with rebound in all quadrants. You review an upright abdominal film taken on admission (Figure 2-116). What is the most likely etiology of her symptoms and signs?

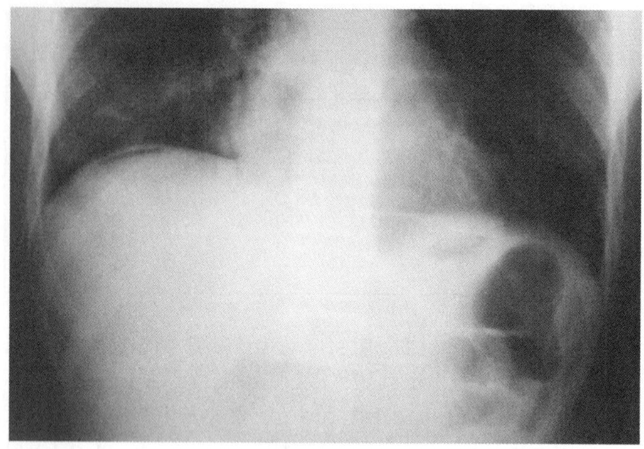

Figure 2-116 • Image Provided by Departments of Radiology and Obstetrics & Gynecology, University of California, San Francisco.

A. Postoperative PID
B. Endomyometritis
C. Appendicitis
D. Ureteral injury
E. Bowel injury

117. A 62-year-old woman is admitted for exploratory laparotomy and debulking procedure for likely ovarian cancer. Upon entering the abdomen, there is bulky disease on every peritoneal surface and surrounding much of the bowel and omentum (a "peek and shriek" case). No further surgical intervention is undertaken, and the patient is closed and subsequently admitted postoperatively to the gynecologic oncology service for her first round of chemotherapy. What should her chemotherapeutic regimen include?

A. CHOP (cyclophosphamide, doxorubicin, oncovin, prednisone)
B. Taxol and carboplatin
C. Melphalan
D. Etoposide and cisplatin
E. CMF (cyclophosphamide, methotrexate, fluorouracil)

118. A 37-year-old woman is undergoing a TAH-BSO for chronic pelvic pain from stage IV endometriosis. There is extensive dissection to free the left adnexa from the bowel and from the pelvic sidewalls. Identification of the ureter on the left side is adequate, but the right ureter is difficult to identify above the pelvic brim. At one point in the procedure, there is a question of right ureteral injury. After the specimen is removed, indigo-carmine dye is given intravenously and spills out of the right ureter approximately 4 cm above the pelvic brim. The distal portion is easily identified and there is no obviously missing portion. What is the best repair for this injury?

A. End-to-end reanastomosis
B. End-to-side reanastomosis
C. Ureteral reimplantation into the bladder dome
D. Ureteral reimplantation into the contralateral ureter
E. Cannot be repaired—place nephrostomy tube

119. A 47-year-old woman undergoes a radical hysterectomy and bilateral salpingo-oophorectomy for stage Ib cervical carcinoma. At the beginning of the procedure, compression stockings and pneumoboots are placed for deep vein thrombosis (DVT) prophylaxis. During the procedure, she has an estimated blood loss of 750 cc. In addition to pneumoboots, which of the following is commonly used for DVT prophylaxis in postoperative patients with cancer?

A. Coumadin
B. Heparin SQ 5000 units TID
C. Low-molecular-weight (LMW) heparin SQ 40 units QD
D. LMW heparin SQ 40 units BID
E. Anticoagulation is not given postoperatively

120. A 32-year-old G_0 woman is undergoing laparoscopy for evaluation of her infertility. A hysterosalpingogram (HSG) showed spillage from the left fallopian tube, but only partial filling on the right. The patient has no history of pelvic pain or dysmenorrhea. In addition, she has regular menses and a positive LH spike on day 13 of her cycle. On entering the abdomen, you notice extensive pelvic adhesions and a 3 cm to 4 cm endometrioma on the right ovary. The right adnexa is adherent to the right pelvic sidewall. When the uterus is injected with indigo-carmine dye, there is spillage from both fallopian tubes—first from the left and then a small trickle from the right. What is the etiology of this patient's infertility?

A. Chronic PID leading to lack of tubal patency
B. Endometriosis leading to lack of tubal patency
C. Endometriosis leading to ovarian dysfunction
D. Endometriosis with uncertain pathophysiology
E. Uncertain etiology leading to lack of tubal patency

121. A 36-year-old G_0 woman presents for operative hysteroscopy and resection of an intrauterine fibroid, which is the presumed cause of her infertility. During the case, the uterus is sounded to 7 cm. During dilation, you notice that dilation is quite difficult until suddenly the 7 French dilator passes easily, but to a distance of 10 cm. Presumably, you have perforated the uterus. What is the next step in this patient's management?

A. Continue with the case
B. Proceed to exploratory laparotomy
C. Continue with the case and treat with antibiotics
D. Follow vital signs and order a pelvic US
E. As most of these perforations are not associated with morbidity, allow the patient to go home

122. A 26-year-old G_1 woman with pregestational type 1 diabetes mellitus presents to labor and delivery for planned induction at 39 weeks GA. Her first prenatal visit was at 7 weeks GA. An US at that time was consistent with a certain LMP. The patient has been monitoring her blood sugars and self-administering insulin since the age of 13, enjoyed good glycemic control before and during this pregnancy, and brings meticulous records to each prenatal visit. An US last week showed growth consistent with dates and normal amniotic fluid. Biophysical profile score was 10/10. On admission, the patient's blood pressure is 105/80. Urine dipstick shows trace glucose and no protein. She is without complaint, but after seeing the impact of pregnancy on her blood sugars, she is concerned about how her disease will affect her labor, delivery, and recovery. How are this patient's insulin requirements most likely to change in the intrapartum and postpartum periods as compared to her third trimester of pregnancy?

A. Increased intrapartum, increased postpartum
B. Increased intrapartum, decreased postpartum
C. Decreased intrapartum, increased postpartum
D. Decreased intrapartum, decreased postpartum
E. Decreased intrapartum, no change postpartum

The next two questions (items 123 and 124) correspond to the following vignette.

A 23-year-old G_1 woman at 33 weeks GA is sent from the clinic to labor and delivery for evaluation of preeclampsia. She was healthy prior to pregnancy, and did not have any elevated blood pressures or proteinuria in her pregnancy until this afternoon. When she presented for her routine prenatal visit (after missing her last two appointments), her blood pressure was 150/98 and urine dipstick revealed 2+ proteinuria. She denied symptoms of preeclampsia. On arrival to labor and delivery, a 24-hour urine collection is started, blood pressures are carefully monitored, and an US is performed.

123. Which of the following, if true, would classify her preeclampsia as severe, rather than mild?

A. Blood pressures are measured in the range 145–150/95–100
B. 1500 mg protein is collected over 24 hours
C. Ultrasonography estimates fetal weight at the 13th percentile
D. The patient is experiencing swelling of her hands
E. The patient is experiencing right upper quadrant pain and tenderness, and has an elevated aspartate transaminase (AST) level

124. Based on the initial assessment, mild preeclampsia is suspected in this patient. A plan to administer corticosteroids and initiate expectant management is discussed with her. Immediately after this discussion, the laboratory calls to report AST = 220 U/L, ALT = 190 U/L, and platelets = 75,000/μL. How does this information change your management of this patient?

A. No change in management
B. Immediate cesarean delivery
C. Initiate tocolysis to allow time for 48 hours of corticosteroids
D. Continue corticosteroids and move toward vaginal delivery
E. Continue expectant management, but begin magnesium sulfate

End of Set

125. A 28-year-old G_5P_3 woman presents to labor and delivery 20 minutes following vaginal delivery of a full-term infant in the ambulance en route to the hospital. She told the paramedics that she had ruptured her membranes 6 hours before calling 911. The patient is admitted and a secondary vaginal laceration is repaired. During the exam and repair, multiple vesicular vulvar and perineal lesions are noted. The patient is very uncooperative and refuses to answer questions about her obstetrical or medical history. Review of her prenatal chart is notable for culture-confirmed herpes simplex virus (HSV-2) 5 days prior; no other antenatal issues are noted. The pediatrics service is now attempting to assess the risk of disseminated neonatal herpes infection. Which of the following, if found in the patient's prenatal chart, would increase your concern for disseminated HSV infection?

A. The patient reported three outbreaks of lesions prior to this pregnancy
B. The current outbreak began in the second trimester
C. The patient has a history of oral HSV-1 infection since childhood
D. A maternal anti-HSV IgG titer drawn 5 days ago was negative
E. Acyclovir was started at 36 weeks GA

The next three questions (items 126, 127, and 128) correspond to the following vignette.

Thirty-six hours after delivery of a viable female infant, a 32-year-old G_2P_1 woman develops a temperature of 38.6°C and shaking chills. Her labor was induced at 42 0/7 weeks GA with oxytocin. The first stage of labor lasted 37 hours, the second stage lasted 4.5 hours, and the third stage lasted 24 minutes. Artificial rupture of membranes was performed 19 hours prior to delivery. An episiotomy was performed with a third-degree extension. Estimated blood loss was 450 cc. The patient received an epidural for analgesia. She was afebrile during her labor. Her prenatal labs were all normal and included a negative GBS culture and HIV test.

126. What is the most common puerperal infection after a vaginal delivery?

A. Infected vaginal hematoma
B. Endomyometritis
C. Thrombophlebitis
D. Pyelonephritis
E. Pneumonia

127. Which of the following tests should be performed first?

A. Chest X-ray
B. Bimanual exam
C. Pelvic US
D. Lower-extremity Doppler
E. Sputum culture

128. An aerobic culture reveals gram negative rods. Which of the following is the most likely to be the etiologic organism in a puerperal infection after vaginal birth in this culture?

A. *Staphylococcus epidermidis*
B. *Escherichia coli*
C. *Enterococcus* species
D. *Bacteroides fragilis*
E. *Chlamydia trachomatis*

End of Set

The next two questions (items 129 and 130) correspond to the following vignette.

A 22-year-old G_1P_1 woman is 14 hours after a vaginal delivery of a healthy baby girl. The patient has tried to breastfeed, but thus far is discouraged because she has not produced very much breast milk. You encourage her and discuss with her the physiology of breastfeeding as well as its long-term benefits.

129. Compared to mature milk, colostrum contains:

A. More fat
B. Fewer minerals
C. More protein
D. More sugar
E. The exact same contents, but in a more concentrated form

130. The release of which hormone is responsible for the milk "let down" reflex?

A. Estrogen
B. Prolactin
C. Oxytocin
D. Placental lactogen
E. Stimulactogen

End of Set

131. You are asked by your chief resident to counsel a new mother regarding breastfeeding versus formula feeding for her new baby. Before going to talk to the patient, you review the literature on the benefits of breastfeeding. You tell her that the benefits of breastfeeding her infant will include which of the following?

A. Increased childhood allergies
B. Decreased infantile ear infections
C. Decreased postpartum maternal weight loss
D. More rapid weight gain for her infant
E. Decreased rates of autism

132. A 28-year-old G_1P_0 woman at 38 1/7 weeks GA with poorly controlled gestational diabetes has been completely dilated and pushing for more than 2 hours. You are called for the delivery and notice prolonged crowning of the head followed by the "turtle" sign. After delivery of the head, you apply gentle downward traction on the head but the shoulders do not easily deliver. What is your next step to deliver this infant?

A. Persistent strong downward traction of the head
B. Attempt a vacuum-assisted vaginal delivery
C. Attempt a forceps-assisted vaginal delivery
D. Sharply flex the maternal hips and apply moderate suprapubic pressure
E. Apply forceful pressure on the uterine fundus

133. A 30-year-old G_1 woman at 32 3/7 weeks GA presents to labor and delivery with uterine contractions and cervical change consistent with preterm labor. She is admitted and placed on magnesium sulfate for tocolysis. What is the most likely benefit from this tocolysis?

A. Prolonging pregnancy for an additional 48 hours to allow for treatment with antibiotics
B. Prolonging pregnancy for an additional 48 hours to allow for treatment with steroids
C. Stopping uterine contractions and increasing the likelihood of a term delivery
D. Decreasing the rate of maternal and neonatal seizures
E. There is no benefit of magnesium sulfate tocolysis in this patient

134. A 29-year-old G_2P_1 woman at 28 2/7 weeks GA presents with a single episode of bright red, painless vaginal bleeding soaking a large towel. She denies uterine contractions, loss of fluid, trauma, or recent intercourse, and describes normal fetal movement. Abdominal exam reveals a nontender uterus. Speculum exam is notable for a moderate amount of bright red blood in the vagina and a visually closed, normal-appearing cervix. Fetal heart tracing is reassuring and no uterine contractions are demonstrated on tocometry. US is obtained (Figure 2-134). What is the most likely etiology for antepartum hemorrhage in this patient?

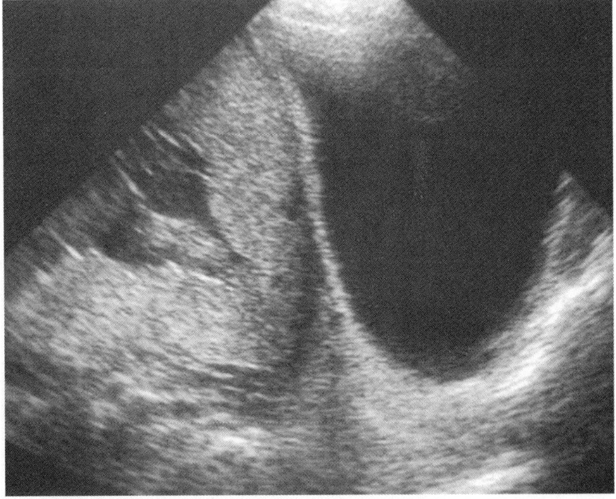

Figure 2-134 • Image Provided by Departments of Radiology and Obstetrics & Gynecology, University of California, San Francisco.

A. Placental abruption
B. Placenta previa
C. Cervical cancer
D. Preterm labor
E. Hemorrhoids

135. You are seeing a 28-year-old G_2P_1 woman at 37 1/7 weeks GA with multiple complaints including shortness of breath, fatigue, sneezing, congestion, nausea, and vomiting. Her blood pressure is 103/77, her pulse is 110, her respiratory rate is 22, and room air saturation is 90%. The patient's urinalysis reveals 3+ ketones and a specific gravity of 1.030. You perform a physical exam and several laboratory tests including a CBC, electrolytes, and arterial blood gas. Of the following results, which is the most concerning?

A. Blood urea nitrogen of 4 and creatinine of 0.5
B. WBC count of 15 million/mL
C. Arterial blood gas with a P_{CO2} of 44 mm Hg
D. Hematocrit of 33%
E. Mean corpuscular volume (MCV) of 78

136. A 34-year-old G_3P_0 woman at 18 3/7 weeks GA without complaints was sent to labor and delivery by the US department because on US her cervix was 1.5 cm long with funneling. She notes fetal movement and denies contractions, leakage of amniotic fluid, and vaginal bleeding. The patient reports that she has a history of cervical dysplasia treated with conization. On her chart, you note a history of two second-trimester losses occurring without painful contractions. The FHR tracing is reactive, and the tocometer shows no uterine activity. Her cervix is closed at the external os, 1.5 cm long, and 50% effaced. An US image of her cervix is obtained (Figure 2-136). You diagnose her with incompetent cervix and recommend which of the following measures?

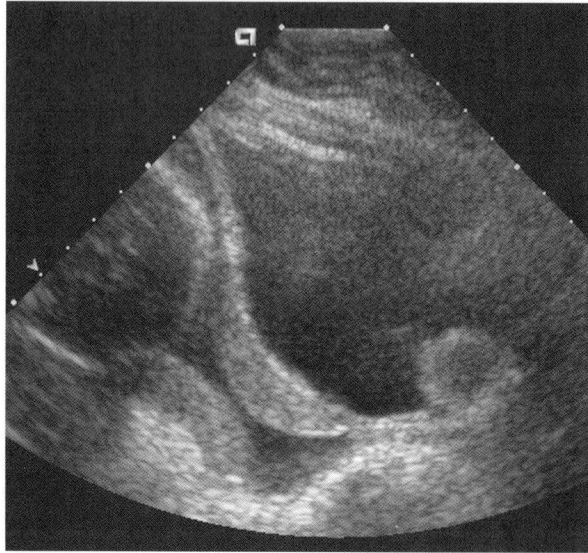

Figure 2-136 • Image Provided by Departments of Radiology and Obstetrics & Gynecology, University of California, San Francisco.

A. Bedrest and betamethasone
B. IV antibiotics
C. Trendelenburg position
D. Cervical cerclage
E. Tocolysis

137. A 22-year-old G_1P_0 woman at 37 3/7 weeks GA is referred for elevated blood pressure in the clinic. Her blood pressure is 147/93. Her urinalysis is significant for 3+ protein. The patient has been seeing "spots" in her visual field since she woke up this morning. You decide to admit her to the labor unit and induce her labor. You examine her cervix and monitor the fetus and the patient's contractions. Her fetus has a reactive FHR tracing, she is not having contractions, and her cervix is unfavorable. You plan to use PGE_1 (misoprostol) for cervical ripening. You check the amniotic fluid index (AFI), which is 7 cm. You obtain further maternal medical history and decide that it is unsafe to use misoprostol. What are the maternal contraindications to prostaglandins?

A. Hypertension and asthma
B. Asthma and glaucoma
C. Hypertension and uterine contractions every 4 minutes
D. Hypertension and an AFI less than 10 cm
E. Glaucoma and preeclampsia

138. You are managing the labor of a 25-year-old G_2P_1 woman with preeclampsia. She is in spontaneous active labor and making adequate progress with uterine contractions every 3 to 4 minutes. She is currently 8 cm dilated and 0 station. The FHR tracing reveals minimal variability (Figure 2-138). You perform a fetal scalp stimulation. The FHR tracing reveals no acceleration in response. You then decide to perform a fetal scalp pH. Which of the values below is matched with the appropriate action?

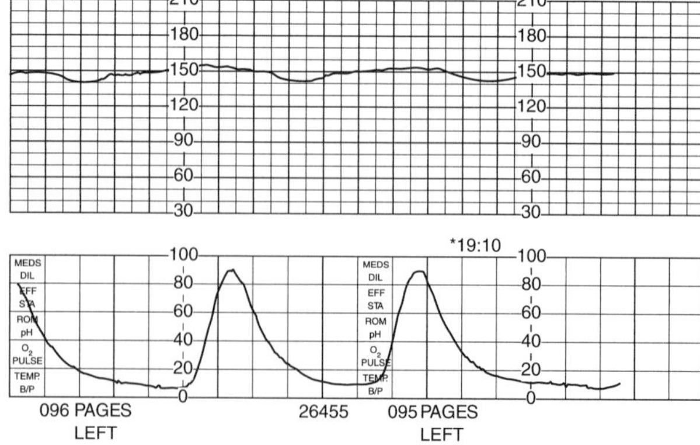

Figure 2-138 • Reproduced from Callahan TL, Caughey AB. Blueprints Obstetrics & Gynecology, 4th ed. Baltimore: Lippincott Williams & Wilkins, 2007. Fig. 4-7B, p. 43.

A. Fetal scalp pH 7.30—expectant management
B. Fetal scalp pH 7.10—resample
C. Fetal scalp pH 7.15—expectant management
D. Fetal scalp pH 7.55—cesarean section
E. Fetal scalp pH 7.22—cesarean section

The next two questions (items 139 and 140) correspond to the following vignette.

A 26-year-old G_2P_1 woman at 40 2/7 weeks GA has been in the active phase of labor for 7 hours. She is receiving a Pitocin infusion of 16 mU/min for uterine contractions and is contracting every $2^1/_2$ to 4 minutes. Her pain is controlled via epidural analgesia. The FHR tracing falls to the 90 beats/min range (Figure 2-139). Despite maternal repositioning and delivery of O_2 by face mask, the deceleration persists for $4^1/_2$ minutes. You perform a vaginal exam and find that the patient's cervix is completely dilated and the fetal vertex is occiput anterior and −1 station with no other findings.

139. What is the most likely cause for the prolonged deceleration?

A. Cord compression
B. Placenta previa
C. Tetanic contraction
D. Cord prolapse
E. Precipitous delivery

140. Considering the most likely cause of the FHR deceleration, which of the following is the most appropriate course of action?

A. Emergent cesarean section
B. Forceps-assisted vaginal delivery
C. Stop the Pitocin infusion and administer terbutaline subcutaneously
D. Elevation of the fetal vertex
E. Scalp pH sampling

End of Set

141. A 23-year-old G_2P_1 woman at 41 2/7 weeks GA reports a history of a normal spontaneous vaginal delivery at 35 weeks. She is in active labor and her labor course has been protracted. Currently, she has been at 7 cm for 4 hours. You augmented her labor with amniotomy and oxytocin. An IUPC was placed 6 hours ago, and her uterine contractions are now occurring every 3 minutes, each approximately 70 Montevideo units. The FHR tracing has a baseline in the 120s with moderate variability, rare accelerations, and occasional variable decelerations. Which of the following is the appropriate next step in this patient's management?

A. Perform a cesarean section for fetal indications
B. Perform a cesarean section for active-phase arrest with adequate forces
C. Perform a cesarean section for prolonged second stage
D. Perform a cesarean section for active-phase arrest without adequate forces
E. Perform a cesarean section but only after 3 more hours of active-phase arrest

142. A 17-year-old G_1P_0 woman at 34 weeks GA by LMP presents with decreased urine output, dyspnea, and blood pressure of 145/110. Her urinalysis shows 2+ proteinuria. You diagnose her with preeclampsia and admit her to the ward for labor induction. Additionally, you administer a 4 g loading dose followed by a 2g/h infusion of magnesium sulfate for seizure prophylaxis. While checking on the patient later in the day, you notice that her magnesium sulfate drip is running at 10g/h rather than 2g/h. You quickly stop the IV and check the patient's magnesium level. As magnesium levels rise, which is the first side effect seen?

A. Loss of deep tendon reflexes
B. Cardiac arrest
C. Seizures
D. Pulmonary suppression
E. Cortical blindness

143. A 39-year-old G_3P_2 woman at 32 weeks GA is hospitalized for treatment of a solitary pulmonary nodule, which was confirmed on biopsy to be primary adenocarcinoma of the lung. Which of the following is true regarding cancer in pregnancy?

A. Metastasis to the fetus occurs
B. Chemotherapy is contraindicated throughout pregnancy
C. Survival is higher when breast cancer is diagnosed during pregnancy compared to the nonpregnant state
D. Radiation treatment is a recommended therapy in pregnancy
E. Termination of pregnancy improves cancer prognosis

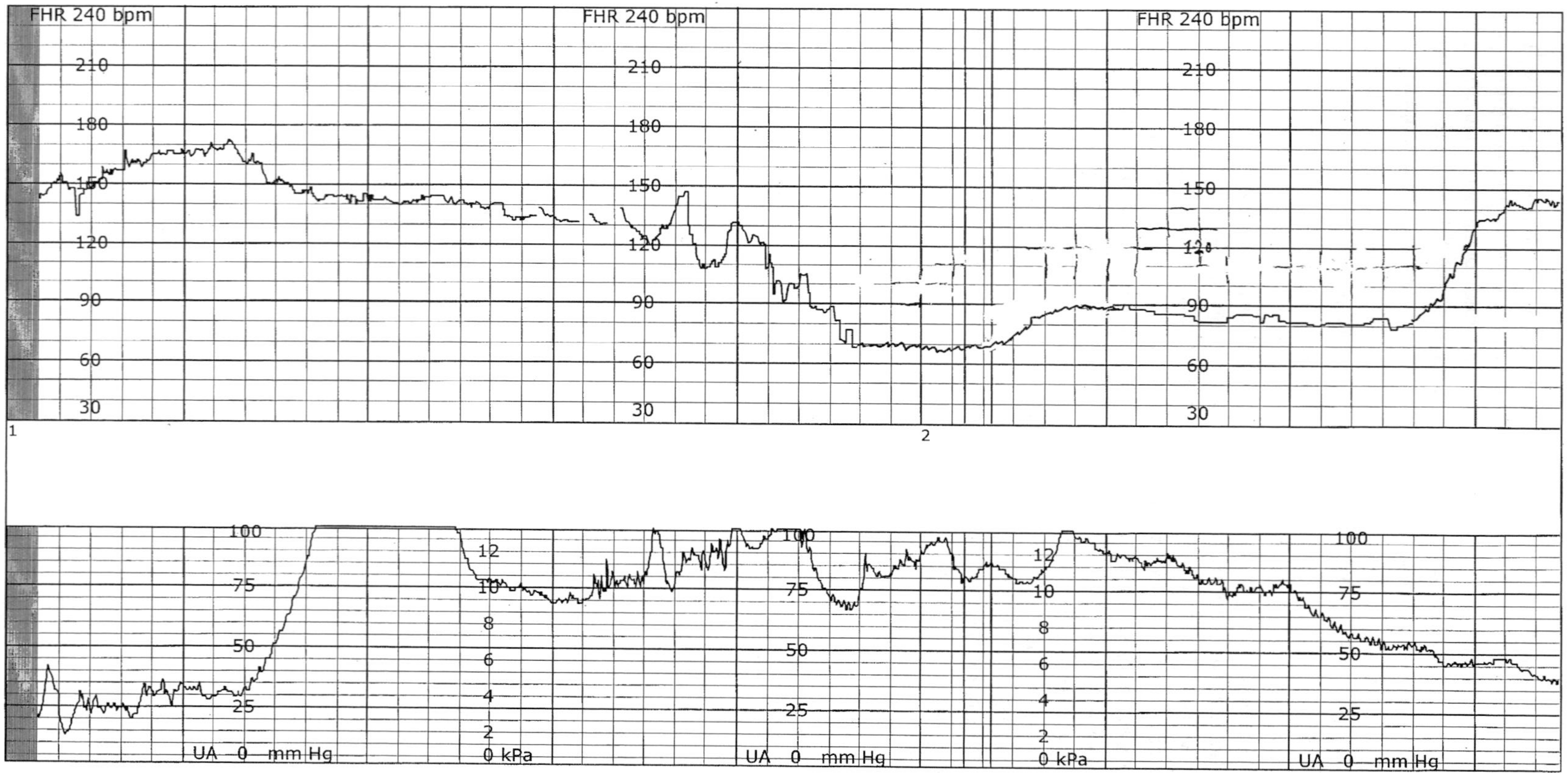

Figure 2-139 • Image Provided by Department of Obstetrics & Gynecology, University of California, San Francisco.

144. A 15-year-old G_0 female is undergoing exploratory laparotomy for an 8 cm complex left ovarian mass that was diagnosed last week when she presented to the ED with symptoms concerning for ovarian torsion. Doppler US revealed no evidence of acute torsion, and the patient was discharged home with strict torsion precautions as well as a consultation appointment with gynecologic oncology. Which of the following tumors is accurately paired with the appropriate tumor marker?

A. Choriocarcinoma and alpha-fetoprotein (AFP)
B. Dysgerminoma and AFP
C. Embryonal carcinoma and hCG and AFP
D. Endodermal sinus tumor and CA-125
E. Immature teratoma and hCG

The next two questions (items 145 and 146) correspond to the following vignette.

A 40 year-old woman is admitted from the ED with severe menorrhagia and symptomatic anemia (hematocrit = 15) for observation and blood transfusion. An US is obtained (Figure 2-145).

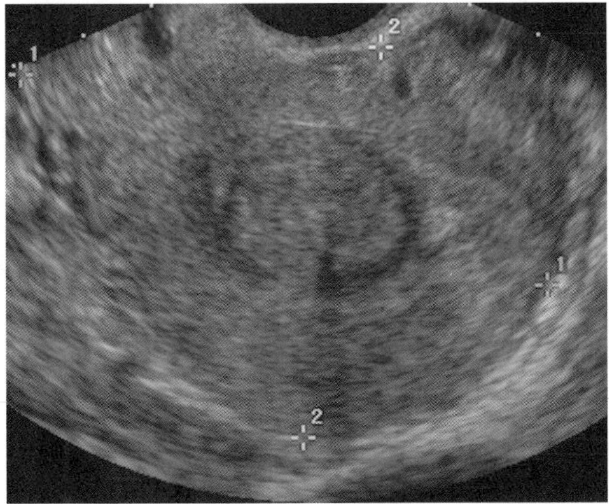

Figure 2-145 • Image Provided by Departments of Radiology and Obstetrics & Gynecology, University of California, San Francisco.

145. What is her diagnosis and the likely source of her menorrhagia?

A. Cervical cancer
B. Submucosal fibroid
C. Ovarian cancer
D. Endometrial polyp
E. Tubo-ovarian abscess (TOA)

146. Given her diagnosis, which of the following is an appropriate treatment option?

A. Thermal balloon ablation
B. LEEP
C. Cone biopsy
D. Hysteroscopic resection
E. Total abdominal hysterectomy with bilateral salpingo-oophorectomy (TAH-BSO)

End of Set

147. You are called to see a 54-year-old patient who is postoperative day 2 status post an uncomplicated total abdominal hysterectomy (TAH) for fibroids. The patient now has a temperature of 100.8°F. She is on Demerol and an antiemetic and has no significant past medical history. You arrive to find an obese patient in no apparent distress. She reports feeling slightly warm but denies cough, shortness of breath, pain, difficulty ambulating, dysuria or hematuria, problems with her incision, or passage of flatus since surgery. She has ambulated once today after removal of her Foley catheter, stating she was too tired to do more. On exam, her incision appears clean, dry, and intact, with staples in place, and her abdomen is soft and nontender. Bowel sounds are decreased but present in all four quadrants. Her lungs are clear but breath sounds are decreased at the bilateral bases. Her calves are nontender. What is the most likely diagnosis and appropriate management of her postoperative fever?

A. Urinary tract infection—initiate antibiotic therapy
B. Wound cellulitis—initiate antibiotic therapy
C. Atelectasis—incentive spirometry, ambulation, and observation of temperatures
D. Deep vein thrombosis (DVT)—lower-extremity Doppler US
E. Postoperative infection—check blood cultures, urine culture, and chest x-ray; initiate antibiotic therapy

148. A 37-year-old woman is 6 hours status post an exploratory laparotomy and right salpingo-oophorectomy for a large adnexal cyst involving so much of her ovary that a cystectomy could not safely be performed without resulting in a large amount of bleeding. The estimated blood loss (EBL) from the procedure was 1000 mL. When you perform a postoperative check on her now, you notice that she is lying in bed and appears pale. Her blood pressure is 100/62, pulse is 132, respiratory rate is 16, and temperature and oxygen saturation are both normal. The patient's urine

output has been approximately 280 mL since her surgery, but over the last hour, she has made only 15 mL of urine. She reports that her pain is controlled, but when you palpate her abdomen, it is somewhat distended and surprisingly tender to the patient. You hear very faint and rare bowel sounds. Exam of her dressing reveals a large amount of bloody drainage, but the incision and fascia are intact. What is the most appropriate next step in management of this patient?

A. Abdominal X-ray
B. Remove her Foley catheter and have her void spontaneously
C. Check a stat hemoglobin/hematocrit
D. Exploratory laparotomy
E. Remove her staples and probe her wound

149. A 49-year-old G_1P_1 woman is postoperative day 2 following a total abdominal hysterectomy (TAH) for chronic pelvic pain and large fibroids. Her surgery was made difficult by dense pelvic and bowel adhesions due to endometriosis, requiring extensive lysis of adhesions. You are called to see her for severe nausea and vomiting that is refractory to antiemetics. She had minimal bowel sounds on exam this morning and denied passage of flatus. At that time, she had only minimal nausea and her diet was advanced to clear liquids. The patient's medications include a morphine sulfate patient-controlled analgesia (PCA) device, which she has used liberally since surgery, as well as ondansetron for nausea and vomiting. She has ambulated only once since this morning. On exam, she has rare bowel sounds and her abdomen is mildly diffusely, tender to palpation, distended, and tympanic, but without rebound or guarding. Her incision is clean, dry, and intact, with staples in place. You obtain an abdominal film (Figure 2-149). What is the best treatment for this patient?

A. Advance diet as tolerated
B. NPO, IV hydration
C. Take back to the operating room for exploratory laparotomy
D. NPO, nasogastric tube
E. Milk of magnesia

150. A 57-year-old G_0 postmenopausal woman is undergoing exploratory laparotomy, total abdominal hysterectomy, bilateral salpingo-oophorectomy, and staging for suspected ovarian malignancy. The patient originally presented complaining of abdominal bloating for 6 months along with an 8 lb weight loss achieved without dieting. A pelvic US revealed massive ascites and bilateral 6 cm complex adnexal masses (Figure 2-150). Which of the following statements is true regarding the major types of ovarian tumors?

A. Germ cell tumors are the most common.
B. Sex-cord stromal tumors include granulosa-theca and Sertoli-Leydig tumors.
C. Epithelial cell tumors are more frequent among women in their twenties.
D. Germ cell tumors are more frequent among women in their late fifties.
E. Germ cell tumors include mucinous and endometrioid tumors.

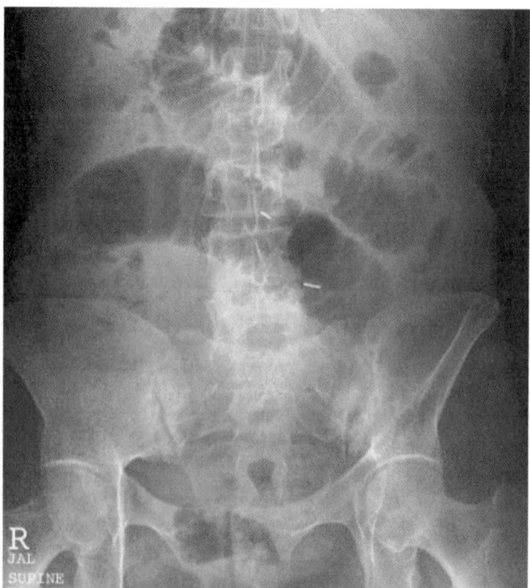

Figure 2-149 • Image Provided by Departments of Radiology and Obstetrics & Gynecology, University of California, San Francisco.

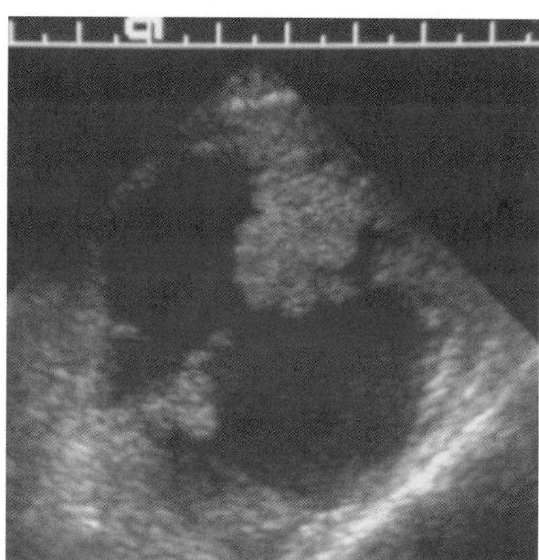

Figure 2-150 • Image Provided by Departments of Radiology and Obstetrics & Gynecology, University of California, San Francisco.

A Answers and Explanations

101. B
102. A
103. C
104. D
105. C
106. E
107. B
108. C
109. B
110. E
111. B
112. B
113. C
114. A
115. B
116. E
117. B
118. A
119. B
120. D
121. D
122. D
123. E
124. D
125. D
126. B
127. B
128. B
129. C
130. C
131. B
132. D
133. B
134. B
135. C
136. D
137. B
138. A
139. C
140. C
141. B
142. A
143. A
144. C
145. B
146. D
147. C
148. C
149. B
150. B

101. **B. A low forceps delivery is defined as at least +2 station, meaning that the fetal skull is at least 2 cm below the ischial spines. An outlet forceps is when the fetal scalp is visible without separating the labia. A mid forceps is when the head is between 0 and +2 station and engaged. Anything above a mid forceps is a high forceps, which is no longer practiced in the United States because of its association with fetal injury.**

A. Adequate anesthesia is necessary for an operative vaginal delivery. Often it will consist of an epidural, but it can also be a pudendal block or (rarely) spinal anesthesia.

C. Fetal macrosomia is a relative contraindication to operative vaginal delivery because it is associated with shoulder dystocia, which is associated with higher risk of perinatal morbidity and mortality. However, this fetus does not meet any criteria of fetal macrosomia, which ranges in definition from 4000 g to the most commonly used 4500 g threshold. If anything, the fact that the patient successfully delivered a prior fetus who was thought to be larger than this fetus is reassuring.

D. The fetal position is LOA, so it meets the criteria for a nonrotation. While knowledge of the fetal position is imperative for operative vaginal delivery, the actual position itself is rarely a contraindication. However, it may change the skill level needed from the clinician and the designation of the type of forceps delivery. For example, if the fetal position is LOT, to perform a forceps delivery, a 90° rotation will need to be performed. LOT position would be a contraindication for clinicians not trained to perform rotations.

E. Maternal exhaustion is actually an indication for elective operative vaginal delivery.

102. **A. Classically, to diagnose active-phase arrest of labor or failure to progress in labor, adequate forces of labor must be demonstrated. The strength of contractions can be measured with an IUPC, as the external tocometer simply measures the frequency and duration of contractions. The units used most commonly to describe the forces of labor are Montevideo units. They are calculated by measuring the difference between the baseline and peak intrauterine pressures of the individual contractions summed over a 10-minute period. Adequate forces are greater than or equal to 180 to 200 Montevideo units. Failure to progress in labor is usually defined when (1) adequate forces are demonstrated and (2) the patient has no change in cervical dilation or station over a period of 2 hours in the active phase. At this point, cesarean delivery is commonly offered. Of note, one recent study suggests that waiting for 4 rather than 2 hours may lead to another 60% of patients delivering vaginally (Rouse DJ, Owen J, Savage KG, Hauth JC. Active phase labor arrest: revisiting the 2-hour minimum. Obstet Gynecol 2001;98:550–554).**

B. On the Friedman curve, a cervical dilation of at least 1 cm per hour is expected in the active phase, which is actually the 5th percentile of cervical change. That is, 95% of all patients will dilate at 1 cm per hour or faster.

C. Commonly, if the forces of labor as measured are inadequate, oxytocin is begun and increased until contractions are considered adequate. Many patients will achieve adequate labor on their own and will not need oxytocin augmentation. Alternatively, if a patient is not making adequate progress, she is often begun on oxytocin augmentation prior to receiving the IUPC.

D. Active-phase arrest of labor is diagnosed when, in the setting of adequate forces of labor as measured by an IUPC, no change in dilation or station occurs during a 2-hour period.

E. The duration of the active phase of labor differs between multiparous and nulliparous patients. The total length is not actually used to make the diagnosis of failure to progress. One reason for this is that a patient with inadequate labor may undergo slow cervical change for several hours before augmentation is begun, thus increasing the total length of labor.

103. **C. Late and variable FHR decelerations are generally a sign of acute decrease in oxygen, which leads to vagal stimulation and a decrease in the FHR. The decelerations described here are associated with contractions, begin after the contraction begins, and end after the contraction is over. This is a description of late decelerations, which are associated with uteroplacental insufficiency. Uteroplacental insufficiency itself can be caused by decreased maternal perfusion of the uterus secondary to anemia, hypoxia, or hypotension, as well as by poor gas exchange across the placenta secondary to increased placental resistance or abruption.**

A. Early decelerations begin and end with contractions and are thought to be due to fetal head compression.
B. Variable decelerations are not necessarily associated with contractions. They are sudden in onset, and the FHR reaches its nadir within 15 to 30 seconds. These decelerations are thought to occur secondary to umbilical cord compression.
D. Late decelerations are not caused by head compression.
E. A nuchal cord—that is, an umbilical cord that is wrapped around the fetal neck—is seen in 10% to 15% of pregnancies. As the fetus descends, the nuchal cord can be pulled and compressed, leading to variable decelerations.

104. **D. Uterine atony is the most common etiology of postpartum hemorrhage. This patient has multiple risk factors for postpartum hemorrhage due to uterine atony, including chorioamnionitis, use of magnesium sulfate, and a macrosomic fetus. In addition to uterine massage, uterine atony is treated with uterotonic agents such as oxytocin, PGF2α (Hemabate), and methylergonovine (Methergine).**

A. A cervical laceration is not an uncommon cause of a postpartum hemorrhage. This patient has one risk factor for cervical laceration—a macrosomic fetus. Other risk factors include a fast labor and pushing against a cervix that is not fully dilated. Cervical laceration is still much less likely than uterine atony.
B. A vaginal laceration, particularly one into the pelvic sidewall, can bleed quite impressively. Vaginal lacerations are more likely in the setting of an operative vaginal delivery.
C. Ruptured hemorrhoidal vessels are an uncommon source of blood loss after delivery.
E. Retained POCs, such as a placental cotyledon or a succenturiate lobe, may lead to uterine atony and postpartum hemorrhage. On exam, this patient's placenta was intact, and there was no evidence of a succenturiate lobe. In this setting, uterine exploration for retained POCs is indicated only after all other treatments have failed.

105. **C. The liver transaminases, AST and alanine transaminase (ALT), are commonly checked as a part of routine preeclampsia labs. Substantial elevation—particularly twice the normal level—is consistent with HELLP syndrome, in the absence of other hepatic pathology. HELLP syndrome is a severe variant of preeclampsia and always demands delivery regardless of GA.**

A. Creatinine is essential to assess renal function. Creatinine levels in pregnancy should be low, certainly less than 0.7, because the glomerular filtration rate (GFR) is increased. A mildly elevated creatinine level is often abnormal. However, a creatinine abnormality is not a part of HELLP syndrome.
B. The hematocrit can identify the degree of hemoconcentration, which is another feature of preeclampsia. With HELLP, the hematocrit should be falling secondary to hemolysis. Because of the two effects of hemoconcentration and hemolysis, better diagnostic tests for hemolysis are lactate dehydrogenase (LDH) or peripheral blood smear.
D. Uric acid levels have been noted to be elevated in patients with preeclampsia, but have not been formally added to the diagnostic criteria or even the screening criteria. One study did show that this measure can be used to screen for preeclampsia among patients with renal disease and/or chronic hypertension who have normal baseline serum uric acid levels. In these high-risk patients, a uric acid level that is increasing or that is higher than 6.0 is good screening tool for preeclampsia.
E. A low platelet count (less than 150,000) is needed for the diagnosis of HELLP syndrome. However, this finding can be misleading because 8% of pregnant women at term may have a platelet count between 100,000 and 150,000.

106. **E. Twin pregnancies can be dizygotic (two initial zygotes) or monozygotic (one initial zygote that splits into two at some point). Dizygotic twins will always be dichorionic and diamnionic (di/di)—two placentas and two amniotic cavities. Monozygotic twins can be di/di, mono/di, mono/mono, or conjoined (known by laypersons as "Siamese") depending on when the zygote splits. At delivery, twin pregnancies can present in a variety of ways. Each fetus can be cephalic (head first), breech (buttocks first), or transverse, creating nine possible presentations. If the presenting fetus is**

cephalic, and the twins are concordant, a TOL with cephalic delivery or breech extraction of the second twin is reasonable.

A. Vaginal delivery of a breech-presenting twin followed by a cephalic twin is usually not allowed. In addition to the usual risks of delivering the breech-presenting twin, there is a risk of interlocking twins, wherein the second twin's head comes through the pelvis before the first twin's head.

B. After the delivery of the first twin, the uterus rapidly decreases in size, which increases the risk for abruption of the second twin's placenta. Augmentation with high-dose oxytocin is likely to increase the risk of abruption and tetanic contractions and, therefore, is contraindicated. Classically, the occurrence of an undiagnosed twin is the reason oxytocin is not given until after delivery of the placenta.

C. Forceps should never be applied when the cervix is not fully dilated.

D. If both twins are cephalic presenting, there is no indication for cesarean delivery.

107. **B. The decision to attempt a TOL in the setting of a breech presentation is one that needs careful counseling. Common requirements include a fetus between 2500 and 4000 g, a flexed fetal head, no fetal or uterine anomalies, and an adequate maternal pelvis as determined by clinical or CT pelvimetry. A recent prospective, randomized, multicenter trial demonstrated that women randomized to TOL had higher rates of fetal trauma. However, because this trial included centers that did not have fetal monitoring and did not use CT pelvimetry, it has been criticized. Because the diameters of the head are minimized with flexion, the head of a breech-presenting fetus undergoing a TOL should be flexed to avoid head entrapment.**

A. Generally, the fetus undergoing breech delivery should be less than 4000 g or not macrosomic. Some practitioners will use a lower cutoff of 3800 g because of the inaccuracy of US and Leopold maneuvers.

C. While it is frequently suggested to the patient that she have adequate anesthesia, often via an epidural, lack of epidural anesthesia is not an absolute contraindication to a vaginal breech delivery. However, because of the likely need for piper forceps and possible need for emergent cesarean delivery, patients undergoing a TOL for a breech presentation are recommended to have epidural anesthesia.

D. While a prior vaginal delivery, considered a "proven pelvis," is desirable, the absence of such is not a contraindication.

E. Few studies have examined breech vaginal delivery after prior cesarean section. In those rare studies conducted on this issue, there was no obvious increase in complications other than those from a breech vaginal delivery.

108. **C. Betamethasone or dexamethasone is given to patients between 24 and 34 weeks GA at acute risk for preterm delivery. Several prospective, randomized, controlled trials (conducted as early as 1972) showed that these agents decrease the risk of respiratory distress syndrome and increase the rate of survival. Later studies demonstrated decreased rates of intraventricular hemorrhage and necrotizing enterocolitis.**

A, D. This patient is in preterm labor (i.e., regular uterine contractions that cause cervical change) and should be tocolyzed to prevent preterm delivery. Magnesium sulfate is commonly used for tocolysis in preterm labor. Other agents used for tocolysis include terbutaline, ritodrine, indomethacin, and nifedipine. The principal benefit of these tocolytic agents has been to increase the length of pregnancy by 48 hours. Fortunately, that is the amount of time necessary to gain the benefits from betamethasone. While tocolysis is an important aspect of this patient's care, administration of antenatal corticosteroids to promote fetal lung maturity is more important. Terbutaline is another tocolytic agent.

B. Erythromycin is used in conjunction with ampicillin in patients with preterm premature rupture of the membranes to promote prolonged latency period (time from rupture of membranes to delivery). However, erythromycin is not commonly used for prophylaxis in patients with intact membranes, like the patient in this case.

E. IV penicillin is commonly used in preterm labor or term labor in women who are documented GBS carriers. Its widespread use has decreased the rate of neonatal sepsis. However, its effectiveness in a preterm patient pales in comparison to that of betamethasone.

109. B. There is evidence from a large, randomized, controlled trial in patients with PROM at term. Of note in examining that study's results, "premature" refers to rupture of membranes prior to the initiation of uterine contractions; in contrast, "preterm" refers to rupture of membranes occurring in a fetus of less than 37 weeks GA. In that investigation, patients who underwent immediate induction of labor with either oxytocin or prostaglandins delivered sooner than those who underwent expectant management. The length of labor, rate of operative delivery, and use of epidural anesthesia were roughly the same for both groups. The rates of maternal infection were higher in the expectant management group. Thus the most commonly recommended course of management for patients with term PROM is induction of labor.

A, E. It is not common practice to discharge patients with term PROM to home. However, some patients strongly prefer spontaneous onset of labor and will want expectant management at home. In these patients, frequent temperature checks and daily visits to the hospital for fetal nonstress tests are an important component of management. No protocol suggests implementing this management for longer than 72 hours, at which time induction should be strongly suggested.

C. In patients with preterm PROM, antibiotics are given to increase the time until labor ensues. At term, antibiotics are used prophylactically only in patients who are GBS positive.

D. Betamethasone is only used in patients until 34 weeks GA.

110. E. The most common cause of ambiguous genitalia is congenital adrenal hyperplasia (CAH). Three common enzyme deficiencies can lead to CAH: (1) 3-β-hydroxy-steroid dehydrogenase, (2) 11-β-hydroxylase, and, most commonly, (3) 21-hydroxylase. 21-Hydroxylase deficiency leads to accumulation of 17-hydroxyprogesterone and a deficiency of cortisol and the mineralocorticoids. Testosterone is slightly elevated, but progesterone and estrogen levels are usually normal. As a consequence, male fetuses usually have an entirely normal appearance, but female newborns may have ambiguous genitalia. Medical treatment involves replacement of the missing steroid hormones.

A. Corrective surgery should be deferred for at least several months to allow for adjustment to medical therapy, but should be performed before the child can remember the gender confusion. Parents may push to have the surgery as soon as possible.

B. Estradiol is usually normal.

C. Progesterone will be either normal or slightly elevated, and does not need replacement.

D. Testosterone is likely elevated in this newborn, leading to the ambiguous genitalia.

111. B. This patient has experienced a prolapsed umbilical cord, which is an obstetric emergency requiring immediate cesarean delivery. In the setting of an emergent cesarean delivery, it is reasonable to utilize spinal anesthesia as long as it can be administered quickly and there is no evidence of abruption, uterine rupture, or ongoing fetal hypoxia. In this case, given the reassuring FHR once the fetal head is elevated off of the umbilical cord, spinal anesthesia is preferred.

A. Epidural anesthesia takes longer to reach a surgical level and is less often successful than spinal anesthesia. Epidural anesthesia is excellent for labor because continuous administration and titration for less neuromuscular block are possible.

C. In a true emergent cesarean delivery, if the anesthesiologist does not normally place many spinals, general anesthesia is commonly used. This patient may not be a good candidate for intubation, given her history of scleroderma. Ideally, the patient and her airway will have been evaluated by anesthesia at the time of her admission.

D. Occasionally, if anesthesia is unavailable, a cesarean section will be performed under local anesthesia with conscious sedation. This is certainly not an optimal way to perform surgery and, given the presence of an obstetric anesthesiologist in this case, is unnecessary here.

E. Pudendal anesthesia may be administered by an obstetrician prior to performing an operative vaginal delivery with vacuum or forceps but is not appropriate for cesarean delivery.

112. B. While variable decelerations and even prolonged decelerations are relatively common phenomena during labor, the sudden change of the fetal station from +2 to unpalpable and

high is abnormal and highly concerning. In this setting of a patient undergoing a TOL after having had a prior cesarean delivery, the most likely diagnosis is a uterine rupture. Other common signs and symptoms associated with uterine rupture include a maternal "popping" sensation in the abdomen, extreme abdominal pain, palpation of fetal parts outside of the uterus, gush of vaginal bleeding, and maternal hypotension secondary to intra-abdominal bleeding. Even though the FHR returns to baseline, a rapid cesarean delivery is indicated.

A. Fetal scalp pH is likely to be relatively reassuring because there is still good FHR variability. Nevertheless, in this scenario, delivery should be facilitated.
C. Forceps cannot be used with a fetal head this high or a cervix that is not fully dilated.
D. Expectant management would be reasonable if uterine rupture did not appear to be the likely diagnosis. If the head were still at +2 station and there were no recurrences of the prolonged decelerations, the patient would ideally be completely dilated soon and could be delivered vaginally.
E. As with expectant management, if you did not suspect uterine rupture, you would restart the Pitocin about 20 to 30 minutes after the prolonged deceleration.

113. **C. Wound infections are the most common complication of abdominal and pelvic surgery. They can consist of a simple cellulitis, a wound abscess, or a fasciitis; the last complication carries a relatively high rate of mortality. The next step in this patient's management is to further assess the wound. The simplest way to do so is at the bedside with local anesthesia. The incision should then be opened 1 to 2 cm to allow for exploration of the wound with a cotton swab. If the abscess is local and without much depth, the wound can be irrigated and packed with cotton gauze. Otherwise, consideration should be given to irrigation and debridement in the operating room.**

A. The patient may require intravenous antibiotics depending on the extent of the wound infection. If she is admitted with a fasciitis, broad-spectrum antibiotics should be given. However, with a small wound abscess that is opened and packed, continuing the oral antibiotics for the accompanying cellulitis should be adequate.
B. If the infection is found to be quite extensive, or if the patient does not tolerate examination under local anesthesia, exploration in the OR may be necessary.
D. The wound should be irrigated, but not until it is explored.
E. A CT scan is sometimes used if a wound is closed and without obvious fluctuance but the cellulitis does not resolve after treatment. It can identify any enclosed areas of fluid or an intra-abdominal abscess.

114. **A. This patient is likely intravascularly depleted. The first step in dealing with her oliguria is to give IV fluid. Patients who undergo abdominal surgery have large insensible losses. This patient also had approximately 4 L of ascites drained, is likely quite dry, and should receive aggressive hydration.**

B. While this patient is likely down several liters of total fluid, a 2000 cc bolus is a bit aggressive in this situation and can cause pulmonary edema.
C. Salt-poor albumin (SPA) may be useful for this patient if several boluses of crystalloid fail to produce adequate urination. Patients with ovarian cancer often have low oncotic pressure secondary to low albumin, and boluses of colloid can improve intravascular volume at least temporarily.
D, E. Only if the patient normally takes a diuretic should one be given in the first 24 hours postoperatively for oliguria. While the patient is likely to show a response, the diuretic may leave her with even less intravascular fluid and may increase the risk of acute renal failure.

115. **B. The average female patient has between 4 and 4.5 L of intravascular volume. Because this patient is larger than average, she may have as much as 5 L. Her blood loss during the case was approximately one-third of her total blood volume. In addition, she was given a large fluid bolus to replace the volume. Now, 6 hours postoperatively, she has re-equilibrated most of the fluids. Appropriately, her hematocrit is approximately two-thirds of her starting hematocrit.**

A. In this stable patient with normal urine output, there is no reason to check serial hematocrits unless concern arises that she may have continued intra-abdominal bleeding.

C. In this stable patient, there is no reason to re-explore.
D. With a hematocrit of 28 and a stable patient, there is no need to transfuse blood. Occasionally, cancer patients or cardiac patients are transfused for hematocrits lower than 30 to prepare for chemotherapy or to maximize oxygen-carrying capacity.
E. There is no reason at this point to suspect a coagulopathy. If one was suspected, a better screening test is to check for fibrin split products such as the D-dimer.

116. **E. Laparoscopic injuries to the bowel are rare and dangerous complications. The bowel can be injured during insertion of the Veress needle, insertion of the trochars, operative dissection using sharp instruments, and use of electrocautery—particularly unipolar electrocautery, as it can lead to arcing of sparks. Patients may present immediately or several days postoperatively with symptoms related to bowel perforation. In this patient with an acute abdomen and septic physiology, a bowel injury leading to a perforation is the most likely diagnosis. Of note, the free air seen on the upright abdominal film is concerning for ruptured viscus. However, it could also be secondary to remaining gas in the abdomen after surgery (as long as 7 days postoperatively).**

A. Postoperative PID alone is unlikely in this patient, as it is usually seen in patients after the release of a hydrosalpinx that is filled with contaminated material. This patient's signs and symptoms indicate a systemic problem and are more consistent with the rupture of a viscus.
B. Endomyometritis should not create such widespread abdominal symptoms.
C. Appendicitis can present like this patient's signs and symptoms, but given the timing of the recent surgery, bowel injury is more likely. In either situation, consultation with general surgery and immediate abdominal exploration constitute the next step.
D. It is unlikely that ureteral injury would present with signs of infection and subsequent progression to sepsis.

117. **B. Currently, first-line combination chemotherapy for patients with epithelial ovarian carcinoma consists of Taxol and carboplatin. Carboplatin has replaced cisplatin as the primary platinum-based alkylating agent because it is associated with fewer side effects.**

A. CHOP is most commonly used to treat non-Hodgkin's lymphoma.
C. Melphalan was once a commonly used single agent to treat ovarian cancer. It is still used in patients who are less likely to survive combination therapy because it is well tolerated.
D. Etoposide and cisplatin are most commonly used to treat oat cell lung cancer.
E. CMF combination chemotherapy has been used to treat breast cancer, with and without tamoxifen.

118. **A. With a ureteral transection above the pelvic brim, the best repair is to reapproximate the two ends over a stent. The stent helps to prevent stenosis from scarring during the healing process.**

B. End-to-side reanastomosis is unusual in ureteral repair. It is used more commonly in bowel reanastomosis to prevent stenotic sites.
C. If a distal ureteral injury has occurred, reimplantation may be used over reanastomosis. In this case, the injury is too proximal to be reimplanted on the bladder.
D. End-to-side anastomosis may be used in ureteral repair when implanting the ureter into the contralateral ureter. This procedure is performed rarely in instances where the distal ureter has been resected and there is no way to bridge the distance between the ureter and the bladder.
E. When the ureter has been damaged to such an extent that there is not enough distance to implant into the bladder or contralateral ureter, a nephrostomy tube will be placed; it allows the kidney to continue functioning.

119. **B. Heparin SQ dosed 5000 units BID or TID is most commonly used for DVT prophylaxis perioperatively. The original studies examined the TID dosing, which should be used in patients at highest risk (e.g., those with cancer). The BID dosing is commonly used in patients who are healthy and likely to mobilize quickly.**

A. Coumadin has a slow onset and a long half-life. As a consequence, it is not used for perioperative prophylaxis.
C. LMW heparin such as Lovenox can be used for DVT prophylaxis, dosed at 40 units QD.

However, because it has a longer half-life than unfractionated heparin, it is not usually used perioperatively.

D, E. See the explanations for A, B, and C.

120. **D. The patient's infertility in this case is most likely related to her endometriosis. However, with good tubal patency on the left and some spillage on the right, it is impossible to say for certain that tubal factor is implicated. Patients with infertility secondary to endometriosis will have increased fertility with the fulguration of implants that are seemingly unrelated to the adnexa.**

A. With pelvic adhesions, chronic PID is in the differential diagnosis. With an endometrioma, endometriosis is the most likely diagnosis.

B. While this is a possible etiology, it is unlikely to be the diagnosis in this patient as good tubal patency has been demonstrated on the left.

C. This patient with regular menses and documented ovulation does not have ovarian dysfunction.

E. This is incorrect on both accounts because there is both a clear etiology (i.e., endometriosis) and tubal patency.

121. **D. Although most uterine perforations go unnoticed and are not associated with morbidity or mortality, recognition of a uterine perforation requires that one evaluate the patient for stability and intra-abdominal bleeding. The least invasive way to do so is to perform a pelvic US to look for blood or other fluid in the pelvis. In this case, because the hysteroscopy had not begun, minimal fluid should be present in the pelvis. Occasionally, if the patient is showing signs of cardiovascular instability, laparoscopy is performed to look for ongoing bleeding.**

A. If a uterine perforation is recognized, it is unsafe to proceed with hysteroscopy because the fluid under pressure is likely to pass in large amounts into the abdomen through the perforation site. In addition, placement of the hysteroscope may further dilate or damage the perforation site.

B. Laparotomy is not needed, unless there is evidence of intra-abdominal bleeding from the perforation site. Laparoscopy could be performed if the concern for bleeding was quite high.

C. As noted in the explanation for A, the case should not be continued. Antibiotics are a reasonable addition to expectant management—usually broad-spectrum agents similar to those used for PID.

E. While most uterine perforations are not associated with long-term morbidity, it is still wise to admit the patient overnight for observation.

122. **D. The patient will most likely require less insulin during labor, and certainly less after delivery, relative to her antepartum requirements. During pregnancy, placental products (e.g., human chorionic somatomammotropin and placental growth hormone) increase maternal resistance to insulin, thus increasing insulin requirements for patients with pregestational diabetes, and sometimes generating a new requirement for exogenous insulin in gestational diabetics. In the active intrapartum period, these requirements usually decrease secondary to the increased glucose metabolism by the uterus and other physiology of labor. It is important to carefully monitor the patient's blood sugars, as maintaining adequate control can be tough. Most pregestational diabetics will require a continuous insulin infusion to keep tight blood sugar control. After delivery, insulin requirements drop even further with the expulsion of the placenta and the loss of its counterregulatory products (which have short half-lives). For this reason, long-acting insulin is to be avoided near delivery, if possible, out of concern for inducing postpartum hypoglycemia. On discharge from the hospital, insulin is typically restarted at 66% to 100% of prepregnancy levels for overt diabetics. For gestational diabetics, insulin is usually withheld altogether, and a glucose tolerance test should be repeated at 6 weeks postpartum.**

A, B, C, E. See the explanation for D.

123. **E. Preeclampsia is formally diagnosed by proteinuria (equal to or greater than 300 mg proteinuria/24 h, or persistent dipstick of 1+ or greater) and hypertension (BP greater than 140 mm Hg systolic or 90 mm Hg diastolic on two occasions at least 6 hours apart). Severe preeclampsia can be diagnosed based on increased thresholds for these values (protein level exceeding 5000 mg/24 h, or BP higher than 160/110), patient symptoms (e.g., severe**

headache, visual disturbances, RUQ pain), laboratory values (e.g., elevated liver transaminases, thrombocytopenia), or clinical assessment of oliguria or pulmonary edema. In this patient, RUQ pain and an elevated AST would make the diagnosis of severe preeclampsia.

A. This level of hypertension meets the criteria for mild, but not severe, preeclampsia.
B. This level of proteinuria meets the criteria for mild, but not severe, preeclampsia.
C. IUGR (fetal weight less than the 10th percentile), when combined with hypertension and proteinuria, is a particularly ominous sign for the fetus, reflecting uteroplacental insufficiency. In fact, some authors have proposed using IUGR as a criterion for severe preeclampsia; however, this choice remains debatable. In this case, the 13th percentile is of concern but does not merit immediate intervention if other fetal testing is reassuring.
D. Nondependent edema can be seen in both severe and mild preeclampsia. In addition, assessment of type or degree of edema is of limited utility in the diagnosis of preeclampsia, as it is rather nonspecific.

124. **D. This patient shows evidence of HELLP syndrome and immediate delivery is indicated. At 31 weeks, most obstetricians would manage this patient expectantly if her preeclampsia was mild, gaining additional time for fetal maturation until 35 to 36 weeks GA. With stable severe preeclampsia diagnosed only by elevated BPs or proteinuria, and with BPs controllable with medications, the most common choice is expectant management, at least until a full course of corticosteroids can be given. However, in the setting of HELLP syndrome, the risk to the mother (and the fetus) is too great to delay delivery. Corticosteroids should be continued, as evidence suggests that they may improve neonatal outcomes. It is also reasonable to attempt a trial of induction of labor to achieve a vaginal delivery. In any event, careful maternal and fetal monitoring is imperative, and cesarean delivery rates are certainly higher in these patients than in most patients undergoing a trial of induction of labor. Magnesium sulfate seizure prophylaxis should also be initiated.**

A. See the explanation for D.
B. Cesarean delivery is generally reserved for obstetrical indications. In this patient, these indications may develop as nonreassuring fetal monitoring or rapidly changing maternal lab tests or other indications of maternal decompensation.
C. Tocolysis to gain time for steroid administration is a common obstetrical strategy in the setting of preterm labor, but would be of no benefit in the setting of HELLP syndrome.
E. This would be a reasonable strategy with the diagnosis of severe preeclampsia. In the setting of HELLP syndrome, magnesium sulfate should be initiated for seizure prophylaxis. However, expectant management is not appropriate.

125. **D. Evidence that this outbreak is a primary infection, indicated by the absence of maternal anti-HSV IgG antibodies, elevates concern for disseminated disease in the neonate. Primary herpes infections carry a far greater risk of transmission to the fetus (as high as 50% if lesions are present at delivery) than do recurrent infections (less than 5%), and the risk of severe adverse neonatal outcomes is markedly increased. This higher risk is believed to be due to higher viral loads and the lack of protective transplacental maternal antibodies. A negative IgG titer indicates that the infection is primary, recent, and dangerous. Although infections may be limited to local lesions (e.g., sores on the skin and mouth), disseminated HSV (viral sepsis, pneumonia, encephalitis) is associated with a mortality rate greater than 50%. If this patient had not delivered in the ambulance, current guidelines would dictate cesarean delivery. Placental transmission of HSV is rare, and the vast majority of infection occurs through exposure to maternal lesions and viral shedding in the birth canal, which can be minimized with cesarean delivery.**

A. The patient's prior outbreaks would suggest that this outbreak represents a secondary infection, which carries a much lower risk of transmission and disseminated disease.
B. The knowledge that this outbreak occurred in the second trimester does not help distinguish between primary and secondary infection. If this is indeed a primary infection, infection remote from delivery carries a lower risk of adverse neonatal outcome, as there is more time for protective maternal antibody formation.

C. A history of oral HSV-1 does not help distinguish between primary and secondary infection. If this is indeed a newly acquired HSV-2 infection, previous HSV-1 infection does mitigate the risk of adverse neonatal outcome; such an infection is known as a "nonprimary first infection." Cross-reactive HSV-1 antibodies, present in maternal serum, reduce the risk of transmission, and neonatal infections are generally less severe and shorter in duration.

E. Acyclovir beginning at 36 weeks GA has been shown to reduce positive culture rates and viral shedding. Although a benefit of reducing transmission rates has not been definitively demonstrated, acyclovir therapy would be reassuring, if anything, against the risk of disseminated disease.

126. **B. Endomyometritis, commonly known as "childbed fever," is the most common cause of puerperal fever and involves infection of the decidua and superficial myometrium. Puerperal infection is defined as a temperature to 38.0°C (100.4°F) or higher for 2 of the first 10 days postpartum, exclusive of the first 24 hours. The single greatest risk factor for puerperal infection is the route of delivery, with cesarean delivery conferring a higher risk. Additional risk factors for postpartum uterine infection include chorioamnionitis, multiple cervical exams, prolonged rupture of membranes, internal fetal monitoring, and lower socioeconomic status.**

A. Infection of a vaginal hematoma presents with exquisite pain in the vaginal area and is less commonly associated with a high fever and rigors. Vaginal hematomas are detected by physical exam and the presence of a firm, tender mass. Large vaginal hematomas require drainage.

C. Deep vein thrombosis (DVT) most commonly occurs in the lower extremities and is associated with puerperal temperature elevations. Classic puerperal deep vein thrombophlebitis, also known as phlegmasia abla dolens (milk leg), has a rapid onset and is associated with a painful and edematous leg and thigh. Doppler studies should be ordered when a lower-extremity DVT is of concern. Thrombophlebitis of the pelvic venous plexuses also occurs and should be considered if fever spikes continue despite adequate antibiotic therapy and exclusion of an abscess.

D. Pyelonephritis can present with fever and rigors in the postpartum period; unilateral lower back pain is often a concomitant complaint. Costovertebral angle tenderness on physical exam also increases one's suspicion for pyelonephritis. A urine analysis with microscopy should be performed as well as culture with sensitivities. Pregnant women are at increased risk for pyelonephritis secondary to mass compression of the ureters and bladder. Bladder catheterization is a risk factor for urinary tract infections.

E. Pneumonia also can present with a fever and rigors in the postpartum period, but a cough is often present with this diagnosis. In the absence of intubation, as for an emergent cesarean delivery, postpartum pneumonia is rather uncommon. Intubation increases one's risk for aspiration pneumonia, most commonly in the right lower lobe. Unilobar rales are often present on physical exam. A chest radiograph should be ordered if pneumonia is under serious consideration. A major cause of pneumonia in pregnancy is preceding pyelonephritis.

127. **B. The first steps in evaluation of a patient with a fever should be a review of the patient's course, a brief patient interview, and a physical exam. In this patient, a bimanual exam should be performed as part of the physical exam. The external perineum and vagina should be inspected for hematoma formation, episiotomy infection/dehiscence, and evidence of necrotizing fasciitis. The cervix should be assessed for cervical motion tenderness and masses concerning for a cervical hematoma. The uterine body and parametria should be assessed for tenderness, size, and masses. Return of malodorous lochia or clot should be noted. The work-up of a puerperal fever also includes a urine analysis and, depending on the clinical scenario, a CBC and blood cultures.**

A. Chest X-ray should be ordered only if there is a heightened clinical suspicion of a respiratory process, such as pneumonia or pulmonary edema.

C. A pelvic US may be useful if a bimanual exam raises concern for an infected hematometrium (blood in the uterus) or other pelvic mass. A pelvic US is not diagnostic for endomyometritis.

D. Before ordering a lower-extremity Doppler, one should first perform a physical exam. Typical findings with a lower-extremity DVT include asymmetric edema (if asymmetry is unclear, one should measure the circumference of each calf with a measuring tape), tenderness to palpation of the calf, presence of a palpable cord in the lower extremity, erythema, and a positive Homan's sign (calf pain elicited by dorsiflexion of the foot). Of note, Homan's sign is present in 50% of cases where a DVT is confirmed as well as 50% of cases where a DVT is excluded. Although its clinical utility is as good as flipping a coin, it is nonetheless a favored diagnostic criterion on standardized exams.

E. Sputum culture is rarely helpful in any clinical setting, with the exceptions being evaluation of tuberculosis and ventilated patients.

128. **B. *E. coli* is a gram negative rod that grows under aerobic conditions that is a common cause of pelvic infections.**

A. *S. epidermidis* is a skin flora that is not a common cause of pelvic infection.

C, D, E. In addition to *E. coli*, these are common pathogens of puerperal pelvic infections. The causal factor is that they are bacteria that normally reside in the bowel and commonly colonize the perineum, vagina, and cervix. Although routinely sterile, the uterus can become colonized by ascending pathogens after rupture of the amniotic membranes. Common pathogens include: Group A, B and D Streptococcus, Enterococcus species, gram-negatives (*E. coli* and *Klebsiella*), *Staphylococcus aureus*, *Peptostreptococcus*, *Bacteroides fragilis*, *Clostridium species*, *Chlamydia trachomatis*, and *Neisseria gonorrheae*. However, *Enterococcus* is a gram positive cocci, *B. fragilis* is an anaerobic organism, and *C. trachomatis* is an intracellular organism that is difficult to culture and most commonly detected by DNA tests.

129. **C. Colostrum is the initial yellow liquid produced by the breast as a result of pregnancy. Colostrum production occurs during the first 5 postpartum days and then gradually converts to mature milk production over the course of approximately 4 weeks. Compared to mature milk, colostrum has more protein. It also carries immunoglobulin A, which is thought to confer early protection again enteric pathogens to the breastfed neonate.**

A. Colostrum contains less fat than mature milk

B. Colostrum contains more minerals than mature milk

D. Colostrum has less sugar than mature milk

E. See the explanations for A, B, C, and D.

130. **C. Oxytocin, released from the posterior pituitary, is responsible for the milk "let down" reflex. This reflex mechanism may be provoked by nipple stimulation, such as suckling, or the cry of an infant. Stress and fright may inhibit the reflex.**

A. Estrogen plays a role in breast maturation but does not directly cause milk ejection.

B. Prolactin, released by the anterior pituitary gland, stimulates milk production, not milk "let down."

D. Placental lactogen does not cause milk let down and is produced only by the placenta; thus, after the third stage of labor, it is no longer produced.

E. There is no hormone called stimulactogen.

131. **B. Infants who are breastfed have a lower incidence of ear infections as compared to formula-fed infants. This difference is attributed in part to the passive maternal antibodies contained in breast milk, which provide the infant with passive immunity to many neonatal and infantile infections.**

A. Breastfed infants have fewer allergies, both as infants and subsequently as adults, than do formula-fed infants.

C. Women who breastfeed their infants lose their "pregnancy weight" faster than women who bottle-feed their babies. Breastfeeding consumes, on average, 500 kilocalories per day, while pregnancy requires only an additional 300 kilocalories per day.

D. Typically, infants who are fed formula gain weight more rapidly and tend to continue to be heavier as compared to infants who are fed breast milk. Some speculate that the increased weight (and percentage of body fat) of formula-fed infants sets their metabolism such that they are more prone to becoming obese as adults.

E. It has been reported that breastfed infants gain unique protection from Crohn's disease, ulcerative colitis, certain lymphomas, diabetes, pneumonia, and meningitis. However, no studies to date suggest lower rates of autism in breastfed infants.

132. **D. Prolonged crowning of the fetal head followed by the "turtle" sign (incomplete delivery of the fetal head followed by retraction into the vagina after pushing) is suggestive of shoulder dystocia. Gestational diabetes and prolonged second stage are risk factors. Other risk factors include fetal macrosomia, previous dystocia, maternal obesity, and post-dates delivery. A series of maneuvers exist for delivering an infant with shoulder dystocia, including the following: (1) McRoberts maneuver (Figure 2-132), a sharp ventral rotation of both maternal hips bringing the pelvic inlet and outlet into a more vertical alignment, and facilitating delivery of the fetal shoulders; (2) suprapubic pressure, to dislodge the anterior shoulder from behind the pubic symphysis; (3) Rubin maneuver; (4) Wood's corkscrew maneuver; and (5) delivery of the posterior arm/shoulder. These maneuvers may be repeated if they prove unsuccessful the first time. If the infant is still undelivered, episiotomy or fracturing the fetal clavicle may be indicated for delivery.**

A. Gentle downward traction alone is often insufficient initial management of shoulder dystocia. Strong, jerking, downward traction of the head is never appropriate, as it can lead to fetal injury.

B, C. Vacuum-assisted and forceps-assisted deliveries are contraindicated when shoulder dystocia is suspected, as both are associated with a slightly increased rate of shoulder dystocia. In this patient, because the head has already delivered, neither of these devices offers any benefit.

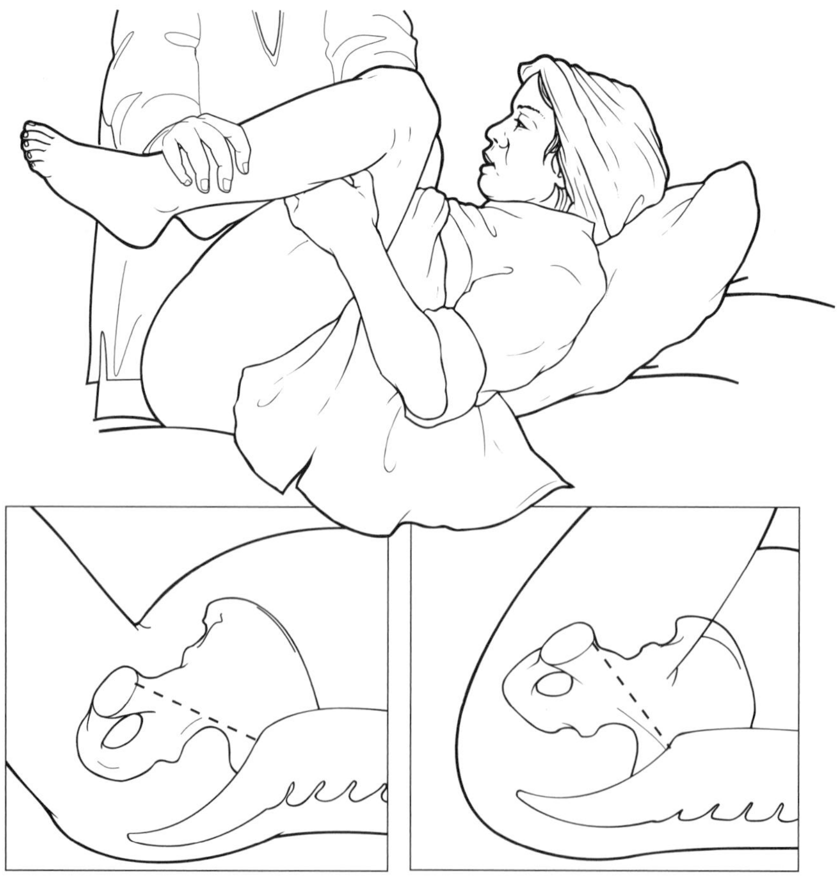

Figure 2-132 • Reproduced from Callahan TL, Caughey AB. Blueprints Obstetrics & Gynecology, 4th ed. Baltimore: Lippincott Williams & Wilkins, 2007. Fig. 6-7, p. 80.

E. Uterine fundal pressure is contraindicated in the event of shoulder dystocia, as it will lead to further impaction of the shoulder behind the pubic symphysis.

133. **B. The principal benefit of prolonging pregnancy for an additional 48 hours is that it allows treatment with steroids. Betamethasone, a glucocorticoid, has been shown to decrease the incidence of respiratory distress syndrome and other complications from preterm delivery.**

A. No evidence exists that treatment of preterm labor with antibiotics prolongs pregnancy. Strong evidence, however, indicates that the use of antibiotics in PPROM leads to a longer latency period prior to the onset of labor.

C. Although magnesium sulfate has been shown to stop contractions in small placebo-controlled trials, it has not been shown to change the GA at delivery. Many of the tocolytics used have been shown to make a difference only by prolonging gestation for 48 hours.

D. Intravenous magnesium sulfate is also used in pregnant patients with preeclampsia to decrease the risk of seizures. This patient does not have preeclampsia, so it would not be used for this reason.

E. See the explanation for B.

134. **B. Sudden onset of profuse, painless vaginal bleeding is indicative of placenta previa. Risk factors for placenta previa include history of prior placenta previa or cesarean section, multiparity, multiple gestation, erythroblastosis, smoking, and increasing maternal age. As most patients who receive prenatal care in the United States undergo a second-trimester US, placenta previa is usually diagnosed prior to the classic presentation that this woman has experienced.**

A. The classic presentation of placental abruption is vaginal bleeding associated with severe abdominal pain, typically occurring in the third trimester. Physical exam often reveals a firm, tender uterus. Small, frequent uterine contractions are usually seen on tocometry. Additionally, fetal monitoring may be nonreassuring secondary to uteroplacental insufficiency. Risk factors for placental abruption include history of prior placental abruption, hypertension, substance use, trauma, and multiple gestation.

C. Cervical cancer may cause vaginal bleeding in its advanced stages. The classic presentation of advanced cervical cancer is postcoital bleeding. Other signs and symptoms that may accompany cervical cancer include abnormal vaginal bleeding, watery discharge, pelvic pain or pressure, and rectal or urinary symptoms. On speculum exam, an exophytic lesion on the cervix may be visible. Given that women are routinely screened prenatally via Pap smears and that cervical cancer is generally a slowly progressing cancer, occurrence of advanced-stage cervical cancer during pregnancy is rare.

D. While labor can cause some vaginal bleeding, it is rarely a large amount and more often is described as "bloody show," or bloody mucus. Preterm labor is defined as uterine contractions that cause a cervical change prior to 37 weeks GA. This patient is not experiencing contractions.

E. Hemorrhoids do lead to rectal bleeding that can be confused with vaginal bleeding antepartum. However, the bleeding is generally greatest at the end of pregnancy, is associated with bowel movements, and rarely would be heavy enough to soak a towel.

135. **C. Many changes in the pulmonary, renal, and hematologic systems occur during pregnancy. In this scenario, the patient has many complaints but the most concerning lab result is her hypercarbia, indicating pulmonary compromise. In pregnancy, the tidal volume increases by approximately 40% while the respiratory rate remains unchanged, leading to an increase in the minute ventilation. An increase in the minute ventilation produces increases in the alveolar and arterial O_2 levels and decreases in the alveolar and arterial CO_2 levels (normal $PaCO_2$ in pregnancy is 30 mm Hg). This patient is retaining CO_2, which is abnormal and concerning.**

A. The glomerular filtration rate increases by approximately 50% in pregnancy, leading to lower BUN and creatinine levels. Additionally, the renin-angiotensin system creates elevated levels of aldosterone, which keeps serum sodium levels normal.

B. The WBC count increases in pregnancy, with the upper limit of normal being 16. In fact, the WBC count is often 20 million/mL during labor.

D. Pregnancy-related changes in hemoglobin and hematocrit occur, as the plasma volume increases by 50% but the RBC volume increases by 25%, leading to a lower hematocrit during pregnancy.
E. Many pregnant women experience an iron-deficiency anemia secondary to the increase in RBC mass.

136. **D. This patient has recurrent cervical incompetence and may have benefited from a cervical cerclage at an earlier GA (12 to 14 weeks). However, with her history of past losses and the current cervical exam, it is reasonable to offer a cerclage now. A cerclage is a permanent suture placed at the cervical–vaginal junction (McDonald) or at the internal os (Shirodkar) to close the cervix. The complications from its placement can be disastrous, including infection and preterm premature rupture of membranes. Typical management of previable cervical incompetence is cerclage placement (if cervical dilation and effacement are not too great), expectant management, or elective termination.**

A. In the setting of incompetent cervix with the membranes pushing down through the cervix (prolapsing membranes), strict bedrest is a less interventional modality that may be offered. Betamethasone for fetal lung maturity would not be utilized until the fetus reached viability (24 weeks GA).
B. Antibiotics are not efficacious in the management of cervical incompetence. They are used commonly in the setting of preterm premature rupture of the membranes to increase the time period from rupture of membranes to the onset of labor (latency).
C. As noted in the explanation for A, bedrest in the Trendelenburg position may be employed in the setting of advanced cervical dilation with prolapsing membranes. In theory, this positioning with the maternal head below the pelvis allows gravity to facilitate the membranes moving back up the cervix, thereby reducing the forces on the cervix. However, a cerclage is more likely to be beneficial to this patient.
E. Tocolytics are administered when a patient has uterine contractions, but they are rarely used in the previable fetus.

137. **B. Asthma and glaucoma are contraindications for the use of prostaglandins. Obstetric contraindications include uterine contractions as frequent as every 5 minutes and prior cesarean delivery or other uterine scar. Relative contraindications include oligohydramnios (AFI less than 5 cm at term) and IUGR, but prostaglandins can still be used in these settings if a negative contraction stress test with oxytocin precedes their use.**

A, C, D, E. See the explanation for B. Hypertension (including the hypertension of preeclampsia) is a contraindication to the use of Methergine (methylergonovine), a medicine employed to treat uterine atony as an etiology for postpartum hemorrhage. However, prostaglandins may be used in the setting of hypertension.

138. **A. Fetal scalp sampling for pH is rarely used, but it is a direct measure to assess possible fetal acidemia. The clinical setting in this case is one in which fetal scalp sampling is useful. There is nothing reassuring about the FHR tracing and with a failed fetal scalp stimulation, the next step is often immediate delivery. However, in a multiparous patient who may be an hour or so from delivery, a reassuring fetal scalp sample buys enough time to expectantly manage the patient. A fetal scalp sample that is greater than 7.25 is reassuring, so expectant management is appropriate.**

B, C. A fetal scalp pH of less than 7.20 is nonreassuring, and in such a case the fetus should be delivered via cesarean section or assisted vaginal delivery. At a pH of 7.10, delivering the fetus rather than taking the time to resample is the appropriate action. Similarly, a pH of 7.15 also merits delivery rather than expectant management.
D. A scalp pH of 7.55 should alert the practitioner to contamination, possibly with amniotic fluid, and should lead to resampling rather than moving immediately to delivery.
E. When the scalp pH is between 7.20 and 7.25, the fetus is slightly below normal and the scalp pH should be resampled within a short period of time (less than 30 minutes) if the indication for assessing fetal pH persists. A cesarean section for a pH of 7.22 is unnecessary.

139. C. The most likely cause of the FHR deceleration is a tetanic contraction (contraction lasting more than 2 minutes). The long contraction squeezes venous blood out of the uterus and limits arterial perfusion. The placental unit is subsequently affected, the fetus becomes hypoxic, and the heart rate falls for a prolonged period of time—$4^1/_2$ minutes in this case. Tetanic contraction can be diagnosed by palpation of a firm, contracting uterus that does not relent. The length of the contraction can also be seen in the tocometer portion of the FHT shown (see Figure 2-139).

A. Cord compression is a possible cause of prolonged decelerations. In this setting, given the prolonged uterine contraction and no resolution secondary to patient manipulation, the tetanic contraction is the more likely etiology.

B. Placenta previa would present in the early stages of labor with profuse vaginal bleeding. Patients with placenta previa must have a cesarean delivery for maternal and fetal safety.

D. Cord prolapse can result in prolonged deceleration or bradycardia but is exceedingly uncommon when the fetal vertex is engaged. Furthermore, a cord prolapse is usually noted on vaginal exam, with the cord looping down past the fetal head and into the vagina.

E. A precipitous delivery may rarely be associated with a prolonged deceleration due to head or cord compression. However, in this instance, the fetus is at –1 station.

140. C. Discontinuation of the Pitocin infusion with administration of 0.25 mg terbutaline subcutaneously will likely resolve the prolonged uterine contraction, allowing for perfusion of the placental unit. Tetanic uterine contraction or hypertonus is diagnosed by palpating the contracted uterus, verifying the prolonged contraction of the external monitor, or IUPC.

A. If the FHT does not recover within a few moments or the preceding measures do not resolve the tetanic contraction, an emergent cesarean section must be performed.

B. The cervical exam confirming that the vertex is at –1 station eliminates forceps-assisted vaginal delivery as an option.

D. In the setting of cord prolapse, elevation of the fetal vertex is important to keep the umbilical cord from being occluded. In this setting, however, it has no utility.

E. Scalp pH sampling is helpful when long-term metabolic changes are expected (i.e., after 30 minutes of an abnormal FHT).

141. B. When a patient's cervical exam remains unchanged for 2 hours despite adequate forces (180 to 200 Montevideo units during contractions over 10 minutes), the diagnosis of active-phase arrest is made. It is an indication for cesarean section.

A. The fetal heart tracing (FHT) overall is reassuring and not an indication for cesarean section.

C. This patient is still in the active part of the first stage of labor. The second stage begins with complete cervical dilation.

D. The uterine forces are adequate by the 200 Montevideo unit convention.

E. There is no need to continue labor based on the adequacy of uterine contractions, as the patient's cervix is unlikely to change.

142. A. A normal magnesium level in healthy individuals ranges from 1.5 to 3 mg/dL. At 4 to 7 mg/dL, the level is therapeutic for seizure prevention. One will begin to see EKG changes from 5 to 10 mg/dL, loss of the deep tendon reflexes at 8 to 12 mg/dL, warmth and flushing at 9 to 12 mg/dL, and somnolence and slurred speech at 10 to 12 mg/dL. However, muscle weakness/paralysis or respiratory difficulty does not manifest itself until 15 to 17 mg/dL. Cardiac arrest is also a real danger of magnesium overdose, although it does not occur until levels approach 25 to 30 mg/dL or higher.

B, D. See the explanation for A.

C. Increased magnesium levels decrease the rate of seizures.

E. While diplopia and blurry vision are common side effects from elevated magnesium levels, blindness is not associated with magnesium use and should be attributed to the underlying preeclampsia.

143. A. Metastasis to the placenta and, more rarely, to the fetus have been reported. Although extremely uncommon, the greatest risk for

metastasis to either mother or baby is seen with melanoma, leukemia, lymphoma, and breast cancer.

B. Chemotherapeutic agents are contraindicated in the first trimester, during organogenesis, because they may be teratogenic and mutagenic. They are relatively safe later in pregnancy.
C. Breast cancer diagnosed during pregnancy is no different than that diagnosed in the non-pregnant state, but the diagnosis is usually delayed during pregnancy due to physiologic changes in the breast, resulting in a more advanced stage and poorer survival rate at diagnosis.
D. Radiation therapy is contraindicated during pregnancy. It may cause spontaneous abortion, growth restriction, and mental retardation.
E. Termination of pregnancy may be needed to proceed with treatment such as radiation therapy, but it does not change the course of the malignancy.

144. C. Embryonal carcinomas may produce hCG, AFP, and CA-125.

A. Choriocarcinoma is a germ cell tumor, also a form of gestational trophoblastic disease, which secretes hCG, not AFP.
B. Dysgerminoma, a germ cell tumor of the ovary affecting predominantly girls and young women, is remarkable for its secretion of LDH as a tumor marker. Germ cell tumors of the ovary arise from totipotential cells. Patients commonly present with a rapidly enlarging adnexal mass and abdominal pain. Functioning germ cell tumors of other types may produce tumor markers including AFP, hCG, and CA-125.
D. Endodermal sinus tumors may produce AFP.
E. Immature teratomas, or immature dermoid cysts, may produce CA-125.

145. B. This image shows a submucosal fibroid. Menorrhagia is a common symptom of fibroids, particularly submucosal fibroids, which can distort their overlying endometrium and erode into the endometrial cavity.

A. This image does not show cervical cancer, which is better characterized on CT scan (although CT scan is not a formal part of the staging process). While cervical cancer lesions can bleed, they rarely lead to acute blood loss and anemia of this magnitude.
C. This image does not show an adnexal mass. Additionally, ovarian cancer does not typically lead to menorrhagia. If the mass secretes such large amounts of estrogen that the endometrium is stimulated, vaginal bleeding can occur, but is unlikely to be severe.
D. Endometrial polyps can are difficult to diagnose on US unless fluid is instilled into the uterine cavity (known as a water or saline US). They are best identified on hysteroscopy or endometrial biopsy. Typically, they cause metrorrhagia rather than severe menorrhagia.
E. This image does not show a TOA. Also, TOAs are not associated with menorrhagia.

146. D. Hysteroscopic resection is a minimally invasive treatment option for removal of lesions in the endometrial cavity such as fibroids and endometrial polyps.

A. In thermal balloon ablation, the endometrial lining is destroyed by heat in an effort to treat dysfunctional uterine bleeding once malignancy has been ruled out. It is not an appropriate treatment option for submucosal fibroids.
B, C. LEEP is an office procedure utilized to excise cervical abnormalities such as LSIL and HSIL. Similarly to LEEP, cone biopsies are performed in the setting of cervical rather than intrauterine abnormalities.
E. While hysterectomy is used in the treatment of fibroids, it is usually implemented after more conservative options such as medical therapy have failed. Of note, hysteroscopic resection is appropriate only for fibroids accessible via the endometrial cavity (i.e., submucosal fibroids). If hysterectomy were to be performed, one must take into account the patient's age and determine whether it would be appropriate to perform a bilateral salpingo-oophorectomy at the same time. In this patient who is likely quite remote from menopause (average age of menopause is 50 years), excision of the ovaries would likely be inadvisable given the premature surgical menopause that would result.

147. C. **Postoperative sources of fever include atelectasis, urinary tract infection, deep vein thrombosis, medications, and infection of the wound, lungs, or abdomen. With a relatively low-grade temperature (less than 101°F) and decreased breath sounds, the most likely diagnosis is atelectasis. Appropriate management involves encouragement of incentive spirometry and ambulation, both of which will help re-expand the lungs. The patient's temperatures should be observed, as true infections will continue to cause fevers.**

A. Without complaints of dysuria or hematuria and without an indwelling catheter, the likelihood of urinary tract infection is low. However, this possibility could easily be investigated with a urinalysis and urine culture.
B. There is no wound erythema or drainage, making a wound cellulitis or infection unlikely.
D. While this patient is at increased risk of thromboembolic events such as DVT due to her obesity and immobility postoperatively, her exam does not reveal any palpable cords, nor does she complain of difficulty ambulating.
E. Postoperative infections can arise from the wound, lungs, urine, and (rarely) retained foreign bodies such as laparotomy sponges. If a patient mounts significant temperatures and exam is suggestive of a pulmonary or urinary tract etiology, appropriate studies should be obtained. In particular, if a patient has signs and symptoms concerning for a pulmonary embolus (e.g., tachycardia, shortness of breath, decreased oxygen saturation), a spiral CT scan should be obtained. If there is concern for sepsis, blood cultures can be sent. Additionally, the patient can be symptomatically treated with acetaminophen while awaiting diagnostic evaluation. This patient's exam is suggestive of atelectasis, so a full infection work-up is not necessary at this time.

148. C. **This patient's exam is concerning for continued blood loss with a likely intra-abdominal source. The first step would be to check a stat hemoglobin/hematocrit to see whether it is consistent with her reported EBL and subsequent intravenous fluid hydration. Intravenous fluids should be continued, and a fluid bolus should be administered to see whether urine output increases in response, which would be suggestive of decreased intravascular volume. In the setting of large bloody drainage from the wound, decreased urine output, and vital signs concerning for decreased intravascular volume, if the blood count is lower than expected, consideration should be given to taking the patient back to the operating room for repeat exploratory laparotomy. Another diagnostic option that was not an answer choice is a bedside US to look for large amounts of intra-abdominal fluid suggestive of intra-abdominal bleeding.**

A. While abdominal X-ray might show findings suggestive of increased abdominal fluid concerning for continued blood loss, it is not the best method to explore this possibility.
B. Occasionally, decreased urine output is falsely demonstrated secondary to a clogged or kinked Foley catheter. In this setting, using a syringe to inject saline into the bladder to unclog or unkink the catheter ("flushing the Foley") is usually reasonable. Removing the catheter would be unwise, as you are using urine output as a crude assessment of renal perfusion.
D. See the explanation for C.
E. If you do remove the patient's staples so soon postoperatively, her wound will separate. This may be part of an exploratory laparotomy, but it would not be the initial step in assessment.

149. B. **This patient has a postoperative ileus, as evidenced by her symptom of nausea, signs of vomiting, abdominal distention, and the KUB image with air-fluid levels. Such a patient should remain NPO until she begins to pass flatus. While NPO, she must also receive IV hydration. In the case of a prolonged ileus, total parenteral nutrition (TPN) is used in addition to hydration. Of note, risk factors for ileus in this patient include extensive bowel manipulation during surgery, minimal postoperative mobility, and liberal use of narcotics.**

A. In this patient with a postoperative ileus, she should be made NPO, rather than advancing her diet.
C. If such a patient has evidence for acute hemorrhage or a ruptured or torsed viscus, then exploratory laparotomy may be necessary.

Hemorrhage would be suspected in the case of unstable vital signs or decreased urine output. Bowel injury will usually lead to an acute abdomen with peritoneal signs, which are not seen in this patient.

D. While the patient should be made NPO, nasogastric decompression of the ileus is usually unnecessary in gynecologic surgery unless aggressive manipulation of the bowel occurs during the procedure. Although the use of a nasogastric tube is not wrong, it certainly is less important than the IV hydration.

E. In the case of an ileus, oral bowel stimulants such as milk of magnesia (MOM) or Golytely are likely to exacerbate the problem. By stimulating the bowel proximal to the ileus, greater distention and abdominal pain will be caused. Some physicians will use suppository agents such as Dulcolax or even enemas to stimulate the distal bowel in an attempt to relieve some of the symptoms. However, these methods have not been studied in prospective trials and little evidence supports their use in the case of an ileus.

150. B. The major types of sex-cord stromal tumors include granulosa-theca and Sertoli-Leydig cell tumors, as well as gonadoblastomas.

A. Epithelial cell tumors (rather than germ cell tumors) are the most common and give rise to benign and malignant tumors. Major categories of epithelial tumors include serous and mucinous tumors, endometrioid clear cell tumors, undifferentiated carcinomas, and Brenner tumors.

C, D. While epithelial cell tumors can affect women at any age, they occur most frequently among women in their late fifties. Germ cell tumors generally affect girls and women ages 0 to 25 years. Like all tumors, however, they may be seen at any age.

E. Mucinous and endometrioid tumors are considered epithelial cell neoplasms. Germ cell tumors include teratomas, dysgerminomas, endodermal sinus tumors, and choriocarcinomas. Ovarian neoplasms are classified by the cell type of origin: surface epithelial, germ, and sex-cord stromal cells.

SETTING 4: EMERGENCY DEPARTMENT

Generally, patients encountered here are seeking urgent care; most are not known to you. A full range of social services is available, including rape crisis intervention, family support, child protective services, domestic violence support, psychiatric services, and security assistance backed up by local police. Complete laboratory and radiology services are available.

151. A 32-year-old G_2P_1 woman at 33 1/7 weeks GA presents to the ED complaining of severe, nonradiating, right-sided abdominal pain that worsens with movement. She has not eaten since last night due to recurrent nausea and vomiting that started this morning, and her last bowel movement was yesterday. She denies travel, sick contacts, or food poisoning. The pregnancy has been uncomplicated. Physical exam is significant for a temperature of 101.0°F, abdominal guarding, rebound, and tenderness to palpation over the right middle abdomen. The patient's cervix is closed and not effaced on vaginal exam. Contractions are not detectable on tocometer, and fetal heart tracing is reassuring. Laboratory studies reveal a WBC count of 20,000 with a left shift. Urinalysis reveals only mild ketones. What is the appropriate diagnosis and treatment for this patient?

    A. Diverticulosis—stool softeners
    B. Preterm labor—tocolysis
    C. Nephrolithiasis—hydration and pain control
    D. Placental abruption—immediate delivery
    E. Appendicitis—exploratory laparotomy

152. A 19-year-old G_1P_0 woman at 39 2/7 weeks GA presents complaining of constant epigastric pain and severe nausea and vomiting that started this afternoon. She has been receiving regular prenatal care and reports that the pregnancy has been uncomplicated. On further questioning, she states that she has also had a headache all day, but no visual disturbances. Physical exam is significant for normal temperature and BP, tenderness to palpation in the right upper quadrant of the abdomen, hyperreflexia, and 2+ lower-extremity edema as well as mild hand and facial edema. Vaginal exam reveals a cervix that is 2 cm dilated and 90% effaced. Tocometer reveals occasional contractions, and fetal heart tracing is reassuring. Urine dip reveals 1+ proteinuria. What is the most important next step in diagnosis and treatment of this patient?

    A. IV fluids and pain control
    B. Check preeclamptic labs, initiate magnesium prophylaxis, and move toward delivery
    C. Tocolysis
    D. Right upper quadrant US and pain control
    E. Urgent cesarean section

153. A 23-year-old nonpregnant woman presents to the ED with sudden-onset, severe left-sided abdominal pain that is now mildly improved. She reports moderate pelvic discomfort over the past week, but denies fever, vomiting, vaginal discharge or bleeding, or bowel or bladder abnormalities. Her LMP was normal and occurred 2 weeks ago. She is sexually active, uses condoms, and has never had a STD. On physical exam, she has normal vital signs, is moderately tender to palpation in the left lower quadrant, has no cervical motion tenderness, and has no palpable adnexal or uterine masses. A urine pregnancy test is negative, and CBC shows a normal white count and hematocrit of 39. US is performed (Figure 2-153). What is the appropriate next step in this patient's management?

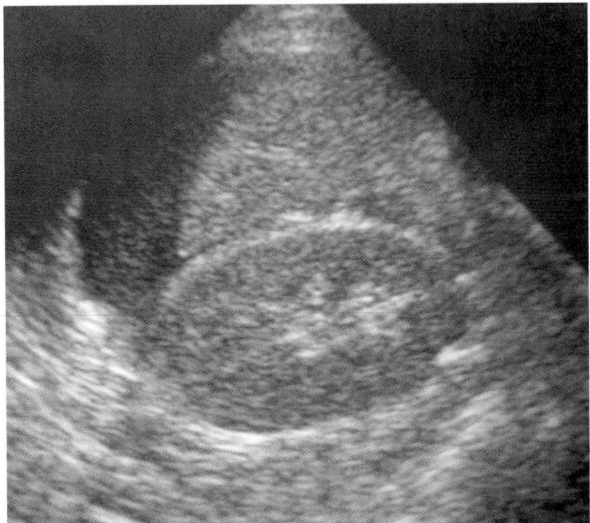

Figure 2-153 • Image Provided by Departments of Radiology and Obstetrics & Gynecology, University of California, San Francisco.

    A. Diagnostic laparoscopy
    B. IV antibiotics
    C. Abdominal/pelvic CT scan
    D. Pain relief and discharge home with precautions and outpatient follow-up
    E. D&C

The next two questions (items 154 and 155) correspond to the following vignette.

A 17-year-old nonpregnant woman presents to the ED complaining of suprapubic pain of 3 days duration. She has decreased her fluid intake because she is urinating so frequently, which worsens the pain and also causes a burning sensation. She denies fever, discharge, or GI symptoms. She just became sexually active and recently started using birth control pills. On physical exam, she is afebrile and has moderate tenderness to palpation in the suprapubic region. Bimanual exam reproduces the suprapubic discomfort, but is otherwise within normal limits.

154. Which of the following combination of urinalysis abnormalities is most consistent with her symptoms and likely diagnosis?

A. WBCs, lipids
B. WBCs, calcium deposits
C. RBCs, renal epithelium
D. Nitrites, WBCs, renal epithelium
E. Nitrites, WBCs, leukocyte esterase, RBCs

155. Which of the following measures is appropriate management of this patient?

A. Decrease fluid intake
B. Foley catheter
C. Urine culture and sensitivity
D. IV antibiotics
E. Low protein diet

End of Set

156. A 17-year-old G_0 woman with a history of dysmenorrhea and menorrhagia presents to the ED complaining of gradual-onset lower abdominal pain and heavy vaginal bleeding that has soaked five pads over the past 12 hours. The patient is not sexually active. Her vital signs are stable, and she is afebrile. Physical exam reveals normal bowel sounds and mild lower abdominal tenderness to palpation, but no peritoneal signs or palpable masses. On pelvic exam, you note a small amount of blood in the vaginal vault, but no evidence of active bleeding, and no cervical motion tenderness or adnexal masses. Pelvic US is performed (Figure 2-156). The patient's hematocrit is 31. In addition to starting iron supplementation, which of the following measures would be appropriate management of this patient?

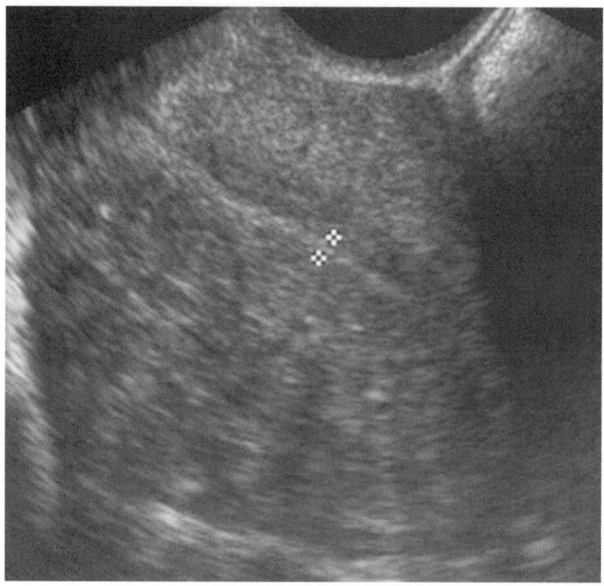

Figure 2-156 • Image Provided by Departments of Radiology and Obstetrics & Gynecology, University of California, San Francisco.

A. D&C
B. Cyclic OCPs
C. Gonadotropin-releasing hormone (GnRH) therapy
D. Endometrial ablation
E. Progestin trial (Depo-Provera)

157. A 47-year-old G_3P_3 woman with a history of menorrhagia and fibroids presents to the ED with a 5-day history of severe vaginal bleeding and complaining of weakness and dyspnea on exertion. Physical exam reveals a pale woman with tachycardia and orthostatic hypotension. Speculum exam is significant for a small amount of bleeding from the cervical os, and bimanual exam reveals an 8-week-sized uterus. The patient's hematocrit is 16.1. You obtain an US (Figure 2-157). What is the next step in treatment?

A. Administer depot Lupron
B. Blood transfusion
C. Observation
D. Hysterectomy
E. Endometrial ablation

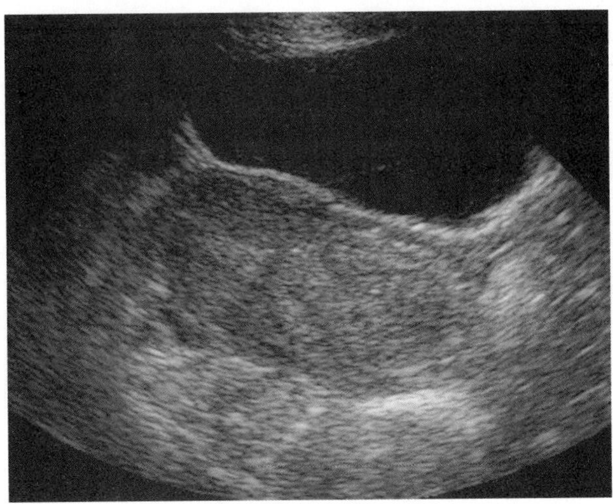

Figure 2-157 • Image Provided by Departments of Radiology and Obstetrics & Gynecology, University of California, San Francisco.

158. A 32-year-old G_2P_1 at 31 5/7 weeks GA presents with painless vaginal bleeding that started today while she was walking. She reports soaking a hand towel with bright red blood, but denies leakage of fluid, contractions, trauma, intercourse, history of abnormal Pap smears, hematuria, hemorrhoids, or bleeding per rectum. On further questioning, she recalls being told at her 18-week US that her placenta was "over" her cervix, but failed to keep subsequent follow-up US appointments. Fetal heart tones are reassuring, and tocometer shows rare uterine contractions. The patient is hemodynamically stable and no longer having vaginal bleeding. Bedside abdominal US confirms complete placenta previa. What is the most appropriate next step in treatment?

A. Immediate delivery
B. Blood transfusion
C. Amniocentesis for fetal lung maturity
D. Administration of IV estrogen
E. Observation and administration of corticosteroids

159. A 22-year-old nonpregnant woman presents to the ED with bilateral groin pain and fever for several days. She is sexually active with two partners and uses the birth control patch for contraception. Her past gynecologic history is significant for hospitalization at age 19 for PID and treatment of chlamydia last year. On exam, she has enlarged inguinal lymph nodes bilaterally, but her abdomen is benign, and she does not have cervical motion tenderness or vaginal discharge. Which of the following statements is true regarding lymphogranuloma venereum (LGV)?

A. It is caused by the L serotypes of *Chlamydia trachomatis.*
B. It typically starts out with a painful lesion in the genital region.
C. Treatment involves a 3-week course of doxycycline and surgical exploration of lymph nodes.
D. Involvement is usually limited to the lymph nodes.
E. It is not sexually transmitted.

160. A 30-year-old G_1P_1 comes to the ED complaining of progressive difficulty walking over the past day due to vaginal pain. She was discharged from the hospital the previous day after undergoing precipitous vaginal delivery of a 9 lb infant during which she sustained a second-degree vaginal laceration that was repaired. Physical exam is significant for mild tachycardia; neurologic exam is normal. The vaginal laceration repair is intact, but you note a tense and tender 7cm left vaginal wall hematoma. A CBC is normal except for a hematocrit of 22.2 (down from her predelivery hematocrit of 36). What is the most appropriate next step in this patient's management?

A. Blood transfusion
B. Incision and drainage of the hematoma with ligation of vessels and/or packing of the wound
C. Sitz baths and iron replacement
D. Administration of Pitocin
E. Uterine artery embolization

161. A 16-year-old patient presents with intense genital itching for several days. She is sexually active with a new partner and otherwise healthy. She is afebrile, but exam reveals the specimen shown in Figure 2-161. You prescribe lindane shampoo and lotion, which successfully treats her infection. Which of the following genital infections is correctly matched to its causative agent?

A. Crabs—*Sarcoptes scabiei*
B. Condyloma acuminata—human papillomavirus (HPV)
C. Chancroid—L serotype of *Chlamydia trachomatis*
D. Scabies—*Phthirus pubis*
E. Syphilis—*Haemophilus ducreyi*

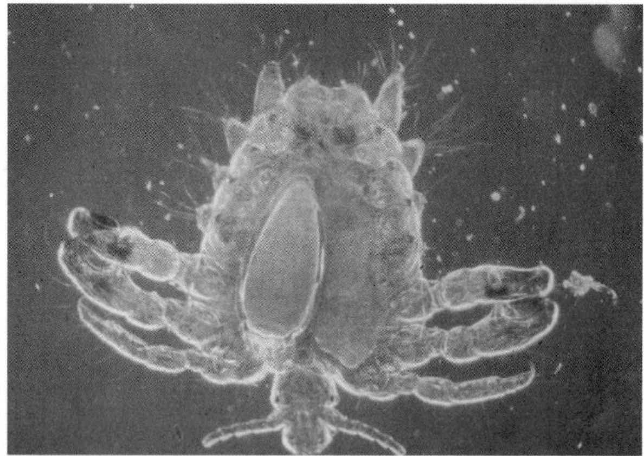

Figure 2-161 • Image Courtesy of D.A. Burns, MB BS, FRCP, FRCP (Edin), Consultant Dermatologist and Honorary Senior Lecturer in Dermatology, Department of Dermatology, Leicester Royal Infirmary, Leicester, England.

162. A 27-year-old G_2P_2 who is postoperative day 5 from an uncomplicated, elective repeat low transverse cesarean section presents to the ED reporting copious light pink discharge from her wound. She denies fever or significant pain but is very anxious that the incision may be infected, as her husband noticed a small area where the wound seems to be separating. Physical exam is significant for an obese woman with a normal temperature and benign abdomen. However, the incision is quite moist and does appear to be separating on the right. You remove the steristrips and find that the wound separates with gentle probing, releasing moderate serosanguinous fluid. There is no erythema and moderate tenderness to your exam. Exploration of the wound reveals that the fascia is intact and the open wound tracks 3 cm to the left, is 4 cm deep, and is 4 cm long. What is the next best step in managing this woman's wound seroma?

A. Irrigate the wound and pack it with moist dressings
B. Administer antibiotics
C. Irrigate the wound and use steristrips to close it
D. Take her to the operating room for surgical closure of the wound
E. Expectant management

163. An obese 16-year-old girl presents to the ED complaining of diffuse abdominal pain of 6 hours duration. There is no associated nausea, vomiting, fever, chills, or anorexia. She denies any significant past medical or surgical history. You discover on exam that she is pregnant and contracting. On further questioning, she denies knowledge of the pregnancy and states that her LMP was "sometime last year." She denies substance use or trauma. Cervical exam reveals that she is 8 cm dilated with a bulging bag of water. You are able to visualize fetal cardiac motion on bedside US, confirm that the fetus is cephalic in presentation, and obtain fetal biometry that is consistent with approximately 38 weeks GA. Which of the following steps is appropriate for subsequent management of this patient?

A. Corticosteroids should be administered to promote fetal lung maturity
B. Magnesium tocolysis should be administered to stop labor
C. You should perform amniocentesis to assess fetal lung maturity
D. You should send the patient for formal US to get a better EGA
E. You should transfer the patient to labor and delivery for impending delivery

164. A 23-year-old G_1P_0 woman at 36 1/7 weeks GA presents to labor and delivery complaining of severe headache and visual changes. She has had an uneventful pregnancy until today. On exam, she appears mildly edematous and her BP is 159/91. She does not have any visual field defects and is slightly hyperreflexic. Fetal heart tones are reassuring, and there are no signs or symptoms of labor. Which of the following tests would assist in the diagnosis of mild preeclampsia?

A. CBC
B. Uric acid
C. Lactate dehydrogenase
D. Creatinine
E. 24-hour urine protein

165. An anxious 29-year-old nonpregnant woman comes to the ED reporting a 2-day history of copious, foul-smelling vaginal discharge that is green and frothy. She reports unprotected intercourse several days ago and is worried that she has contracted a STD. She is afebrile on exam and has a benign abdomen. Sterile speculum exam reveals an erythematous, punctate-appearing cervix and a large amount of discharge. You prepare the wet mount shown in Figure 2-165. There is no cervical motion tenderness, and the patient's uterus and adnexa are within normal limits. What is the diagnosis and appropriate management for this patient?

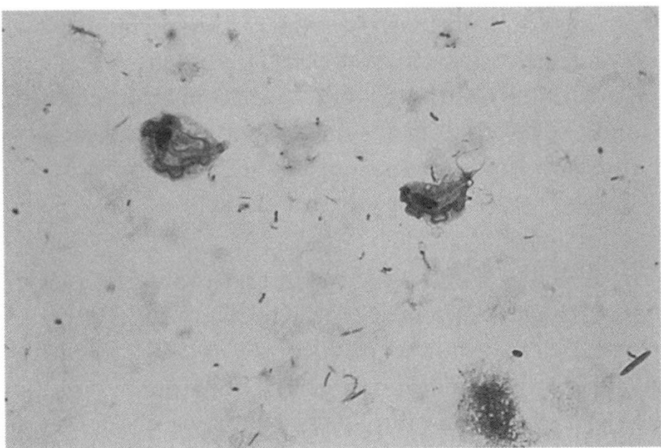

Figure 2-165 • Reproduced with permission from Axford J. Medicine, 2nd ed. Blackwell Publishing, 2004: Fig. 3.17, p. 87.

A. Bacterial vaginosis—metronidazole
B. Bacterial vaginosis—miconazole cream
C. Trichomonas—metronidazole
D. Trichomonas—miconazole cream
E. Candida vaginitis—miconazole cream

166. A 35-year-old G_3P_1 nonpregnant woman presents to the ED with fever and severe pelvic pain for 2 days. She is also experiencing mild nausea, but no emesis, dysuria, hematuria, anorexia, or changes in bowel movements. Significant past gynecological history includes sexual activity with a relatively new partner, sporadic condom usage, chlamydia as a teenager, hospitalization for PID several years ago, two elective first-trimester terminations, and one uncomplicated spontaneous vaginal delivery 7 years ago. She denies any other medical or surgical history. Her temperature is 101.0°C, and she is in mild discomfort. Speculum exam is unremarkable, but bimanual exam reveals moderate cervical motion tenderness and a tender adnexal mass on her left side. Her WBC count returns as elevated with a left shift. You send the patient for US, which shows a somewhat loculated fluid collection/indistinct mass in the region of her right ovary and fallopian tube. What is the most likely diagnosis and appropriate next step in management?

A. Toxic shock syndrome (TSS)—inpatient IV antibiotics
B. Ovarian cancer—exploratory laparotomy and complete surgical staging
C. Tubo-ovarian abscess (TOA)/complex (TOC) — inpatient IV antibiotics
D. Tubo-ovarian abscess/complex—outpatient oral antibiotics
E. Endometritis—outpatient oral antibiotics

167. A 32-year-old G_0 woman presents to the ED with moderately severe left pelvic pain for 1 day. She denies fever, chills, trauma, weight changes, dysuria, or hematuria, but has experienced some mild nausea. She is about to start menstruating and reports that the same pain occurred at the beginning of her last few cycles. In addition to this worsening dysmenorrhea, her past gynecological history is significant for normal Pap smears and no STDs. She is sexually active with her husband, has mild dyspareunia, and does not use birth control as they have been trying unsuccessfully to conceive for approximately 1 year. A serum pregnancy test is negative, and she is afebrile with normal vital signs. Pertinent physical findings include a mildly tender lower abdomen, normal speculum exam, and bimanual exam revealing mild uterosacral nodularity and a small left adnexal mass that is tender to palpation. You send her for US, which reveals a 3 cm left adnexal mass that has a "ground glass" appearance (Figure 2-167). The remainder

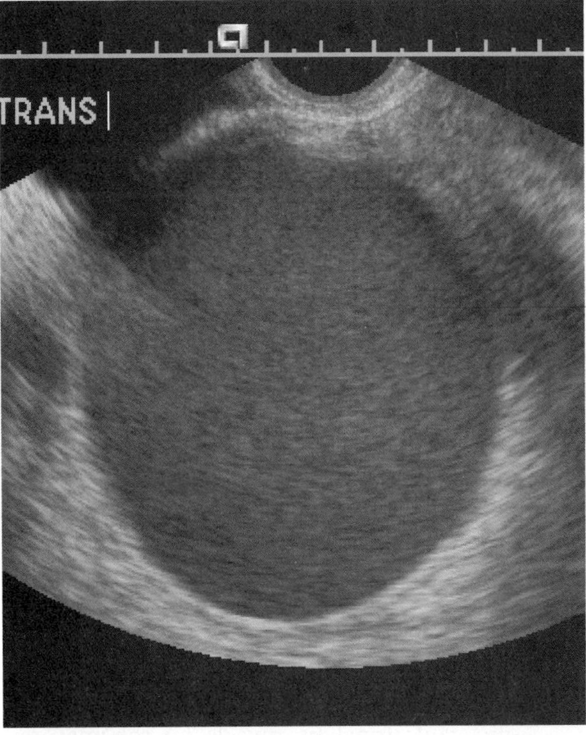

Figure 2-167 • Image Provided by Departments of Radiology and Obstetrics & Gynecology, University of California, San Francisco.

of the US is within normal limits. What is this patient's most likely diagnosis and how should she be treated?

A. Endometriosis—expectant management and initiation of infertility evaluation
B. Endometriosis—OCPs
C. Ovarian cancer—exploratory laparotomy and complete cancer staging
D. Mittelschmerz—NSAIDs
E. Fibroids—hysterectomy

`168. A 19-year-old G_1P_0 at 19 4/7 weeks GA presents to the ED with leakage of clear fluid noted upon awakening. She denies contractions, vaginal bleeding, fever, chills, or trauma. Pregnancy history is significant for entry into prenatal care at 17 weeks GA and diagnosis of chlamydia infection at that time, which was subsequently treated. Physical exam reveals a thin woman with normal temperature and nontender uterine fundus palpable 1 cm below the umbilicus. Sterile speculum exam shows pooling of vaginal fluid that is nitrazine positive and exhibits ferning under the microscope. Bedside US shows a live fetus in breech presentation. Which of the following measures would be appropriate management of preterm premature rupture of membranes (PPROM) in this patient?

A. Administration of corticosteroids for fetal lung maturity
B. Tocolysis
C. Administration of antibiotics
D. Induction of labor
E. Continuous fetal monitoring

169. A 33-year-old G_2P_1 woman at 29 2/7 weeks GA presents with severe right back pain radiating to her abdomen that began suddenly today. She denies prior episodes of pain, leakage of fluid, vaginal bleeding, fever, dysuria, hematuria, trauma, or drug usage. However, she does report some nausea and vomiting as well as mild contractions every 6 to 8 minutes. On exam, she is pacing the room, unable to stay still because of the pain. She is afebrile but with significant right CVAT. Fetal heart tones are reassuring, and tocometer reveals contractions every 5 to 8 minutes, but her cervix is closed, long, and high. A WBC count is within normal limits and urinalysis reveals microhematuria. What is the likely diagnosis and next step in management?

A. Nephrolithiasis—extracorporeal shock wave lithotripsy to break up large stones
B. Nephrolithiasis—IV hydration, pain control
C. Pyelonephritis—outpatient oral antibiotics
D. Pyelonephritis—inpatient IV antibiotics
E. Preterm labor—tocolysis

170. A 31-year-old G_1P_0 woman at 38 5/7 weeks GA with previously normal BPs reports to the ED after home monitoring reveals a BP of 158/98. She reports that the prenatal course has been uncomplicated. A repeat BP taken upon her arrival to the ED is 140/92, and the patient's urine dips 2+ proteinuria. Fetal heart rate (FHR) monitoring is reassuring. You draw the appropriate preeclamptic labs. As you await their return, the nurse informs you that the patient is having a seizure. Upon your arrival to the bedside, the patient is confused, but no longer seizing. Physical exam is within normal limits, and the lab results are still pending. An FHR tracing is obtained (Figure 2-170). Which of the following steps is the best management at this point?

A. Administer phenytoin
B. Administer diazepam
C. Administer phenobarbital
D. Administer magnesium sulfate
E. Emergent cesarean delivery

171. A 42-year-old G_2P_2 woman comes to the ED reporting severe, burning pain in the genital area of 2 days duration. She has never experienced this pain before. Additionally, she reports a flu-like illness several days ago. Past medical and surgical histories are noncontributory. Her gynecological history is significant for two vaginal deliveries, regular menses, and normal Pap smears. She is sexually active with her boyfriend of 2 months and reports 100% condom usage. On exam, she is afebrile and does not have inguinal lymphadenopathy. You note several crops of vesicles and some ulcerated lesions on her perineum and labia majora that are exquisitely tender (Figure 2-171). What is the likely diagnosis and appropriate treatment?

A. Genital warts—imiquimod
B. Genital warts—metronidazole
C. *Molluscum contagiosum*—trichloroacetic acid
D. Genital herpes—hydrocortisone cream
E. Genital herpes—acyclovir

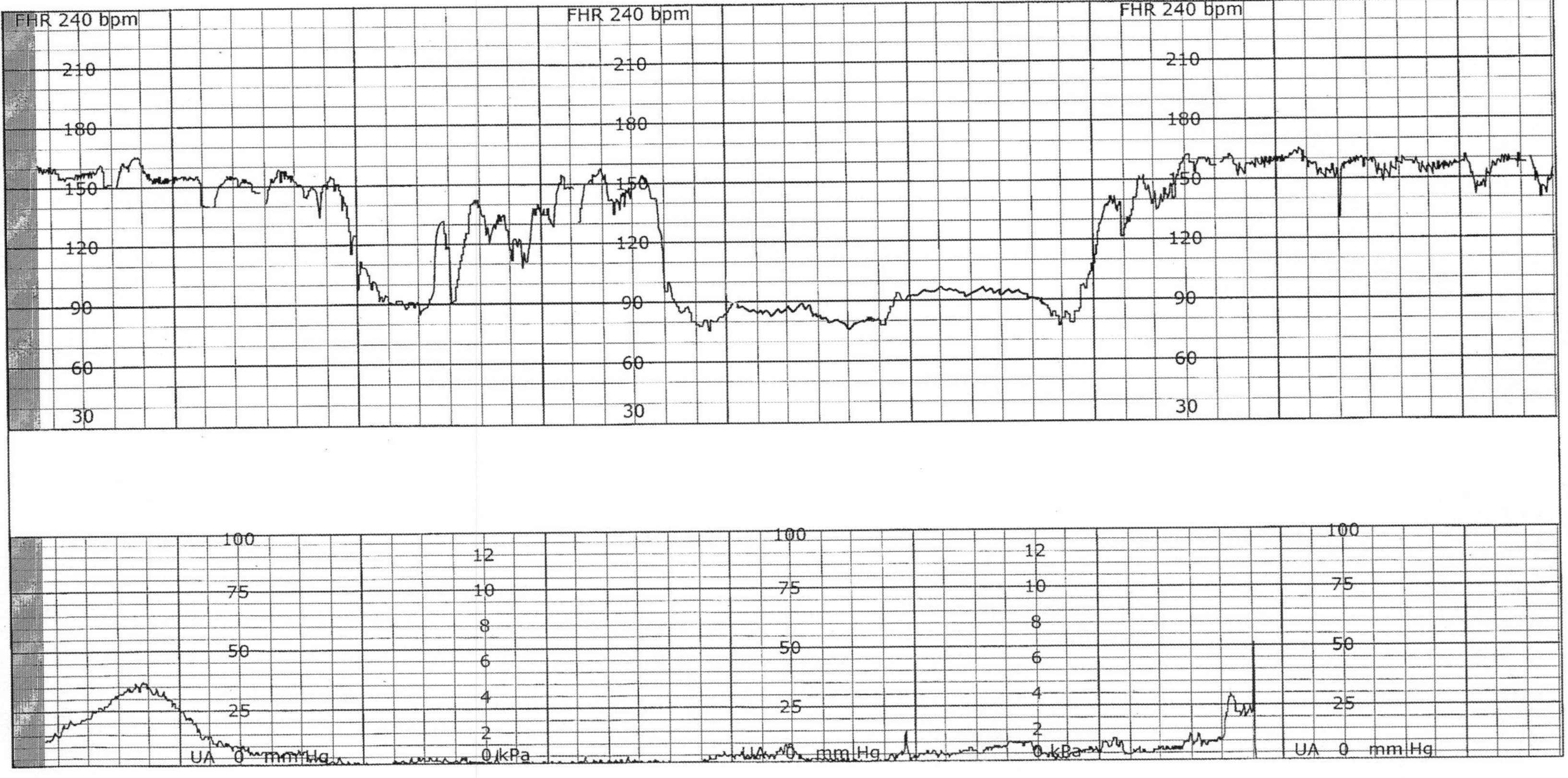

Figure 2-170 • Image Provided by Department of Obstetrics & Gynecology, University of California, San Francisco.

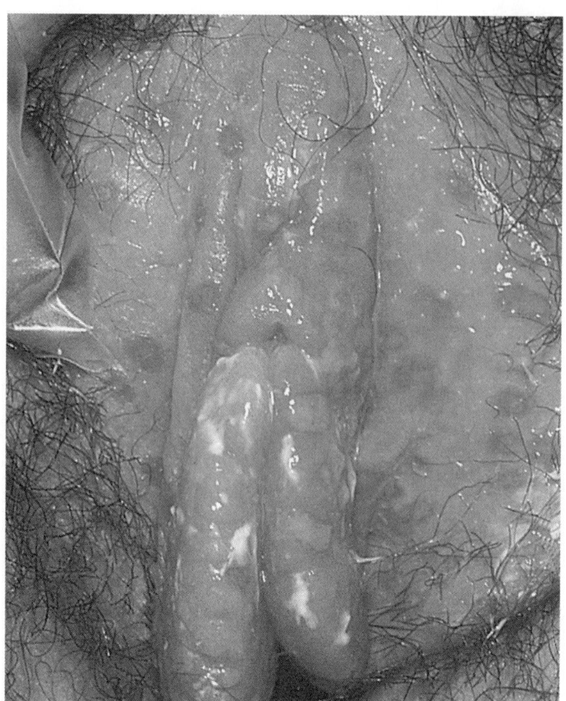

Figure 2-171 • Reproduced from Callahan TL, Caughey AB. Blueprints Obstetrics & Gynecology, 4th ed. Baltimore: Lippincott Williams & Wilkins, 2007. Fig. 16-2, p. 177.

172 A 21-year-old G_1P_0 woman is brought to the ED by her friend, who reports that the patient has been experiencing persistent, severe vaginal bleeding since undergoing pregnancy termination 2 days prior via D&E of a 15-week gestation. She denies fever, chills, nausea, or vomiting, but does report painful cramping. The patient appears pale and is tachycardic with normal BP and temperature on exam. Her abdomen is benign, but speculum exam reveals a moderate amount of bleeding from her cervix, which appears to be open but intact. Bimanual exam is significant for a mildly tender 12-week-sized uterus, no cervical motion tenderness, and no adnexal masses or tenderness. You perform a bedside US and see that the uterus has a thick, heterogeneous endometrium (Figure 2-172), there is no free fluid in the pelvis, and both adnexa are within normal limits. What is the most likely diagnosis and appropriate treatment for this patient?

A. Retained POCs—suction curettage
B. Retained POCs—expectant management
C. Normal exam—expectant management
D. Cervical laceration—operative repair
E. Uterine perforation—diagnostic laparoscopy

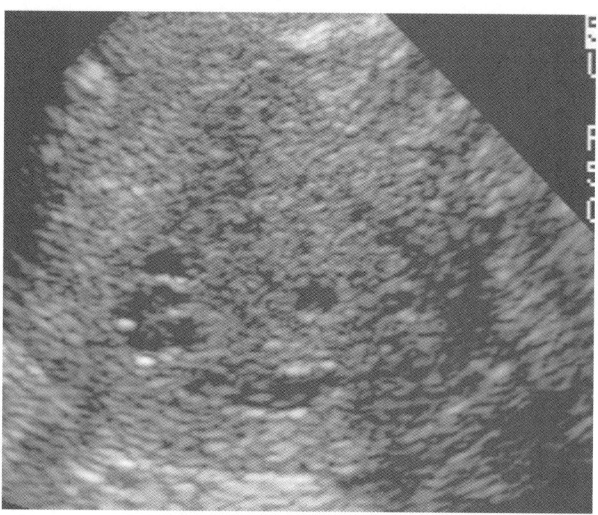

Figure 2-172 • Image Provided by Departments of Radiology and Obstetrics & Gynecology, University of California, San Francisco.

173. A 28-year-old G_1P_0 woman at 19 0/7 weeks GA presents to the ED complaining of pelvic pressure and increased vaginal discharge. She denies cramps or contractions, leakage of fluid, vaginal bleeding, or fever. Her pregnancy has been uncomplicated thus far. She had two prenatal visits at 8 and 14 weeks and is scheduled to see her provider again after her routine US appointment scheduled for tomorrow. Her past gynecological history is significant for a cone biopsy of the cervix at age 23 for persistent high-grade squamous intraepithelial lesion (HSIL). All subsequent Pap smears have been within normal limits. Speculum exam reveals a cervix that is approximately 2 cm dilated with visible amniotic membranes. You also notice a pool of fluid in the vagina, which is nitrazine and fern positive. Which of the following statements is true regarding the management of this patient's incompetent cervix?

A. Her risk factors for incompetent cervix include her Pap smear in the first trimester.
B. Treatment options include emergent cerclage placement.
C. Patients with a history of incompetent cervix can be offered a prophylactic cerclage in subsequent pregnancies that should be placed prior to conception.
D. Treatment options include pregnancy termination.
E. Her incompetent cervix could have been diagnosed by US at 14 weeks.

174. A 70-year-old demented woman is sent from her nursing home to the ED when she is found to have vaginal bleeding. Review of her medical records reveals that she has hypertension and suffered a cerebrovascular accident 2 years prior with subsequent speech and motor deficits, necessitating full-time care. She never had any children and became menopausal at age 52. On exam, she is awake, but demented and unable to communicate. Gynecological exam reveals a large, necrotic, bleeding sore on her left vulva. Additionally, she has left inguinal lymphadenopathy. Her uterus is not palpable on bimanual exam, but you confirm its presence as well as the absence of adnexal masses on US. The vaginal tissue is atrophied but otherwise within normal limits for her age. You suspect a vulvar malignancy. Which of the following statements is true regarding cancer of the vulva?

A. Vulvar cancer is one of the most common gynecologic malignancies.
B. Symptoms of vulvar cancer include bleeding, pain, pruritus, ascites, and bloating.
C. Malignant melanoma is the most common subtype of vulvar cancer.
D. Treatment of squamous cell cancer of the vulva involves wide local excision with lymph node dissection.
E. Staging of vulvar cancer can be performed via biopsy of the mass and palpation of the inguinal lymph nodes.

175. A 33-year-old G_3P_2 woman who had an uncomplicated delivery of an infant 3 weeks ago presents to the ED complaining of right breast pain and fever for 2 days. On physical exam, you note an area of focal tenderness, warmth, and erythema on the right breast. The patient is found to have a temperature of 101.2°C and an elevated WBC count of 12,000. Which of the following is appropriate treatment for mastitis?

A. Symptomatic treatment of pain with acetaminophen only
B. Stop breastfeeding until completion of antibiotic course
C. Oral dicloxacillin
D. IV antibiotics
E. Oral doxycycline

176. A 23-year-old G_0 woman presents with acute-onset, severe right lower quadrant pain and mild nausea. She denies fever, chills, or vaginal bleeding or discharge. The patient reports feeling this pain twice in the last 6 months, with this time being the worst it has ever been. On physical exam, she is afebrile, appears extremely uncomfortable, and has severe RLQ tenderness, but does not have any peritoneal signs. Pelvic exam is significant for a tender right adnexal mass and cervical motion tenderness. Pelvic US reveals minimal fluid in the cul-de-sac and a 6 cm right adnexal mass with no Doppler flow (Figure 2-176). The patient's WBC count and hematocrit are normal, and a urine pregnancy test is negative. Which of the following is the most likely diagnosis?

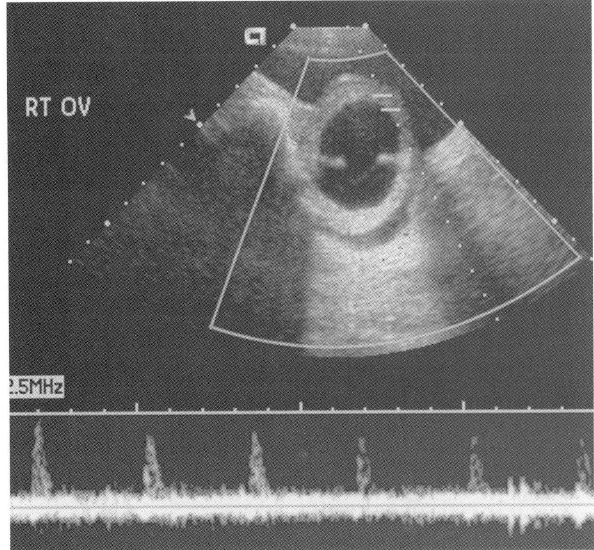

Figure 2-176 • Image Provided by Departments of Radiology and Obstetrics & Gynecology, University of California, San Francisco.

A. Acute appendicitis
B. Early ectopic pregnancy
C. Torsion of adnexa
D. PID
E. Ruptured hemorrhagic ovarian cyst

177. A 27-year-old woman presents to the ED with complaints of heavy vaginal bleeding and painful abdominal cramping that started this morning. She reports that she stopped taking birth control pills approximately 3 months ago in an effort to conceive and that she had some light spotting a month later but no normal menstrual period since then. Her blood type is O positive, and her hematocrit is 39.2. A urine pregnancy test in the ED is positive. On physical exam, you note mild lower abdominal tenderness in

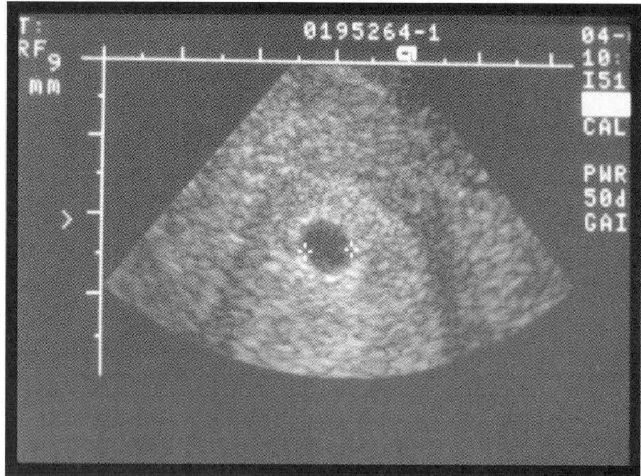

Figure 2-177 • Image Provided by Departments of Radiology and Obstetrics & Gynecology, University of California, San Francisco.

the midline, but an otherwise benign abdominal exam. On speculum exam, you note a large amount of bright red blood in the vaginal vault and an open cervical os containing large blood clots. Endovaginal US (Figure 2-177) confirms the presence of a gestational sac in the uterus consistent with a 6-week gestation, but no yolk sac is visible. What is the correct diagnosis and management of this patient?

A. Ectopic pregnancy—emergent surgery
B. Threatened abortion—D&C
C. Incomplete abortion—expectant management
D. Inevitable abortion—D&C
E. Complete abortion—expectant management

178. A 20-year-old G_1P_1 woman presents to the ED complaining of nausea, vomiting, and lower abdominal pain for the past 2 days. She reports intermittent condom usage with her partner of 3 months. Her vital signs are within normal limits, with the exception of a temperature of 100.2°C. On exam, you note abdominal, adnexal, and cervical motion tenderness, but no peritoneal signs. Mucopurulent discharge is apparent at the cervical os. A urine pregnancy test is negative, and the patient's WBC count is 13,700/mm^3. A wet mount shows numerous leukocytes. Which of the following are absolute indications for inpatient treatment of PID?

A. Age greater than 18
B. Age less than 40
C. Severe nausea and vomiting
D. Adnexal tenderness
E. Penicillin allergy

179. A 28-year-old G_3P_0 woman is brought to the ED shortly after passing out. She is conscious on arrival, but appears to be in acute distress and severe pain. She reports vaginal bleeding and worsening left lower abdominal pain that became sharp and severe just prior to her loss of consciousness. She had a positive urine pregnancy test 4 weeks ago and is certain that her LMP was 8 weeks ago. Past medical history is significant for PID that was treated 5 years ago. Her vital signs are BP 92/60, pulse 118, respiration 26, and temperature 97.2°F. Urine pregnancy test is positive. The patient has a normal WBC count and a hematocrit of 32.3. On physical exam, she has diffuse lower abdominal pain and exhibits guarding and rebound. Pelvic exam reveals cervical motion tenderness and significant tenderness to palpation in the left adnexal region. Transvaginal US (Figure 2-179) shows a large amount of free fluid in the cul-de-sac, but no masses and no intrauterine pregnancy. What is the most appropriate next step in managing this patient?

A. Uterine curettage to definitively exclude ectopic pregnancy
B. Perform a culdocentesis
C. Obtain a quantitative β-hCG level to determine whether medical or surgical treatment is indicated
D. Administer methotrexate and follow serial quantitative β-hCG levels for appropriate decline
E. Stabilize the patient and take her emergently to the operating room

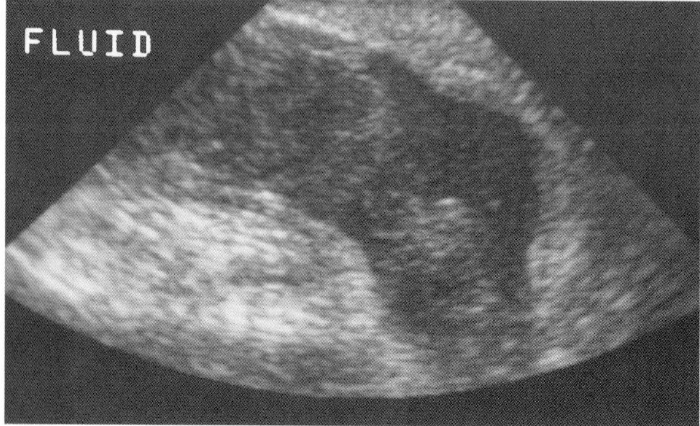

Figure 2-179 • Image Provided by Departments of Radiology and Obstetrics & Gynecology, University of California, San Francisco.

180. A 20-year-old G_0 woman presents to the ED in tears. She reports being sexually assaulted by three men unknown to her while attending a party this evening. You obtain a history from her, which is difficult because she is visibly shaken and upset. She doesn't believe any of the assailants used a condom and is unsure whether they ejaculated. There was no oral or anal penetration. On speculum exam, you obtain swabs from the vagina for evidence and for microscopic exam. You do not see any evidence of spermatozoa, trichomonads, or bacterial vaginosis. Which of the following steps would be appropriate management of this patient?

A. Start oral contraceptive pills immediately
B. Azithromycin 1 g PO and ceftriaxone 250 mg IM × 1
C. Do not contact police if the patient does not want to press charges
D. Reassure her that she has no risk of pregnancy
E. Reassure her that she has minimal risk of contracting HIV if there was no ejaculation

181. A 17-year-old G_0 woman is brought to the ED by her mother, who is concerned that the patient has been experiencing fevers, rigors, nausea, vomiting, and myalgias since this morning. She is not sexually active, and her LMP began 5 days ago. Her vital signs are BP 84/46, temperature 103.1°C, pulse 122, and respiration 24. On physical exam, the patient appears acutely ill, has a diffuse erythematous rash, and exhibits mild, diffuse abdominal tenderness, but no nuchal rigidity. After removal of a blood-saturated tampon, pelvic exam reveals a small amount of blood in the vaginal vault but no cervical motion tenderness or vaginal discharge, and the uterus and adnexa are within normal limits. Laboratory studies are significant for a WBC count of 21,000, platelets of 93,000, and elevated BUN and creatinine. Which of the following statements about this patient's diagnosis is true?

A. It is caused by *Streptococcus agalactiae.*
B. It has been associated with polycystic ovarian syndrome (PCOS), vaginal infections, vaginal and cesarean delivery, and postpartum endometritis.
C. Blood cultures are often positive.
D. Treatment may include admission to an intensive care unit for management of hypotension.
E. There are approximately 1500 cases per year in the United States.

182. A 27-year-old G_2P_1 woman at 35 1/7 weeks GA presents to OB triage and anxiously states that she has not felt the baby move for the past 5 hours. She denies vaginal bleeding, rupture of membranes, or uterine contractions. The pregnancy is complicated by poorly controlled gestational diabetes mellitus requiring insulin administration. The patient began twice-weekly antepartum testing at 32 weeks gestation, but has missed several appointments. Physical exam is significant for an obese woman with a random blood glucose of 154. Her cervical exam is 1 cm dilated, 50% effaced, and –3 station. Nonstress testing is performed (Figure 2-182). What is the most appropriate next step in the management of this high-risk patient with decreased fetal movement?

A. Administer insulin to decrease the patient's glucose level
B. Vibroacoustic stimulation (VAS) of the fetus followed by US to look for gross and fine fetal movements
C. Administer betamethasone to promote fetal lung maturity in anticipation of possible premature delivery
D. Begin induction of labor with a prostaglandin agent
E. Emergent cesarean section

183. A 32-year-old G_3P_3 woman presents to the ED complaining of persistent fevers and abdominal pain that have worsened over the past day and are only temporarily relieved by ibuprofen. She is postpartum day 7 after a vaginal delivery of a term infant male weighing 3500 g. The delivery was complicated by a postpartum hemorrhage requiring manual extraction of the placenta. The patient's vaginal bleeding has decreased since discharge from the hospital, requiring two to four pad changes per day. Her vital signs are BP 108/72, temperature 102.6°C, pulse 96, and respiration 20. On physical exam, she has fundal tenderness but no peritoneal signs. Pelvic exam confirms uterine tenderness and reveals scant vaginal bleeding as well as a minimal amount of purulent discharge. The laceration repair is intact and hemostatic. Laboratory studies reveal a hematocrit of 34.4 and a WBC count of 18,000 with a left shift. What is the appropriate diagnosis and treatment for this patient?

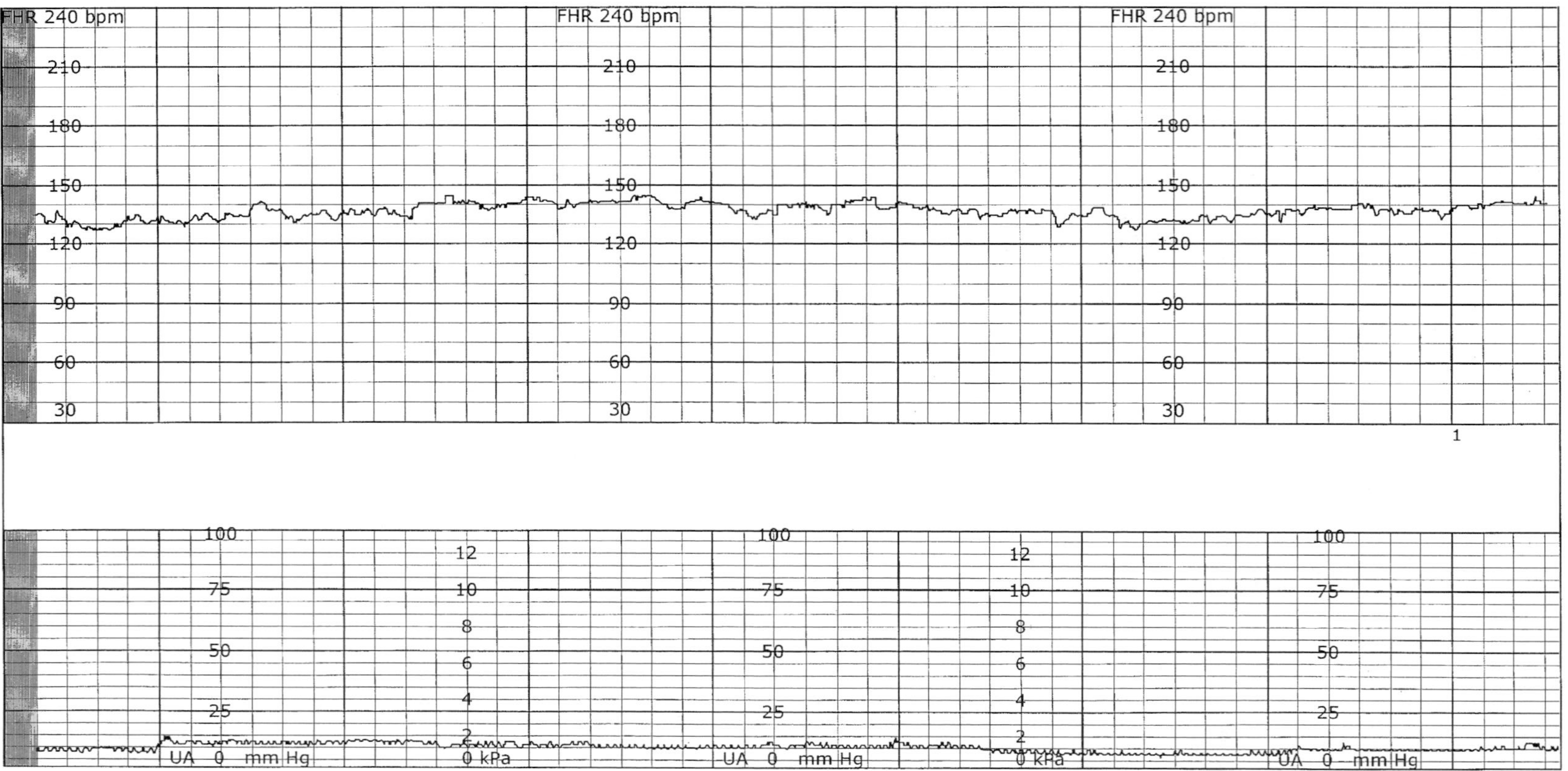

Figure 2-182 • Image Provided by Department of Obstetrics & Gynecology, University of California, San Francisco.

A. Delayed postpartum hemorrhage—D&C
B. Placenta accreta—exploratory laparotomy
C. Undiagnosed vaginal hematoma—ligation of the offending blood vessel
D. Endomyometritis—clindamycin and gentamicin
E. Endomyometritis—D&C

184. A 30-year-old G_0 woman presents to the ED after an episode of postcoital bleeding that soaked a pad over the last 2 hours. She reports four to five prior episodes of postcoital bleeding over the last few months that were less severe. She denies any significant past medical history. Her menses occur every month and are regular. She has not had a Pap smear since age 18, when she first became sexually active. At that time, she was found to have chlamydia, for which she underwent treatment. The patient reports multiple current sexual partners, and she uses condoms intermittently. Her hematocrit is 40.1. Vital signs and physical exam are within normal limits. Pelvic exam reveals a minimal amount of blood and watery discharge in the vaginal vault, as well as a 2 cm × 3 cm exophytic mass on the cervix that does not appear to involve the upper vagina or fornix. The uterus and adnexa are within normal limits. You biopsy the lesion, which returns 1 week later as cervical cancer invasive to 7 mm. The patient undergoes staging, which reveals negative cystoscopy, proctoscopy, and IV pyelogram (IVP). What is the stage and appropriate treatment of her disease?

A. Ib1—cone biopsy to preserve fertility
B. Ib1—radical hysterectomy or radiation therapy
C. Ib2—radical hysterectomy or radiation therapy
D. IIa—radical hysterectomy
E. IIb—radiation therapy

185. A 34-year-old G_4P_3 woman at 33 4/7 weeks GA presents to the ED complaining of a gush of vaginal bleeding as well as the onset of severely painful uterine contractions. The patient denies history of abdominal trauma, recent intercourse, or cocaine usage and has a history of three prior vaginal deliveries. Her vital signs are BP 162/99, temperature 98.4°C, pulse 114, and respiration 18. Physical exam reveals a woman in moderate distress with a firm and tender uterus. The fetal heart rate (FHR) tracing is initially formally reactive, with a baseline rate of approximately 145 beats per minutes (bpm). US exam confirms that there is no evidence of placenta previa. On sterile speculum exam, a moderate amount of blood is seen in the vaginal vault. Cervical exam reveals 1.5 cm dilation, 50% effacement, and –3 station. As you are writing the patient's note, the nurse informs you that the FHR tracing now shows a prolonged deceleration of 5 minutes duration to approximately 80 bpm with no signs of spontaneous recovery to baseline (Figure 2-185). The nurse has already turned the patient to her left side, given O_2 by face mask, and checked her BP, which is now 158/102. What is the most appropriate next step in this patient's management?

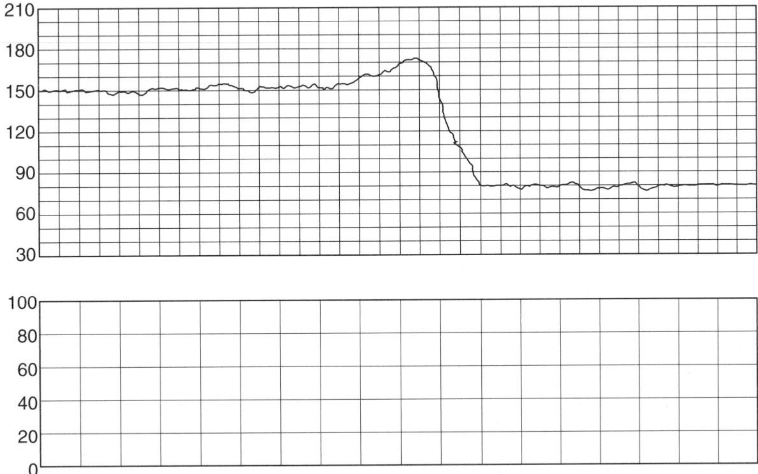

Figure 2-185 • Reproduced from Caughey A. Blueprints Q&A Step 3 Obstetrics & Gynecology. Blackwell Science, 2002: Fig. 89, p. 55.

A. Transfuse 2 units of packed red blood cells (PRBC) immediately and have the lab type and cross 2 additional units
B. Administer betamethasone to promote fetal lung maturity in anticipation of preterm delivery
C. Administer magnesium sulfate tocolysis to alleviate the fetal distress from contractions
D. Initiate induction of labor for nonreassuring FHR tracing
E. Move to the operating room (OR) for cesarean section for nonreassuring FHR tracing

186. A 36-year-old G_2P_2 woman presents to the ED with acute-onset shortness of breath and chest pain. She is 1 day postpartum following a cesarean delivery and left the hospital prior to the recommended day of discharge (generally, postoperative day 2 or 3) due to childcare issues. Of note, the patient is not breastfeeding. She denies a history of trauma. Her past medical history is significant for obesity, and her vital signs are BP 116/74, temperature 100.0°C, pulse 112, respiration 28, and O_2 saturation 91% on room air. On physical exam, she is in moderate distress, is tachypneic, and has rales and mildly decreased breath sounds in the left lung. Pelvic exam reveals a minimal amount of blood in the vaginal vault but is otherwise within normal limits. Chest X-ray is negative, but EKG reveals sinus tachycardia and nonspecific ST-T wave changes. A blood gas drawn on room air reveals an a-A gradient of 43. You order a ventilation/perfusion (V/Q) scan, which is read as inconclusive. At this point, a pulmonary arteriogram is performed (Figure 2-186). Which of the following would be the most appropriate treatment for this patient?

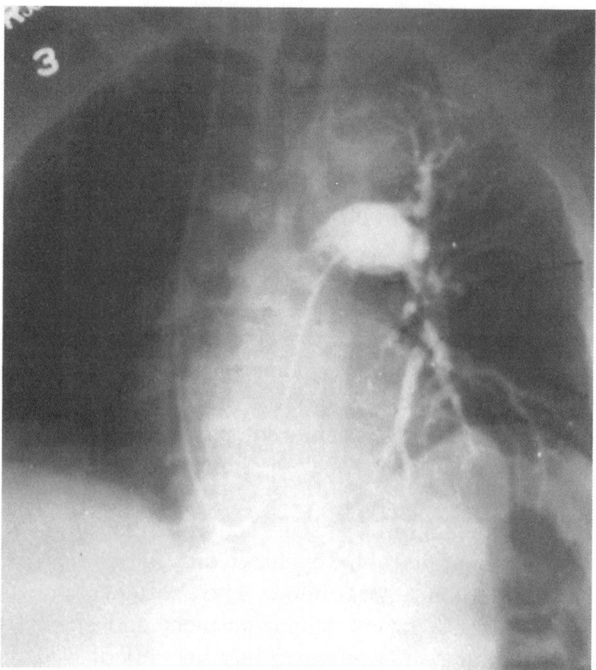

Figure 2-186 • Reproduced with Permission from Dildy G. Critical Care Obstetrics. Blackwell Science, 2004: Fig. 20-7, p. 284.

A. Supplemental oxygen by nasal cannula
B. IV heparin
C. Low-molecular-weight heparin
D. Oral warfarin therapy
E. IV furosemide

187. A 68-year-old G_0 woman with a history of stage IIIc ovarian cancer presents to the ED with persistent nausea and vomiting for several days. She has not had anything to eat or drink for 2 days. Additionally, she has not had a bowel movement or passed gas in 5 days. Approximately 7 months ago, she underwent TAH-BSO, complete staging work-up, and 6 cycles of chemotherapy for her ovarian cancer. Her vital signs are BP 114/72, temperature 100.8°C, pulse 108, and respiration 18. On physical exam, she is a thin, obtunded woman with dry mucous membranes and skin tenting. Abdominal exam reveals distention, absent bowel sounds, severe tenderness, and peritoneal signs. Laboratory studies are significant for a hematocrit of 45.2 and WBC of 15,000. You send the patient for an abdominal X-ray series, which reveals numerous air-fluid levels and a sliver of hyperlucency below the diaphragm. What is the next step in the management of this patient?

A. Insert a nasogastric tube (NGT) and expectant management
B. Begin total parenteral nutrition (TPN)
C. Laparoscopy to look for residual disease
D. Administer broad-spectrum antibiotics and plan laparotomy when her signs of infection have resolved
E. Proceed to the operating room (OR) for exploratory laparotomy

188. A 36-year-old G_0 woman presents to the ED complaining of severe pelvic pain for 2 days. The patient is well known to you and has endometriosis confirmed by laparoscopy. She denies history of current or past physical or sexual abuse and does not desire future fertility. Over the past 3 years, she has tried various treatment regimens, including both cyclic and continuous OCPs. The latter yielded a 4-month pain-free period. The patient admits to recent discontinuation of the continuous OCPs secondary to concern regarding amenorrhea. Her vital signs are stable, and she is afebrile. Physical exam reveals normal bowel sounds, mild pelvic tenderness, but no masses or peritoneal signs. On pelvic exam, the patient has diffuse pelvic tenderness and uterosacral nodularity on rectovaginal exam. There are no adnexal masses or vaginal discharge or bleeding. Pelvic US is within normal limits. Which of the following steps is the most appropriate treatment for this patient?

A. Resume cyclic OCPs
B. Resume continuous OCPs
C. Trial of progestin treatment
D. Trial of GnRH agonist treatment
E. Exploratory laparoscopy

189. An 18-year-old G_1P_0 woman at 14 4/7 weeks GA presents to the ED complaining of weight loss and severe nausea and vomiting for 3 days. This is her fifth visit to the ED for this problem, and she has had two prior short-term hospitalizations. She has tried vitamin B_6, Reglan (metoclopramide), Tigan (trimethobenzamide), and Compazine (prochlorperazine), but obtained only temporary relief. She has no significant past medical history but is currently in an abusive relationship with the father of the baby. Her vital signs are BP 102/68, temperature 96.8°C, pulse 96, and respiration 16. On physical exam, she appears uncomfortable, has dry mucous membranes, and shows poor skin turgor. Pelvic exam is within normal limits. Laboratory studies reveal hypokalemia, hypochloremia, alkalemia, hematocrit of 48, and a BUN/creatinine ratio exceeding 20:1. Urinalysis reveals ketones and high specific gravity. Which of the following components of this patient's management should be used only when the others have failed?

A. Hospitalization for IV hydration and repletion of electrolytes
B. Social work consultation
C. Zofran (ondansetron) 4 mg IV, then 8 mg PO TID when tolerating oral intake
D. Initiation of total parenteral nutrition (TPN)
E. Placement of a nasogastric feeding tube

190. A 31-year-old G_2P_2 woman presents to the ED complaining of severe abdominal pain and vaginal spotting. She denies fever, chills, nausea, and vomiting. Over the past 6 months, she has noticed that the duration and amount of her regular menses have diminished. This is coincident with the fact that approximately 6 months ago, she underwent a loop electrosurgical excision procedure (LEEP) for cervical dysplasia. Her vital signs and physical exam are within normal limits. On pelvic exam, you note a slightly enlarged, tender, anteverted and anteflexed uterus with cervical motion tenderness and no cervical, uterine, or adnexal masses. What is the most likely diagnosis and appropriate treatment?

A. Pelvic abscess—CT-guided drainage
B. Endometriosis—diagnostic laparoscopy
C. Progression of residual cervical dysplasia to cancer—hysterectomy
D. Cervical stenosis—OCPs
E. Cervical stenosis—cervical dilatation

191. A 24-year-old G_1P_0 woman who had a positive urine pregnancy test 9 weeks ago presents to the ED complaining of severe nausea, vomiting, and painless vaginal bleeding. She has not had her initial prenatal exam yet. She denies any significant past medical history. On physical exam, she has no abdominal tenderness, but her fundus is palpable just below the umbilicus. Pelvic exam reveals a small amount of tissue at the cervical os, but no lesion, discharge, or active bleeding. Quantitative β-hCG is 117,000. US is performed (Figure 2-191). Which of the following statements is correct regarding this patient's diagnosis and management?

A. Tissue evacuated from the uterine cavity is likely to have a 46,XX karyotype.
B. Treatment should be expectant management.
C. Treatment should be hysterectomy.
D. Treatment should be immediate single-agent chemotherapy.
E. There is a 25% risk of recurrence with subsequent pregnancies.

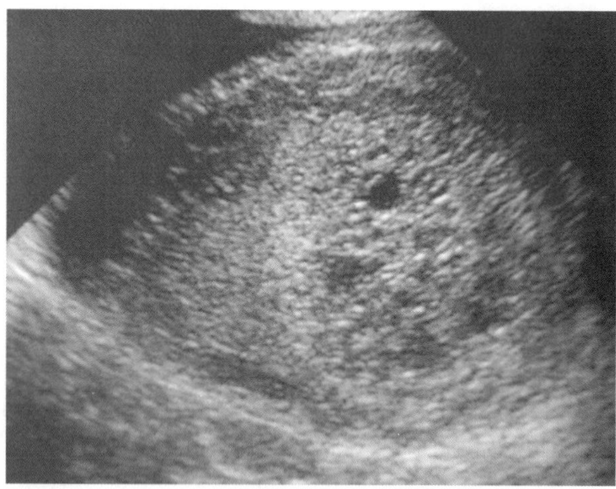

Figure 2-191 • Image Provided by Departments of Radiology and Obstetrics & Gynecology, University of California, San Francisco.

192. A 62-year-old G_3P_3 woman presents to the ED 5 days after undergoing a laparoscopic Burch culposuspension procedure for stress urinary incontinence. She reports that she has been able to micturate only small volumes over the past 6 hours despite constant urgency. Additionally, she is experiencing mild nausea and increasing midline lower abdominal pain without radiation, but denies vomiting, fever, chills, constipation, or loose stools. Her past medical history is noncontributory. Vital signs are within normal limits. On physical exam, you note mild suprapubic pain, normal bowel sounds, and no peritoneal signs. Pelvic exam reveals discomfort with uterine manipulation, but no cervical motion tenderness, no vaginal discharge or bleeding, and no uterine, cervical, or adnexal masses. Rectal exam is nontender with normal tone. You collect a 20 cc urine specimen, which gives the following results on urine dipstick: specific gravity 1.010, no RBCs, negative leukocyte esterase, 2 to 5 bacteria/high-power field, and 1 to 3 squamous cells/high-power field. Which of the following is the most appropriate next step in management of this patient?

A. Outpatient treatment of UTI
B. Hospitalization for IV antibiotic treatment
C. Straight catheterization to obtain a clean sample for urinalysis
D. Placement of a Foley catheter
E. Surgical exploration/repair

193. You are called by an ED resident to evaluate a 26-year-old G_4P_2 woman presenting with epigastric pain and severe nausea. On arrival to the ER, her BP is 155/110, her heart rate is 72, and her temperature is 37.6°C. The patient reports that she has missed her last three menstrual periods (and normally has very regular cycles). A urine pregnancy test is positive, and urine dipstick demonstrates 2+ protein but is otherwise normal. A CBC with platelets, LFTs, amylase, and lipase were sent immediately and were all within normal limits. Abdominal US in the ER showed no evidence of appendicitis or cholestatic disease. The resident is not sure what she is seeing when scanning the uterus. Before hanging up, she asks if any laboratory values should be added on to her original orders to help evaluate this patient. Serum levels of which *one* of the following would be *most* valuable in the diagnosis of this patient?

A. CA-125
B. Quantitative β-hCG
C. Magnesium
D. Alpha-fetoprotein (AFP)
E. Thyroxine (T_4)

194. A 38-year-old G_1P_0 woman presents to the ED at 9 weeks GA with 2 days of vaginal bleeding. She is very upset about the possibility of miscarriage, as this is a highly desired pregnancy achieved with intrauterine insemination. An US at 7 weeks was thought to show a normal intrauterine pregnancy. Pelvic exam in the emergency room reveals vesicles protruding from the cervical os and a small amount of active bleeding. Pelvic US reveals a thickened placenta with multiple cysts and a fetus consistent with her dating. Quantitative β-hCG is 183,000. If suction evacuation is performed, what will be the most likely karyotype of the tissue recovered?

A. 46,XX
B. 47,XXY
C. 47,XX+18
D. 47,XX+21
E. 69,XXY

195. A 30-year-old G_0 female comes into the ED complaining of extreme pelvic pain. The pain began insidiously over the last few days. The patient reports a prior history of similar pain, but this time the pain is worse. It seems to coincide with her periods, and she has noticed increasing pain with intercourse. The patient has been married for

4 years and, despite not using contraception, has been unable to conceive. A urine serum pregnancy test is negative. The patient's pelvic exam is unremarkable except for diffuse pain of both adnexa. A pelvic US reveals a normal midline uterus with a slightly thickened endometrium consistent with current menstruation. Also, two 6 cm well-circumscribed masses with low attenuation are identified, one in each adnexa. The patient tells you that she has spoken with her doctor in the past about a diagnostic laparoscopy to evaluate the etiology of this pain. Which of the following potential intraoperative findings is the most likely cause of her pain?

A. Corpus luteum cyst
B. Scant powder-burn lesions
C. Bilateral endometriomas (chocolate cysts)
D. Peritoneal tuberculosis implants
E. Tubo-ovarian abscess (TOA)

196. You are called from the ED about a pregnant patient in the first trimester presenting with a febrile illness and history of a recent new sexual contact. The physician's assistant asks about the risk of transmission of various infections during pregnancy while the lab work is pending. You inform him that which of the following infections has been shown to be unlikely to be transmitted across the placenta?

A. Toxoplasmosis
B. HIV
C. *Neisseria gonorrhoeae*
D. Varicella zoster virus
E. Parvovirus

197. A 19-year-old G_0 woman presents to the ED several hours after experiencing a sudden sharp pain in the left lower quadrant that has subsided over the last few hours and become more diffuse. Her LMP was approximately 2 weeks ago. She reports similar prior episodes of pain on the right side 2 to 3 months ago, has been sexually active with the same partner for 2 years, and denies vaginal discharge. She is afebrile, has a normal white count, and has a negative urine pregnancy test. On physical exam, she has mild diffuse abdominal pain, but no peritoneal signs. Pelvic exam is within normal limits with no cervical motion tenderness. What is the most likely diagnosis?

A. Mittelschmerz
B. PID
C. Adnexal torsion
D. Ruptured ectopic pregnancy
E. Appendicitis

198. A 17-year-old G_3P_1 woman at 32 5/7 weeks GA presents to the ED complaining of moderately painful uterine contractions every 5 minutes for the past hour. Significant prenatal issues include obesity (prepregnancy weight of 253 lb), history of a prior preterm delivery at 32 weeks gestation, and history of a therapeutic abortion at 11 weeks gestation 3 years ago. Her vital signs are stable, and the patient is afebrile. On physical exam, she is an obese woman in moderate discomfort but with an otherwise negative exam. Sterile speculum exam and wet mount reveal abundant pseudohyphae, and cervical exam reveals 3 cm dilation and 75% effacement. Which of the following is this patient's biggest risk factor for preterm delivery?

A. Prior preterm delivery
B. Prior therapeutic abortion (TAB)
C. Vaginal candidiasis
D. Prepregnancy weight
E. Maternal age

199. A 31-year-old woman presents to the ED complaining of gradual-onset left lower quadrant pain. She denies nausea, vomiting, fever, chills, constipation, or loose stools. However, she notes an 8 lb weight gain over the past month. Her gynecological history is significant for current infertility treatment by ovulation induction with gonadotropins. During her infertility workup, a hysterosalpingogram revealed an occluded left tube, and laparoscopy revealed stage 3 endometriosis. The patient reports that she has continued to have unprotected intercourse throughout her current treatment. However, her urine pregnancy test is negative. Her vital signs are within normal limits. On physical exam, you note mild abdominal distention, tenderness to palpation in the left lower quadrant, and a left adnexal mass. No blood or discharge is apparent in the vaginal vault, and exam fails to show any cervical motion tenderness. US exam reveals an enlarged ovary approximately 7 cm × 8 cm in size that is composed of numerous enlarged follicles. There is a moderate amount of free fluid in the cul-de-sac. The patient's hematocrit is 42 and her WBC count is 8000. What is this patient's most likely diagnosis?

A. Adnexal torsion
B. Ovarian hyperstimulation (OHSS)
C. Early ectopic pregnancy
D. Endometrioma
E. PID

200. A 29-year-old G_2P_0 woman at 10 2/7 weeks GA by a sure LMP presents to the ED reporting cramping that started this afternoon. She is very anxious because she had a miscarriage with her last pregnancy and this pregnancy is highly desired. The patient denies vaginal bleeding, usage of an IUD, history of pelvic infections, smoking, or ectopic pregnancy. On exam, she is tearful but otherwise appears well with normal vital signs. Her abdomen is soft, nontender, and without masses. On speculum exam, no blood is seen in the vaginal vault. Bimanual exam reveals a mildly enlarged, nontender uterus, no cervical motion tenderness or dilation, and no adnexal masses or tenderness. A bedside US (Figure 2-200) reveals an intrauterine gestational sac with a fetal pole consistent in size with a 6-week gestation but no cardiac motion and no adnexal masses or free fluid in the cul-de-sac. A quantitative β-hCG is 13,327. Which of the following statements is true regarding this patient's diagnosis and treatment?

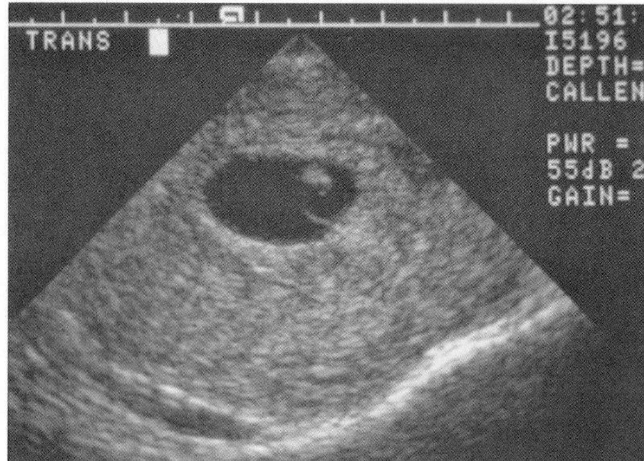

Figure 2-200 • Image Provided by Departments of Radiology and Obstetrics & Gynecology, University of California, San Francisco.

A. She has experienced a complete abortion.
B. Expectant management is not appropriate.
C. She can be given a prostaglandin to induce uterine evacuation.
D. Rhogam should be administered.
E. She should be evaluated for recurrent pregnancy loss.

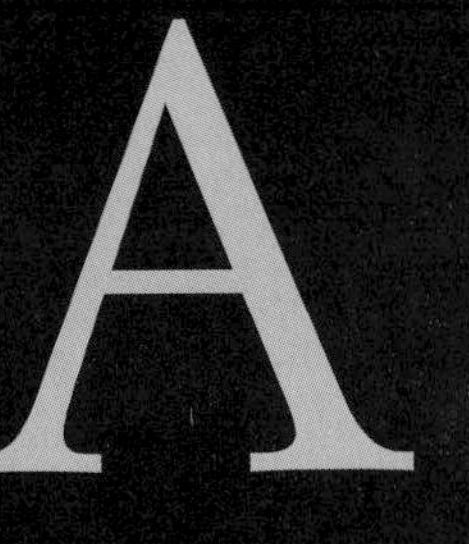

Answers and Explanations

151. E
152. B
153. D
154. E
155. C
156. B
157. B
158. E
159. A
160. B
161. B
162. A
163. E
164. E
165. C
166. C
167. A
168. D
169. B
170. D
171. E
172. A
173. D
174. D
175. C
176. C
177. D
178. C
179. E
180. B
181. D
182. B
183. D
184. B
185. E
186. B
187. E
188. B
189. D
190. E
191. A
192. D
193. B
194. E
195. C
196. C
197. A
198. A
199. B
200. C

151. **E. Appendicitis is the diagnosis most consistent with this patient's clinical history, acute abdomen, fever, and leukocytosis. Of note, the enlarged uterus can displace the appendix, making McBurney's point an unreliable landmark in pregnant women. Exploratory laparotomy is the most appropriate treatment for suspected appendicitis in pregnancy, as laparoscopy would be unsafe and technically difficult with the gravid uterus.**

A. Diverticulosis is generally a condition of older age and occurs uncommonly in women of child-bearing age. Additionally, diverticuli do not cause an acute abdomen and are typically symptomatic only when inflamed (i.e., diverticulitis). Treatment would involve dietary changes and stool softeners.

B. This patient is having focal abdominal pain, which is inconsistent with contractions. While it is important to rule out the diagnosis of preterm labor, this patient has no identifiable contractions on tocometer and a closed cervix that is not effaced. At 33 weeks GA, treatment of preterm labor would involve tocolysis and administration of corticosteroids to promote fetal lung maturity.

C. In general, patients with pain due to nephrolithiasis (i.e., renal colic) are constantly moving, whereas patients with an acute abdomen lie as still as possible. Such patients will often have microscopic or gross hematuria on urinalysis. The more important diagnosis to rule out in this patient with fever, vomiting, abdominal pain, and leukocytosis is pyelonephritis. The lack of bacteria and WBCs on urinalysis and no CVAT make this a less likely diagnosis.

D. Placental abruption, which involves the premature separation of the normally implanted placenta, can result in severe hemorrhage and fetal death. It typically occurs in the third trimester and involves vaginal bleeding associated with severe abdominal pain and/or frequent contractions; bleeding can also be concealed, however. This patient is not having any vaginal bleeding, contractions, or evidence of nonreassuring fetal status. Immediate delivery would be indicated in the event of massive placental abruption.

152. **B. This patient's symptoms are concerning for HELLP syndrome (hemolysis, elevated liver enzymes, low platelets), which is a subcategory of severe preeclampsia. Affected patients can also develop disseminated intravascular coagulation. Unlike in mild and severe preeclampsia, hypertension and proteinuria are not always present in HELLP syndrome. Diagnosis is therefore made via clinical suspicion and a finding of the lab abnormalities that make up the syndrome's name. HELLP syndrome is uncommon, but can involve rapid maternal and fetal deterioration. Treatment involves magnesium sulfate seizure prophylaxis and delivery. In this patient at term and already in early labor, vaginal delivery would be the optimal choice.**

A, D. Epigastric pain, nausea, and vomiting can be suggestive of pancreatitis or some other GI etiology, in which case IV fluids and pain control would likely be appropriate initial therapy. However, this patient's pain is not related to food intake. GI etiology can be considered, but the more important diagnosis of HELLP syndrome must first be ruled out.

C. Tocolysis is not indicated in this patient at term whose signs and symptoms are concerning for severe illness.

E. See the explanation for B. The optimal mode of delivery would be vaginal rather than surgical in a patient with a potential for hemodynamic instability and coagulopathy. In the event of rapid deterioration remote from delivery, however, operative delivery may be necessary.

153. **D. US shows mild to moderate amounts of free fluid in the pelvis, but no evidence of adnexal (not shown) or uterine masses. This patient's sudden pain occurring in the midluteal phase that is now resolving in the setting of essentially normal physical exam and lab studies is most consistent with a ruptured ovarian cyst. Her abdominal discomfort is most likely due to peritoneal irritation by the free fluid. In a hemodynamically stable patient, treatment involves pain relief and outpatient follow-up. It is also reasonable to observe the patient with serial blood counts to confirm that she is not having continued bleeding. Follicular cysts are common functional cysts found in women of reproductive age. They result from the failure of a developing follicle to rupture and generally resolve within 60 days. However, they can grow to a size of 8 cm and are subject to torsion as well as rupture, both of which can cause pain.**

A. Diagnostic laparoscopy is not indicated in a patient without an acute abdomen.
B. This patient does not show evidence of infection or findings consistent with PID or tubo-ovarian abscess. Antibiotics are therefore not indicated.
C. A GI etiology is unlikely in this patient without any GI symptoms and an US exam consistent with a ruptured ovarian cyst.
E. This patient is not experiencing vaginal bleeding or other signs or symptoms that would necessitate a D&C of the uterus.

154. **E. This patient's symptoms are suggestive of a UTI, which is one of the most common infections of the lower GU tract. UTIs occur more commonly in women than in men due to the relatively shorter length of the urethra in women. All of the items listed in this answer choice are possible findings in the setting of UTI. Nitrites are produced by bacteria. The presence of WBCs is suggestive of infection, and leukocyte esterase is suggestive of the presence of WBCs. RBCs can be present in urine due to inflammation and irritation of bladder or urethral mucosa.**

A. While WBCs can be seen in UTIs, lipids are not a typical component of a urinalysis (or UTIs).
B. WBCs and calcium deposits might be seen with nephrolithiasis or renal stones.
C, D. Renal epithelium can be seen in urine specimens in the setting of renal disease, but are generally not present with an uncomplicated lower UTI.

155. **C. This patient appears to have an uncomplicated UTI. She is afebrile and does not have any CVAT, which might be suggestive of pyelonephritis. Treatment for UTIs should include oral antibiotics and increased fluid intake. UTIs are often caused by GI organisms such as *E. coli, S. saprophyticus, and Enterococcus.* Common oral regimens for UTIs include Macrodantin (nitrofurantoin), Bactrim (trimethoprim-sulfamethoxazole), Keflex (cephalexin), and ampicillin. Additionally, urine should be cultured to identify the infectious organism and assess its sensitivity to antibiotics to ensure appropriate treatment.**

A. Fluid intake is an important part of maintaining adequate hydration and ensuring that antibiotics reach the lower urinary tract.
B. There is no indication for a Foley catheter. Occasionally in patients who have primary genital HSV infection, the dysuria is so great that they will need a catheter placed. This patient's symptoms can be treated with phenazopyridine (Pyridium), which acts as a topical analgesic by becoming concentrated in the urine.
D. If a patient has signs and symptoms concerning for pyelonephritis and cannot tolerate oral intake, she should be admitted for IV antibiotics. Otherwise, oral antibiotics will rapidly and adequately treat uncomplicated UTIs.
E. In patients with particular types of renal stones as well as gout, a low-protein diet may be used. It has no role in patients with UTIs.

156. **B. Cyclic OCPs are the best treatment option for this patient with menorrhagia and dysmenorrhea. Over a period of 6 months, her symptoms should diminish. Eventually, women who cycle on OCPs will have minimal bleeding because of the endometrial atrophy that develops with OCP administration.**

A. In the absence of ongoing vaginal bleeding (soaking more than 1 pad per hour), D&C is not indicated.
C, E. Neither GnRH nor progestin therapy is an appropriate treatment option for this patient.
D. Although endometrial ablation would likely stop the patient's bleeding, it would also compromise her future fertility and, therefore, is not the best treatment option.

157. **B. The etiology of this woman's hemorrhage is most likely her submucosal fibroid, shown beginning to prolapse into the vagina. She has already lost enough blood to cause significant symptoms of anemia. While she will likely need definitive treatment in the form of a hysterectomy, she is currently hemodynamically unstable and should first be stabilized with a blood transfusion. Emergent hysterectomy or uterine artery embolization could be performed if bleeding was refractory to hormonal treatment. Once the patient is stable, the fibroid can likely be removed vaginally by grasping it with a toothed tenaculum and twisting. If it is not prolapsed through the cervix, then it can be removed with hysteroscopic resection.**

A. Depot Lupron (leuprolide) is a GnRH analog that inhibits gonadotropin release and essentially creates a chemical menopause, causing fibroids to stop growing and possibly shrink in size. At this time, it is not employed as a long-term treatment for fibroids because its prolonged use can lead to bone density loss. Lupron is administered in some women in anticipation of surgery (i.e., hysterectomy) to make surgery safer by decreasing the fibroid bulk and diminishing the potential for blood loss. Patients will often be placed on concurrent iron replacement to increase the hematocrit prior to surgery. While certainly an option for this patient, administration of Lupron is not the most appropriate next step in her treatment.

C. This woman is experiencing symptomatic anemia, making observation an inappropriate option. If she refused blood transfusion, she should be intravenously hydrated at minimum.

D. Hysterectomy would be definitive treatment in this patient. Before this procedure is performed, however, other causes of bleeding (e.g., endometrial cancer) as well as ovarian and cervical abnormalities (e.g., malignancy) should be evaluated, because such findings could alter the nature of the hysterectomy (e.g., radical hysterectomy versus simple hysterectomy, preservation of ovaries versus bilateral salpingo-oophorectomy).

E. Endometrial ablation is a process in which the endometrial lining is destroyed, usually via thermal means, to stop dysfunctional uterine bleeding. While this method might reduce the patient's bleeding, it would not address the most likely cause of her bleeding (i.e., fibroids).

158. **E. Placenta previa is the abnormal implantation of the placenta over the cervical os. Depending on how much of the cervix is covered by the placenta, placenta previa is further classified as complete, partial, or marginal. As the lower uterine segment grows, placental attachments can be disrupted, leading to bleeding that ranges from spotting to profuse hemorrhage. One in 200 births is affected by placenta previa, which accounts for 20% of antepartum hemorrhage. Management of placenta previa varies, but most providers will agree that the patient should be placed on pelvic rest (i.e., no intercourse). Bleeding episodes warrant admission for observation to monitor fetal and maternal well-being, and administration of corticosteroids for fetal lung maturity if appropriate (24 to 34 weeks GA).**

A. Immediate delivery is warranted only in the event of nonreassuring fetal status, life-threatening hemorrhage, or unstoppable labor. Otherwise, patients are delivered at 36 weeks via cesarean section, usually after confirmation of fetal lung maturity via amniocentesis.

B. Blood transfusion is warranted in situations involving severe blood loss and anemia. Such is not the case in this hemodynamically stable patient.

C. At 33 5/7 weeks GA, fetal lung maturity is unlikely. Thus, if delivery were warranted at this GA, amniocentesis would not be useful.

D. Hormonal management has no role in bleeding in placenta previa, as this kind of bleeding is related to placental detachment rather than endometrial abnormalities.

159. **A. LGV is caused by the L serotypes of *Chlamydia trachomatis.***

B. The classic LGV lesion is a painless—not painful—papule or shallow ulcer in the genital region that can be transient. This patient has advanced to the inguinal stage.

C. LGV is treated with a 3-week course of doxycycline, which may be repeated if the disease is persistent. Surgical exploration of lymph nodes is not part of therapy.

D. The third stage of LGV, known as anogenital syndrome, involves proctocolitis, rectal stricture, or rectovaginal fistula.

E. LGV is a sexually transmitted infection.

160. **B. Vaginal wall hematomas can result from injury to a blood vessel in the vaginal wall that does not disrupt the overlying epithelium. They are usually diagnosed while the patient is still hospitalized, as affected patients often experience severe vaginal pain, difficulty walking, or larger than expected drops in hematocrit. However, hematomas that develop slowly can be missed until after discharge, when the patient eventually becomes symptomatic. Management can be expectant unless the hematoma is expanding or tense, in which case it should be evacuated. The**

wound frequently has to be packed, because bleeding vessels cannot always be identified for ligation.

A. While this is a large drop in hematocrit for a vaginal delivery, the patient is asymptomatic. In the absence of cardiac risk factors, most young, healthy patients can withstand a hematocrit of 22, making the risks of transfusion greater than the benefits in this situation.

C. While iron replacement is warranted, the patient should not be discharged home without evacuation of the hematoma because the hematoma is symptomatic, tense, and possibly expanding. On rare occasions, concealed hemorrhage can be life-threatening if severe. Sitz baths are not appropriate therapy for vaginal/vulvar hematomas.

D. Pitocin has no role in the case of vaginal wall hematoma. It is helpful only in cases involving bleeding due to decreased uterine tone.

E. Uterine artery embolization is not appropriate treatment for a vaginal wall hematoma, because the bleeding is not uterine in origin and such treatment could potentially lead to decreased fertility. The injured vessel and its surrounding vaginal tissue must be addressed.

161. **B. Condyloma acuminata, or genital warts, are caused by HPV. (Different serotypes of HPV are responsible for cervical cancer.) Genital warts can occur throughout the anogenital region. Treatment regimens vary and include topical medicines, cryotherapy, laser vaporization, and local excision.**

A. This patient has pubic lice, or crabs, which is caused by infection with *Phthirus pubis*. Treatment involves application of lindane to affected areas.

C. Chancroid is caused by infection with *Haemophilus ducreyi* and is characterized by a painful ulcer with possible inguinal lymphadenopathy. Diagnosis is made clinically, because *Haemophilus ducreyi* is difficult to culture. Multiple treatment regimens exist, including ceftriaxone 250 mg intramuscularly once; single dose of azithromycin 1 g; or erythromycin 500 mg QID for 7 days.

D. Scabies is caused by infection with the itch mite *Sarcoptes scabiei*. It is similar to infection with pubic lice, but the distribution occurs throughout the body and characteristic burrows can often be identified. Treatment also involves lindane application to affected areas.

E. Syphilis is caused by infection with *Treponema pallidum*. This systemic disease progresses through three stages if left untreated. Primary syphilis is characterized by a painless chancre. Secondary syphilis involves a maculopapular rash, appearing characteristically on the palms and the soles of the feet. Tertiary syphilis is characterized by neurologic manifestations (e.g., tabes dorsalis), aortitis, and gummas (granulomas) of skin and bones. Diagnosis of syphilis is made via nonspecific antibody tests: rapid plasma reagin (RPR) or Venereal Disease Research Laboratory (VDRL). Positive results are confirmed with either the microhemagglutination assay for antibodies to *T. pallidum* (MHATP) or the fluorescent treponemal antibody absorption (FTA-ABS) test. Treatment of early syphilis consists of a one-time dose of 2.4 million units of penicillin G given intramuscularly. This therapy is repeated weekly for 3 weeks in cases of syphilis persisting for longer than 1 year. Because neurosyphilis is more severe, treatment involves 2 to 4 million units of penicillin G every 4 hours for 10 to 14 days.

162. **A. Wound seromas can result in wound separation when pockets of serosanguinous fluid become trapped beneath the surface of the skin and lead to poor wound healing. Obesity is a risk factor for the development of seromas. Treatment involves exploration of the wound to disrupt any subcutaneous loculations, followed by irrigation and debridement. Finally, the wound should be packed with moist dressings and allowed to close via secondary intention. Dressing changes should be performed twice a day during the healing period, and the patient should be instructed regarding daily wound care.**

B. If evidence of a cellulitis (e.g., erythema) was found, oral antibiotics to cover skin flora could be prescribed. Otherwise, the wound needs to heal by secondary intention.

C. While irrigation and debridement are part of care, a wound that has a 3 cm track and is 4 cm deep is unlikely to heal if the overlying skin is merely reapproximated with steristrips. Once the wound has sufficiently healed by secondary intention and is shallow, consideration can be given to steristrip closure.

D. One study of surgical reclosure of disrupted cesarean section wounds as compared to healing by secondary intention showed that wound healing time could be significantly shortened by performing such reclosure. However, all wounds were first managed via irrigation and debridement for a minimum of 4 days before closure was considered. While this is an option for this patient, current practice supports healing by secondary intention.

E. Expectant management is not appropriate in the setting of wound seromas.

163. **E. A patient who arrives to the hospital with painful contractions and 8 cm dilated is in the active phase of labor, and delivery should be considered imminent. In the absence of prenatal care and with a poor history, it is difficult to assess GA, which is important in terms of preparing and caring for the newborn. Tocolysis at 8 cm dilation is unlikely to be successful, as well as being unnecessary in this patient, who is probably at term or near to it based on bedside US measurements consistent with a term fetus. Routine prenatal labs as well as a urine toxicology screen should be obtained because the patient did not have prenatal care and to assess for possible substance-induced preterm labor. Otherwise, the patient should be managed like all other laboring patients.**

A. Antenatal corticosteroids have been shown to improve fetal outcomes by promoting fetal lung maturity and decreasing the incidence of intraventricular hemorrhages. However, their benefits have been proven only in fetuses who have achieved viability (greater than 24 weeks GA) and in those less than 34 weeks GA, beyond which the incidence of respiratory distress syndrome (RDS) is low (but not insignificant). Additionally, benefit is generally seen only if the fetus is exposed for at least 24 to 48 hours.

B. See the explanation for E.

C. Amniocentesis to assess fetal lung maturity is not appropriate because delivery is imminent.

D. While formal US can estimate fetal age, this patient will likely deliver before she goes for the study. A bedside US for estimated fetal weight and GA can be performed quickly to advise the nursery. Of note, the margin of error in US varies with GA: It can be off by 1 week in the first trimester, 2 weeks in the second trimester, and 3 weeks in the third trimester. Thus this patient could be anywhere between 35 and 41 weeks GA.

164. **E. The diagnosis of preeclampsia is made with three findings: (1) elevation of the BP above 140/90 at least two times, 4 to 6 hours apart; (2) significant proteinuria, exceeding 300 mg in a 24-hour urine collection; and (3) nondependent edema of the face and hands.**

A. The CBC helps rule out the diagnosis of severe preeclampsia. A low platelet count can be seen in the setting of HELLP syndrome. Elevation of the hematocrit secondary to hemoconcentration can be seen in preeclampsia, but is not part of the diagnostic criteria.

B, D. Glomerular filtration rate (GFR) and creatinine clearance can be decreased in preeclampsia, resulting in decreased uric acid excretion and elevated serum levels. However, these findings are not part of the diagnostic criteria for preeclampsia. The GFR's only diagnostic use is in patients with baseline proteinuria and hypertension in whom the diagnosis is difficult to make.

C. Severe preeclampsia can lead to RBC hemolysis, which would elevate lactate dehydrogenase (LDH) levels.

165. **C. This patient has the classic findings of trichomonas, which is caused by infection with *Trichomonas vaginalis,* a unicellular protozoan that is sexually transmitted. Signs and symptoms include profuse, frothy, foul-smelling discharge and a "strawberry" cervix (i.e., erythematous, punctate cervical epithelium). Diagnosis is made by visualization of the motile organisms on wet mount. Treatment consists of a single 2g dose of metronidazole. Clotrimazole cream for 7 days is another treatment alternative.**

A, B. The wet mount does not show the classic clue cells of bacterial vaginosis (BV)—namely, vaginal epithelial cells that are covered with bacteria, thus making the cell's borders appear indistinct. BV is often associated with a fishy-smelling discharge. Treatment for BV includes oral metronidazole 500 mg BID for 7 days or clindamycin 300 mg TID for 7 days. These antibiotics can also be used in gel or cream form intravaginally. Miconazole cream is not an appropriate therapy for bacterial vaginosis.

D. See the explanation for C. Miconazole cream is not an appropriate therapy for trichomonas.
E. Wet mounts for suspected yeast infections should be prepared with potassium hydroxide (KOH) rather than saline to evaluate for the characteristic branching pseudohyphae of *Candida albicans.* Yeast vaginitis typically produces a thick, white, pruritic discharge. Treatment relies on any of the azole creams (e.g., miconazole, terazole) or a single 150 mg dose of oral fluconazole (Diflucan).

166. **C. The adnexal mass identified on the physical and US exams is most likely a TOA, also referred to as a TOC when it is not walled off as in the case of abscesses. TOAs/TOCs typically result from persistent PID and involve the fallopian tube and adjacent ovary. This patient exhibits classic signs and symptoms of pelvic infection (e.g., fever, leukocytosis with left shift, cervical motion tenderness), and the diagnosis is confirmed with US. Blood cultures should be obtained to rule out sepsis. Treatment involves inpatient IV broad-spectrum antibiotics such as cefoxitin and doxycycline or triple antibiotics until 48 hours afebrile, followed by a 10- to 14-day course of oral antibiotics upon her discharge home. If clinical improvement is not achieved with antibiotics, surgical removal (usually via unilateral salpingo-oophorectomy) may be necessary.**

A. This patient does not have TSS, which is caused by the toxic shock syndrome toxin-1 (TSST-1) produced by *Staphylococcus aureus.* Historically, TSS has been associated with vaginal infections caused by tampon usage. Signs and symptoms include high fever, hypotension, late-onset desquamation of palms and soles, erythematous rash, and thrombocytopenia. Patients can become very ill, necessitating inpatient management, which consists mostly of supportive care and use of pressors as needed to maintain BP. IV antibiotics have not been shown to decrease the length of acute illness because symptoms are caused by the exotoxin.
B. The adnexal mass in this young patient with symptoms of infection is unlikely to be an ovarian malignancy. She is not having any symptoms of cancer, nor do imaging studies support such a diagnosis (e.g., no omental cake, solid and cystic mass).
D. See the explanation for C. Outpatient management is not appropriate in the acute setting.
E. Endometritis is an intrauterine infection seen most commonly after cesarean section, vaginal delivery, dilation and curettage, and IUD placement. When it involves the myometrium, it is called endomyometritis. While endometritis can present with symptoms similar to those seen with TOAs/TOCs, it is not associated with an adnexal mass. Treatment consists of inpatient IV antibiotics until the patient has been afebrile for 48 hours.

167. **A. This patient has some of the classic signs and symptoms of endometriosis: dysmenorrhea, dyspareunia, uterosacral nodularity, likely endometrioma, and infertility. Endometriosis is a chronic condition in which endometrial tissue occurs outside of the uterus (typically on pelvic organs such as the ovary, cul-de-sac, or uterus). Endometriosis implants can become cyclically painful. They can also take the form of endometriomas, known as "chocolate cysts," which are ovarian endometriosis cysts filled with dark, old blood. They are not malignant, but can be painful and are at risk for torsion if large. Endometriosis is associated with infertility, possibly resulting from adhesions, scarring, and alteration of normal pelvic anatomy. Endometriosis can only be truly diagnosed by visualizing endometriosis implants within the pelvis, which is usually achieved via laparoscopy. Implants can be excised or ablated during surgery. OCPs and NSAIDs are appropriate medical treatment for endometriosis. Because this patient is trying to conceive, however, OCPs are not the optimal choice. Of note, because the patient has been trying to conceive for 1 year, an infertility evaluation should be initiated. If this evaluation returns negative, consideration should be given to diagnostic laparoscopy, whereby a diagnosis of endometriosis can be formally made and, if present, implants can be excised or ablated in an attempt to improve fertility.**

B. See the explanation for A.
C. Ovarian cancer is rare in a 32-year-old patient. She is not experiencing any concerning symptoms (e.g., early satiety, bloating, weight changes, fatigue). Additionally, the US findings do not support an ovarian malignancy.

D. Mittelschmerz is midcycle pain thought to be due to ovulation. This patient's pain occurs at the start of her cycle.

E. No fibroids are identified on this patient's physical or US exams. Additionally, fibroids do not typically cause pain unless they are degenerating. Note that not all fibroids are managed via hysterectomy, especially in women desiring preservation of fertility.

168. **D. The fetus is considered previable until 24 weeks GA. Unfortunately, rupture of membranes before viability means the end of the pregnancy. If rupture of membranes occurs before the onset of labor, it is called premature rupture of membranes. This case is an example of PPROM (less than 37 weeks GA). At 19 weeks GA, the chance of the pregnancy lasting until viability is slim to none. Once rupture of membranes occurs, the potential for labor and/or infection increases. In fact, it is thought that PPROM occurs as a result of subclinical infection. As such, tocolysis has no role here, as maintenance of an infected pregnancy increases the risk of maternal infection and sepsis. After appropriate counseling and discussion, management of PPROM typically involves termination of the nonviable pregnancy via labor induction. Although expectant management is an option while awaiting onset of spontaneous labor, the risk of infection increases with time so most providers will advocate a more active approach (e.g., labor induction).**

A. Corticosteroids are not administered to promote fetal lung maturity unless a fetus is viable.

B. See the explanation for D. Some institutions will administer tocolysis for 48 hours in the absence of signs or symptoms of infection in an effort to administer antenatal corticosteroids to promote fetal lung maturity.

C. While PPROM may result from infection and may subsequently lead to worsening infection, administration of antibiotics is not appropriate in an effort to prolong the pregnancy in the setting of a previable fetus. In the setting of overt infection, administration of antibiotics and labor induction should be initiated as soon as possible.

E. Fetal monitoring is not done on a continuous basis on previable fetuses. Certainly in the case of pregnancy termination, it is not necessary and even cruel to monitor the fetus during labor induction.

169. **B. Colicky back/abdominal pain with CVAT and hematuria are highly suspicious for nephrolithiasis. It is not unusual for patients with nephrolithiasis or other abdominal pain to experience contractions, but these contractions are more consistent with uterine irritability than with labor. Treatment of nephrolithiasis in pregnancy is expectant with IV fluids and pain control. If imaging studies reveal large calculi resulting in significant hydronephrosis or hydroureter, or persistent infection/pyelonephritis, consideration should be given to placement of a nephrostomy tube to drain the kidney.**

A. Pregnancy is a contraindication to extracorporeal shock wave lithotripsy (ESWL).

C, D. In the absence of fever, urinalysis consistent with infection, and leukocytosis with left shift, this is unlikely to be a pyelonephritis. Nevertheless, this diagnosis is important to consider because pregnancy does increase urinary stasis both by relaxation of smooth muscle and through compression of ureters by the enlarging uterus. In the event of pyelonephritis, initial treatment of pregnant patients should always be as inpatients with IV antibiotics so that maternal and fetal well-being can be monitored in the early stages.

E. Despite regular contractions, this patient is not dilating her cervix and is therefore not in preterm labor. However, serial cervical exams should be performed at least initially to rule out labor.

170. **D. Magnesium sulfate has been shown to be the most effective agent in preventing recurrent seizures in eclamptic patients. It can also be effective in interrupting the event, and can usually be given as a 10g IM load to patients without an IV placed.**

A, C. Until recently, phenytoin represented the drug of choice to prevent recurrent seizures in eclampsia in much of the world. Several studies have since demonstrated magnesium sulfate's efficacy. Like phenytoin, phenobarbital may help to prevent recurrent seizures, but does not seem to be as effective in randomized trials.

B. If the patient is actively seizing, diazepam or another short-acting benzodiazepine is commonly used to break the ongoing seizure activity.

E. The fetal heart rate tracing is currently reassuring. While the patient should be transferred to labor and delivery for labor induction, emergent delivery is unnecessary.

171. **E. This patient has the classic signs and symptoms of genital herpes and is likely suffering from a primary outbreak, which can often be preceded by a flu-like illness. Herpes is caused by infection with herpes simplex virus (HSV). There are two strains of this virus: HSV-1, which tends to cause oral herpes, and HSV-2, which tends to cause genital outbreaks. However, both types can be found in either region. Because it is a viral infection, herpes can recur after the initial outbreak, with the frequency of recurrences varying between individuals. Diagnosis is usually via visualization of the characteristic cropped vesicles and ulcers, but confirmation can be achieved with viral culture or Tzanck smear to evaluate for multinucleated giant cells. Treatment for herpes relies on acyclovir to shorten the course of the outbreak. People who suffer from frequent recurrences can also take daily acyclovir for suppression therapy. Of note, because lesions can occur throughout the genital area and are transmitted by direct contact, condom usage cannot prevent transmission of herpes.**

A. Genital warts are caused by infection with certain serotypes of human papillomavirus (HPV), a sexually transmitted pathogen. Warts, also known as *condyloma acuminata*, are typically painless, raised, and papillomatous or spiky in appearance. Treatment involves excision, cryotherapy, laser ablation, and a variety of topical medications (e.g., trichloroacetic acid, podophyllin, 5-fluorouracil, imiquimod, and podofilox). This patient's lesions are not characteristic of genital warts.

B. Metronidazole is not appropriate therapy for genital warts.

C. *Molluscum contagiosum* is spread via direct contact with an affected area. The infectious organism is a pox virus, which results in the characteristic lesion, a 1 mm to 5 mm domed papule with an umbilicated center. Lesions are typically painless. Treatment involves expectant management, as lesions generally resolve on their own. Lesions can also be treated with excision, cryotherapy, or application of trichloroacetic acid.

D. This patient does have genital herpes, but hydrocortisone cream is not an appropriate therapy for this STD.

172. **A. Persistent vaginal bleeding after pregnancy termination is concerning for a complication such as retained POCs, uterine perforation, or cervical laceration. After complete uterine evacuation, the endometrium should appear thin on US. The fact that this patient's endometrial cavity is thick and heterogeneous is suspicious for incomplete uterine evacuation. The most efficient way to stop her bleeding is suction curettage. This procedure can be performed under US guidance to ensure complete uterine evacuation. While the same effect might be achieved with administration of agents that promote uterine tone and contractions (e.g., methergine, misoprostol), incomplete evacuation would necessitate further suction curettage.**

B. Expectant management is not appropriate in this patient, who has symptoms consistent with anemia. The uterus will continue to bleed until it is completely evacuated.

C. A thick endometrial complex on US is not normal after D&E.

D. Cervical laceration is not relevant here, as the cervix appears intact on exam. However, because cervical trauma can occur during D&E, it should be considered in the differential diagnosis for persistent vaginal bleeding. Careful exam at the end of the procedure is important.

E. Uterine perforation is a rare but serious complication of D&E. Fortunately, it is unlikely in this patient, who has no GI symptoms, a benign abdomen, and no free fluid on US. Moreover, the patient has an obvious and more common explanation for her persistent bleeding (i.e., retained POCs). If bleeding persists after the uterus is completely evacuated or the patient develops an acute abdomen, consideration should be given to diagnostic laparoscopy to visualize the uterus and possibly repair any damage.

173. **D. Incompetent cervix entails painless dilation of the cervix occurring in the second trimester. While it should be differentiated from preterm labor, which consists of cervical dilation in response to uterine contractions, this distinction**

can be difficult to make at times because advanced cervical dilation can lead to contractions, in addition to infection or premature rupture of membranes that can also lead to contractions. Incompetent cervix tends to occur in the second trimester before fetuses reach viability, so it often leads to pregnancy loss. Treatment for pregnancies beyond 24 weeks is similar to treatment for preterm labor: magnesium sulfate tocolysis and administration of corticosteroids for fetal lung maturity. Treatment options vary in previable fetuses depending on the degree of dilation. Most patients with advanced dilation are managed expectantly to see whether labor will ensue. Because of the possibility of delivering a previable neonate at 23 to 25 weeks, termination of pregnancy is offered. An attempt can be made to place an emergent cerclage, which is a permanent suture placed around the cervix at the level of the cervical–vaginal junction (McDonald cerclage) or the internal cervical os (Shirodkar cerclage) in an effort to prevent further dilation. If successful, the cerclage is removed at approximately 36 to 38 weeks in anticipation of spontaneous labor. However, the cerclage should be removed at any time that unstoppable labor occurs (even if it is preterm), as cervical trauma can be sustained if a woman is allowed to labor with a cerclage in place. In this patient who has rupture of membranes in addition to an incompetent cervix remote from viability (i.e., 24 weeks GA), the prognosis is grim. Cerclage should not be offered, and termination via either D&E or induction of labor should be strongly encouraged. If the patient wishes expectant management, it should be done only with the understanding that if she develops any signs of infection, termination of pregnancy should proceed at that time.

A. Risk factors for cervical incompetence include uterine anomalies, multiple prior D&E procedures, cervical surgery, and maternal diethylstilbestrol (DES) exposure. Most cases of cervical incompetence happen to women with no identifiable risk factors. Pap smear screening has not been associated with any complications of pregnancy.
B. See the explanation for D.
C. If a patient has experienced a prior delivery/fetal loss due to incompetent cervix, a prophylactic cerclage should be offered in subsequent pregnancies and placed between 12 and 14 weeks GA.
E. Incompetent cervix commonly occurs beyond 17 to 18 weeks of gestation, so a 14-week US would not be a good diagnostic tool for cervical incompetence.

174. **D. Vulvar cancer is primarily treated with surgical excision with wide margins. Additionally, exploration of lymph nodes is critical. For disease beyond stage I, the contralateral groin lymph nodes should also be evaluated. In poor surgical candidates, such as this patient, as well as in patients with disease recurrences, pelvic radiation can be used to decrease tumor bulk. Prognosis is directly related to the number of lymph nodes involved, with 5-year survival rates as follows: more than 90% with one positive lymph node, 75% to 80% with two positive lymph nodes, and less than 15% with three or more positive lymph nodes.**

A. Vulvar cancer is actually quite uncommon, accounting for only 5% of the various gynecologic malignancies. Risk factors include advanced age (average age of diagnosis is 60), diabetes, hypertension, obesity, low socioeconomic status, and prior vulvar disorders.
B. Symptoms of vulvar cancer tend to be local at the site of the mass. Bleeding, pain, and pruritis are common, but ascites and bloating are not characteristic of vulvar cancer.
C. Some 85% to 90% of vulvar cancer entails squamous cell carcinoma (SCC), which can appear as a fungating mass or an indurated ulcer. It spreads primarily via lymphatics but can also spread via direct extension. Malignant melanoma accounts for 5% to 10% of vulvar cancers. Unlike in SCC, the depth of invasion determines prognosis in melanoma. Basal cell carcinoma accounts for 2% to 3% of vulvar cancers. The remaining 1% comprises very rare types of vulvar cancers (e.g., leiomyosarcomas, fibrous histiocytomas).
E. Vulvar cancer is surgically staged and mere palpation of the lymph nodes is insufficient. In fact, 27% of patients with positive lymph nodes do not have palpable nodes on physical exam. Staging is based on size, extent of spread, and nodal involvement.

175. **C. Mastitis can be treated by oral antibiotics that will cover maternal skin flora or the infant's oral flora. First-generation cephalosporins or dicloxacillin are commonly used. Admission for IV antibiotics is rarely necessary, and only in cases where oral antibiotics have failed to resolve symptoms or the patient cannot tolerate oral medications.**

A. Breast pain due to mastitis can be treated symptomatically with NSAIDs or occasionally with acetaminophen and codeine. There is no reason that acetaminophen needs to be used alone, although in very mild cases it may afford some pain relief.

B. It is important to continue breastfeeding or pumping breast milk during the acute phase of the infection to prevent the intraductal accumulation of infected material. Patients should be reassured that because most cases of mastitis are caused by the patient's skin flora or the infant's oral flora, it is not harmful to continue breastfeeding.

D, E. See the explanation for C.

176. **C. Adnexal torsion is the twisting of the ovary or adnexa around the ovarian pedicle, resulting in vascular obstruction. Although uncommon, it is an emergency and requires operative intervention. Patients occasionally report prior occurrences of similar pain as the offending cyst or neoplasm enlarges and intermittently undergoes torsion. It can be associated with a mild fever, normal WBC count, nausea, and vomiting. Diagnosis can be confirmed by US, which typically shows an enlarged ovary that is uniformly echogenic with decreased Doppler flow.**

A. Although this patient has pain localizing to the RLQ, acute appendicitis generally presents with anorexia, fever, leukocytosis, and, not uncommonly, an acute abdomen. With an identifiable adnexal mass, the etiology of the pain is unlikely to be due to other causes.

B. The patient has a negative pregnancy test.

D. Salpingitis typically presents with fever, elevated WBC count, vaginal discharge, and cervical motion tenderness.

E. Although certainly more common than adnexal torsion, ruptured ovarian cysts typically produce pain that is bilateral and begins at or after ovulation. If this case truly involved rupture of an ovarian cyst, the patient would usually experience more diffuse pelvic pain. Also, the patient might have presented with a decreased hematocrit if bleeding were severe. US would show free fluid in the cul-de-sac and is less likely than torsion to reveal the presence of an enlarged adnexal mass.

177. **D. In an inevitable abortion, the patient will experience vaginal bleeding and a dilated cervix in a pregnancy less than 20 weeks GA but no expulsion of POCs. Although the use of prostaglandins to promote the expulsion of the POCs is an option, D&C is preferential in the setting of heavy bleeding. Expectant management is also an option for patients not anxious about bleeding and cramping at home. Of note, if this patient were Rh D (–), Rhogam administration would be necessary to prevent alloimmunization in subsequent pregnancies.**

A. In any pregnant woman presenting with vaginal bleeding and abdominal pain, ectopic pregnancy must be ruled out. The presence of an intrauterine gestational sac makes the likelihood of a concurrent extrauterine pregnancy highly unlikely, but ectopic pregnancy must still be excluded by history, physical exam, labs, and a careful survey of the lower pelvis by US.

B. A threatened abortion is defined by vaginal bleeding in a pregnancy less than 20 weeks GA in the presence of a closed cervical os and no expulsion of POCs. In the setting of a desired pregnancy, the patient should be given instructions for pelvic rest and followed for continued bleeding rather than proceed prematurely to definitive procedures such as D&C.

C. An incomplete abortion involves the partial expulsion of POCs prior to 20 weeks gestation. It can be allowed to complete on its own, or the patient can be offered D&C or D&E.

E. A complete abortion involves the complete expulsion of all POCs prior to 20 weeks gestation. Patients should be followed for signs of infection and recurrent bleeding.

178. **C. Outpatient treatment of uncomplicated PID has been promoted over the past decade. To qualify for this treatment, the patient must have no signs of pelvic abscess (adnexal masses or abscesses seen on US) or perihepatitis (liver**

transaminase elevations or RUQ tenderness). Furthermore, patients must be nonpregnant and reliable. Severely ill patients not tolerating oral intake are unlikely to comply with medication regimens and will need hospitalization for parenteral therapy.

A, B. Because untreated PID can lead to infertility, hospitalization is generally recommended but not required for reproductive-age patients. Conversely, it is highly recommended that adolescents or any patients in whom compliance may be an issue be hospitalized for treatment.

D. Adnexal tenderness is part of the diagnostic criteria of PID, and is not particularly an indication for hospitalization.

E. Patients with a penicillin allergy can either be treated without penicillins and cephalosporins, or be treated with a cephalosporin in the ED with the knowledge that there is only a 10% to 15% cross-allergic response. In patients with a history of anaphylaxis to penicillin, adequate coverage can be obtained with oral levofloxacin and clindamycin.

179. **E. This patient is diagnosed with a ruptured ectopic pregnancy based on the fact that she has no identifiable intrauterine pregnancy at a GA where one should easily be found by US. Additionally, she has free fluid in the cul-de-sac suggestive of rupture and a history of PID, which is a known risk factor for ectopic pregnancy. The decision to take the patient emergently to the operating room is based on the high probability for a ruptured ectopic pregnancy and the fact that the patient has an acute abdomen and appears hemodynamically unstable.**

A, B. Uterine curettage or culdocentesis is unnecessary as the diagnosis is highly likely given the US findings.

C, D. Although serial quantitative β-hCG levels would have been helpful in diagnosis prior to rupture, obtaining a value now does not affect the patient's management. Medical management is not appropriate once the ectopic pregnancy has ruptured.

180. **B. The patient should be treated empirically for chlamydia and gonorrhea. Azithromycin 1 g PO covers *Chlamydia trachomatis,* and ceftriaxone 250 mg IM covers *Neisseria gonorrhoea.***

A. Simple initiation of OCPs at this time will not ensure pregnancy prevention. Instead, the patient should be tested for preexisting pregnancy and offered emergency contraception. If she does not have menses within 21 days, she should be advised to see her gynecologist for follow-up.

C. Even if the patient objects to having this crime reported, it is nevertheless a reportable crime. Often, the nursing staff in the ED will already have done so, but it is important that the physician seeing the patient follows up and makes sure that the crime has been reported. Along these lines, evidence of the crime needs to be collected as well. The patient can then decide whether to give a report to the police once they become involved.

D, E. Despite no initial visual evidence of sperm on a wet prep slide, it is still possible that intravaginal ejaculation did occur. As a consequence, the patient should be offered emergency contraception, baseline HIV testing, and AZT prophylaxis.

181. **D. This patient has a presentation that is worrisome for TSS, which carries a high mortality rate; all patients with this condition should be hospitalized. In severe cases, pressors may be required to stabilize BPs. With aggressive supportive management, it is likely that mortality can be reduced.**

A. TSS is caused by *Staphylococcus aureus* exotoxin. Its systemic absorption leads to fever, rash, and desquamation of palms and soles.

B. No data exist that support an association between PCOS and TSS. The other potential causes provide portals of entry for infection. One of the most commonly associated findings with TSS was a highly absorbent tampon.

C. Because the exotoxin is absorbed through the vaginal wall, blood cultures are usually negative.

E. Fewer than 300 cases of TSS have been reported annually since 1984.

182. **B. Although the fetal heart tracing (FHT) is not reassuring because it is nonreactive, there is no evidence of acute fetal insult (FHT decelerations or absent variability) that would necessitate emergent delivery at this time. Attempts should be made to achieve reassuring fetal testing by alternative means—for example, by using vibroacoustic**

stimulation (VAS) to achieve a reactive tracing or by using US to obtain a biophysical profile (BPP). Another method that is used in labor to obtain fetal response as measured by fetal heart rate acceleration is the fetal scalp stimulation.

A. Although elevated, the patient's glucose level does not warrant administration of additional insulin at this time. There is no reason to react to a blood sugar less than 200 in this setting.

C. Assuming the GA is accurate, there is no evidence of fetal benefit from administration of betamethasone beyond 34 weeks of gestation.

D, E. Delivery is not indicated in this patient unless the FHT becomes nonreassuring. If that were the case, the decision regarding route of delivery would depend on the severity of the nonreassuring FHT as well as fetal presentation. If induction of labor were indicated rather than emergent cesarean section, a prostaglandin agent would be appropriate in this patient with an unfavorable cervix.

183. **D. Because of her history of manual placenta extraction, this patient is at increased risk for development of endomyometritis, which is a polymicrobial infection of the uterine lining and wall. Diagnosis is made by the presence of fever, uterine tenderness, and elevated WBC count. Treatment consists of broad-spectrum antibiotics. D&C is indicated only if retained POCs are suspected, which is not the case in this patient whose lochia has decreased appropriately.**

A. Given her history of decreased vaginal bleeding, stable vital signs, and hematocrit, this patient does not have a delayed postpartum hemorrhage.

B. Placenta accreta (abnormal adherence of the placenta to the uterine wall) would be manifested as continued vaginal bleeding unresponsive to contractile agents and is more likely to be diagnosed immediately postpartum rather than 1 week later.

C. The patient shows no evidence of a vaginal hematoma, which occurs when the trauma of delivery injures a blood vessel without disrupting the overlying epithelium. Such hematomas can be managed expectantly, unless the patient is hemodynamically unstable, in which case surgical exploration and ligation of the disrupted vessel(s) may be required.

E. See the explanation for D.

184. **B. A lesion that is confined to the cervix, more than 5 mm invasive, and less than 4 cm wide is a stage Ib1 lesion. Approximately 40% of cervical cancer is stage Ib at diagnosis; cancer at this stage has an 85% cure rate regardless of whether radical hysterectomy or radiation therapy is used. For bulky stage Ib to IVa disease, primary treatment with cisplatin-based chemotherapy in conjunction with radiation therapy can prolong disease-free survival when compared to radiation therapy alone.**

A. This is stage Ib1 disease; cone biopsy is appropriate only in microinvasive disease (stages Ia1 and Ia2).

C. Stage Ib2 lesions are more than 4 cm wide.

D, E. Stage II lesions extend beyond the cervix but not to the sidewall, with vaginal involvement in the upper two-thirds only. Stage IIa lesions do not involve the parametria, whereas stage IIb lesions have obvious parametrial involvement. Radical hysterectomy is beneficial treatment only for stage IIa or earlier disease. Radiation therapy is indicated once the cancer has spread to the parametria or beyond (stage IIb or later). Primary chemotherapy can be beneficial for both stage IIa and IIb disease.

185. **E. This patient is most likely having a placental abruption secondary to her elevated BPs and possible preeclampsia. Although the patient is hemodynamically stable and the fetus is premature, emergent delivery by cesarean section is indicated because of nonreassuring fetal status. It is reasonable to check the fetal heart rate in the OR to verify that it is still decreased; such a finding will help determine the rapidity with which the delivery needs to occur.**

A. This patient may require blood transfusion because the volume of blood loss in a placental abruption is often underestimated due to concealed bleeding. However, this is not the most appropriate next step given the nonreassuring FHT.

B. Although the fetus is premature and would likely benefit from the administration of betamethasone, immediate delivery is indicated. Thus there would not be sufficient time to benefit from corticosteroids.

C. The use of tocolytics to prolong the pregnancy until fetal lung maturity can be achieved might be indicated in a stable abruption, which is not the case here. If the patient is having a tetanic contraction, it is reasonable to give terbutaline 0.25 mg SQ to promote uterine relaxation.

D. Induction of labor is inappropriate because emergent delivery is indicated.

186. **B. In this patient with a pulmonary embolus who is 24 hours status post an abdominal surgery, IV heparin is the best initial management because it has a short half-life, leads to rapid anticoagulation, can be stopped immediately, and can be reversed with protamine sulfate.**

A. Supplemental oxygen should be provided, but it should not be the only treatment administered to the patient—she will also require medical therapy. Patients who require supplemental oxygen because of shunting should usually be placed on it by means of a nonrebreather face mask. Many patients on nasal cannula will simply breathe through their mouth, decreasing the efficacy of such treatment.

C. Treatment of an acute DVT or PE is now often accomplished with low-molecular-weight heparin. If this patient had delivered vaginally or was a few more days out from her delivery, this therapy would be a reasonable option (see the explanation for B).

D. Eventually, this patient can be converted to warfarin therapy. However, this agent is not a good initial treatment because it often takes several days of therapy to achieve adequate anticoagulation.

E. Furosemide (Lasix) is commonly used in patients with pulmonary edema to facilitate diuresis. It has no role in this patient.

187. **E. Based on her history and physical, the patient has a small bowel obstruction (SBO). Her abdominal X-rays confirm this fact and are further worrisome for bowel perforation with evidence of free air. This patient needs IVs placed for rehydration and immediate exploration in the OR. She should be asked to give informed consent for possible bowel resection, ileostomy, and/or colostomy.**

A. In patients with SBO who are stable, NGT placement and NPO are reasonable plans for management.

B. Although this patient may require TPN at a later time, she has a SBO that has likely perforated and requires emergent laparotomy prior to management of her malnutrition.

C. Laparoscopy is now being utilized for second-look operations for confirmation of absent disease in ovarian cancer. This possibility is not the issue in this patient.

D. In a patient with appendicitis or cholecystitis, this approach is sometimes taken. However, this patient has a perforated viscous and needs to go to the OR immediately.

188. **B. Because continuous OCPs have proven to be effective for this patient, she should be restarted on them. The patient should be informed that she can withdraw from the OCPs approximately twice a year and that it is acceptable to not have regular menses given the cyclical nature of endometriosis pain.**

A. This regimen has proven to be ineffective for the patient in the past, and there is no reason to believe that resuming it now would provide pain relief for her.

C. Although menstrual suppression by progestin treatment (usually medroxyprogesterone depot injection) is effective treatment for some women with endometriosis, it is preferable to resume an effective treatment rather than experiment with new regimens in this patient.

D. GnRH agonists are effective in treating chronic endometriosis pain in 75% to 90% of women. However, their use is generally limited to 6 months due to the side effects associated with estrogen deficiency (bone loss and vasomotor symptoms). Although "add back" regimens have been utilized successfully to counter these side effects, their effectiveness is tempered by the inconvenience and cost of taking additional medications.

E. There is no indication for operative treatment in this patient with endometriosis responsive to medical treatment and no desire for future fertility.

189. **D. The goals of management in patients with severe hyperemesis gravidarum include maintenance of hydration and nutritional status, as well as symptom relief. Achievement of these goals requires a team approach and often includes consultation with social work and nutrition services. Although many patients will**

respond to IV hydration and antiemetics, a small percentage may require prolonged hospitalization. If oral intake cannot be tolerated in this setting, it is reasonable to place a pediatric feeding tube, which is usually well tolerated. TPN should be considered only after attempting every other form of nutrition and hydration.

A. Hospitalization will be required if the patient cannot tolerate oral intake.

B. Many patients with hyperemesis gravidarum are conflicted about the pregnancy. A social services consult can provide the added social support they may need.

C. Zofran has been used in pregnancy in these patients for several years with no known teratogenic effects. It is commonly reserved for nausea and vomiting refractory to other first-line antiemetic agents.

E. If the patient cannot tolerate oral intake, a feeding tube should be placed. The feeding tube's tip should be placed in the duodenum, making the feeds more easily tolerated. This is the preferred method of feeding over TPN.

190. **E. The patient is experiencing dysmenorrhea secondary to outflow obstruction. She has cervical stenosis, which is a known complication of LEEP and other cervical surgeries. The most appropriate treatment for her is cervical dilation, as OCPs will merely decrease the amount of her menstrual flow but will not eliminate the underlying problem. Unfortunately, many patients with cervical stenosis will experience recurrences of the disorder, requiring repeat cervical dilations.**

A. Although the patient has a history of instrumentation, she does not have any evidence of infection, making pelvic abscess an unlikely etiology for her symptoms.

B. Although dysmenorrhea is a common symptom of endometriosis, the rest of the patient's history is inconsistent with such a diagnosis, which can only be truly made by diagnostic laparoscopy.

C. Given the typically slow progression of cervical cancer, it is highly unlikely that the patient would develop cervical cancer after being diagnosed with cervical dysplasia and undergoing LEEP only 6 months ago. Additionally, cervical cancer often presents as painless postcoital vaginal bleeding rather than dysmenorrhea.

D. See the explanation for E.

191. **A. Complete moles result from the fertilization of an empty ovum by a normal sperm, which is then thought to duplicate itself. Thus the most common karyotype for complete moles is 46,XX. A partial mole is the fertilization of an ovum with two sperm; its most common karyotype is 69,XXY.**

B, C, D. Treatment of complete moles involves immediate suction evacuation of the uterus and gentle curettage. They cannot be managed expectantly, and a hysterectomy would be too extreme. Chemotherapy is indicated only if malignant transformation occurs, which is confirmed by persistently elevated β-hCG levels after uterine evacuation.

E. The risk of developing GTD in subsequent pregnancies is only 5%.

192. **D. This patient is experiencing urinary retention. Given her recent history of urogynecological surgery, the likely etiology is overcorrection of her urinary incontinence with resultant urinary outflow obstruction. The appropriate treatment is placement of a Foley catheter to relieve the obstruction. Surgical exploration and repair are not indicated at this time.**

A, B, C. Although the patient's urine sample was not an ideal specimen, the lack of leukocyte esterase and nitrites on urine dipstick makes the diagnosis of UTI unlikely. If clinical suspicion for infection is high, the urine should be cultured. A straight catheter specimen is not necessary, and a single catheterization will not correct this patient's problem. However, once the Foley catheter is placed, antibiotic suppression against UTIs can be considered.

E. The patient may eventually need a repeat surgery to relax the suspension of the bladder neck. This procedure should not happen immediately, nor should it occur without another trial of voiding.

193. **B. Quantitative serum β-hCG will help indicate the most likely diagnosis: molar pregnancy. This patient presents with marked proteinuria and hypertension in the late first trimester. Most preeclampsia is not seen before 20 weeks (and usually not until the third trimester), except in the setting of molar pregnancy. Epigastric pain and severe nausea should also prompt consideration of gastroenteritis, cholestatic disease, pancreatic disease, and hepatitis. However, this**

patient is afebrile, has normal GI lab values, and proteinuria, moving molar pregnancy to the top of the differential diagnosis. Molar pregnancies have elevated hCG, with levels occasionally exceeding 1 million. The diagnosis will be confirmed by an US that reveals an enlarged uterus filled with hydropic trophoblastic tissue (complete mole) or a fetus with a thickened, hydropic placenta (incomplete mole).

A. CA-125 is a nonspecific tumor marker expressed in many ovarian neoplasms. Ovarian cancer typically presents with vague abdominal complaints, not the acute presentation described here.

C. Serum magnesium levels will not be useful in diagnosing this patient. If she does have preeclampsia secondary to a molar pregnancy, magnesium therapy may be used for seizure prophylaxis.

D. Maternal serum alpha-fetoprotein is, in fact, lower than expected based on GA in molar pregnancies. This finding is not very specific, however; it can result from overestimated GA, chromosomal abnormalities such as trisomies 18 and 21, or maternal obesity. Elevated serum β-hCG is a far more useful diagnostic test in this case.

E. Serum thyroxine is often elevated in molar pregnancy, due to the structural homology of hCG and thyrotropin (thyroid-stimulating hormone, or TSH). Clinical hyperthyroidism is rare, however, and this value, while useful, is not beneficial in the diagnosis of this patient. It would be essential information in the medical and surgical management of this patient.

194. **E. The most likely diagnosis is incomplete (partial) molar pregnancy, which results when a normal ovum is fertilized by two sperm. The karyotype is typically triploid, most commonly (80%) 69,XXY. An incomplete mole is more likely because of the presence of embryonic tissue.**

A. 46,XX is the most common karyotype for a complete mole, which forms when an empty ovum is fertilized by one sperm. No embryonic/fetal tissue is present. All chromosomes are paternally derived. (46,XX is, of course, the karyotype for a normal female.)

B, C, D. 47,XXY, 47,XX+18, and 47,XX+21 are the karyotypes for Klinefelter's, Edward's, and Down syndromes, respectively. These aneuploidies all increase rates of spontaneous abortion, but the elevated β-hCG level, when combined with the vesicles seen on exam and characteristic sonographic findings, make gestational trophoblastic disease the likely diagnosis. Elevated maternal serum β-hCG is seen in trisomy 21, but not to the level observed in this patient.

195. **C. This patient likely has endometriosis, which can be definitively diagnosed only by direct visualization (e.g., diagnostic laparoscopy). Endometriosis is the presence of endometrial cells outside of the endometrial cavity. Several theories have been promulgated regarding the origin of endometriosis. The Halban theory proposes that endometrial cells travel through the lymphatic system to different sites in the pelvis, where they then cause symptoms. Meyer's theory purports that multipotential cells in the peritoneum undergo metaplastic transformation into working endometrium. Sampson theorizes that retrograde menstruation of endometrial cells through the fallopian tubes results in pelvic implants and the symptoms of endometriosis. Endometrial implants can appear as powder-burn, mulberry, or blueberry lesions anywhere in the pelvis. Occasionally, an inverse relationship exists between the amount of disease present and the severity of symptoms.**

A. A corpus luteum cyst results from the rupture of the ovarian follicle that resulted in ovulation. It is extremely rare to have bilateral corpus luteum cysts.

B. Scant powder-burn lesions may be present with endometriosis, but the etiology of this patient's pain is most likely due to her sizable bilateral masses, which are probably blood-filled endometriomas, giving the low-attenuation appearance on US.

D. Peritoneal tuberculosis is an extrapulmonary manifestation of tuberculosis characterized by abdominal pain, fever, weight loss, and ascites. It is the leading cause of infertility worldwide, but it is an unlikely source of this patient's cysts and adnexal pain.

E. TOA would be suspected in a patient with cervical motion, uterine, and adnexal tenderness. TOAs are often associated with fever and risk factors for STDs.

196. **C. Gonococcal (GC) infections are transmitted at the time of delivery and can cause disseminated illness in the neonate. There is also a theoretical concern that they can cause ascending infections in pregnancy, leading to higher rates of preterm labor and delivery. For this reason, GC infections are treated aggressively in pregnancy.**

A. Transmission of toxoplasmosis is most common during the third trimester, but the neonatal complications tend to be milder than those seen with early-pregnancy transmission.
B. HIV transmission can occur transplacentally, but this virus is transmitted more commonly during birth from exposure to blood and vaginal secretions.
D. Varicella zoster virus (VZV) can cause both spontaneous abortions and a fetal infection that can lead to neurologic disease and cutaneous lesions. Patients who are not VZV immune should avoid exposure during pregnancy. If exposed, they should be given immunoglobulin prophylaxis, or VZIG, to decrease the chances of becoming infected.
E. Parvovirus B-19 causes Fifth disease in children and occasionally adults. In the fetus, it can lead to myelosuppression, manifested by anemia and fetal hydrops.

197. **A. Mittelschmerz (from German; literally, "middle pain") is pain due to the rupture of an ovarian follicle during ovulation, resulting in intraperitoneal fluid or blood that can produce localized or diffuse abdominal pain. The easiest way to prevent future bouts of mittelschmerz is to place the patient on OCPs to suppress ovulation.**

B. PID is most commonly seen in young, sexually active women with multiple partners. In addition to being in a long-term monogamous relationship, this patient is unlikely to have PID because she is afebrile, has a normal WBC count, and exhibits no cervical motion tenderness or vaginal discharge.
C. Mittelschmerz can frequently be confused with adnexal torsion. The timing and nature of the symptoms in this patient make mittelschmerz a more likely diagnosis. One would expect a more protracted course with adnexal torsion, usually with concomitant nausea and vomiting. A pelvic US might be helpful in the evaluation if the clinical picture were more confusing.
D. The patient has a negative pregnancy test.
E. Left-side pain can occur uncommonly in acute appendicitis. This patient does not have other signs or symptoms that are consistent with appendicitis.

198. **A. Although numerous risk factors exist for preterm delivery, the biggest risk factor is history of a prior preterm delivery. Other risk factors for preterm labor include multiple gestations, polyhydramnios, being African American, bacterial vaginosis, uterine anomalies, preterm rupture of the membranes, preeclampsia, and some maternal medical conditions.**

B. While it has been theorized that multiple TABs increase the risk of incompetent cervix, no studies to date have correlated history of one prior TAB with preterm delivery.
C. Bacterial vaginosis has been associated with preterm labor, but no such association exists with vaginal candidiasis.
D. A prepregnancy weight of less than 50 kg is a risk factor for preterm delivery, but no such association exists with obesity.
E. While it is true that maternal age less than 20 is associated with preterm delivery, it is not this patient's biggest risk factor.

199. **B. This patient has a mild case of OHSS, a rare but potentially life-threatening complication of ovulation induction with gonadotropins. In addition to ovarian enlargement, affected patients experience weight gain and abdominal distention. In severe cases, patients can present with ascites, pleural effusion, electrolyte imbalance, hypovolemia, and oliguria. The syndrome is managed by hospitalization, discontinuing gonadotropins, correcting fluid and electrolyte imbalances, and supportive therapy.**

A. While adnexal torsion is relatively common in OHSS, this patient's exam and history are not consistent with such a diagnosis. With a diagnosis of adnexal torsion, one would expect nausea, vomiting, and a more concerning pelvic exam.
C. Ectopic pregnancy should be considered in the differential diagnosis of any sexually active woman of child-bearing age who presents with lower abdominal pain. However, the negative pregnancy test and large ovarian mass on US exam make such a diagnosis

unlikely. Because the possibility of an early ectopic pregnancy exists, a quantitative β-hCG would assist in confirming the diagnosis.

D. While the patient may have an endometrioma in the pelvis, her acute symptoms and history are more consistent with OHSS.

E. The patient's history of an occluded left fallopian tube might make the diagnosis of PID more likely. However, with the exception of abdominal pain, she has no physical signs or symptoms of PID.

200. **C. With a sure LMP and an US showing a smaller than expected gestational sac without cardiac motion, this patient is most likely starting a spontaneous abortion of a nonviable pregnancy. Misoprostol is a prostaglandin that can be administered vaginally or orally to induce cervical dilation and uterine contractions to empty the uterus. It is used for labor induction both at term and in the setting of intrauterine fetal demise. Various protocols exist for its use in early miscarriage in women who do not wish to wait for miscarriage to occur spontaneously (expectant management) or who wish to avoid instrumentation (i.e., D&C).**

A. With a closed cervix and a nonviable intrauterine pregnancy (no cardiac motion at a GA when it would certainly be expected), this patient has experienced a missed abortion. If cardiac motion was detected in the setting of vaginal bleeding and cramping but no cervical dilation, this case would be considered a threatened abortion. If the cervix was dilated, and particularly if tissue was present in the cervical os, it would be considered an inevitable abortion. A complete abortion refers to a situation in which a previously pregnant patient has already passed all the pregnancy tissue from the uterus such that the uterus appears empty on US.

B. See the explanation for C.

D. Generally, any pregnant woman who experiences vaginal bleeding should have the blood type and Rh checked so that Rhogam can be administered if she is Rh negative. Rhogam should be considered even if the amount of vaginal bleeding is small, because the risks and consequences of Rh isoimmunization can be quite serious while the risks of Rhogam administration are minimal (e.g., allergic reaction). While this patient is likely to eventually experience vaginal bleeding as the pregnancy spontaneously aborts or she undergoes a medical or surgical evacuation, she currently has not had any vaginal bleeding. Thus Rhogam is not indicated at this time.

E. In general, recurrent pregnancy loss is not diagnosed or evaluated until after three consecutive abortions. In women of advanced maternal age (AMA, 35 years or older), evaluations may sometimes commence after two consecutive abortions. However, this patient is not considered to be of AMA.

Section

3 Pediatrics

SETTING 1: COMMUNITY-BASED HEALTH CENTER

You work at a community-based health facility where patients seeking both routine and urgent care are encountered. Many patients are members of low-income groups; many are ethnic minorities. Several industrial parks and local businesses send their employees to the health center for treatment of on-the-job injuries and employee health screening. There is a facility that provides x-ray films, but CT and MRI scans must be arranged at other facilities. Laboratory services are available.

1. The left pupil of a 12-month-old girl has been noted to be white by the parents. Recently, she has been rubbing that eye and squinting when exposed to bright light. A full ophthalmic exam is performed, but the retina is poorly visualized even after dilation of the pupil. A massive outpouring of white blood cells is seen in the anterior chamber, and fibrous strands are noted to extend from the iris to the lens consistent with uveitis. The remainder of her physical exam is normal. Which of the following is the most appropriate first step in the management of this patient?

   A. CT scan of the orbits
   B. The avoidance of steroid eye drops
   C. Blood samples for acute and convalescent titers of CMV, toxoplasmosis, syphilis, and toxocara
   D. The avoidance of dilating eye drops
   E. Titers of anti-nuclear antibody (ANA)

2. A 5-year-old boy is brought into the clinic with a history of "white spots on his face" for 2 weeks. The lesions are nonpruritic and appear to have a fine scaly uniform texture (Figure 3-2). Under Wood's light exam there is no specific fluorescence. The mother thinks they have become worse since the return from his camping trip. Which of the following is the most appropriate management option?

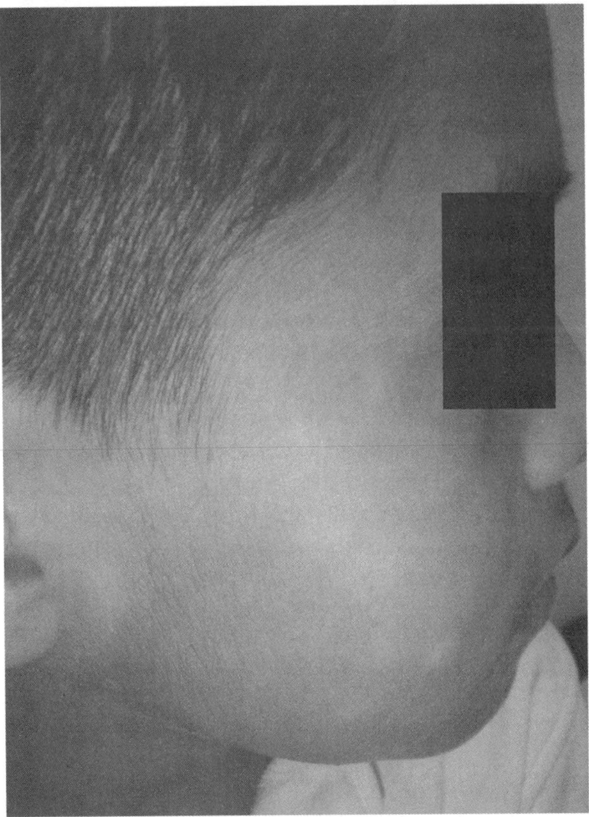

Figure 3-2 • Image Courtesy of the Phoenix Children's Hospital, Phoenix, Arizona.

A. Dermatology referral
B. Griseofulvin
C. Low-potency topical corticosteroid
D. Topical selenium sulfide
E. Diphenhydramine (Benadryl)

3. A 2-year-old boy comes to your clinic for a checkup. He is well except that he walks with a slight in-toed gait. When you place him prone on the examination table with his knees flexed and measure the angle formed by the axis of the thigh and the axis of the foot, you note that the foot is internally rotated. You diagnose internal tibial torsion. The best management for this condition at this age is:

A. Refer to a pediatric orthopedic surgeon for serial casting
B. Obtain leg radiographs to measure the thigh-foot angle
C. Suggest high-top, straight last shoes with arch supports
D. Send patient to be fitted for a Denis-Brown bar
E. Reassure parents that no treatment is needed at this age

4. You are seeing a 12-year-old girl in the clinic because she has ptosis and muscle weakness after repetitive use. You suspect a diagnosis of myasthenia gravis. The best next test to confirm the diagnosis would be:

A. EMG
B. EEG
C. Anti-acetylcholine receptor antibodies assay in the serum
D. Muscle biopsy
E. Serum creatine phosphokinase (CPK) level

5. You are seeing a 9-month-old boy for a well-child exam. This is his first visit to the clinic since the age of 2 months because his parents are homeless and have been living in multiple shelters. He has been bottle fed and reportedly began solids around 6 months of age. The mother does not report any excessive spitting-up, feeding problems, or undercurrent illnesses. On exam, he is alert and interactive, but markedly thin. The rest of the physical exam is normal. His growth chart reveals that his head circumference and length have dropped from the 90th to the 75th percentile, while his weight has dropped from the 75th to less than the 25th percentile. CBC, lead level, urinalysis, CMP, thyroid function, HIV, and sweat tests are all normal. The best next step in management would be:

A. Contrast head MRI
B. Contrast head CT
C. Nuclear medicine gastric emptying study
D. Colonoscopy with biopsies
E. Hospitalization for observed feedings and calorie count

6. You are seeing a 12-year-old obese female in your clinic for the first time. The mother reports that her daughter had a low glucose as a newborn and was very floppy. She had feeding difficulties and grew poorly, requiring nutritional supplements as an infant; she is now overweight. Her mother reports that she is obsessed with food, hides food, and sneaks into the refrigerator at night. She is very behind in school and is in special education classes. On physical examination, she has blue, almond-shaped eyes, and blond hair. She has very small hands and feet. Her speech is nasal in quality. She is quite obese, with her weight above the 99th percentile, and is short for her age. Due to your suspicions, you order a chromosomal evaluation. The result shows an abnormality of chromosome 15. Which of the following is accurate counseling about this patient's syndrome?

A. Hypotonia is progressive, leading to respiratory failure
B. Mental retardation is uncommon
C. Ataxia is commonly seen in older children
D. Obesity and sleep apnea are common in older patients
E. Cardiac and skeletal defects are common

7. A 6-year-old boy who is in first grade is brought to your clinic because his parents are quite upset about his encopresis. The patient had been successfully toilet trained at 3 years of age, but the mother reports the boy now goes several days without having a bowel movement. His stools are so large in size that there is pain with bowel movements. About three times a week, the patient has loose stool that leaks into his underwear. This is causing great problems with teasing at school. On physical examination, you find a large amount of stool in the rectum. The best next step in the management of this patient is:

A. Institute a low-fiber diet
B. Prescribe enemas or laxatives to evacuate retained stool
C. Have child sit on toilet for at least 30 minutes (or until bowel movement) daily
D. Order a barium enema
E. Refer patient to a child psychiatrist

8. A 3-year-old boy is seen in your clinic because of an apparent ataxia that has been progressive for the past year. Recently he has also developed "bloodshot" eyes, which is not associated with eye drainage. His other significant history shows that he suffers from rather severe and resistant sinopulmonary infections and otitis media. Examination reveals bilateral telangiectasis of the conjunctiva. You are concerned about an immunodeficiency syndrome. Which of the following is the most accurate information to give to the family?

   A. This condition is transmitted as an autosomal dominant trait; therefore a parent should have this condition, or it is a result of a genetic mutation
   B. Agammaglobulinemia frequently accompanies this condition
   C. Thymus hypoplasia is associated with this condition
   D. The ataxia which occurs is usually a static condition and not progressive
   E. T-cell function is abnormal, and therefore lymphoproliferative disorders are usually of very low incidence

9. A 2-month-old boy is seen at a clinic well-child checkup and is noted to have a head size greater than the 95th percentile. His height and weight are both near the 50th percentile. His head control is poor, and his anterior fontanelle is also quite large. His cranial sutures are slightly separated. A head ultrasound is ordered (Figure 3-9). Which one of the following statements applies to this patient?

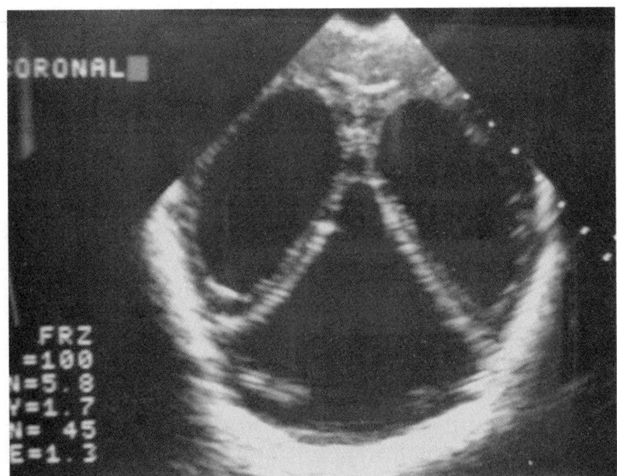

Figure 3-9 • Image Courtesy of the Department of Radiology, Phoenix Children's Hospital, Phoenix, Arizona.

   A. The ultrasound examination reveals hydranencephaly
   B. The ultrasound is most consistent with a Dandy-Walker cyst
   C. A ventricle peritoneal shunt would offer no benefit to this patient
   D. This abnormality is generally associated with myelomeningocele
   E. This benign condition needs only long-term observation

10. A 3-year-old girl presents with a history of coke-colored urine and periorbital edema. She has previously been well, but was noted to have URI symptoms and a sore throat with fever about 2 weeks ago. These symptoms appeared to resolve spontaneously. Her presumed diagnosis is poststreptococcal glomerulonephritis (PSGN). Which one of the following statements is consistent with this diagnosis?

   A. Thinning of the glomerular basement membrane
   B. Late development of hypertension
   C. Elevated serum antistreptolysin O (ASO) titer, but a negative anti-DNAase titer
   D. Decreased renal tubular function
   E. A low serum C3 complement

11. You are seeing a term infant in the clinic for the first time. The infant was born to a mother who abused cocaine throughout her pregnancy. Which of the following is an associated complication of in-utero cocaine exposure that you might expect in this patient?

   A. Ventricular septal defect
   B. Postterm delivery
   C. Hydrocephalus
   D. Placenta previa
   E. Hearing loss

12. A 6-year-old child is being seen in your clinic for the evaluation of scalp itching. On further exam you notice that the boy's hair reveals evidence of head lice. Which of the following would be appropriate advice for this boy's parents?

   A. Head lice are highly contagious as they can jump from person to person
   B. Head lice carry contagious diseases
   C. Infestation can often occur after sharing clothing or helmets
   D. The one-time application of permethrin 1% is inadequate treatment
   E. The child should be allowed to return to school once all nits are gone

13. An 8-year-old male is being evaluated in your clinic for obesity. He is in the second grade and has otherwise been healthy and developing appropriately. His body mass index is 32. Which of the following most likely applies to this patient's obesity?

    A. His exam is likely to yield normal findings
    B. Sleep apnea is a potential complication
    C. TSH levels are expected to be abnormal
    D. A dietary history will be noncontributory
    E. The patient is at a decreased risk for slipped capital femoral epiphysis

14. A 2½-year-old male being seen in the clinic develops an urticarial rash and facial swelling after tasting peanut butter for the first time. He has had no previous history of urticaria, but does have a history of mild atopic dermatitis. Treatment with diphenhydramine improves the symptoms and they gradually clear with continued diphenhydramine administration. The parents are extremely anxious and have a number of questions. Which of the following would be correct information to give to the family?

    A. Peanut allergy will be lifelong
    B. Peanut allergy is more common in adults than in children
    C. Risk factors for peanut allergy include a history of atopy
    D. The prevalence of peanut allergy is decreasing
    E. Peanut allergy is an IgA-mediated phenomenon

15. A 2-month-old with jaundice is seen in your clinic for the first time. The total and direct bilirubin levels are elevated and you are concerned about the possibility of biliary atresia. Which of the following statements about your suspected diagnosis is true?

    A. The condition is usually due to obliteration of the entire extrahepatic biliary tree
    B. Biliary atresia is much more common than neonatal hepatitis
    C. In biliary atresia, an abdominal ultrasound often shows a large gall bladder
    D. A liver biopsy cannot differentiate biliary atresia from neonatal hepatitis
    E. Success of the Kasai procedure is highest if performed after 6 months of life

16. An 18-month-old boy is seen in the clinic for a checkup. You note that he has severe dental decay. The mother is concerned about her son's caries but has heard "many different things about cavities." Which of the following is accurate information to tell this child's mother?

    A. Caries are caused by an overgrowth of *Staphylococcus aureus*
    B. Dental bacterial colonization occurs when a baby is born
    C. The most likely source of bacterial colonization is the mother's oral flora
    D. Children of mothers with high rates of caries are not at greater-than-average risk for developing caries
    E. Dental decay is equally common in rich and poor families

17. A 6-year-old girl is brought to your clinic because of poor weight gain, chronic cough, and intermittent diarrhea. She has a history of asthma and over the last 2 years she has had four bouts of pneumonia that required hospitalization and antibiotic treatment. She takes an inhaled steroid daily, but is on no other medication. What would you do next?

    A. Refer the patient to a nutritionist for a calorie count
    B. Start a leukotriene inhibitor for better asthma control
    C. Obtain a CT scan of the sinuses
    D. Order a sweat chloride test
    E. Refer the patient to a gastroenterologist to rule out Crohn disease

18. A 2-month-old baby comes to your clinic for a checkup. The mother is concerned that the baby has had noisy breathing since shortly after birth. The baby is taking the bottle well and has been gaining weight adequately. On physical examination the baby looks comfortable but has some intermittent inspiratory stridor, which is worsened in the supine position. Which statement about this condition is most accurate?

    A. It is a common cause of expiratory wheezing in young infants
    B. Symptoms usually appear around 6 months when chest muscles are getting stronger
    C. The airway noise is due to collapse of the supraglottic structures during inspiration
    D. Even in severe cases of upper airway obstruction, bronchoscopy is not necessary
    E. Because symptoms rarely resolve spontaneously, most infants require tracheostomy

19. 14-year-old girl is seen at your clinic because of significant pain and swelling of her knees and ankles for the past 2 weeks. She has also had intermittent fevers. There is no family history of arthritis. A rheumatoid factor (RF) is negative, an ASO titer is negative, her sedimentation rate is 80, and an ANA is significantly positive. Which one of the following statements is accurate regarding this girl's illness?
   A. There is sufficient evidence in the information given to make the diagnosis of systemic lupus erythematosus (SLE)
   B. The positive ANA has a low sensitivity but a high positive predictive value for the diagnosis of SLE
   C. The presence of a malar rash and a positive anti-DNA antibody test in addition to the findings described will make the diagnosis of SLE
   D. In children and adolescents with SLE, renal disease is uncommon and does not usually contribute to long-term morbidity as it does in adults
   E. Lupus patients usually produce a variety of anti-nuclear antibodies, but it is unusual to find other autoantibodies

20. A 7-year-old boy is referred to you because he is found to have problems concentrating in school. His teacher also notes that his cognition is near the bottom of the class. You take a thorough history and determine that the patient has been exposed to lead in the home. A blood lead level is 30 μg/dL (normal is <10 μg/dL). The next most appropriate step in managing this patient includes:
   A. Immediate chelation therapy with bronchoalveolar lavage (BAL) and 2,3-dimercaptosuccinic acid (DMSA)
   B. Removal from the source of exposure
   C. Admission to the hospital for observation and repeat lead levels
   D. Calling child welfare to apprehend the child
   E. Performing x-rays of the long bones

21. A 12-year-old girl is seen in your clinic for a preschool checkup. She is found to have a blood pressure of 135/90. She is at the 75th percentile for height and weight. Her femoral pulses are good. She has no cardiac murmurs. Her examination is normal. A urinalysis is also normal. You confirm the blood pressure readings several times in your clinic, and the blood pressures remain about the same. You also check that the cuff size is normal. You consult the tables for normal blood pressure and find that, for her height and age, the 95th percentile for systolic is 126 and for diastolic is 82. Your next step would be:
   A. Prescribe a mild diuretic
   B. Place her on a low-sodium diet
   C. Obtain a renal ultrasound
   D. Advise her that this blood pressure is at the upper limits of normal for her age
   E. Use a home blood pressure monitor for 24 to 48 hours

22. 9-year-old boy is seen in your clinic with a skin rash he's had for the past 2 days. The rash is mostly on his trunk, and seems to come and go. The rash is red and slightly raised, appears to migrate, and is nonpruritic. He gives a history of having had a sore throat about 2 weeks ago, and has had some low-grade fevers and joint pains. An ASO titer is 1:625. Which one group of findings would confirm the diagnosis of acute rheumatic fever?
   A. Arthralgia, no fever, and a rash resembling erythema multiforme
   B. Subcutaneous nodules, fever, and arthralgia
   C. Erythema multiforme, arthralgia, and prolonged PR interval
   D. Arthralgia, fever, no rash, and erythrocyte sedimentation rate (ESR) = 120
   E. Arthritis, no fever, and ESR = 10

23. A 13-year-old slender early adolescent girl has been complaining of right hip discomfort for several weeks. An examination reveals significant discomfort when that hip is rotated, and she prefers to keep her hip slightly flexed and externally rotated. Which one of the following is the most accurate information to give to the family?
   A. Endocrine dysfunction need not be considered as causative factor in slipped capital femoral epiphysis
   B. Slipped capital femoral epiphysis occurs most often in obese adolescent girls
   C. About 50% of cases of slipped capital femoral epiphysis in girls occur after puberty
   D. A simple anterior-posterior (AP) pelvis x-ray may not demonstrate a slipped capital femoral epiphysis
   E. Slipped capital femoral epiphysis is not commonly bilateral

24. A 2-year-old boy presents to the clinic and has pallor on exam. His mother states that he drinks 45 ounces of cow's milk a day. A CBC reveals a hemoglobin of 8.2 and a mean corpuscular volume (MCV) of 65. Which of the following indices is compatible with this patient's diagnosis?

    A. Decreased red blood cell distribution width (RDW)
    B. Increased serum ferritin
    C. Increased total iron binding capacity (TIBC)
    D. Increased reticulocyte count
    E. Increased serum iron level

25. A 15-month-old boy is seen in your clinic because of vomiting and diarrhea. He had two episodes of vomiting earlier today, but now he is able to drink small amounts of fluid without emesis. On physical examination, you find the baby to be mildly dehydrated, but the remainder of the examination is completely within normal limits. Rather than hospitalizing the baby for IV fluids, you decide to treat with oral rehydration solution at home. The composition of the oral rehydration solution should be:

    A. 20–30 mEq of sodium per liter; 2% glucose
    B. 40–50 mEq of sodium per liter; no glucose
    C. 50–90 mEq of sodium per liter; no glucose
    D. 50–90 mEq of sodium per liter; 10% to 12% glucose
    E. 50–90 mEq of sodium per liter; 2% glucose

26. A 6-year-old boy is brought to your clinic because of fever and a painful, swollen eye. His mother thinks he may have been bitten by a mosquito on his face yesterday. The inflamed, tense eyelid swelling, which was first noted about 18 hours ago, has progressed so that you are not able to examine the globe adequately. You order a CT scan of the orbit (Figure 3-26). How will you manage this patient?

    A. Admit to the hospital for observation and pain control
    B. Administer subcutaneous epinephrine and initiate oral corticosteroids
    C. Begin oral administration of amoxicillin and see patient in clinic tomorrow
    D. Start oral antihistamine and application of ice directly to the eye every 4 to 6 hours
    E. Admit patient to the hospital to start IV antibiotics and obtain surgical consultation

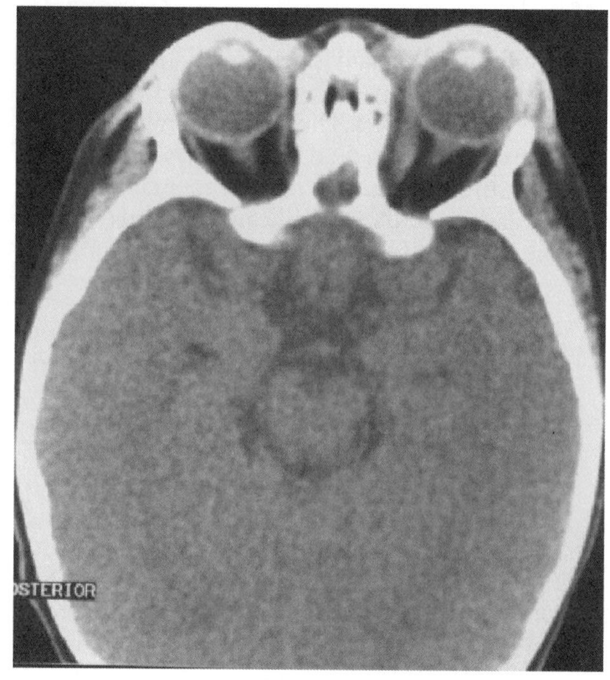

Figure 3-26 • Image Courtesy of Dr. Bangert, Department of Radiology, University Hospitals of Cleveland, Cleveland, Ohio.

27. A 2-month-old boy is brought to your clinic because of nonbilious, projectile vomiting for 3 days. His parents have noted decreased stool frequency. On physical examination, you see peristaltic gastric waves. Which of the statements about this patient's condition is true?

    A. Because of the vomiting, most patients develop metabolic acidosis
    B. A palpable, olive-sized mass can sometimes be palpated in the mid-abdomen
    C. The presence of jaundice is inconsistent with this condition
    D. The diagnosis almost always requires an upper GI series
    E. This is a surgical emergency that requires emergent surgery to prevent perforation

28. A 5-month-old African-American baby is brought to your clinic for a checkup. He has been growing well and his physical examination is normal aside from a large umbilical hernia. Which of the following statements about umbilical hernias is true?

    A. They usually require surgical repair at some time before the child is 1 year old
    B. They are rare in African-American babies
    C. Strangulation occurs more often than with inguinal hernias

D. They may be associated with hypothyroidism and mucopolysaccharidoses
E. Taping a coin over the hernia will result in faster resolution

29. A 16-year-old adolescent comes to you concerned and embarrassed about the dark facial hair she is developing. You also note the tendency to excessively dark hair on her arms and legs. On further questioning, she admits to having some on her chest between her breasts and around her nipples. You note that she is obese and is developing dark, velvety, rugated skin on the back of her neck. You are concerned that she may have, or be at risk for, other associated medical problems. Which one of the following is a common misdiagnosis associated with this condition?

A. Poor hygiene and self-care due to her self-consciousness and possible depression
B. Chronic fatty infiltration of the liver and cirrhosis
C. Diabetes mellitus type II
D. Polycystic ovarian syndrome
E. Hypothyroidism

30. A 4-year-old boy has recently moved to your town. At his first well-child visit with you, his mother expresses concern about her child's short stature. His previous growth chart is shown (Figure 3-30). The patient's father was short as a child, but he is of average adult height. The child is eating and acting well and his development is normal. What is the most appropriate management of this patient?

A. Referral to an endocrinologist
B. Increase caloric intake and check height again in 3 months
C. Order a CBC, electrolytes, urinalysis, sedimentation rate, and thyroid tests
D. Order radiographs of the hands and wrists to determine the bone age
E. No tests or treatment is needed at this time

31. A 6-month-old boy is brought to your clinic because of URI with rhinorrhea, low-grade fever, and cough. When he cries, the mother says she can hear a high-pitched respiratory sound when he takes a breath in. His cry also sounds hoarse to her. The patient has been able to drink well and appears adequately hydrated. He seems active and happy and is neither tachypneic nor dyspneic. The patient does have a mild barky cough when you examine him. What would be the best next step in the management of this patient?

A. Order a radiograph of the neck (AP and lateral views)
B. Prescribe amoxicillin for 10 days
C. Instruct the parents to use a cool mist vaporizer; encourage oral hydration; no medication needed at this time
D. Give oral dexamethasone (Decadron); send the patient to the ER for racemic epinephrine treatments
E. Send the patient to the hospital for admission and airway management

32. A 9-month-old girl is seen in your clinic because her mother reports she is having intermittent abdominal pain associated with vomiting and low-grade fever for the past 24 hours. The baby's stools are noted to contain mucus and blood. On physical examination, you feel a sausage-shaped mass in the right upper quadrant. Which of the following statements about this girl's illness is true?

A. It is most commonly seen in school-age children
B. "Currant-jelly" stools (blood and mucus) are seen in almost all cases
C. The younger the child, the more likely there will be a lead point
D. Most cases are ileocolic
E. Barium or air enema will cause reduction in only about 10% to 20% of cases

33. A 1-month-old baby is brought to your clinic for a regular checkup. The examination is completely normal but the mother is concerned that her baby's feet are crooked. The forefoot is deviated medially and there is a prominence at the base of the 5th metatarsal. The forefoot can be easily manipulated into the normal position. In discussing this child's condition with the mother, which is the most accurate information to discuss?

A. The condition is usually unilateral
B. Radiologic evaluation should be performed early
C. Most cases will resolve spontaneously without treatment
D. Even if the foot is flexible, casting is needed if the foot is not straight by 2 to 3 months
E. Surgery is required in about half of cases

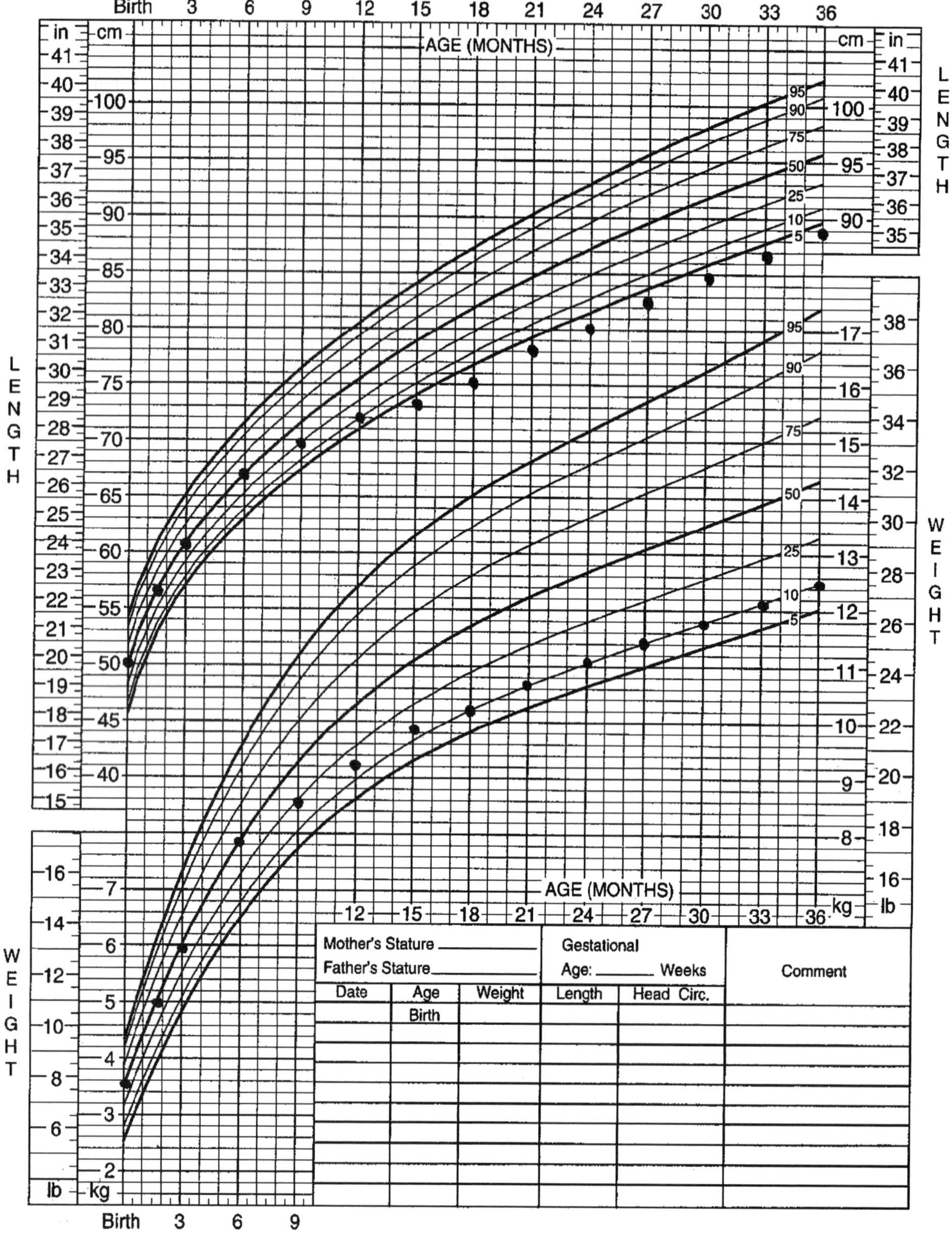

Figure 3-30 • Image Courtesy of the Phoenix Children's Hospital, Phoenix, Arizona. Source: Developed by the National Center for Health Statistics in collaboration with the National Center for Chronic Disease Prevention and Health Promotion (2000). http://www.cdc.gov/growthcharts

34. A 12-year-old boy developed sudden onset of grossly bloody urine. He has been a well child, and there have been no serious illnesses in the past. His examination is normal, and he has a normal blood pressure. His urine, indeed, is grossly bloody and there is also 3+ protein. An older brother also has had intermittent gross hematuria. A maternal uncle, age 22, is hard of hearing. Your initial evaluation of this patient would include which one of the following?

   A. Audiogram, examination of the patient's urine, and serum chemistries including blood urea nitrogen (BUN) and creatinine
   B. Reevaluate this patient in 1 month
   C. Schedule for a renal biopsy
   D. Examination of the mother's and uncle's urine
   E. ASO titer

35. A 2-year-old boy is seen with a mild productive cough of 2 weeks' duration. There has been an intermittent low-grade fever, and mild anorexia. There has been no foreign travel, but a grandmother lives in the same house and she has a chronic productive cough. You have some concern that this boy could have tuberculosis (TB). A TB skin test (Mantoux) test is performed, and you decide to also obtain a chest x-ray (Figure 3-35). Which one of the following would apply?

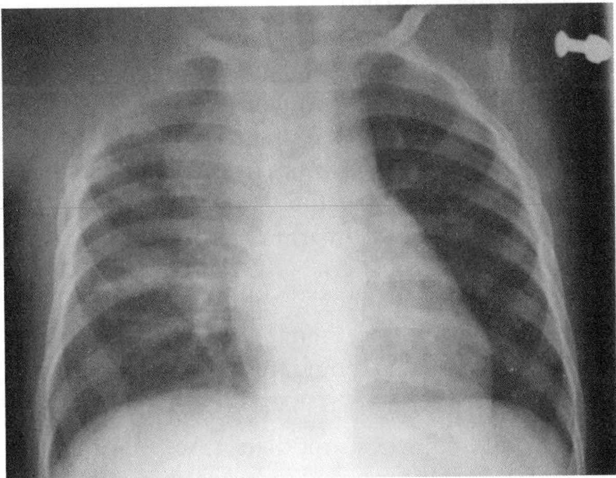

Figure 3-35 • Image Courtesy of the Department of Radiology, Phoenix Children's Hospital, Phoenix, Arizona.

   A. Await results of the TB skin test for further action
   B. Admit to the hospital for sputum collection for acid fast bacilli (AFB)
   C. Start the patient on isoniazid (INH) pending further evaluation
   D. Admit to the hospital for nasogastric (NG) aspirate collection for AFB
   E. Continued observation and follow-up chest x-ray in 1 month

36. A 12-year-old boy returns home from summer camp. After 2 days he develops frequent watery diarrhea and a mild fever. He is seen in your clinic on the third day of his illness. He looks to be mildly dehydrated and stool examination shows no evidence of blood or white blood cells. His mother is worried that he may have swallowed some water when swimming in the camp lake. The physician discusses the possibilities with the mother and together they decide on a treatment plan. Which of the following would likely be part of that plan?

   A. A 3-day trial of erythromycin
   B. Admission to the hospital for IV fluids and culture of stool
   C. A trial of metronidazole while awaiting giardia antigen
   D. Oral rehydration, continued diet, and reevaluation in the next couple of days
   E. A call to the local health board requesting investigation of the camp's lake

37. You are seeing a 2-year-old boy in your clinic for evaluation of potential speech delay. The mother states that he has five words and appears to understand all of her commands. After detailed birth history and physical exam with special attention to the head, eyes, ears, nose, and throat (HEENT) exam, you are concerned about a hearing deficit. The best next step in evaluation of a hearing deficit would be:

   A. Audiogram
   B. Head MRI
   C. EEG
   D. Speech therapy referral
   E. Head CT with special attention to the inner ear structures

38. You are seeing a 6-year-old boy in your clinic for evaluation of headaches. He reports two to three headaches over the past 2 months that are accompanied by the onset of blurry vision followed by severe pounding-type pain. During these headaches his mother states that he lies in

a dark room to feel better. You suspect the child is having classic migraines. Which of the following is the best preventative pharmacologic treatment for this child's condition?

A. Sumatriptan (Imitrex)
B. Acetaminophen with codeine
C. Over-the-counter (OTC) analgesia
D. Propranolol
E. There is no effective preventative treatment

39. A 5-year-old boy presents with a history of generalized dependent edema over the past 3 weeks. According to his mother, the patient appears to have gained weight and is using the bathroom less frequently. His examination reveals a distended abdomen with ascites without hepatomegaly, and 3+ pitting edema of the ankles is noted bilaterally. His urinalysis reveals 4+ protein, trace blood, and specific gravity 1.035. Which one of the following is consistent with the diagnosis of minimal change nephrotic syndrome?

A. Low C3 complement level
B. High serum cholesterol and normal triglycerides
C. No immunoglobulin deposition along the glomerular capillary walls
D. Unresponsiveness to glucocorticoid therapy
E. Normal electron microscopy

40. A 4-year-old boy presents to your clinic with fever to 103.4°C and cough. On exam there are crackles present over the left lower lobe region. He has no wheezing. He has been previously healthy. The chest radiograph shows a consolidative infiltrate in the left lower lobe behind the heart, consistent with pneumonia. Which of the following statements about this patient is most likely to be correct?

A. The most likely bacterial etiology is *Streptococcus pneumoniae*
B. The most likely infectious etiology is respiratory syncytial virus (RSV)
C. This cannot be *Mycobacterium tuberculosis* because the pneumonia is in a lower lobe
D. This is characteristic of foreign body aspiration
E. This patient will likely develop a pleural effusion

41. You are seeing an 8-month-old child with an undescended testis in your clinic. This patient is managed most appropriately with:

A. Monitoring only; testis is likely to descend within the next 6 months
B. Trial of hormone therapy if no descent by 12 months
C. Ultrasound evaluation to identify an intra-abdominal testis
D. Referral to a urologist for further management
E. MRI evaluation to identify an intra-abdominal testis

42. You are seeing a newborn infant in the clinic for the first time. The infant's first-time parents are anxious and concerned about the baby's movements and are worried that something is wrong. Which of the following reflexes is normally absent in a newborn?

A. Startle (Moro)
B. Hand grasp
C. Crossed adductor
D. Toe grasp
E. Protective equilibrium

43. A 6-year-old boy is seen in your clinic for a 4-cm oval polymorphic macular rash located over the lower mid-abdominal skin. The most likely diagnosis is:

A. Scabies
B. Henoch-Schönlein purpura (HSP)
C. Poison ivy
D. Nickel dermatitis
E. Psoriasis

44. A 4-year-old girl is brought to your clinic with the complaint of persistent rhinorrhea for the past 2 months. Her mother also notes red itchy eyes. On physical examination, you find that the patient is mouth breathing and has dark circles under the eyes. There is a watery nasal discharge and edematous, boggy, bluish mucous membranes with no erythema. Which of the following statements about this condition is most accurate?

A. Children whose mothers smoke heavily are not at greater risk for allergic rhinitis
B. A horizontal skinfold over the bridge of the nose is sometimes seen
C. Neutrophils are seen on a nasal smear
D. It is okay for dogs and cats to remain in the home
E. Oral antihistamines and intranasal corticosteroids are generally ineffective

45. A 4-year-old girl presents with a chief complaint of hair loss. On exam, she has a 5-cm area of alopecia on the scalp over her left ear. This is also seen to a lesser degree on the right side of her head. Closer examination of the skin of the scalp in these areas reveals smooth and shiny skin, with no evidence of tiny broken hairs or irritation of the underlying scalp. What is this patient's most likely diagnosis?

A. Tinea capitus
B. Traction alopecia
C. Trichotillomania
D. Alopecia areata
E. Contact dermatitis to a hair product

46. A 1-month-old boy presents to your clinic with feeding intolerance, poor weight gain, and a large tongue. On exam, you notice a large posterior fontanelle and umbilical hernia. Your next step in making the diagnosis would be:

A. Abdominal radiograph
B. CBC and blood culture
C. Barium swallow
D. Follow-up on newborn screen results
E. Admit to the hospital for failure-to-thrive (FTT) work-up

47. An otherwise healthy girl comes to your clinic for evaluation of a bright red facial rash and a lacy, reticulated rash on her chest (Figure 3-47). The girl has been acting and eating normally. She is afebrile and non-toxic appearing. The best management for this situation is:

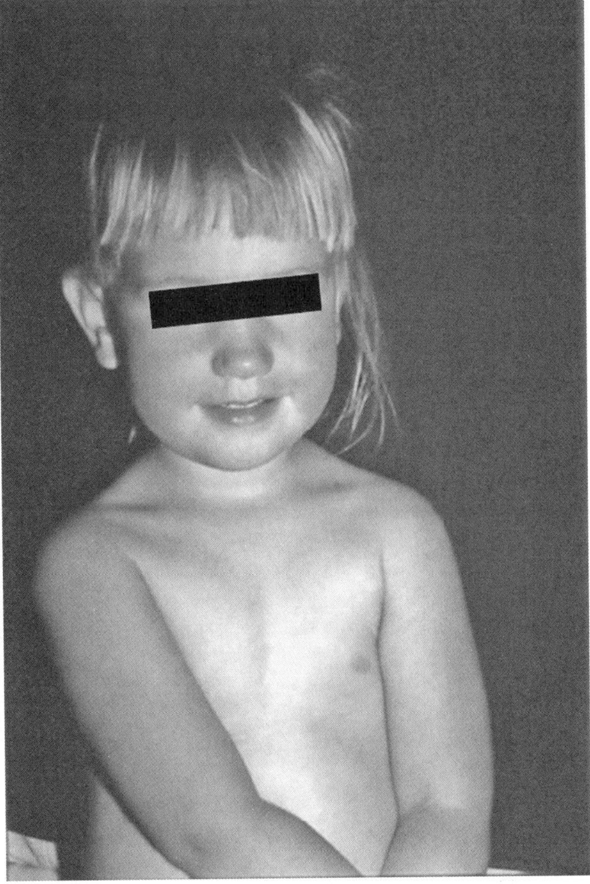

Figure 3-47 • Image Courtesy of the Phoenix Children's Hospital, Phoenix, Arizona.

A. Give the patient amoxicillin for 5 days
B. Keep the patient home from school for 1 week
C. Hospitalize the patient and administer IV gammaglobulin
D. Give all of the patient's classmates parvovirus vaccine
E. The patient needs no treatment; her classmates need no postexposure prophylaxis

48. A 16-year-old female is seen in your clinic with a complaint of irregular periods. She started menstruating at age 12 but has only intermittent periods, about every 3 to 4 months, some very heavy and some very light. Her mother is concerned that she may be pregnant. Her physical examination is significant for obesity, mildly increased facial hair, and pigmentation behind her neck at the hairline and in the axilla. Which of the following lab values would help you confirm the diagnosis?

A. Elevated TSH
B. Low testosterone levels
C. Decreased LH/FSH ratio
D. Elevated serum dehydroepiandrosterone sulfate (DHEA-S)
E. Normal lipid profile

The next 2 questions (items 49-50) correspond to the following vignette.

A 13-year-old female complains of heavy menses. Menarche occurred 3 months ago. Her periods are irregular and consist of bleeding for 5 to 7 days. She denies passing any blood clots. She has to change her pad once during the night and 4 to 5 times during the day. There are no bleeding disorders in her family. Her hemoglobin is 10.

49. What is the most likely etiology of her menometrorrhagia?

    A. Pregnancy
    B. Idiopathic thrombocytopenic purpura (ITP)
    C. Cervical polyp
    D. Foreign body
    E. Immature hypothalamic-pituitary-ovarian axis

50. Which of the following would be the most appropriate management of the patient above with dysfunctional bleeding?

    A. Observe
    B. Start iron therapy
    C. Initiate oral contraceptives
    D. Ibuprofen during menses
    E. Transfuse with 15 cc/kg of packed red blood cells
    F. Start iron therapy and initiate oral contraceptives
    G. Start iron therapy, initiate oral contraceptives, and administer ibuprofen during menses
    H. Transfuse with 15 cc/kg of packed red blood cells, and administer ibuprofen during menses

End of Set

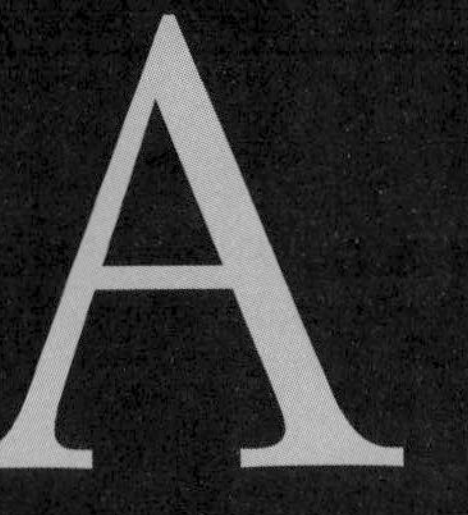

Answers and Explanations

1. A
2. C
3. E
4. A
5. E
6. D
7. B
8. C
9. B
10. E
11. A
12. D
13. A
14. C
15. A
16. C
17. D
18. C
19. C
20. B
21. E
22. B
23. D
24. C
25. E
26. E
27. B
28. D
29. A
30. E
31. C
32. D
33. C
34. A
35. D
36. D
37. A
38. D
39. C
40. A
41. D
42. E
43. D
44. B
45. D
46. D
47. E
48. D
49. E
50. G

1. **A. One of the more dangerous conditions that may present as leukocoria in this age group is retinoblastoma. Retinoblastoma should be ruled out before an extensive further work-up is initiated, particularly in the otherwise asymptomatic child. In addition to a full eye exam, radiographic evaluation of the globe for calcification is critical. Because an MRI may miss the calcification, a CT scan is considered the imaging study of choice.**

   B. With careful monitoring by an ophthalmologist, aggressive steroid use is the key to reducing this uveitis.
   C. The more common infectious, or peri-infectious causes of leukocoria include CMV, toxoplasmosis, syphilis, and toxocara. These entities should be considered *after* retinoblastoma has been ruled out. Tuberculosis and rubella can also create this form of inflammation. There are hundreds of other infectious agents that can be underlying the uveitis, but clinical suspicion must guide evaluation.
   D. In order to prevent papillary occlusion with 360° scarring of the iris border to the lens, dilation of the pupillary sphincter is performed. The strength and frequency of the agent used depends on the degree of inflammation and presence of iris adhesions.
   E. This particular patient has no other symptoms of fever, arthritis, or rash to suggest the initial diagnosis of juvenile rheumatoid arthritis (JRA). Although JRA is unusual at this age, it certainly occurs, and must be considered in the evaluation *after* retinoblastoma has been ruled out. Pauciarticular, rheumatoid factor (RF)-negative, ANA-positive patients need to be screened about every 3 months because their uveitis can have such an insidious onset.

2. **C. The patient in this picture has pityriasis alba, a common skin disorder that presents with discrete areas of hypopigmentation typically on the face, neck, and upper trunk. The underlying etiology is unknown but the lesions appear or are often worsened by sun exposure. Topical corticosteroids and lubrication have been shown to help with resolution of the lesions.**

   A. There is no need for dermatology referral at this point, although vitiligo should be considered in the differential diagnosis.
   B. Griseofulvin would be indicated for the treatment of tinea corporis.
   D. Topical selenium sulfide shampoo would be useful for the treatment of tinea versicolor, another entity to consider in the differential. Tinea versicolor is typically more widespread on the trunk, upper extremities, and occasionally on the face; the lesions are also more prominent following sun exposure. They would be expected to have a copper-orange or bronzed appearance under Wood's light.
   E. Diphenhydramine (Benadryl) would be indicated to control pruritis.

3. **E. Reassure the parents that internal tibial torsion is a common condition that causes an in-toed gait.**

   A, C, D. The condition resolves spontaneously and requires no casts, special shoes, bars, or braces.
   B. Radiographs are not necessary. As in this case, the diagnosis is made from the physical examination.

4. **A. The EMG results in myasthenia gravis are more specific than a muscle biopsy. The muscle potentials would be expected to fall quickly in amplitude with repetitive stimulation.**

   B. An EEG will not reveal any information regarding muscle function.
   C. Anti-acetylcholine antibodies are not always demonstrated in the serum.
   D. Muscle biopsies are generally not helpful in patients with myasthenia gravis.
   E. CPK level should be normal in patients with myasthenia gravis.

5. **E. Nonorganic failure to thrive, as suspected in this scenario, can both be diagnosed and treated with observed feedings and a calorie count within a supervised inpatient setting.**

   A, B, C, D. Any further radiographic or invasive diagnostic procedures should be reserved until it is firmly established that the child does not gain weight on adequate calories.

6. **D. This patient has Prader-Willi syndrome, which is associated with interstitial deletion of chromosome 15. Typical features include severe hypoglycemia and hypotonia in the newborn period. Infants usually have feeding difficulties and grow poorly. Older children commonly develop an excessive appetite and can become morbidly obese, which further contributes to sleep apnea.**

A. The hypotonia can be very severe in infancy but usually abates between 6 months and 6 years.
B. Mental retardation is seen in virtually all patients with Prader-Willi syndrome. Retardation is mild in 63%, moderate in 31%, and severe in 6%.
C. Ataxia is not a feature of Prader-Willi syndrome.
E. Cardiac and skeletal defects are not part of Prader-Willi syndrome.

7. **B. Encopresis (passage of feces into inappropriate places) is a complication of chronic constipation. In encopresis, loose stool usually leaks out around the large, hard, retained stool in the rectum. The most important initial step in the treatment of chronic constipation is complete evacuation of any retained stool in the rectum. As long as the rectum is dilated, rectal tone will remain low and regular stooling will not be achieved. Use of hypertonic phosphate enemas is usually tried first. If enemas are unsuccessful, NG administration of hypertonic electrolyte solutions with polyethylene glycol may be needed. Patients with chronic constipation will also need therapy to prevent reaccumulation of stool. This is often done with lubricants (mineral oil) or mild laxatives (senna). High-fiber diets are recommended. Bowel training and behavioral therapy are also very important.**

A. As in the explanation for B, high-fiber diet is recommended.
C. On a daily basis, on awakening and after dinner, the child should sit on the toilet and attempt to have a bowel movement. However, an excessive amount of time, such as 30 minutes, spent on the toilet can have a negative effect.
D. Most patients with chronic constipation and encopresis will not require a barium enema. However, a history of delayed passage of meconium/stool in the first 48 hours, or chronic constipation since birth would be suspicious for Hirschprung disease and mandate further investigation with a barium enema and subsequent rectal biopsy.
E. Patients who do not respond to medical treatment or who have obvious emotional stressors may benefit from seeing a child psychiatrist. Biofeedback techniques have also been helpful in many cases. The prognosis is usually good and many patients are better in 4 to 6 months.

8. **C. This patient's syndrome is ataxia-telangiectasia (Louis-Barr syndrome). Thymic hypoplasia with poor organization and lack of Hassall corpuscles is a common feature.**

A. Ataxia-telangiectasia is transmitted as an autosomal recessive trait. The abnormal gene is located on chromosome 11, and the gene product is a DNA-dependent protein kinase involved in mitogenic signal transduction.
B. Gammaglobulin abnormalities are associated with ataxia-telangiectasia, but agammaglobulinemia is not present. IgG is usually low, and IgA is frequently absent. IgM may be of low molecular weight.
D. The ataxia in ataxia-telangiectasia is progressive, and these patients are usually confined to a wheelchair in middle or late childhood.
E. In ataxia-telangiectasia, CD3 and CD4 T-cells are moderately reduced. These patients are at increased risk of lymphoreticular cancers, and even adenocarcinomas.

9. **B. This ultrasound reveals a large fluid-filled cyst in the posterior fossa, with proximal dilatation of the ventricular system. A Dandy-Walker cyst results from developmental failure of the roof of the fourth ventricle during embryogenesis. The resulting dilatation of the fourth ventricle results in a cystic appearance, and most of these infants develop hydrocephalus and progressive neurological impairment. Shunting procedures will help reduce the neurological sequelae.**

A. In hydranencephaly there are only remnants of the cerebrum and cerebral cortex, and the remainder of the cranium is filled with fluid.
C. A shunting procedure would relieve the increasing hydrocephalus and allay much of the neurological impairment in Dandy-Walker malformation.
D. The hydrocephalus related to myelomeningocele is generally associated with elongation of the fourth ventricle and kinking of the brain stem, with displacement of the pons and medulla into the cervical canal. The fourth ventricle is not usually cystic. Shunting procedures are used to allay the affects of increasing hydrocephalus.
E. Most Dandy-Walker malformations are not benign and will require shunting.

10. E. While the C3 can be normal, it is low in about 90% of cases. This is the only listed feature which would be expected.

A. Endocapillary proliferation of mesangial cells and polymorphonuclear infiltration in the glomeruli are characteristic pathologic findings in PSGN. Basement membranes are not thin in this disease.
B. Hypertension is expected, most often secondary to fluid retention, and occurs early.
C. The immunologic response to streptococcal antigens is usually seen early in PSGN, but is not limited to ASO. Other anti-strep titers such as anti-streptokinase, anti-DNAase, and anti-NADase are also elevated.
D. Tubular function is often spared. Glomerular filtration is impaired secondary to the proliferative process and immune complex deposition that occurs in the glomeruli.

11. A. In utero exposure to cocaine has been associated with a number of complications that include cardiac defects, intracranial hemorrhage, necrotizing enterocolitis, placental abruption, as well as low apgars, prematurity, fetal distress, intrauterine growth retardation, and genitourinary malformations. Long-term sequelae include behavioral problems, attention and concentration deficits, and an increased probability of learning disabilities.

B. Preterm, rather than postterm, delivery is associated with intrauterine cocaine exposure.
C. Microcephalus, rather than hydrocephalus, is associated with intrauterine cocaine exposure.
D. Placental abruption, rather than placenta previa, is associated with intrauterine cocaine exposure.
E. Hearing loss has not specifically been shown to be related to cocaine exposure.

12. D. Following the one-time treatment of permethrin 1% rinse for head lice, it is suspected that about 20% to 30% of the eggs will still remain. For this reason it is recommended that retreatment occur approximately 7 to 10 days later.

A. Head lice are transmitted usually by direct contact with an infected human source. They cannot fly or jump as commonly thought.
B. Head lice themselves do not carry infectious diseases. Secondary staphylococcal or streptococcal infections may occur following excessive scalp itching.
C. Head lice require a human host to survive. Without a host, they typically die within 1 day. The theoretic risk of transmission from inanimate objects is therefore thought to be extremely rare.
E. The American Academy of Pediatrics (AAP) recommends that a healthy child should not be excluded from school for head lice. Much controversy exists over "no nit" policies and it is believed that by the time the diagnosis of head lice has been made, more than a month of infestation has probably been ongoing.

13. A. Obesity is becoming more of a problem in the younger pediatric population. In a majority of cases, a thorough dietary history of increased caloric intake, coupled with the lack of physical activity and positive family history of obesity, will be essential in arriving at the diagnosis. The physical exam will be normal in most cases as will laboratory testing.

B, E. Obesity increases the risk factor for further development of insulin resistance and hence diabetes, as well as complications of hyperlipidemia, sleep apnea, slipped capital femoral epiphysis, and a variety of other disorders.
C. Although screening for hypothyroidism in circumstances of excessive weight gain is certainly reasonable, there are no other symptoms such as dry hair, hypothermia, or bradycardia to suggest this diagnosis.
D. As in the explanation for A, a dietary history of excessive caloric intake would be expected in this child. Further dietary modifications and possible consultation with a nutritionist would be essential in the management of an obese child.

14. C. Risk factors for peanut allergy include family history, atopy, maternal exposure to peanuts in the diet, soymilk exposure, and peanut oil exposure to the skin. It would be useful to educate the family regarding future potential exposures and have them educated in first aid and CPR. In case of emergencies, a prescription for an Epipen Jr and instructions on its use is essential.

A. Up to 25% of children will outgrow peanut allergy.
B. Peanut allergy is one of the most common types of food allergy in children.
D. The prevalence of peanut allergy is actually increasing.
E. Peanut allergy is mediated by IgE.

15. A. While biliary atresia can occasionally be due to intrahepatic obstruction, 85% of cases are due to obliteration of the extrahepatic ducts.

B. Biliary atresia is seen in 1 in 10,000 to 15,000 births, while neonatal hepatitis is found in 1 in 5,000 to 10,000 births.

C. The gall bladder may be small or absent in bilary atresia, but the same ultrasound findings can be seen with neonatal hepatitis, cystic fibrosis, or total parenteral nutrition.

D. A percutaneous liver biopsy is the best test to differentiate biliary atresia from neonatal hepatitis. Biliary atresia is characterized by bile duct proliferation, bile plugs, portal edema, or fibrosis, with the basic hepatic lobular architecture remaining intact. By contrast, in neonatal hepatitis there is severe hepatocellular disease with inflammatory cells and focal necrosis, but with little change in the bile ductules.

E. It is important to consider the diagnosis of biliary atresia early in any child with direct hyperbilirubinemia; the success of the Kasai procedure is highest if performed in the first 8 weeks of life. Delay in diagnosis and surgical management of cholestasis will lead to progressive bile duct obliteration and cirrhosis.

16. C. The most common source of dental flora is the mother or another intimate care provider. Caries should be considered an infectious and preventable disease that is vertically transmitted from mothers or other intimate caregivers to infants. Prevention of maternal dental decay will decrease the likelihood of caries in the baby.

A. Dental caries result from an overgrowth of normal bacterial flora (*Streptococcus mutans*, Lactobacillus).

B. Babies become colonized between 6 and 30 months of life.

D. The mother's dental history has a direct correlation on the development of caries in the baby. If the mother has frequent sugar intake, low fluoride exposure, poor oral hygiene, active decay or multiple fillings, and/or infrequent dental visits, the baby is more likely to have caries. Dental flora can be inhibited and caries prevented by fluoride intake, good hygiene, and avoidance of sugary foods. Children who sleep with bottles or breastfeed throughout the night are more likely to get dental decay.

E. Low socioeconomic status has also been identified as a risk factor for caries.

17. D. A child with poor weight gain, diarrhea, and multiple bouts of wheezing and pneumonia should be evaluated for cystic fibrosis (CF) with a sweat chloride test. CF is an autosomal recessive transmitted disease caused by a mutation of the CF transmembrane regulator (CFTR) gene on chromosome 7. Typical clinical findings in CF include acute or persistent respiratory symptoms, failure to thrive with malnutrition, malabsorption and/or abnormal stools, rectal prolapse, nasal polyps, sinus disease, and chronic liver disease.

A. Inadequate caloric intake is rarely a cause of poor growth in a child of this age.

B. The diagnosis of asthma may be incorrect in this case, especially given the history of poor weight gain. Patients with CF will often wheeze and present as uncontrolled asthmatics.

C. Sinusitis has been shown to cause wheezing and patients with CF often get sinusitis. In this case, however, there are no signs or symptoms of sinusitis, except for chronic cough.

E. CF is associated with malabsorption due to pancreatic insufficiency. The strong respiratory history is more typical of CF than of Crohn disease.

18. C. The noisy breathing in cases of laryngomalacia results from soft airway cartilage and the resultant collapse of supraglottic structures during inspiration.

A. Laryngomalacia is the most common congenital laryngeal abnormality and the most frequent cause of stridor in infants. Laryngomalacia does not cause expiratory wheezing.

B. The symptoms appear within 2 weeks of life and increase in severity for up to 6 months.

D. Because some cases are associated with other airway structural abnormalities, bronchoscopy may be indicated in more severe cases. A patient with swallowing dysfunction will require a contrast swallow study and esophogram. Among other conditions that must be considered in an infant with stridor are congenital and acquired subglottic stenosis, papillomas, vocal cord paralysis, and congenital laryngeal webs and atresia.

E. In most cases, the stridor disappears as the child becomes older. Tracheostomy is rarely needed.

19. **C. A malar rash and a positive anti-DNA antibody test (immunologic disorder) are both diagnostic criteria for lupus. The arthritis and positive ANA that this patient has are two more criteria. *Therefore, this patient has the necessary four* of the 11 criteria to make the diagnosis of SLE. The other seven criteria are discoid rash, photosensitivity rash, oral ulcers, serositis, nephritis, neurologic disease, and hematologic disorder.**

A. This patient has arthritis and a positive ANA, both major criteria in the diagnosis of lupus. However, four of 11 criteria are needed to confirm the diagnosis and this patient is exhibiting only two.

B. In addition to lupus, a positive ANA can occur with certain drugs, JRA, other collagen vascular diseases, infectious mononucleosis, chronic active hepatitis, and normal individuals. The absence of ANA in childhood lupus is rare. Therefore, an ANA has high sensitivity (percentage with disease who will test positive) and a low positive predictive value (percentage of those with a positive test who will have the disease).

D. Lupus nephritis in children and adolescents is a major cause of long-term morbidity, and frequently culminates in chronic renal failure.

E. Lupus patients have a very active immune system and frequently produce a variety of autoantibodies such as anti-phospholipid, anti-thyroid, anti-coagulant, and Coombs antibodies. Such antibodies are responsible for some of the protean manifestations in lupus patients.

20. **B. Aggressive environmental intervention is important for lead levels between 25 and 45 μg/dL. With a blood lead level of 30 μg/dL, the first step would be to have the local public health authorities perform a home visit to determine the risk factors within the home and to take steps to remove the child from exposure. At this lead level, environmental intervention to remove lead from the home is the most appropriate approach.**

A. Chelation therapy is recommended for lead levels between 45 and 70 μg/dL.

C. Admission to the hospital for observation and repeat lead levels is not necessary unless chelation is planned.

D. A referral to public health authorities, rather than child welfare services, is more appropriate in this setting.

E. X-rays of the long bones can show dense bands at the metaphyses that occur after months to years of exposure. However, normal x-rays do not rule out lead exposure. The most important approach to managing this patient is eliminating the source of lead.

21. **E. Studies have shown that ambulatory blood pressure monitoring can identify significant hypertension much better than intermittent measurements. It is the best way to rule out "white coat" hypertension.**

A. Any treatment for high blood pressure is not appropriate until significant hypertension is confirmed. Significant hypertension is defined as BP readings consistently above the 95th percentile for height and age.

B. Sodium restriction would be recommended if the blood pressure was confirmed to be in the hypertensive range.

C. A renal ultrasound would be useful once significant hypertension has been confirmed by ambulatory monitoring.

D. Advising that this blood pressure is in the upper normal range for her age would suggest you do not know the definition of hypertension.

22. **B. Using Jones criteria, subcutaneous nodules is a major criterion, and fever and arthralgia are minor criteria. One major, two minors, and evidence of recent group A streptococcal infection makes the diagnosis. The major Jones criteria include migratory polyarthritis, carditis, subcutaneous nodules, erythema marginatum, and Sydenham chorea. The minor criteria include fever, arthralgia, elevated ESR/C-reactive protein (ESR/CRP), and prolonged PR interval.**

A. Arthralgia is a minor criterion and erythema marginatum is a major criterion. Required are two majors, or one major and two minors, plus evidence of a preceding group A streptococcus infection. There is not enough evidence for the diagnosis.

C. Using Jones criteria, there is no major manifestation of rheumatic fever here. Arthralgia and prolonged PR interval are minor manifestations, and erythema multiforme is neither a major nor a minor manifestation. See explanation for B for the full diagnostic criteria.

D. Arthralgia, fever, and elevated ESR/CRP are three minor criteria. See explanation for B for the full diagnostic criteria.

E. Arthritis is a major criterion, but there are no minor manifestations. Even though there is evidence of a recent group A streptococcus infection, there is not enough evidence for the diagnosis.

23. **D. In early slipped capital femoral epiphysis (SCFE) the AP radiograph may not demonstrate the abnormality. A frog lateral is the best x-ray view and should be obtained in all suspected cases of SCFE.**

A. SCFE can be seen as a complication of an underlying endocrine disease, such as hypothyroidism. When SCFE occurs before puberty, an investigation for a systemic disease or endocrine disorder is warranted.
B. SCFE occurs more commonly in obese adolescent patients with a 3:1 male predominance, but it does occur also in tall thin adolescents with a recent growth spurt and delayed skeletal maturation.
C. SCFE is not commonly seen in females beyond puberty.
E. Patients with SCFE have a 30% incidence of occurrence on the other side.

24. **C. The patient suffers from iron deficiency anemia secondary to microscopic GI blood loss from excessive milk ingestion; 18 to 20 ounces of milk per day would be more appropriate. The total iron binding capacity is increased with iron deficiency anemia as iron binding sites are more available.**

A. The RDW measures variations in the size of RBCs and increases with iron deficiency.
B. Serum ferritin levels decline and are the earliest marker of iron deficiency. Serum ferritin is also an acute phase reactant that can become elevated in the presence of inflammation.
D. The reticulocyte count measures circulating immature RBCs and decreases with iron deficiency.
E. Decreased serum iron levels would be expected as iron stores in the bone marrow are depleted.

25. **E. Many babies who are not seriously dehydrated can be treated with oral solutions, thus avoiding hospitalization and complications of IV fluid therapy. Rehydration fluids should contain a high sodium content (50–90 mEq/L) and a small amount of glucose (2.0% to 2.5%). Oral rehydration uses a process called cotransport, in which a molecule of glucose promotes the absorption of a molecule of sodium from the small intestine. As sodium is rapidly absorbed from the intestine, water absorption follows.**

A. This solution does not contain enough sodium to promote adequate water absorption from the gut lumen.
B, C. A small amount of glucose is needed for the cotransport process.
D. Solutions high in glucose have a high osmotic load and will draw water into the lumen of the intestine, rather than promoting sodium and water absorption, potentially worsening the diarrhea. Juices, soft drinks, and punches are not appropriate for oral rehydration because they lack sodium and have a high glucose content.

26. **E. The CT scan of the orbit demonstrates the presence of purulent material in the orbit, typical of orbital cellulites. Orbital cellulitis may be associated with decreased or painful ocular movement, proptosis (protrusion of eye), or chemosis (edema of the bulbar conjunctiva due to poor venous or lymphatic drainage). Commonly, the lids are so swollen that an adequate examination is impossible and a CT scan is needed to evaluate the orbital contents. Infection often is secondary to sinusitis. Empiric antibiotic coverage should provide activity against *S. aureus, Streptococcus pyogenes, S. pneumoniae, H. influenza, M. catarrhalis,* and anaerobic bacteria of the upper respiratory tract. Ampicillin-sulbactam would be a good choice. If there is a large, well-defined abscess, complete ophthalmoplegia, or vision impairment, surgical drainage of the abscess and the adjacent sinus may be necessary.**

A. Orbital cellulitis is a dangerous condition that requires immediate IV antibiotic administration and surgical evaluation.
B. A swollen eye due to an allergic reaction from a mosquito bite is not usually painful and tense. The CT scan would show periorbital swelling, but the orbit would appear normal. Periorbital (preseptal) cellulitis may also cause a swollen eye with a normal orbital scan. This condition requires antibiotic administration, but does not generally need surgical consultation.
C. Amoxicillin would not provide adequate treatment for the organisms that commonly cause orbital cellulitis.
D. Antihistamines and local application of ice are not appropriate treatments for this child.

27. **B. In cases of pyloric stenosis, there may be a palpable, hard, mobile, nontender mass in the epigastrium, just to the right of the midline. Visible peristaltic waves may be seen, especially just after the baby has been fed.**

   A. With persistent vomiting there is loss of potassium as well as hydrogen ion and chloride, resulting in the classic presentation of a hypokalemic, hypochloremic metabolic alkalosis.
   C. Jaundice can been seen with pyloric stenosis and other forms of intestinal obstruction.
   D. When accompanied by the typical history of projectile vomiting after feeding, the presence of the two physical findings of peristaltic gastric waves and a palpable olive-sized mass makes further diagnostic studies unnecessary.
   E. Pyloric stenosis is a medical emergency, not a surgical emergency. Bowel necrosis and perforation are not complications of pyloric stenosis. Electrolyte abnormalities should be corrected prior to surgery.

28. **D. Umbilical hernias are often seen in low-birth weight babies and in babies with certain metabolic abnormalities, such as hypothyroidism and mucopolysaccharidoses.**

   A. Umbilical hernias usually resolve spontaneously. Because strangulation is extremely rare, surgical correction is not usually recommended unless the hernia persists past age 4 or 5 years, or if the abdominal wall defect is very large (greater than 2 cm).
   B. Umbilical hernias are much more common in African-American babies.
   C. Strangulation of umbilical hernias is rare and much less common than with inguinal hernias.
   E. Taping a coin over the abdominal wall defect in order to keep the hernia from protruding is not effective and may actually delay spontaneous closure.

29. **A. The dark, velvety, rugated skin on the back of her neck is acanthosis nigricans (AN) and is not due to poor hygiene as is sometimes misdiagnosed.**

   B, C, D, E. Although AN is most commonly associated with type II diabetes mellitus, it can be associated with all of the other disorders listed as well: chronic fatty infiltration of the liver and cirrhosis, polycystic ovarian syndrome, and hypothyroidism.

30. **E. This child's growth pattern is typical of constitutional growth delay. The birth height is normal, the child's height velocity drops off at about 1 year of age, and the child is growing at a normal rate again by 3 years of age. Commonly, the parent of the same gender had short stature as a child but attained normal height as an adult. The growth pattern and family history in this case are typical of constitutional growth delay; no further tests are needed. Of course, if normal growth had not resumed by 3 years of age, further evaluation would have been needed.**

   A. Referral to an endocrinologist is expensive and unnecessary.
   B. The child is eating an adequate diet. Excessive caloric intake could cause obesity.
   C. These tests would be valuable in the determining the cause of short stature due to an organic disease. This child's growth pattern should be considered a normal variant.
   D. The bone age in patients with constitutional growth delay will be less than their chronological age. *The discrepancy between bone age and chronological age can be used to counsel parents* that their child has the potential for catch-up growth. Typically, when other children stop growing in late adolescence, teens with constitutional growth delay continue to grow and catch up to their peers.

31. **C. In this case, the history and physical examination are very typical of viral croup (laryngotracheobronchitis). Croup occurs primarily in the fall and winter and is most often caused by parainfluenza and respiratory syncytial viruses. Patients usually have signs and symptoms of upper respiratory tract infection, a characteristic barky cough, and inspiratory stridor. Viral croup is common in children under age 3. Most children with viral croup can be managed as outpatients with supportive care, oral hydration, humidified air, and parental reassurance.**

   A. The typical radiographic finding in croup is subglottic edema with the classic "steeple sign"; however, most patients do not need radiographic studies unless there is concern about epiglottitis, foreign body aspiration, or other causes of sever upper airway obstruction.
   B. Because croup is a viral illness, antibiotics are not necessary.

D. In moderately severe cases, hospitalization can sometimes be avoided by the use of racemic epinephrine inhalation treatments and a single dose of dexamethasone given via the IM, IV, or oral route.
E. The most severe cases of croup should be hospitalized and may even require endotracheal intubation and management in a pediatric intensive care unit. As the patient in this scenario is well hydrated without any signs of respiratory distress, hypoxia, or resting stridor, outpatient management is more appropriate at this time.

32. **D. An intussusception is the telescoping of a part of the bowel into an adjacent part of the bowel. Almost 90% of cases of intussusception are ileocolic, but ileoileal and colocolic types do occur.**

A. Intussusception can be seen at any age, but is most common in infants 6 to 12 months old.
B. The classic presentation is intermittent abdominal pain and vomiting with blood and mucus in the stools, however, the classical "currant-jelly" stools are seen in only half the cases, so intussusception must be considered even if stools are normal.
C. A lead point is commonly found in children over 5, but rarely in children under 2 years old. Several structures can serve as a lead point, including a polyp, lymphoma, hematoma from Henoch-Schönlein purpura (HSP) or hemophilia, hemangioma, and duplication cysts.
E. Reduction of an intussusception by barium or air enema can be achieved in about 75% of cases. If these procedures fail to reduce the intussusception, immediate surgery is required. Delays in diagnosis can lead to severe complications including bowel necrosis, bowel perforation, severe gastrointestinal bleeding, sepsis, and shock.

33. **C. Metatarsus adductus is a very common deformity of the forefoot in which the metatarsals are deviated medially. Most cases will resolve spontaneously without treatment.**

A. This orthopedic condition is due to intrauterine molding and is usually bilateral.
B. Treatment depends on the severity of the deformity. In cases where the forefoot can easily be manipulated into the normal position, passive muscle stretching several times a day may help, but most cases resolve without any treatment. There is no reason for orthopedic referral, radiographs, or special shoes in young babies with flexible metatarsus adductus.
D. If the condition has not resolved by the time the baby needs shoes (~9 months), referral to an orthopedist for casting is appropriate. Referral at 2 to 3 months is not indicated.
E. If, on initial examination, the foot is not flexible and the forefoot cannot be moved into the normal position, referral to an orthopedic surgeon for 6 to 8 weeks of casting is indicated. Surgery is not commonly needed at a young age. Metatarsus adductus in children older than 4 to 6 years of age may require operative correction, but this is an unusual situation.

34. **A. An audiogram demonstrating significant nerve deafness in this patient would support the diagnosis of familial nephritis with deafness. The urine should demonstrate red cell casts and dysmorphic red cells. Familial nephritis in males generally leads to chronic renal failure, which may be insidious and asymptomatic. Blood chemistries are definitely indicated.**

B. There is enough evidence by history to move on with an investigation.
C. A renal biopsy will not be indicated if familial nephritis is demonstrated by other investigation.
D. This patient's mother and his uncle will demonstrate nephritic urine (red blood cells and RBC casts). The mode of transmission of familial nephritis with deafness is most often X-linked dominant and rarely autosomal dominant, and the carrier will have hematuria. The female carrier will frequently have silent microscopic hematuria. Males will develop renal failure and progressive nerve deafness. Hematuria in familial nephritis is due to glomerular bleeding, and therefore the red cells present in the urine are generally abnormal in appearance (dysmorphic), indicative of glomerular bleeding.
E. An ASO titer will not be indicated with the evidence presented.

35. **D. The x-ray demonstrates a rather typical TB primary complex with a parenchymal infiltrate and regional lymphadenopathy. There is a right upper lobe infiltrate with right hilar adenopathy. This is suspicious for primary TB infection and the child should be admitted to the hospital for AFB collection. In younger children who do not have a productive cough, the collection of early morning NG aspirates upon awakening on 3 consecutive days should be performed.**

A. It would not be appropriate to await purified protein derivative (PPD) results in this case. The tuberculin skin test generally is positive 3 weeks to 3 months after the exposure. This patient's x-ray would suggest the inoculation was at least 1 to 2 months ago and is suspicious for active disease. Therefore, the test should be positive. However, about 10% of immunocompetent children will not develop the delayed hypersensitivity for several months.

B. Sputum collection for AFB is reserved for older children and adolescents who generally have a more productive cough.

C. The treatment of TB is with multidrug therapy. The use of INH alone is reserved for patients with TB exposure who have a positive PPD and negative chest x-ray.

E. Simple observation of this patient is not appropriate management.

36. **D. Acute infectious diarrhea is a very common entity in pediatrics. Causes include bacteria, viruses, parasites, and preformed toxins. A conservative approach is appropriate when there are no underlying medical problems that exist and there is no evidence for invasive disease (bloody stools and/or white blood cells). If oral rehydration is possible then admission to the hospital can be avoided and stool for culture can be sent as an outpatient. Antibiotics are not indicated unless a specific organism is found or unless there are critical medical issues, such as sepsis or immunocompromise.**

A, C. Stool studies should be sent and the diagnosis confirmed before antimicrobial or parasitic therapy is initiated.

B. This child is only mildly dehydrated and deserves a trial of oral rehydration therapy before being admitted to the hospital.

E. A health department investigation would be indicated if a sudden epidemic were to occur at the camp.

37. **A. An audiogram will give objective information regarding hearing and is essential in every evaluation for speech delay.**

B, E. Any radiological imaging, particularly a CT of inner ear structures, is not routine or useful in the evaluation of a hearing deficit unless specific physical findings, such as a cholesteatoma, are seen.

C. An EEG will only give brainwave information and not any information regarding hearing.

D. Speech therapists are experts in this area and are highly useful in language acquisition. However, an objective measure of hearing is necessary before any therapy is initiated.

38. **D. The treatment of migraines is aimed at prophylaxis and acute symptomatic treatment. Avoidance of inciting factors and the prophylactic use of propranolol have been shown to help prevent further attacks.**

A. Sumatriptan is not approved for use in children.

B. Narcotics have not been proven beneficial in the management of classic migraines.

C. OTC analgesia, such as ibuprofen, and antiemetics will help with relief during an acute episode but will not prevent further episodes.

E. Effective preventative treatment, as described above, does exist.

39. **C. There is no immunoglobulin deposition in minimal change nephrotic syndrome.**

A. Complement levels are normal in minimal change nephrotic syndrome. Other types of immune-mediated nephrotic syndromes may have low serum complement levels as well as complement deposition in the glomeruli.

B. Minimal change nephrotic syndrome is always accompanied by hyperlipidemia, and all of the lipids are elevated, including cholesterol and triglycerides. This is not specific for this type of nephrosis. Nephrotic syndrome consists of edema, proteinuria exceeding more than 2 g/24 hr, hypoalbuminemia, and hyperlipidemia.

D. About 80% of children with minimal change nephrotic syndrome will respond to glucocorticoid therapy.

E. Other terms for this nephrotic syndrome include minimal change nephrosis, nil disease, and lipoid nephrosis. There is generally a lack of abnormal findings on *light microscopy*. The "minimal change" feature is the fusion or effacement of the podocytes of the epithelial cells along the basement membrane seen by *electron microscopy*.

40. **A. The most common bacterial cause of pneumonia in this age group is *Streptococcus pneumoniae*. Although viral infections are believed to cause over 80% of the pneumonias in children, the described case has features to suggest bacterial infection: segmental infiltrate, high fever, and localized crackles.**

B. RSV is the most common infecting organism in the lower respiratory tract for children less than 1 year of age, causing mostly bronchiolitis and pneumonia.
C. Children usually have primary pneumonia with *M. tuberculosis* rather than reactivation TB seen in adults; therefore, this could be TB.
D. Although foreign body aspiration can present as a left lower lobe infiltrate, the child is a little older than the usual age (about 2 to 3 years) and the radiographic appearance is more commonly isolated overinflation of the segment partially blocked by the foreign body. Foreign bodies occur on the right side more often than the left side.
E. Pneumococcal pneumonia does lead to parapneumonic effusion and empyema, but in less than 20% of pneumonias. Based on the information given, there is no way to predict whether this patient will develop an effusion or not.

41. **D. Referral to a urologist is indicated in this patient with cryptorchidism. Atrophy and delayed testicular development can be seen as early as 1 year in an undescended testis. Exploratory laporatomy with orchioplexy would be indicated once the testis is located.**

A. Most studies show that a testis that has not descended by 12 weeks is unlikely to do so.
B. Hormone therapy is infrequently successful and germ cell loss in the cryptorchid testis can occur as early as 6 months.
C, E. MRI, CT, and ultrasound are not reliable in identifying an intra-abdominal testis, as bowel loops and viscera tend to obscure the testis.

42. **E. The protective equilibrium response results when the child is pushed laterally by an examiner. The child flexes the trunk toward the force in order to regain the center of gravity while at the same time the arm opposite the force extends to protect against a fall. It does not normally appear until 4 to 6 months of age and then persists voluntarily.**

A, B, C, D. The other primitive reflexes listed, including startle, hand grasp, crossed adductor, and toe grasp are all present at birth and then disappear over the first 15 months of life.

43. **D. The most likely diagnosis is nickel dermatitis of the abdominal skin due to contact of the abdominal skin with the metal snap on his jeans; this would account for the central abdominal location of the lesion.**

A. The lower mid-abdomen is the wrong location for scabies in a 6-year-old child. Scabies lesions are intensely pruritic and often present in the interdiginous areas of the hands and feet, as well as creases of the neck and axillae.
B. HSP lesions are purpuric, not polymorphous macules, by definition, and are often located on the lower extremities and areas of dependent pressure.
C. The description of this rash does not fit well with poison ivy, especially the central lesion. Poison ivy contact usually occurs on the extremities.
E. Psoriatic lesions are red with a silvery scale and typically present on the extensor surfaces. However, they can sometimes present on the flexor surfaces or central location as described in this scenario.

44. **B. This patient's examination is typical of allergic rhinitis. The allergic gape (continuous open-mouth breathing) and allergic shiners (dark circles under eyes) are classic findings. Patients may also demonstrate an "allergic salute," an upward rubbing of the nose with an open palm or extended fingers. This maneuver may cause an allergic crease across the bridge of the nose. The watery discharge and nonerythematous mucous membranes are also typical. Many patients with allergic rhinitis will have conjunctival erythema and itching.**

A. Children whose mothers smoke heavily are at higher risk for developing allergic rhinitis. Other risk factors include family history of atopy, early introduction of foods, heavy exposure to indoor allergens, and higher socioeconomic group.
C. In allergic rhinitis, eosinophils are seen on the nasal smear.
D. Dog and cat allergens are a major problem. Secretions from saliva and sebaceous secretions can remain airborne for long periods. Children can also carry cat allergen on their clothes, thus exposing allergic patients even in cat-free environments. The only effective measure for evading animal allergens in the home is the removal of pets.
E. Oral antihistamines can be used for patients with mild, intermittent symptoms. Patients with more severe symptoms may require treatment with intranasal corticosteroids. If these are not effective, referral to an allergist for skin testing and possible immunotherapy (allergy shots) is indicated.

45. D. Only in alopecia areata is the skin characteristically smooth, shiny, not scaly, and devoid of broken hairs.

A, B, C, E. Tinea capitus, traction alopecia, trichotillomania, and contact dermatitis to a hair product would all show broken-off hairs and irritation of the skin.

46. D. The child described in the vignette has congenital hypothyroidism. Its incidence approximates 1 in 4000 and is nearly universally screened for in the United States with newborn screening programs. If children receive treatment by 1 month of age IQ is usually normal, but if treatment is delayed beyond 3 months, then IQ can fall below 70. Symptoms of congenital hypothyroidism can include feeding problems, constipation, prolonged jaundice, enlarged posterior fontanel, tongue thrust, and a hoarse cry.

A, B, C. Abdominal radiograph, CBC, blood culture, and barium swallow studies would all be normal and not aid in the diagnosis of hypothyroidism.

E. Admission to the hospital for an FTT evaluation and monitoring of nutritional status would not yield a diagnosis unless thyroid function tests are obtained.

47. E. The rash shown in the photo is typical of erythema infectiousum, also called Fifth disease. In normal children, this is a mild self-limited illness caused by parvovirus B19. Generally no treatment is needed and no postexposure prophylaxis is required.

A. Amoxicillin is not indicated in the treatment of Fifth disease.

B. Immunocompromised children and children with chronic hemolysis may develop anemia, bone marrow suppression, chronic infection, and intense viremia. Such children should not attend school and should avoid exposing pregnant women to the virus. An infected fetus can develop bone marrow suppression, heart failure, hydrops, and/or death.

C. IVIG has been used to treat some immunosuppressed patients with chronic viremia and bone marrow suppression.

D. There is no parvovirus vaccine available.

48. D. Polycystic ovarian syndrome (PCOS) is characterized by anovulation and menstrual irregularities, as well as signs of androgen excess such as facial hair, acne, and elevated androgens (DHEA-S, testosterone).

A. Hypothyroidism can cause dysfunctional uterine bleeding and menstrual irregularities with a resultant elevated TSH and low free T4 level.

B. Elevated levels of testosterone would be expected.

C. An elevated LH/FSH ratio would be suggestive of PCOS.

E. Patients with PCOS frequently are hyperlipidemic and more than 50% develop insulin resistance characterized by AN on exam.

49. E. The majority of dysfunctional uterine bleeding in adolescents is due to anovulatory cycles from an immature hypothalamic-pituitary-ovarian axis; 50% to 75% of their cycles are anovulatory from menarche to 2 years after menarche.

A. Pregnancy is always a consideration with irregular menstrual bleeding and urine human chorionic gonadotropin (hCG) should be checked. If suspicion is high in a sexually active adolescent and the urine hCG is negative then a quantitative serum hCG should be obtained.

B. ITP typically presents with petechia, bruising, and significant thrombocytopenia following a viral illness. It is more common in younger children.

C. Cervical polyps can occur in adolescents but typically present with intermittent vaginal bleeding.

D. A foreign body, such as a retained tampon, should always be considered with abnormal vaginal bleeding.

50. G. Iron replacement should be initiated for 3 months to replace stores while menorrhagia is being controlled. Ibuprofen can be used to decrease menstrual blood loss by up to 50%. Oral contraceptives can be started once daily if there is no active bleeding. A monophasic pill with 35 μg of ethinyl estradiol is preferable and the patient can be cycled for 1 to 3 months. If bleeding is stabilized during that time, the OCPs can be discontinued. If the patient is actively bleeding at the time of initiating OCPs, a taper can be given to stop the bleeding: use the "4-3-2" rule of one pill four times a day for 4 days, then

one pill three times a day for 3 days, then one pill twice a day for two days, and finally one pill a day until withdrawal bleeding occurs. Antiemetics are often required with this regimen. The patient can then be cycled for 3 to 6 months on OCPs and then discontinued. Frequently this is enough for the hypothalamic-pituitary-ovarian axis to mature and the menstrual cycles will normalize.

A. Observation alone is not preferable in this patient because she is already anemic.
B. Iron therapy alone will not be sufficient treatment for this patient with menometrorrhagia.
C. Oral contraceptives alone will not be sufficient treatment for this patient with menometrorrhagia.
D. Ibuprofen alone will not be sufficient treatment for this patient with menometrorrhagia.
E. A blood transfusion would only be required if she was overtly symptomatic from her anemia with tachycardia, hypoxia, shortness of breath, etc. This typically would occur only if her hemoglobin was less than 6 g/dL. A work-up for a bleeding disorder should also be undertaken in those situations, while IV estrogen can be used to stop the vaginal bleeding.
F. See explanations for B and C. The explanation for G lists what constitutes the most appropriate management strategy.
H. See explanations for D and E. The explanation for G lists what constitutes the most appropriate management strategy.

SETTING 2: OFFICE

Your office is in a primary care generalist group practice located in a physician office suite adjoining a suburban community hospital. Patients are usually seen by appointment. Most of the patients you see are from your own practice and are appearing for regular scheduled return visits, with some new patients as well. As in most group practices, you will often encounter a patient whose primary care is managed by one of your associates; reference may be made to the patient's medical records. You may do some telephone management, and you may have to respond to questions about articles in magazines and on television that will require interpretation. Complete laboratory and radiology services are available.

51. A 5-month-old infant has been referred to a pediatric cardiologist by you for a murmur suspicious for a ventral septal defect (VSD) found during a well-child checkup. The cardiologist noted that the infant falls on the 25th percentile curves for both height and weight. An echocardiogram done during the office visit confirmed the diagnosis of a small muscular VSD. You discuss the results of the consultation with the mother, who is quite distraught and asks for immediate repair as she had a brother who died from congestive heart failure complications as a child. You calmly explain the defect and the cardiologist's plan of treatment, which seems to set the mother at ease. Which of the following statements would likely be part of that plan?

    A. Cardiac catheterization to confirm the diagnosis and measure the pulmonary artery wedge pressures
    B. Referral to pediatric cardiothoracic surgery for surgical repair at the end of winter viral season
    C. Routine evaluations by the cardiologist with the expectation that the septal defect may close spontaneously
    D. Routine evaluations by the cardiologist with the expectation that the patient will need diuretics and digitalis
    E. NG tube insertion education for the parents, so that increased caloric feeds can be given during the night

The next 2 questions (items 52-53) correspond to the following vignette.

A 2-month-old infant presents for his well-child checkup. The mother reports that her child has had a 5-week history of a dry, hacking, persistent cough. He has not had any fevers or other symptoms. The eye discharge she complained about at his 1-month well-child checkup is now gone. His exam shows an afebrile infant with mild retractions and prominent crackles in both lung fields. He has also had poor weight gain, now below the 5th percentile, despite a reliable history of adequate formula intake. Laboratory examination shows a mild elevation in total WBC count with more lymphocytes than neutrophils and a marked eosinophilia. A chest radiograph is obtained (Figure 3-52).

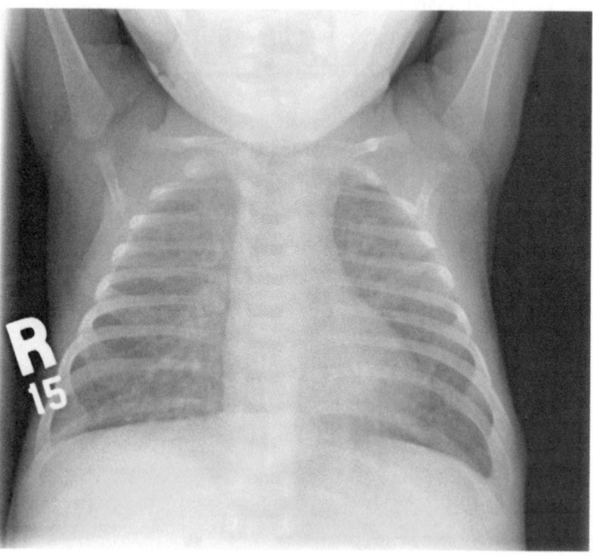

Figure 3-52 • Image Courtesy of the Department of Radiology, Phoenix Children's Hospital, Phoenix, Arizona.

52. Which of the following is the most likely cause of the patient's symptoms?

    A. *Streptococcus pneumoniae*
    B. Group B streptococcus
    C. *Staphylococcus aureus*
    D. *Escherichia coli*
    E. *Bordatella pertussis*
    F. *Chlamydia trachomatis*
    G. *Mycoplasma pneumoniae*
    H. Herpes simplex
    I. Congenital varicella

53. If an infectious work-up were negative, and the mother said the patient's stools were abnormally foul smelling, which of the following metabolic diseases should be considered?

A. Wilson disease
B. Cystic fibrosis (CF)
C. Gaucher disease
D. Galactosemia
E. Hereditary fructose intolerance

End of Set

54. You are seeing a 12-month-old HIV-infected child in your office for his 1-year well-child visit. Upon review of his chart you realize that his immunizations are delayed; he has not received any vaccines since 4 months of age. He has a history of multiple ear infections and recurrent pneumonias. His latest labs show an HIV viral load of 25,000 and a CD4 count of 470/14%. Which of the following vaccines should this child receive?

    A. Pneumovax
    B. *Haemophilus influenzae* vaccine (Hib)
    C. Hepatitis A
    D. Measles, mumps, rubella (MMR)
    E. Varicella

55. A 12-year-old child is being seen in your office for the acute onset of a swollen left testicle. There is no history of trauma. On physical exam you notice an erythematous, swollen, painful left testicle with an absent cremasteric reflex. Which of the following is most consistent with the management of this condition?

    A. Surgical consultation should not be delayed
    B. Surgical consultation should be deferred pending imaging studies
    C. CT scan should be used to confirm the diagnosis
    D. Antibiotics are necessary for proper treatment
    E. Differentiation from epididymitis is easily demonstrated by exam

56. Two weeks after birth, a girl is brought to your office for evaluation of persistent tearing and a fullness between the eye and the bridge of the nose, just below the medial canthus. The skin over the mass is of normal color, and palpation shows the mass to be soft but yields no discharge. The baby's mother has noted the mass since birth and has noted no changes in its size or appearance. The most appropriate regimen for evaluation and treatment includes:

    A. Obtain STAT MRI followed by needle aspiration
    B. Request follow-up at 2 years of age, if the tearing persists
    C. Hospitalize the child and obtain neurosurgical consultation
    D. Request ophthalmology consultation and treatment to occur in the subsequent days
    E. Order x-rays of the sinuses and keep the child NPO for a minimum of 24 hours

57. A 13-year-old male is being seen in your office for follow-up of scoliosis. He has been doing relatively well without any complaints. Your partner had been concerned enough to send the patient for radiographs. The report shows the patient has a measured angle of 18° without any other significant pathology noted. The next step in the management of this patient would be:

    A. Obtain an MRI for further imaging
    B. Referral to an orthopedic surgeon for bracing
    C. Referral to an orthopedic surgeon for surgery
    D. Continued monitoring every 4 to 6 months
    E. No further need to monitor this patient's scoliosis

58. A 4-month-old male infant has been seen on three occasions with febrile illnesses without localizing signs. He is breast fed, and his growth and development have been normal. During weekdays he is in a daycare setting while the mother works, and there are at least five other infants being cared for in that daycare center. The mother is concerned about some sort of immune deficiency that is making her infant susceptible to infections. Which one of the following statements is true?

    A. Hypogammaglobulinemia is a normal occurrence at 4 months
    B. Infants are born with IgG, IgM, and IgA levels near normal adult values
    C. Boys born with X-linked (Bruton) agammaglobulinemia usually develop serious infections before 6 months of age
    D. Infants with hypogammaglobulinemia will generally do poorly with ordinary viral infections
    E. Patients with hypogammaglobulinemia can usually handle infections with encapsulated organisms normally

59. A 14-year-old girl is seen at your office because of significant pain and swelling of her knees, ankles, and finger joints for the past 6 weeks. She is mildly anemic and has had intermittent fevers, with considerable prostration when she has her fevers. There is no family history of arthritis. There are several subcutaneous nodules found over the extensor surface of her elbows. A rheumatoid factor (RF) is positive, an antistreptolysin O (ASO) titer is negative, her sedimentation rate is 80, and an anti-nuclear antibody (ANA) is significantly positive. Which one of the following statements is true?

    A. A positive RF indicates that this girl has IgG antibodies directed against her synovial membranes
    B. More than half of patients with this disease will have a positive ANA
    C. This type of arthritis occurs equally in males and females
    D. Only 10% of these patients will go on to have significant disease as adults
    E. The positive ANA strongly suggests that this girl has lupus

60. A 16-year-old female, last seen in your office 9 months ago, now presents with a 15-pound weight gain and complaints of amenorrhea for 3 months. Menarche occurred at 12 years of age and her periods have been regular until 7 months ago. Her flow decreased and she would have a period every 6 to 8 weeks. She also notes that her stools have been hard for the last 6 weeks and improved with Metamucil daily. On further questioning she describes dry skin and a decreased energy level but has a normal affect. What lab test is most likely to render a diagnosis in this patient?

    A. CBC
    B. Urine β-hCG
    C. FSH level
    D. Prolactin level
    E. TSH

61. You are seeing a 15-month-old boy for a well-child checkup in the office. His mother is concerned about his development. "He is not like the other kids. All of his other friends are cruising and walking already," she states. Which of the following motor milestones should this boy have mastered?

    A. Sitting alone
    B. Rolling over
    C. Cruising
    D. Pulling to a stand
    E. Walking three steps alone
    F. Sitting alone, rolling over, cruising, pulling to a stand, and walking three steps alone
    G. Sitting alone and rolling over only
    H. Sitting alone, rolling over, and cruising only
    I. Sitting alone, rolling over, cruising, and pulling to a stand only

62. You are seeing a 10-year-old female in your office for follow-up of Graves disease. You are discussing the variety of treatment options available for Graves disease with the family. When considering the use of radioactive iodine (^{131}I) therapy for Graves disease in children, it is important to remember the following true statement:

    A. Surgical thyroidectomy has a better cure rate than ^{131}I
    B. Treatment with methimazole or propylthiouracil (PTU) offers a better long-term remission rate and a low incidence of adverse reactions
    C. Surgical thyroidectomy is simple in comparison, and of low risk to the patient
    D. ^{131}I has never been used in children
    E. ^{131}I is a successful therapy for childhood Graves disease

63. A 15-year-old Jewish girl comes to your office following a recent hospitalization. She was admitted for a history of bruising, nosebleeds, fatigue, and intermittent severe leg pain. On physical examination she has marked hepatosplenomegaly. Laboratory evaluation demonstrates anemia and thrombocytopenia, but the leukocyte count and peripheral smear is normal. A liver biopsy was performed (Figure 3-63), which shows cells with a "wrinkled paper" appearance. What is the most appropriate next step in the management of this patient?

    A. Tell the parents that this is an untreatable hereditary condition
    B. Measure the acid β-glucosidase activity
    C. Initiate therapy with corticosteroids
    D. Initiate treatment protocol for acute lymphoblastic leukemia (ALL)
    E. Initiate enzyme replacement therapy

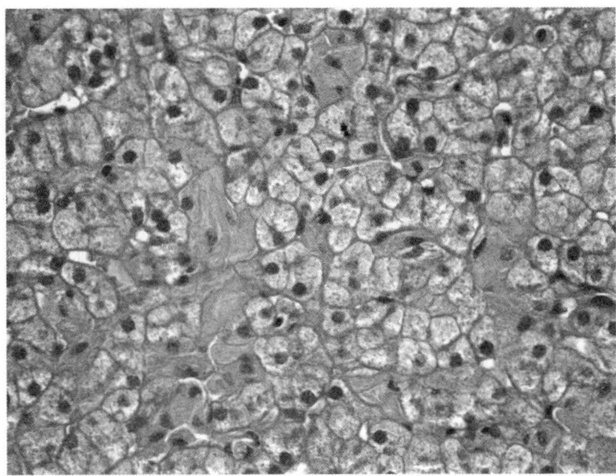

Figure 3-63 • Image Courtesy of the Department of Pathology, Phoenix Children's Hospital, Phoenix, Arizona.

64. You are seeing a 10-year-old boy in your office who presents with the sudden onset of unilateral facial weakness and mouth droop. You suspect that he is suffering from a Bell palsy. His mother is concerned about how this will affect his future. Which of the following best describes the prognosis?

   A. Most cases result in permanent facial nerve paralysis
   B. Twenty-five percent of cases resolve spontaneously with no residual facial weakness
   C. Eighty-five percent of cases resolve spontaneously with no residual facial weakness
   D. Fifty percent of patients are left with residual facial weakness
   E. Fifty percent of cases resolve spontaneously with no residual facial weakness

65. You are seeing a 13-year-old girl who was diagnosed with anorexia nervosa at age 12. She is being managed with antidepressants, counseling with a psychologist, and consultation with a nutritionist. She has a contract with her parents to reward appropriate eating behavior with expanded privileges. Her weight for height has been stable at 19% below ideal body weight for the past 6 months. Today, her weight is at 22% below ideal body weight. She reports no suicidal ideation and her parents agree that she has appeared compliant with the diet and exercise contract. What is the appropriate next step?

   A. Contact her psychologist to reevaluate her antidepressant regimen
   B. Strengthen the behavior contract to include an increase in caloric intake
   C. Admit her to the hospital for nutritional rehabilitation
   D. Maintain the current management regimen and reevaluate in 2 weeks
   E. Maintain the current management regimen and reevaluate in 1 month

66. You are preparing to perform a circumcision on a 2-week-old infant when you notice an undescended testicle and hypospadias. What is the next step in diagnosis and management?

   A. Further genetic and endocrine evaluation
   B. Surgical repair of hypospadias
   C. Review of newborn screen for inborn errors of metabolism
   D. Renal ultrasound
   E. Perform circumcision and reevaluate in 2 weeks

67. You are caring for a 6-month-old baby with chronic cough. You order a sweat chloride test and the results show the chloride is 104 mmol/L (normal is <40) on the right arm and 108 mmol/L on the left arm (with adequate volume of sweat at each site). The next appropriate step is:

   A. Repeat the sweat test for confirmation and refer to your local CF center
   B. Refer to a geneticist for further evaluation
   C. Obtain a stool elastase
   D. Send a hair sample for analysis of mineral deficiency
   E. Repeat the sweat test in 6 months to confirm the diagnosis

68. You receive a call from a nurse at a local high school about a football player who has been practicing in hot, humid weather and now has become confused and combative. His temperature is measured at 41°C. You are concerned about heat stroke. What advice will you give the nurse for initial management until the patient can be brought to the ED?

   A. Give a double dose of aspirin
   B. Avoid giving oral and IV fluids
   C. Sponge the boy with lukewarm water
   D. Remove the boy's clothes and let the body temperature fall slowly
   E. Give ice water bath; administer large amount of IV/oral fluids

69. You are seeing a family for a prenatal consult. The mother is 20-weeks pregnant and has been referred secondary to an abnormally low alpha-fetoprotein (AFP) level. Her pregnancy has otherwise been uncomplicated. Which of the following is/are associated with low levels of maternal AFP?

A. Neural tube defects
B. Twin gestation
C. Trisomy 21
D. Gastroschisis
E. Cystic hygroma
F. Neural tube defects and twin gestation
G. Gastroschisis and cystic hygroma
H. Trisomy 21 and cystic hygroma

70. An 8-year-old girl comes to your office because she has been having episodes where she stops moving and talking, demonstrates a blank facial expression, and rapidly blinks her eyelids. These episodes last about 5 to 15 seconds, after which she returns completely to her normal behavior. A true statement about this form of epilepsy is:

A. The episodes can often be induced by hyperventilation for 3 to 4 minutes
B. The typical EEG pattern is called hypsarrhythmia
C. It usually starts in children less than 5 years old
D. These seizures rarely occur more than once a day
E. This type of seizure is commonly treated with dilantin

71. A 10-year-old boy is seen in your office because of complaints of shortness of breath, cough, and fatigue associated with exercise. The patient has a history of reactive airway disease and has been hospitalized twice in the past year for wheezing episodes. You find that on office spirometry, his forced expiratory volume 1 (FEV1) falls by 15% after 7 minutes of heavy exercise. How will you manage this patient initially?

A. Try to minimize strenuous exercise as much as possible
B. Try to exercise mostly when the air is cold
C. Pretreat with albuterol inhaler prior to all exercise
D. Start an inhaled corticosteroid on a twice-daily basis
E. Start oral antihistamines

72. A 9-year-old boy comes to your office because of nightly bedwetting. He has had this problem since he was a very young child and has never had any prolonged period of dryness at night. He has no history of urinary tract infection. Examination of his external genitalia is normal. He reports a normal urinary stream. The boy's father also wet his bed until he was 10 years old. The treatment that most likely will result in a long-term cure is:

A. Strict fluid restriction prior to bed
B. Behavior modification with star charts and rewards
C. Imipramine
D. Desmopressin
E. Buzzer alarm bladder conditioning device

73. A 2-year-old is brought to your office because she has not been moving her arm since yesterday. Last night, she was taken to a local hospital emergency room where an x-ray of her arm proved to be normal. The mother does not remember any trauma, except that the child tripped yesterday while holding hands and walking with her mother. Examination does not reveal joint effusion or point tenderness, but the child will not bend the elbow. What would be the most appropriate next step in management?

A. Repeat the radiographs of the arm
B. Obtain a CT scan of the elbow
C. Prescribe warm soaks and anti-inflammatory agents
D. Refer the patient to an orthopedic surgeon
E. Perform a maneuver to reduce an elbow dislocation

74. A 3-year-old boy was treated in your office with amoxicillin for right otitis media 2 weeks ago. When he returns for an ear check, you find that his tympanic membrane is retracted and there is some clear fluid with air bubbles behind the drum. His mother reports that there has been a mild problem with his hearing. How will you manage this patient?

A. Refer to otolaryngologist
B. Prescribe an oral decongestant medication
C. Prescribe an antibiotic with wider coverage than amoxicillin
D. Have an audiologist perform an audiogram
E. No treatment now, but see patient again in 1 month

75. A mother calls you at 2 AM to report her 3-year-old child has developed a fever of 38.5°C and rash over the past 3 to 4 hours. The rash is described as "little red dots." On further questioning the mother tells you the pinpoint dots appear more red than pink. Some of them are flat and some are raised. Most dots disappear when compressed, but others do not. You suspect that the most likely diagnosis is a nonspecific viral rash. What is the most appropriate advice to give to this child's mother?

A. Antipyretic for fever, no treatment for rash
B. Antipyretic for fever; see patient in office tomorrow
C. Antipyretic for fever, calamine lotion for rash
D. Tell mother to take child to the ED immediately
E. No antipyretic if child is comfortable; see patient in office tomorrow

76. You have been following a 3-year-old patient with atopic dermatitis. You have tried a low-potency steroid cream and some lubrication lotion. The parents return with the concern that the rash is no better and has actually been spreading to new areas. The child has been itching and crying at night. Which of the following would you change to make the family's treatment of the child's atopic dermatitis more effective?

A. Twice daily soaking followed by lubrication
B. Application of a low- to mid-potency steroid cream several times daily followed by emollient
C. Wearing soft, nonirritating clothing
D. Prescription of an antihistamine at bedtime in high enough dosage to cause somnolence
E. Washing only soiled areas of skin with mild, creamed, nonperfumed soap

77. A 12-month-old male infant with tetrology of Fallot is seen at your office for a presurgical check-up. He has been doing rather well with a minimal number of "blue spells" and surgery is anticipated in a week or two. He is at the 5th percentile for height, and below the 5th percentile for weight. His blood count is as follows: Hb 17.2 g/dL; RBC 5.7; reticulocyte count 1.7%; MCV 66; MCHC 32; MCH 30; and RDW 17.0. Which one of the following is the most important next step in his management?

A. A dietary consultation emphasizing the importance of adequate caloric intake
B. Call the surgeon and recommend immediate surgery
C. Do a partial exchange to reduce the circulating RBCs
D. Immediately begin oral iron therapy
E. Clear this infant for surgery if the extracardiac examination is unremarkable

78. On a routine well-child checkup on a new patient to your practice, you note this 2-year-old girl to have a small hemangioma located over her sacral area in the midline. There is no dimple or hair tufts associated with the lesion. You would recommend for the parents to:

A. Not worry—these lesions usually disappear by age 8
B. Obtain a biopsy of the lesion to rule out a malignant lesion
C. Have the lesion removed by laser treatment to prevent any bleeding or cosmetic problems in the future
D. Get an ultrasound or MRI of the lumbosacral spine to rule out a tethered cord or spinal dysraphism
E. Do nothing, unless the lesion changes in size, color, or thickness

79. A 6-month-old infant boy is seen in your office with failure to thrive. There is a history of child abuse and nutritional deprivation. Your examination reveals significant loss of subcutaneous tissue, growth retardation, and a rachitic rosary is apparent. You make the clinical diagnosis of rickets, and you assume it is secondary to vitamin D deficiency. Regarding this patient, which one of the following will most likely be found?

A. The serum calcium will be normal and phosphorus will be high
B. Alkaline phosphatase will be normal
C. Parathyroid hormone (PTH) will be low
D. Craniotabes may be present in this infant
E. 25 (OH) vitamin D (calcidiol) will be normal

80. A 5-year-old boy is found to have a blood pressure of 120/85. You consult the table of blood pressure norms and find that the 95th percentile for his age and height for systolic and diastolic are 111 and 72, respectively. His physical examination is normal. The blood pressure readings by ambulatory monitoring range between 115 and 125 systolic, and between 80 and 85 diastolic. This blood pressure is consistent with which one of the following?

A. Hypertension
B. High normal blood pressure
C. White coat hypertension
D. Cushing syndrome
E. Adrenogenital syndrome due to 21-hydroxylase deficiency

81. As part of a routine checkup, you order a complete blood count on a 15-month-old African-American boy. His physical examination is normal but he is found to have a hemoglobin level of 8.5 g/dL and a mean corpuscular volume of 66 fL. The lab calls to inform you that red blood cells appear to be abnormal. His blood smear is shown (Figure 3-81). The next step in this child's management should be:

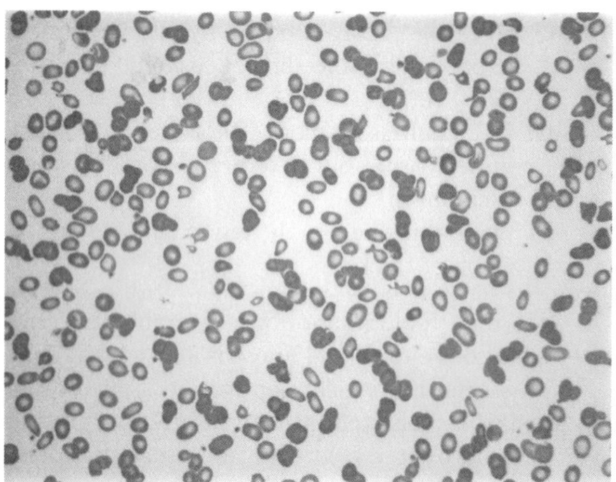

Figure 3-81 • Image Courtesy of the Department of Pathology, Phoenix Children's Hospital, Phoenix, Arizona.

A. Order a serum ferritin level, obtain a dietary history, and initiate oral ferrous sulfate
B. Perform a lead mobilization test with calcium EDTA
C. Order a hemoglobin electrophoresis for α-thalassemia trait
D. Measure the serum folate level
E. Admit the patient to the hospital for packed red blood cell transfusion

82. A 2-year-old boy with an unrepaired ventricular septal defect (VSD) is going to the dentist to have a dental cavity filled. The dentist asks your advice regarding endocarditis prophylaxis. The best advice would be:

A. No prophylaxis is necessary
B. Amoxicillin 50 mg/kg/dose every 6 hours on the day prior to the procedure
C. Amoxicillin 50 mg/kg/dose, one dose given 1 hour prior to the procedure
D. Amoxicillin 50 mg/kg, one dose given 3 hours after the procedure
E. Sulfisoxazole 50 mg/kg/dose, 1 hour before and 1 hour after the procedure

83. A 6-month-old boy is seen in your office because of atopic dermatitis refractory to standard therapy, and only partially responsive to topical steroids. There is a history of prolonged bleeding from his newborn circumcision, and he has had some intermittent bloody diarrhea. He has also had two bouts of otitis media in the past 2 months. Which one of the following disorders is likely to apply to this patient?

A. Wiskott-Aldrich syndrome
B. Ataxia telangiectasia
C. X-linked agammaglobulinemia
D. Severe combined immunodeficiency
E. Hyper-IgM syndrome

84. A 9-year-old boy comes to your office for evaluation of "attention problems" at school. Parents report that he has never had difficulty at school before this year, but is now at risk for failing 4th grade due to his disruptive behavior and refusal to complete his schoolwork. He has been in two fights at school and has recently shown a tendency to dangerously impulsive behavior at home. His parents do not recall any previous problems with behavior or any recent illness. Which of the following would probably be most helpful for this child?

A. Trial of stimulant medication such as methylphenidate (Ritalin)
B. Testing for learning disabilities
C. Psychological evaluation for depression or other psychiatric disorder
D. Thyroid testing
E. Continued observation and reevaluation in 4 to 6 months

85. You are evaluating a 5-year-old Hispanic girl with Turner's syndrome. Her physical exam reveals no evidence of heart murmur, but is significant for a webbed neck, low hairline, and wide-spaced nipples. Which of the following hormonal abnormalities would be expected and necessitate treatment at this time?

A. Low insulin growth factor-1 (IGF-1)
B. Low insulin-like growth factor binding protein 3 (IGFBP3)
C. Estrogen deficiency
D. Growth hormone resistance
E. Adrenocorticotropic hormone (ACTH) deficiency

86. A 1-year-old boy has growth failure over the past several months. Both his weight and height are now below the 5th percentile. Your examination is unremarkable with the exception of his small stature. You decide to investigate the cause of his growth failure. A blood count is unremarkable. Serum electrolytes are Na^+ 140 mEq/L; K^+ 2.5 mEq/L; and Cl^- 117 mEq/L; CO_2 is 12 mEq/L. Serum calcium is 9.0 mg/dL (normal is 8–10 mg/dL), and phosphorus is 2.0 mg/dL. In further investigation, you would expect which one of the following?

A. Significant hypoglycemia
B. Aminoaciduria
C. Elevated BUN and creatinine
D. Urine pH above 6.0
E. Hyperparathyroidism

87. A 15-year-old female presents to your office requesting oral contraceptive pills (OCPs). You counsel her on the complications, benefits, and side effects of OCP usage, which includes which of the following?

A. Increased incidence of anemia
B. Worsening of acne
C. Decreased risk of ovarian cancer
D. Increased risk of endometrial cancer
E. Decreased venous thrombosis

88. A 2-year-old boy who had been walking normally since age 12 months has been noted to have a progressively worsening waddling gait. He falls frequently, has difficulty climbing stairs, and trouble getting up from the floor. On physical examination you note lumbar lordosis and a rubbery feel to his calf muscles. You suspect Duchenne muscular dystrophy. Which of the following is the most accurate information to give to the parents?

A. Enlargement of the calves (pseudohypertrophy) is a classic feature
B. Gross motor skills are often delayed by 2 months of age
C. The creatinine kinase (CK) level becomes elevated at about 2 to 3 years of age
D. The disease affects boys and girls equally
E. The muscle degeneration and fibrosis causes muscle spasms and severe myalgias

89. A 5-year-old boy presents with a history of fever and dysuria. He has a history of having had a urinary tract infection (UTI) when he was 2 years old. He was treated then with an antibiotic and has had no further trouble until now. No investigation was carried out when he had his first UTI. A urinalysis now indicates that he, indeed, has a UTI. There is significant pyuria, and a mid-stream urine grew more than 100,000 *E. coli*. Which one of the following statements is true?

A. It is an acceptable standard to wait for the second UTI in a boy before further urologic investigation
B. UTI often causes significant vesicoureteral reflux
C. Reflux nephropathy rarely leads to end-stage renal disease in children
D. Reflux nephropathy can cause significant hypertension
E. There is no familial incidence of vesicoureteral reflux

90. The parents of a 3-year-old faithfully follow your prescribed treatment for atopic dermatitis. However, the anticubital areas remain wet, weepy, erythematous, and crusted. Which of the following is the most likely explanation for treatment failure in this patient?

A. Secondary bacterial infection
B. Bathing with tepid water
C. Application of steroid cream before the emollient
D. Cool, humid ambient temperatures
E. Excessive use of lubrication

91. You are seeing a 14-year-old boy with prune belly syndrome in your office who has developed chronic renal failure over the past 5 years. Which of the following metabolic abnormalities associated with untreated chronic renal failure is a common finding?

A. Microcytic anemia
B. Delayed bone age
C. Osteosclerosis
D. Hypoparathyroidism
E. Hyperosmolar urine

92. A 17-year-old sexually active female presents to your office with vaginal discharge. The discharge is white and cottage cheese-like and she complains of pruritis. Vaginal pH is less than 4.5 and KOH prep reveals pseudohyphae. Which of the following is the most appropriate therapy?

A. Sitz baths
B. Metronidazole vaginal gel for 5 days
C. Azithromycin 1-g single dose
D. Fluconazole 150-mg single oral dose
E. Metronidazole 2-g single oral dose

93. A 7-year-old female has been evaluated by her pediatrician for short stature and chronic diarrhea. She has not been out of the country and there have been no identified infectious causes. The lab calls her physician with positive anti-transglutaminase and anti-gliadin antibodies suggestive of gluten-sensitive enteropathy (celiac disease). Which of the following is true?

A. There is an increased risk of diabetes type I in this patient
B. There is a higher risk of malignancy with a gluten-free diet
C. Polycythemia is likely to be found on initial labs
D. Often there is a recent exposure to carpet-cleaning solutions
E. The albumin level will be increased

94. A 20-month-old male presents to your office with 5 days of fever to 104°C that reduces minimally with antipyretics. On exam he has a strawberry tongue, edema of the hands and feet, and an erythematous maculopapular rash on his trunk. Which of the following is required to make the diagnosis of Kawasaki disease?

A. Inguinal lymphadenopathy greater than 2 cm
B. Nonexudative bulbar conjunctival injection
C. Oral ulcerations
D. Mitral valve regurgitation on ECHO
E. Scrotal edema

The next 2 questions (items 95–96) correspond to the following vignette.

A 15-year-old male calls his coach's wife, a pediatrician, after the development of some chest discomfort, palpitations, near syncope, and dyspnea while in football practice. The symptoms subsided shortly after discontinuation of exercise and he is calling from the locker room. He is feeling ok at this time. The adolescent is in excellent shape and takes no medication. He has a brother with reactive airway disease, but no other problems in the family are reported.

95. Which of the following advice would be most appropriate?

A. Take two puffs of the brother's albuterol inhaler and call back if no improvement
B. Lay down on the ground with legs elevated for 15 minutes
C. Make an appointment with the office next week and avoid exercise until that time
D. Call his parents so that they can pick him up and take him to be evaluated by a physician today
E. Take his pulse the next time one of these episodes occurs

96. As the adolescent in the previous case hangs up the phone, a smoke alarm sounds and there is a rush to exit the locker room. While trying to exit, the adolescent slips on some water and falls with hands outstretched on the concrete. There is an obvious fracture of the wrist and the boy is transported via ambulance to the ED where he meets his parents. The ED physician orders a chest x-ray and an ECG along with the casting supplies. On examination the physician notes a heart rate of 100, along with a sharp upstroke of the brachial pulses and a late systolic ejection murmur that increases with standing and decreases with squatting. As you are the patient's primary care physician, the ED physician refers him to your office for follow-up treatment. While reviewing the case history, you note that which of the following statements is most likely to be true?

A. Albuterol would have had beneficial effects in this case
B. ECG demonstrates left ventricular hypertrophy
C. ECG demonstrates supraventricular tachycardia (SVT)
D. Echocardiogram and CXR shows dextrocardia
E. Digitalis is frequently used for this problem

End of Set

97. An 18-year-old African-American male is seen before leaving for college. He has been healthy throughout his life and takes no medications. Currently he has been having some diarrhea with abdominal cramping and flatulence. He is beginning a weight program for football practice in the fall and as such has been drinking a high-protein milkshake twice daily. He thinks this coincides with the start of his symptoms. When questioned he relates that his mother never drinks milk but she does have some occasional ice cream. Which of the following would be appropriate information to give to this patient?

    A. Complete elimination of milk products is needed for symptom relief
    B. African-Americans are the most commonly affected individuals
    C. Diarrhea is caused by an enzyme deficiency which interferes with NaCl channels
    D. Calcium supplements will often cause similar symptoms in these individuals
    E. A breath hydrogen study can confirm the diagnosis, but often an appropriate dietary change is all that is needed

98. A newborn male infant is seen shortly after birth. The diagnosis of trisomy 21 is considered and a genetics consult is ordered. The geneticist evaluates the infant the next day and concurs with the diagnosis. High-resolution chromosomes are sent. Nursing reports that there have not been any problems except that there has been no passage of meconium. The anus appears patent. Of the following, which is the most likely reason for the lack of stooling?

    A. Congenital hypothyroidism
    B. Duodenal atresia
    C. Hirschsprung disease
    D. Meckel diverticulum
    E. Tracheoesophageal fistula (TEF)

The next 2 questions (items 99–100) correspond to the following vignette.

The best-corrected visual acuity of the right eye of a 7-year-old boy is noted to be 20/20, while that of his left eye is 20/200. His pupils are equal in size and reactivity. The left eye drifts inward.

99. The most appropriate therapeutic regimen should include:

    A. Wait until puberty to begin therapy
    B. Begin patching the right eye immediately
    C. Advise the parents that their son is too old to begin therapy
    D. Patch the left eye each night at bedtime
    E. Urgent surgery to realign the eyes

100. After detailed description of the disease process, you should ensure a follow-up appointment to reassess the visual acuity within:

    A. One day
    B. Two weeks
    C. Three months
    D. Four years
    E. Follow-up evaluation is not indicated

End of Set

A Answers and Explanations

51. C
52. F
53. B
54. B
55. A
56. D
57. D
58. A
59. B
60. E
61. I
62. E
63. B
64. C
65. C
66. A
67. A
68. E
69. C
70. A
71. D
72. E
73. E
74. E
75. D
76. B
77. D
78. D
79. D
80. A
81. A
82. C
83. A
84. C
85. D
86. B
87. C
88. A
89. D
90. A
91. B
92. D
93. A
94. B
95. D
96. B
97. E
98. C
99. B
100. C

51. **C. In an otherwise healthy infant with a small VSD, no invasive therapy or surgical intervention is needed immediately. However, close monitoring and subacute bacterial endocarditis (SBE) prophylaxis is indicated. Spontaneous closure is likely with small VSDs and muscular VSDs. Often there is a history of congenital defects in the family.**

A. Cardiac catheterization would not be indicated in this scenario, but is useful in helping to manage those patients with complex congenital lesions.
B. As in the explanation for C, spontaneous closure is likely with a small muscular VSD; surgery is not necessary in this scenario.
D. The patient should periodically be followed for spontaneous closure, but the likelihood of developing congestive heart failure from a small VSD is rare.
E. This patient is growing well at the 25th percentile and does not need NG feeds. NG feeds for caloric supplementation would be indicated in cases of poor growth and suboptimal weight gain.

52. **F. *Chlamydia trachomatis* is the most likely cause of this patient's symptoms, which are quite typical, including dry, hacky, classically described as staccato, cough that started in the first month of life, slow progression over weeks with progressive respiratory distress, afebrile, peripheral eosinophilia, eye discharge, and failure to thrive despite adequate formula intake.**

A, B, C, D. The fact that he has had symptoms for several weeks without any fevers makes the more virulent bacterial strains unlikely (Strep, Staph, *E. coli*).
E. Pertussis could cause a cough for a prolonged period and should be considered, but the coughing typically occurs in spasms and is not associated with a peripheral eosinophilia, but a marked lymphocytosis instead.
G. Mycoplasma is a common cause of atypical pneumonia in childhood, but not in infants.
H, I. Herpes simplex and varicella can cause neonatal infections, but they have other associated symptoms, which often will include vesicular skin lesions

53. **B. CF is the only metabolic disease listed that could explain the above patient's symptoms, and should be considered in any infant who has respiratory symptoms and failure to thrive, even if there were not a history of foul smelling stools suggestive of fat malabsorption. The various genetic defects in chloride channels that cause CF result in problems with secretions; the systems most affected are the respiratory and gastrointestinal systems. All the other metabolic diseases listed are not associated with respiratory problems.**

A. Wilson disease affects copper metabolism and presents with liver, neurologic, or psychiatric manifestations much later in childhood.
C. Gaucher disease is a lysosomal storage disease that presents with pathologic fractures, bone pain, hepatosplenomegaly, and/or hematologic problems.
D. Galactosemia comes from an inability to break down galactose found in human and cow's milk and can present in the newborn period with poor weight gain, jaundice, vomiting, irritability, feeding difficulties, or full blown sepsis, often from *E. coli*. However, respiratory distress is not one of its features.
E. Hereditary fructose intolerance presents in infants when they are first fed fruit, fruit juices, or table sugar (sucrose) and symptoms can mimic those of galactosemia. Again, slowly progressive respiratory distress is not part of the clinical picture.

54. **B. All HIV-infected children without evidence of severe immunosuppression or symptomatology should receive all of the following vaccines by 12 months of age: prevnar, Hib, hepatitis B, DTaP (diphtheria, tetanus, acellular pertussis vaccine), and IPV (inactivated polio vaccine). These are all inactivated vaccines and are recommended to be given to all HIV-infected children regardless of their immune status and CD4 counts.**

A. Pneumovax is a 23-valent pneumococcal vaccine that is recommended in children older than 2 years of age who are HIV infected, as well as other selectively immunocompromised or asplenic patients, such as those with sickle cell anemia.
C. Hepatitis A vaccine (HAV) is recommended in high-risk children older than 2 years of age, such as those with HIV, as well as those living in areas with a high prevalence of disease. HAV is also often required before children can be enrolled in Head Start programs.

D, E. As the MMR and varicella vaccines are live attenuated vaccines, they should NOT be given to HIV-infected children who are considered to be severely immunocompromised with CD4 counts less than 15%, such as the child in this scenario.

55. **A. The clinical scenario of scrotal swelling and pain with absence of the cremasteric reflex is consistent with testicular torsion. Testicular torsion occurs more commonly in children younger than 6 years of age, although it is seen through adolescence as well. Testicular survival decreases rapidly after 6 hours and demonstrates the need for prompt surgical intervention.**

    B. Ultrasound with Doppler or isotopic scans can be useful in the diagnosis, but should not delay further surgical consultation or intervention.
    C. CT scan is expensive and not recommended in this clinical situation.
    D. Antibiotics are not indicated in the treatment of testicular torsion.
    E. Epididymitis occurs more commonly in adolescence, but can mimic testicular torsion. A urinalysis will often reveal pyuria in the case of epididymitis and the cremasteric reflex should be present.

56. **D. The diagnosis is dacryocystocele. Tearing and a small mass in the inner corner of the lower eyelid characterize this form of congenital nasolacrimal duct obstruction. It is due to an amniotic fluid distended nasolacrimal sac. In addition to the simpler distal obstruction of most congenital nasolacrimal duct obstructions, a dacryocystocele has a proximal obstruction of the punctae or common canaliculus. Surgical dilatation of the proximal tear system is needed in the first few weeks of life to prevent a life-threatening cellulitis. Distal dilatation can be attempted, but is not always successful.**

    A. Imaging is not needed in this case. The typical findings of this case are consistent with the diagnosis of a dacryocystocele—congenital, tearing, nonprogressive fullness below the medial canthal tendon. The treatment of choice is opening the proximal tear system, not penetrating the skin.
    B. Early diagnosis and treatment is critical for dacryocystocele. Surgical treatment of congenital nasolacrimal duct obstructions is best performed by 1 year, with a 90% cure rate. Surgical treatment of dacryocystocele should be performed in the first year of life.
    C. Hospitalization and systemic antibiotic therapy is needed for an infected dacryocystocele, which has the characteristics of this case plus erythema of the skin overlying the nasolacrimal sac, and a purulent discharge. Neurosurgical evaluation would be helpful if the mass was above the medial canthal tendon and shown to connect with the CNS, such as occurs with an encephalocystocele.
    E. Imaging is rarely indicated, unless nonclassic signs are present. Just prior to the anesthetic and surgical period, an NPO status can be instituted for 4 to 6 hours.

57. **D. Curves that measure less than 25° usually do not require any immediate intervention, but should be monitored every 4 to 6 months for continued progression of curvature. Curves that are greater than 25° should be referred to an orthopedic surgeon for further management.**

    A. Obtaining an MRI in this scenario is unnecessary and expensive. An MRI may be indicated if further pathology were noted on x-ray, such as a compressed disc, or if neurologic symptoms develop.
    B. Bracing for scoliosis is typically reserved for patients with curves from 25° to 45°.
    C. Surgical intervention is required for correction of curves greater than 45°.
    E. The risk of progression of the patient's scoliosis still exists and it would be malpractice to ignore further progression of disease. Of note, premenarchal girls with a curve of 20° or more have a higher risk of disease progression than those with the same curve who are 1 to 2 years postmenarche.

58. **A. Hypogammaglobulinemia is expected at 3 to 4 months when the maternally derived IgG antibodies reach a nadir, and the infant's own IgG production is not yet optimal. A level as low as 200 mg/dL is not unusual. The occasional infant with a benign "transient hypogammaglobulinemia of infancy" may get as low as 100 mg/dL, but recovery in these infants is seen by 6 to 12 months. A normal adult level of IgG is near 1000 mg/dL.**

B. IgG is the smallest immunoglobulin molecule and is readily transferred to the infant in utero. Therefore, infants are born with IgG levels similar to the mother. IgM and IgA, however, do not cross the placenta, and therefore levels of these immunoglobulins are very low in the newborn. Any significant amount of IgM (above 20 mg/dL) in the newborn should make one suspicious of congenital infection.
C. Bruton agammaglobulinemia infants (agammaglobulinemia) generally do well for 6 to 9 months while maternal immunoglobulins are still present. The development of infections with encapsulated organisms becomes problematic in the last half of the first year.
D. Ordinary viral infections generally do not pose problems in infants with agammaglobulinemia, because viral infections are handled more by cellular immune functions. The exceptions are hepatitis viruses and enteroviruses.
E. Those patients with immunoglobulin deficiencies are at increased risk of infection from encapsulated organisms such as *Streptococcus pneumoniae* and *Haemophilus influenzae*.

59. B. About 75% of older children and adolescents with *RF-positive* rheumatoid arthritis have a positive ANA.

A. RF is an IgM antibody directed against the Fc portion of the patient's own IgG.
C. This patient would be classified as having late-onset polyarticular juvenile rheumatoid arthritis (JRA) with onset of disease after 8 years of age and more than four joints affected. Eighty percent of late-onset polyarticular JRA occurs in girls.
D. Late-onset polyarticular RF-positive JRA acts much like the adult disease. About 50% will go on to have significant and frequently disabling disease.
E. The likelihood of lupus in this patient is remote if there is no other confirmatory evidence clinically or by further testing. In late-onset RF-positive JRA, ANA is positive in about 75% of patients.

60. E. This patient's constellation of symptoms is classic for hypothyroidism. She has decreased energy, constipation, weight gain, and amenorrhea. TSH will be elevated with a decreased T4 level.

A. A CBC would be useful in evaluating for anemia with symptoms of fatigue, but there is no history of heavy menstrual bleeding or other symptoms to suggest the patient may be anemic.
B. A urine β-hCG should be obtained on all patients with secondary amenorrhea, but pregnancy does not explain the remainder of her symptoms.
C. FSH levels are helpful for evaluating primary ovarian failure and will be elevated.
D. A prolactin level is elevated in patients with pituitary microadenomas who may present with amenorrhea but frequently have galactorrhea. They may also demonstrate visual field defects on neurologic exam, and an MRI of the brain should be obtained.

61. I. The boy in this scenario should have mastered the following skills by 15 months of age: sitting alone, rolling over, cruising, and pulling to a stand. His mother should not be concerned at this point if he has mastered these skills. Table 3-61 represents the ranges of normal development for the above-listed tasks. Notice that this 15-month-old child is still within the normal range of development even if he is still not walking independently.

TABLE 3-61 Normal Motor Milestones Development Ranges

Rolling over	2 to 5 months
Sitting alone	5 to 7 months
Pulling to a stand	7 to 9 months
Cruising	8 to 13 months
Walking three steps alone	9 to 17 months

A, B, C, D, E, F, G, H. See explanation for I.

62. E. ^{131}I is a controversial but successful therapy for childhood Graves disease. Radioactive ^{131}I has been used to treat children with Graves disease; in fact, it has been used in children as young as 1 year of age. It is a simple, inexpensive, and efficacious therapy (>90% cure rate) that is rarely accompanied by acute side effects. However, long-term studies do not exist, so long-term risks have not been adequately assessed.

A, C. Surgical thyroidectomy offers a similar cure rate to ^{131}I (around 90% if performed by a skilled thyroid surgeon), but has greater immediate risk and cost.

B. PTU and methimazole are commonly used therapies for children with Graves disease; however, both drugs offer a *low* long-term remission rate (<30% to 40%) and a *high* incidence of adverse reactions (20% to 30%), which may be (rarely) fatal.

D. As in the explanation for E, ^{131}I has been used successfully in children.

63. **B. The liver biopsy demonstrates the classic Gaucher cell, engorged with glucocerebroside, giving a "wrinkled paper" appearance. Gaucher disease is the most common lysosomal storage disease and is often seen in Ashkenazi Jews. The condition is due to a deficient activity of acid β-glucosidase, with resultant deposition of glycolipids in cells of the reticoendothelial system. The progressive deposition causes infiltration of the bone marrow, progressive hepatosplenomegaly, and skeletal complications. The liver biopsy findings strongly suggest Gaucher disease, but similar cells can be seen in granulocytic leukemia and myeloma; therefore, suspected cases should be confirmed by measuring acid β-glucosidase activity in leukocytes or cultured fibroblasts.**

C. Corticosteroids have no role in the treatment of Gaucher disease.

D. A bone marrow analysis would be expected to show greater than 30% leukemic lymphoblasts to make the diagnosis of ALL; these lymphoblasts would also be expected to be seen on peripheral smear. This patient, however, has Gaucher disease.

A, E. After confirmation of diagnosis Gaucher disease can be treated with enzyme replacement therapy with IV infusion of recombinant acid β-glucosidase. The organomegaly and abnormal hematologic abnormalities are reversed initially and then, with monthly maintenance doses, bone pain is decreased and growth improves.

64. **C. Bell palsy is an acute facial paralysis caused by facial nerve dysfunction. The etiology is suspected to be viral in a majority of cases. Eighty-five percent of cases will resolve spontaneously with no residual facial weakness.**

A, D. Only 5% are left with permanent facial weakness, while another 10% will have minor residual facial weakness.

B, E. As in the explanation for C, 85% of cases resolve spontaneously with no residual facial weakness.

65. **C. Admit to the hospital for nutritional rehabilitation and psychiatric care. This child is failing maximal outpatient management of anorexia nervosa. Anorexia nervosa is a life-threatening illness with a mortality rate from 2% to 8%; death usually results from a combination of decreased myocardial muscle mass and electrolyte imbalance. Hospitalization is often indicated once the patient's weight drops to 80% (or below) of their ideal body weight.**

A. Antidepressants have not been shown to be markedly helpful in managing anorexia. It is unlikely that a shift in medication will reverse the persistent weight loss and may delay decision making around hospitalization.

B. While both parents and child report compliance with the behavior contract, the persistent weight loss implies that this child is managing to circumvent the contract surreptitiously, a hallmark of anorexic behavior. Changing the contract is unlikely to bring about the desired effect.

D, E. Watchful waiting may bring this child closer to death. She has been in a starvation state for several months already and has failed outpatient management.

66. **A. Further genetic and endocrine evaluation for intersexuality/hermaphroditism is indicated. Because hypospadias is an anatomical anomaly of anterior urethral development, boys with simple hypospadias should have otherwise normal genitalia. Patients with ambiguous genitalia, by contrast, have a more extensive genital anomaly, reflecting the failure of all androgen-dependent development. A useful rule of thumb is to assume that any baby with hypospadias, as well as an undescended testis and/or bifid scrotum, should be investigated for hermaphroditism, with immediate hormonal, chromosomal, and anatomic studies.**

B. Surgical repair of the hypospadias will be necessary, but can wait until the genetic evaluation is complete and a decision is made as to whether orchiopexy will be necessary.

C, D. This combination of hypospadias and undescended testicle is not associated with any particular inborn error of metabolism or renal abnormality.

E. Circumcision at this point is not recommended and should be avoided in patients with hypospadias as the foreskin may be needed for future repair.

67. **A. A sweat chloride value above 60 mmol/L is diagnostic of CF. Because the test requires precise technical performance, all positives are repeated for confirmation. Subsequent DNA analysis is often obtained as well. CF centers specialize in the care of children with CF and outcomes are generally better when the CF center participates in the child's care.**

B. Genetic counseling is appropriate to consider if there is trouble establishing the diagnosis by sweat testing or if there are family-planning issues.
C. Stool elastase may help identify pancreatic insufficiency, but is not diagnostic of CF.
D. Mineral deficiency is not a cause of a positive sweat test nor the cause of CF.
E. Six months is too long to wait to confirm the diagnosis; appropriate therapy will not be initiated if the diagnosis is delayed.

68. **E. Treatment for heat stroke starts with CPR with attention to the ABCs (airway, breathing, and circulation). These patients may be dehydrated and hypotensive. Aggressive cooling with ice water baths, cooling fans, and removal of excess clothing is required to return the body temperature to normal as quickly as possible. Rapid administration of IV fluids is important for the treatment of hypovolemia; in settings where an IV would be difficult or impossible to place, aggressive oral rehydration should be initiated.**

A. Aspirin and other antipyretics work by bringing the body's "thermostat" back to a normal setting. Because the thermostat is not elevated in heat-related illness, aspirin would have no effect on the body temperature in this case.
B. This patient needs rapid administration of fluids.
C, D. Neither lukewarm sponge baths nor removal of clothing alone will bring the body temperature down fast enough.

69. **C. Down syndrome, trisomy 21, is associated with low maternal levels of AFP, as are trisomy 18, intrauterine growth retardation, and incorrect gestational age.**

A, B, D, E. *High* levels of AFP are associated with conditions such as neural tube defects, twin gestation, gastroschisis, cystic hygromas, and polycystic renal disease. AFP levels are typically drawn during 16 to 18 weeks of gestation to serve as a screening tool for the above-listed conditions.

70. **A. The episodes described are typical absence (petit mal) seizures. There is no aura and no postictal state. Sometimes teachers mistake the stare and expressionless face for inattentive misbehavior. Hyperventilation can be used in the office setting to induce onset of an episode.**

B. The classic EEG pattern of absence seizures shows 3 cycles per second spike-wave complexes. Hypsarrhythmia is seen in infantile spasms.
C. Absence seizures are rare under age 5 and are more common in girls than in boys.
D. Children with absence seizures may have countless seizures during a single day.
E. Absence seizures are commonly treated with ethosuximide (Zarontin), not dilantin.

71. **D. This patient has exercise-induced asthma (EIA), which is commonly associated with wheezing, cough, shortness of breath, fatigue, and lack of interest in physical activities. The diagnosis is confirmed with a 10% to 15% fall in FEV1 with an exercise challenge. Although EIA is occasionally an isolated illness, the vast majority of patients with this problem also have poorly controlled underlying persistent reactive airway disease. Because this patient has been hospitalized twice in the last year, it is unlikely he has isolated EIA. For both his persistent asthma and the EIA, an inhaled corticosteroid should be prescribed to control airway inflammation.**

A. The goal should be normal physical activity. Inactivity or reduced exertion should not be accepted.
B. Cold air tends to make EIA worse.
C. Using inhaled albuterol prior to exercise may be useful for patients with pure EIA who do not have underlying persistent asthma. There is some evidence that the effect of albuterol wears off quickly in many patients.
E. Antihistamines are not indicated in EIA.

72. **E. Buzzer alarm conditioning devices take several months to decrease the frequency of bedwetting, but they have the best long-term cure rates for primary nocturnal enuresis. These alarms will help approximately 75% to 80% of enuretics to achieve nighttime dryness. In comparison, the spontaneous cure rate even without any treatment is approximately 15% per year.**

A. Fluid restriction prior to bed is ineffective.
B. Behavior modification with star charts and rewards for dry nights seems to improve cure rates when used in conjunction with other enuresis treatments.
C, D. Medications, such as imipramine and desmopressin, may help some children; however, once the medicine is discontinued the majority of children relapse. Desmopressin is very expensive. While less expensive, imipramine is a dangerous medication that can cause cardiac arrhythmias and convulsions if overdosed. Many pediatricians reserve medications for special situations such as a slumber party or summer camp.

73. **E. A nursemaid's elbow (radial head subluxation) is caused by a sudden, forceful pull on an extended forearm. Commonly, this condition occurs when a child trips while holding a parent's hand, or when the child is being swung by his or her arms. Immediately following the event, the child refuses to use the arm. The elbow appears normal on physical examination and the x-ray is often normal. The primary care physician can attempt reduction by gently flexing the elbow with the palm up until a palpable snap is felt at the lateral elbow.**

A. Radiographs may be needed if there is joint fluid and/or point tenderness that suggest presence of a fracture.
B. A CT scan is expensive and not indicated in this case.
C. Warm soaks and anti-inflammatory agents would delay proper treatment. The longer the elbow stays subluxed, the harder it is to reduce back into the normal position in the joint.
D. Orthopedic consultation would be indicated if the reduction maneuver was not successful. Once the subluxation is reduced, the child will begin using the arm normally almost immediately.

74. **E. A retracted tympanic membrane with an effusion in the middle ear and mild hearing loss suggests that the eustachian tube is blocked. This condition is called otitis media with effusion (OME) and is commonly seen for several weeks following a bout of acute otitis media (AOM). In fact, it is so common as to be considered part of the natural course of AOM. This condition is not due to treatment failure and there is no need for additional expensive antibiotics at this time. Furthermore, most studies have failed to show that oral decongestants are efficacious for preventing or treating OME.**

A. Referral to an otolaryngologist for placement of tympanostomy tubes should be delayed until the effusion has been present for 4 to 6 months.
B, C. As in the explanation for E, neither amoxicillin nor a decongestant is appropriate or useful for the treatment of OME.
D. Current recommendations suggest that audiology evaluation be considered if OME persists for longer than 6 weeks to 3 months.

75. **D. The mother should be instructed to take her child to the emergency room. While a nonspecific viral rash is most likely, you cannot rule out the possibility of meningococcemia. Meningococcal infections in the blood or spinal fluid can be life threatening and require immediate medical attention. Rashes are extremely difficult to diagnose over the phone because parents may have difficulty giving an accurate description of the lesions. Typically, meningococcemia is associated with petechiae, pinpoint spots caused by leakage of blood from capillaries. These lesions are red-purple in color and are either not raised or only slightly raised. When the lesion is compressed or the surrounding skin is stretched, the petechial lesions remain visible. In contrast, a nonspecific viral rash is maculopapular, pink in color, and blanches (disappears) when compressed.**

A, B, C. Although antipyretics may be given for fever, the concern for meningococcemia necessitates that the child be evaluated immediately, rather than in the office tomorrow. Calamine lotion would not be indicated.
E. Delay in treatment of this child until tomorrow would be inappropriate in this scenario.

76. B. The steroid cream needs to be applied before the emollient to be effective.

A. Soaking in plain water (not bathing with soap) to hydrate the skin is helpful before application of steroid cream and emollient.
C. Clothing that is nonirritating, such as cotton and certain synthetics, will cause less pruritis.
D. Antihistamine dosages need to be high enough to cause somnolence to be effective in decreasing pruritis.
E. Judicious use of nondrying soaps in limited areas is now accepted.

77. D. This is iron deficiency in this infant with cyanotic heart disease. Hypoxemia overdrives the erythropoiesis causing the polycythemia. The microcytosis (low MCV) and high RDW indicate that there is iron deficiency. Iron-deficient RBCs are extremely nondeformable (rigid), increasing blood viscosity. These patients are prone to clot and have strokes. Iron therapy is indicated.

A. Dietary advice would also be indicated because this infant is iron deficient, but it would be more important first to begin iron therapy.
B. There is no surgical urgency as long as this infant is doing well. It is probably wise to correct the iron deficiency before surgery.
C. A partial exchange would only reduce this infant's oxygen-carrying capacity.
E. It would be wise to wait a bit for surgery until the iron therapy at least partially corrects the iron deficiency, as long as there is no urgent need for surgery (at least 3 to 4 weeks). Any episode of dehydration could precipitate a stroke.

78. D. Vascular lesions in the midline over the spine can often be associated with spinal and spinal cord abnormalities. These require further imaging to uncover hidden spinal lesions of serious future significance.

A. It is true that many infantile hemangiomas appearing in the first 6 months of life will resolve by 8 years of age. However, further investigation is prudent for ones located over midline structures.
B. A malignant hemangioma is very unlikely. Biopsy also carries some risks of significant bleeding.
C. Investigation for underlying serious pathology should be done before removal of the lesion.
E. Watching for changes is an appropriate approach for nevi and vascular lesions not located in the midline.

79. D. Craniotabes is a thinning of the skull seen in rickets causing a "ping pong" effect to palpation. This may be a physical sign of rickets.

A. While serum calcium and phosphorus may be normal early in vitamin D deficiency, both will be low in manifest cases of vitamin D deficiency rickets.
B. Alkaline phosphatase is high in all forms of rickets, indicating increased osteoblast activity.
C. PTH is stimulated by low serum calcium; therefore, in all forms of rickets associated with low calcium, PTH will be high. Thus, this patient with vitamin D deficiency will have an elevated PTH.
E. 20-hydroxylation of vitamin D takes place in the liver, but in vitamin D deficiency there is lack of substrate, and therefore there will be deficient production of this intermediary product. The most active form of vitamin D (1,25 $[OH]_2$ vitamin D) is produced in the kidney, and this may be normal early, but would be expected to be low in severe cases.

80. A. Clearly, the blood pressure readings are consistently over the 95th percentile. This is true hypertension, not just high normal.

B. The blood pressure readings are consistently over the 95th percentile, which defines true hypertension, not just high normal blood pressure. This is confirmed by ambulatory monitoring.
C. White coat hypertension is generally a finding in older children and adolescents, and is ruled out by ambulatory monitoring.
D. While Cushing syndrome is a cause of hypertension, this is not likely in view of the normal physical examination.
E. The adrenogenital syndrome due to 21-hydroxylase deficiency causes salt wasting and does not cause hypertension. It is the adrenogenital syndrome secondary to 11-hydroxylase that has significant sodium-retaining effects and can cause hypertension.

81. **A. The smear demonstrates microcytic, hypochromic red blood cells, which are typical of iron deficiency anemia. In children, this is most commonly due to inadequate iron intake, often as a result of being fed large amounts of whole milk, which contains little absorbable iron. Patients with iron deficiency anemia have a low MCV and an elevated RDW. The MCV should be at least 70 plus the child's age (in years). Further laboratory evaluation would likely yield an elevated or normal TIBC, and decreased ferritin, iron, and percent saturation.**

B. With lead poisoning, basophilic stippling may be seen in peripheral blood cells. Iron deficiency is often seen in association with lead poisoning, so lead screening is important in children living in older housing. A blood lead level would be done prior to consideration of a lead mobilization test (which is done to determine which children are likely to benefit from chelation therapy).

C. In α-thalassemia trait, the MCV is low but the total number of RBCs is elevated with a normal RDW. Hypochromia is not seen on the blood smear, and laboratory evaluation should reveal a normal iron, TIBC, percent saturation, and ferritin. While hemoglobin electrophoresis can detect β-thalassemias, it does not generally detect α-thalassemia trait except in young infants.

D. In folate deficiency, the red cells are larger than normal, resulting in a hyperchromic anemia with an elevated MCV. Folate deficiency is often seen in babies who are fed goat's milk.

E. Dietary iron deficiency anemia can generally be treated as an outpatient. Blood transfusions and hospital admission are usually reserved for patients who have evidence of hemodynamic instability or excessive fatigue secondary to their anemia.

82. **C. The American Academy of Pediatrics (AAP) recommends that children with congenital heart disease who are undergoing a dental procedure be given antibiotics to prevent endocarditis. The standard prophylaxis regimen is amoxicillin 50 mg/kg, given as a one-time dose an hour before the procedure. Prophylaxis is also recommended for certain respiratory tract, gastrointestinal tract, and genitourinary tract procedures that are likely to cause transient bacteremia. For patients who are allergic to penicillin, the drug of choice is clindamycin.**

A. Patients who do *not* require prophylaxis include those with 1) physiologic or innocent murmurs; 2) an isolated secundum atrial septal defect (ASD); 3) a surgically repaired ASD, ventricular septal defect (VSD), or patent ductus arteriosus (PDA); and 4) mitral valve prolapse without valvular regurgitation. This patient, however, does require prophylaxis.

B, D. These are correct dosages, but administered at incorrect times.

E. This is not the standard prophylaxis regimen recommended by the AAP.

83. **A. This patient probably has Wiskott-Aldrich syndrome, which is an X-linked recessive syndrome consisting of atopic dermatitis, thrombocytopenia, and susceptibility to infection. Patients with Wiskott-Aldrich syndrome have impairment in the formation of antibodies to the polysaccharide capsular antigens. In general IgM is low, IgA and IgE are elevated, and IgG is slightly low.**

B. Ataxia telangiectasia is an autosomal recessive syndrome consisting of thrombocytopenia, progressive ataxia, and variable humoral and cellular immunodeficiency.

C. Patients with Wiskott-Aldrich syndrome have impairment in the formation of antibodies to the polysaccharide capsular antigens, but they are not agammaglobulinemic. In general IgM is low, IgA and IgE are elevated, and IgG is slightly low.

D. Severe combined immunodeficiency patients have severe deficiency of both cellular and humoral immunity. Gammaglobulin levels are extremely low to absent, and absolute leukocyte counts are frequently less than 500/μL.

E. Hyper-IgM syndrome is an X-linked immunodeficiency syndrome consisting of elevated polyclonal IgM, and usually normal T-cell function. These patients develop frequent respiratory infections beginning in the first or second year. Lymphoid hyperplasia is usually present.

84. **C. Psychological evaluation for depression or other psychiatric disorder should be initiated. This child is showing an acute change in**

behavior, more consistent with anxiety or depression, and should be evaluated before symptoms worsen.

A. While this child is showing some of the hallmark characteristics of attention deficit/hyperactivity, part of the diagnostic criteria for ADHD includes presence of symptoms before age 7.
B. Testing for learning disabilities is also warranted, but the acute nature of his behavior change both at home and at school warrants a careful assessment of mood disorder as the initial evaluation.
D. Hyperthyroidism can mimic psychiatric disorders and should be ruled out, but testing should neither delay nor replace psychological evaluation.
E. Simple observation and reevaluation in the future is not acceptable given the evolving severity of behaviors in this child.

85. **D. Turner syndrome is a chromosomal disorder (gonadal dysgensis: XO) resulting in a syndrome characterized by short stature, lymphedema, webbed neck, low posterior hairline, and cubitus valgus; there are often associated cardiac and renal anomalies as well. Growth hormone (GH) therapy is standard care for a child with Turner syndrome. Its use is not for the treatment of GH deficiency, but for the treatment of GH resistance. As a consequence, the dosage of GH used in Turner patients is higher than the patient with GH deficiency. Other associated endocrine conditions in Turner syndrome include glucose intolerance and hypothyroidism. In addition, certain autoimmune disorders are noted in Turner patients, including Hashimoto thyroiditis, celiac disease, inflammatory bowel disease, and JRA.**

A, B. Although GH is used in Turner patients, they do not have GH, IGF-1, and IGFBP3 deficiency, but rather require GH therapy because of GH resistance.
C. Most Turner syndrome patients will have delayed puberty and estrogen deficiency. Estrogen deficiency does not cause the short stature seen in these patients. A 5-year-old girl would be prepubertal and not need estrogen replacement therapy until she is older than 12 years of age.
E. ACTH deficiency is not associated with Turner syndrome.

86. **B. The findings of hyperchloremic acidosis and hypophosphatemia with growth delay suggest this patient has Fanconi syndrome. Aminoaciduria is a feature of Fanconi syndrome, which this patient probably has. The aminoaciduria is not selective because there is a generalized proximal tubular dysfunction.**

A. Glycosuria is a feature of Fanconi syndrome, which is secondary to the inability of the proximal tubules to reabsorb all of the filtered glucose. Blood glucose is generally unaffected.
C. Fanconi syndrome is not likely to be associated with an elevated BUN and creatinine. Other features of Fanconi syndrome include glycosuria and aminoaciduria. The syndrome consists of generalized proximal tubular dysfunction with decreased reabsorption of glucose, phosphorus, amino acids, and bicarbonate. Potassium wasting is also a common feature. In the first year of life, Fanconi syndrome is secondary to cystinosis (lysosomal cystine storage) until proven otherwise.
D. In proximal tubular acidosis, the kidneys can produce acid urine because the problem is in reabsorption of bicarbonate. When acidosis exists, the decreased filtered bicarbonate can all be reabsorbed, resulting in little distal delivery of bicarbonate. The distal tubular acidification can then function normally. Urine is considered "acid" when pH is *below* 6.0.
E. Hypophosphatemic rickets can be the consequence of Fanconi syndrome, especially when it is due to cystinosis. This rickets is generally not associated with hypocalcemia, and therefore PTH is unaffected.

87. **C. Patients who take OCPs have a reduced risk of ovarian cancer that occurs after relatively short-term use (5 years) and persists for 10 to 20 years after their use has been discontinued.**

A, B, D. Benefits of OCPs include a decreased incidence of anemia due to reduction of blood loss at each menses, an improvement in acne due to a decrease in free testosterone, and a reduced risk of endometrial cancer.
E. OCPs can cause venous thromboembolism, resulting in stroke and pulmonary embolus.

88. **A. In Duchenne muscular dystrophy, the calf muscles may feel rubbery and appear enlarged.**

B. While some head control problems may be detected early, the hip-girdle weakness does not appear until the second or third year. Pelvic weakness is detected by a waddling gait, wide-based stance, and a Gower sign (propping hands on thighs to push up to a standing position).

C. The CK level is extremely high, even in the earliest stages of the disease.

D. The disease is X-linked and is found in about 1 in 3600 boys.

E. The muscle degeneration seen with Duchenne muscular dystrophy is a painless process that is not associated with muscle spasm or myalgias. The muscle biopsy shows atrophic and hypertrophic muscle fibers and immunohistochemical staining shows deficient or defective dystrophin. Cardiomyopathy is a constant feature of this disease and repeated cardiac assessment is indicated. Death occurs by age 18, usually due to pneumonia, respiratory failure, or heart failure.

89. **D. Nephropathy secondary to vesicoureteral reflux is one of the most common causes of hypertension in children.**

A. Even the first documented UTI in a boy should be investigated to rule out significant urologic abnormalities. Generally, renal ultrasound and voiding cystogram are indicated. The first UTI in a girl under 4 to 5 years of age should also be investigated further.

B. Significant vesicoureteral reflux has been associated with urinary tract infection. However, it is generally felt that the reflux is more causative, and that *significant* reflux does not result from urinary tract infection. The more severe grades of reflux (grade 3 to 5) are more often associated with urinary tract infection and/or reflux nephropathy.

C. Untreated significant vesicoureteral reflux has been associated with end-stage renal disease. It accounted for 15% to 20% of end-stage kidney disease in the past before greater attention was placed on the management of UTIs and reflux. End-stage disease is less common now in children followed and treated appropriately.

E. Indeed, vesicoureteral reflux is an inherited trait. While the incidence is as high as 30% to 35% in siblings, most are asymptomatic. About 12% of asymptomatic siblings with reflux have evidence of renal scarring.

90. **A. Secondary bacterial infection is a common complication of atopic dermatitis and often results from poorly controlled disease and/or pruritis. Antihistamines should be used as an adjunct to control pruritis, while oral antibiotics, such as cephalexin, are used to treat the concurrent infection.**

B. Short baths with tepid water are recommended for patients with atopic dermatitis. Excessively warm baths or longer baths will further dry the skin and exacerbate the underlying affected skin.

C. Steroid creams used to treat and control the patchy, erythematous skin of atopic dermatitis need to be applied before an emollient.

D. Cooler, humid ambient temperatures will have less of an effect on drying out the skin than warmer, more arid temperatures.

E. Lubrication needs to be used liberally and almost cannot be too liberal.

91. **B. Growth delay is a characteristic of uremia secondary to poor response to growth hormone. Other factors include poor nutrition, acidosis, and renal osteodystrophy. Bone age is therefore generally delayed.**

A. Anemia in chronic renal failure is usually normocytic, and is secondary to deficiency of erythropoietin production in the kidneys.

C. Osteopenia, not osteosclerosis, would be expected. Rickets is a part of the osteodystrophy of chronic renal disease. It is due to the decreased production of 1,20-dihydrocholecalciferol, the active metabolite of vitamin D. The secondary effects of this deficiency are decreased intestinal absorption of calcium, and failure in calcification of the osteoid to form new bone.

D. Hyperparathyroidism, not hypoparathyroidism, in chronic renal failure results from the lack of vitamin D, poor absorption of calcium, and phosphorus retention—all of which stimulate the parathyroid glands.

E. Most often, the urine in patients with chronic renal failure is closer to isotonic with osmolality near 300, and specific gravity near 1.010. There is usually a concentrating defect.

92. **D. Vulvovaginal candidiasis causes a discharge that is classically thick, white, cottage cheese-like, and adherent to the vaginal walls. The discharge usually has no odor. The vaginal pH is normally less than 4.5 and is unchanged with a candidal infection. KOH prep is helpful with visualizing the yeast and pseudohyphae by lysing the epithelial cells. Oral fluconazole offers a single-dose treatment.**

 A. Sitz baths may provide some comfort but will not treat the underlying infection.
 B. Topical azole creams can be used but length of therapy is 7 days and compliance may serve as a barrier in the adolescent population.
 C. Azithromycin as a single dose would be acceptable for the treatment of *Chlamydia trachomatis*.
 E. Metronidazole would be used to treat bacterial vaginosis.

93. **A. Diabetes type I and other autoimmune diseases such as rheumatoid arthritis, thyroid disease, and IgA deficiency are indeed associated with celiac, another autoimmune disease. In those with celiac disease, an autoimmune process takes place after exposure to the protein gluten. This protein is found in wheat, rye, and barley. Normally not the targets of the immune system, portions of this protein are attacked as well as some other human proteins. The immune response leads to inflammation and ultimately damage to the local area.**

 B. Those with strict adherence to a gluten-free diet will have fewer complications, including a reduced chance of GI malignancy.
 C. Polycythemia, or an elevated hematocrit, is not associated with celiac disease. In fact, the opposite is true and anemia is very frequently associated with celiac disease, with the disruption of iron and vitamin B12 absorption.
 D. Cleaning solutions are not associated with celiac disease.
 E. Decreased albumin is another factor pointing to the ongoing malabsorption that takes place in celiac disease.

94. **B. The conjunctival injection with Kawasaki disease is nonexudative and typically involves the bulbar conjunctiva. To meet the criteria for classic Kawasaki disease, there should be evidence of fever for at least 5 days plus four of the following five criteria: 1) bulbar conjunctival injection without exudates, 2) mucosal changes such as dry, fissured lips; strawberry tongue or injected pharynx, 3) unilateral cervical lymphadenopathy, usually, greater than 1.5 cm 4) induration or edema of the hands and feet, and 5) generalized erythematous rash, which can vary from maculopapular to one resembling erythema multiforme. Five days of fever, three of the above criteria, plus coronary artery abnormalities will also confirm the diagnosis of classic Kawasaki disease.**

 A. Cervical lymphadenopathy greater than 1.5 cm is one of the criteria associated with the diagnosis of Kawasaki disease.
 C. Oral ulcerations are a clinical criteria associated with systemic lupus erythematous.
 D. Mitral valve regurgitation is often seen with rheumatic heart disease. Active carditis is one of the major Jones criteria used to make the diagnosis of rheumatic fever. (See the explanation to question 22 for a listing of the Jones criteria.)
 E. Scrotal edema can be seen in Kawasaki disease secondary to an associated hypoalbuminemia that may occur. It is not a clinical criteria used in making the diagnosis of Kawasaki disease. Patients with Henoch-Schönlein purpura (HSP) are often noted to have scrotal edema on exam as well.

95. **D. The symptoms described of chest discomfort, palpitations, near syncope, and dyspnea, in an otherwise healthy patient, are worrisome for serious cardiac and/or pulmonary problems and need immediate evaluation. Although the scenario offers the choice to call the parents to pick up their son, ambulatory transport to an ER would be recommended if the symptoms are severe or persistent.**

 A. It would not be appropriate to try albuterol, as this may have unwanted side effects such as tachycardia.
 B. Placing the patient supine with elevated legs for 15 minutes without any further medical attention would not be appropriate.
 C. Waiting a week for further evaluation given the acute nature of the symptoms would be wholly inappropriate.
 E. Although taking the patient's pulse during another episode may be helpful, future diagnostic evaluation is needed to prevent or establish the etiology for his symptoms.

96. B. This particular exam and symptoms point to the diagnosis of hypertrophic cardiomyopathy. The murmur is typically heard at the lower left sternal border as a systolic ejection grade II-IV/VI murmur. The murmur would be expected to decrease with valsalva maneuvers, such as squatting, and increase with standing. Sharp upstroke of brachial pulses is characteristic. ECG findings of left ventricular hypertrophy would be expected, as would deep Q waves in leads V5 and V6.

A, E. Digitalis and other drugs, such as albuterol, may increase the tone of the heart, resulting in negative effects which can worsen the degree of obstruction.

C. A heart rate of 100 would not be consistent with SVT.

D. There is nothing to suggest dextrocardia in this case.

97. E. Lactase deficiency or lactose intolerance is a very common problem in the United States. The intolerance can be partial to complete and can be associated with other disease processes. There is a breath hydrogen study available for further confirmation.

A. Treatment for partial intolerance may be to restrict lactose until asymptomatic.

B. Those of European descent are affected the least, while those of Asian descent are affected the most. African Americans are very commonly affected.

C. The problem occurs when increased lactose is presented to intestinal bacteria and an osmotic diarrhea ensues.

D. If milk products are reduced significantly then calcium supplements are indicated.

98. C. All of the answers listed—congenital hypothyroidism, duodenal atresia, Hirschsprung disease, Meckel diverticulum, and TEF—are associated with trisomy 21 (Down syndrome). Hirschsprung disease should be considered whenever there has been no passage of meconium in the first 48 hours. In Hirschsprung disease, there is an absence of ganglionic cells in the bowel wall, confirmed by biopsy. The result is delayed passage of meconium or further problems with chronic constipation.

A. Hypothyroidism will cause constipation in time.

B. Duodenal atresia should cause upper GI tract symptoms such as early emesis.

D. Meckel diverticulum should not delay the stooling, and would be expected to present with hematochezia.

E. TEFs do not delay passage of stool and often present with choking during feeds and/or excessive secretions.

99. B. The child has amblyopia of the left eye. Early diagnosis and treatment are crucial to this disease. Amblyopia is characterized by central suppression of the vision of one or both eyes. In a literate child, the best corrected vision of 20/30 or worse in one *or both* eyes, not explained by eye pathology, is diagnostic. Correcting the vision with the appropriate glasses, and occluding or blurring the vision of the better-seeing eye to eliminate suppression of the affected eye, are key therapeutic elements.

A, C. Therapy initiated in teenage years will not typically be successful, and initiating therapy prior to age 8 is best.

D. Patching the left eye is not appropriate, as the child has amblyopia of the left eye.

E. Simply realigning the eye will not force the brain to stop suppressing the eye, so surgery is often deferred until the amblyopia is resolved.

100. C. There are several items to ensure in follow-up evaluations of amblyopia. Assessing degree of vision improvement, and ensuring that the dominant eye has not been weakened, are both critical. Encouragement of the patient and family during this tiresome and stigmatizing treatment is needed. Subsequent exams are scheduled weeks or months apart, depending on the age of the child. The plasticity of the visual system demands that younger children be reevaluated at intervals of no more than 1 week for each month of their age (a 4-month-old should be reassessed no later than 4 weeks after therapy is initiated.). The typical interval for older children is 3 months.

A, B, D. These follow-up times are incorrect. See explanation for C.

E. Follow-up of patients with amblyopia is critical. See explanation for C.

SETTING 3: INPATIENT FACILITIES

You have general admitting privileges to the hospital. You may see patients in the critical care unit, the pediatrics unit, the maternity unit, or recovery room. You may also be called to see patients in the psychiatric unit. A short-stay unit serves patients who are undergoing same-day operations or who are being held for observation. There are adjacent nursing home/extended-care facilities and a detoxification unit where you may see patients.

101. A term infant is born to a mother whose perinatal labs include HIV, nonreactive; RPR– (rapid plasma reagin–); GBS–(group B streptococcus–); hepatitis B–; blood type, O+. The infant is approximately 20 hours old and appears to be jaundiced to the chest. He is exclusively breastfed and clinically has been doing well. The most likely cause of his jaundice is:

    A. Breastfeeding jaundice
    B. Breastmilk jaundice
    C. Biliary atresia
    D. ABO incompatibility
    E. Physiologic jaundice

102. During an initial newborn exam you detect a palpable clunk in the patient's left hip during your Ortolani and Barlow maneuvers. You are concerned for developmental dysplasia of the hip (DDH). Your next course of action would be:

    A. Obtain radiographs of the pelvis and hips
    B. Obtain hip ultrasound
    C. Place the infant in triple diapers
    D. Orthopedic referral
    E. Observe and follow-up in 1 month

103. A 6-year-old boy is admitted with a 1-month history of cervical lymphadenitis that has continued to progress despite outpatient treatment with amoxicillin-clavulanate (Augmentin). The child has been clinically well without any other constitutional symptoms. A previously placed PPD measures 5 mm. His physical exam is pertinent for right cervical lymphadenopathy measuring about 3 to 4 cm with some overlying tenderness and erythema. A needle biopsy of the lymph node is undertaken (Figure 3-103). The most appropriate management of this patient would be:

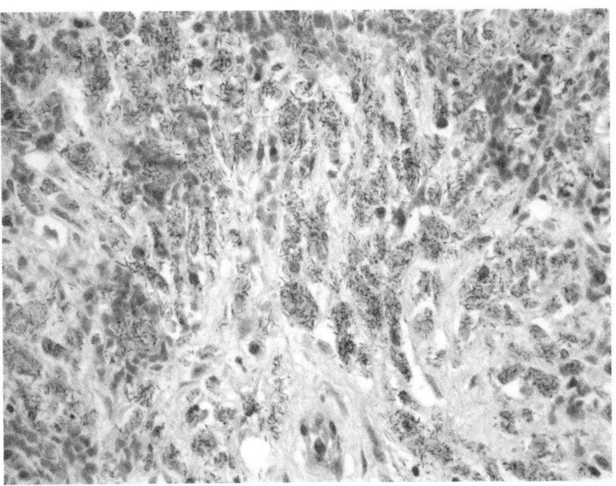

Figure 3-103 • Image Courtesy of the Department of Pathology, Phoenix Children's Hospital, Phoenix, Arizona.

    A. Surgical excision of the lymph node
    B. IV therapy with ampicillin-sulbactam (Unasyn)
    C. Referral to an oncologist
    D. Intralesional injection of corticosteroids
    E. IV therapy with ceftazidime and gentamycin

104. A 2-week-old infant is admitted to the wards with a 3-day history of poor feeding, tachypnea, and vomiting. Her perinatal history is unremarkable. Vitals are T, 37.6°C; P, 150; R, 52; and BP, 80/55, with a physical exam that is remarkable for a slightly sunken anterior fontanelle, tachypnea with clear breath sounds, and mottled skin appearance. Labs obtained in the ER show a normal CBC and differential; Na^+, 135; K^+, 2.6; Cl^-, 89; CO_2, 7; BUN, 16; and creatinine, 0.5. Which of the following would be the most useful step in arriving at a final diagnosis?

    A. Obtaining an ammonia level
    B. Completing a full septic evaluation
    C. Urine for organic acids
    D. 17-OH-progesterone
    E. TSH

105. You are called to the bedside of a 5-day-old preterm infant for increasing respiratory distress. The infant has been on a ventilator since birth. The physical exam is significant for tachypnea, retractions, and some decreased breath sounds noted on the right. You request a STAT x-ray (Figure 3-105). The next most appropriate step in management is:

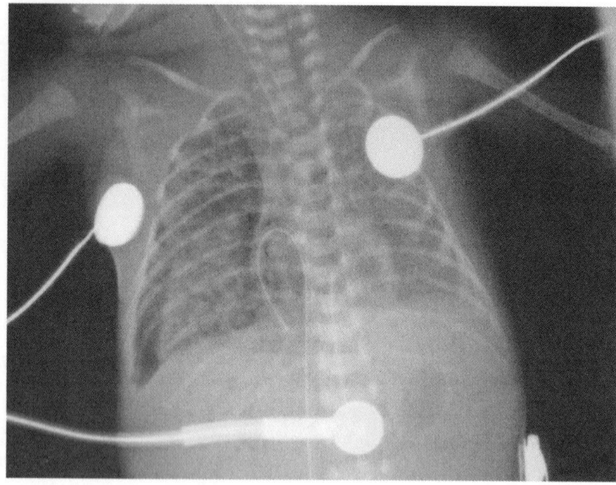

Figure 3-105 • Image Courtesy of the Department of Radiology, Phoenix Children's Hospital, Phoenix, Arizona.

A. Immediate broad-spectrum antibiotics
B. Confirmatory left lateral decubitus radiograph
C. Placement of a chest tube
D. Confirmatory ultrasound or CT
E. Immediate albuterol treatment

106. The housestaff presents a case of a 13-year-old female with chronic abdominal cramping to their attending physician. Their thorough history and physical exam demonstrates a Tanner stage 2 female with flattening of the growth curve over the last 2 years and a right lower quadrant mass. In discussing the differential diagnosis of these problems, a senior resident states that inflammatory bowel disease is high on the list. A discussion then ensues about the differences between Crohn disease and ulcerative colitis. Which of the following statements would be most accurate to share with the patient and her family?

A. Extra-intestinal manifestations occur in both diseases, and include problems such as peripheral arthritis, erythema nodosum, and anemia
B. Colectomy is advised in all patients with ulcerative colitis within 2 years of diagnosis
C. Ulcerative colitis patients typically have more difficulty with fissures and fistulas
D. Skip lesions are required for the diagnosis of Crohn, but are common in ulcerative colitis as well
E. Esophageal and stomach involvement is quite rare in Crohn and if found would suggest eosinophilic gastroenteritis as a comorbid condition

107. A 15-year-old male with Burkitt lymphoma in remission is transferred to the PICU with active seizures. The patient is currently taking antibiotics for pneumonia. His physical examination is nonfocal and the patient does not appear to be dehydrated. Serum electrolytes reveal a serum sodium of 112 mEq/L. What would be the most appropriate action at this time?

A. Infusion of 3% hypertonic saline to acutely raise the serum sodium to 120 to 125 mEq/L
B. Furosemide (Lasix) at 1 mg/kg IV
C. Fluid restriction to 80% maintenance fluid
D. Acute correction of serum sodium to 140 mEq/L
E. Phosphenytoin 18 mg/kg IV load

108. A 4-week-old ex-34-week preemie is admitted with retractions, tachypnea, and an oxygen saturation of 80% on room air. The respiratory rate is 70 breaths/min and wheezes are heard diffusely in all lung fields. A nasal-pharyngeal wash demonstrates the presence of respiratory syncytial virus (RSV). The parents ask you what you can do in the PICU to help their child and relieve his respiratory distress. You respond:

A. Steroids can be administered but will take 6 to 12 hours before we begin to see an effect
B. Supportive care is the mainstay of bronchiolitis therapy
C. Antibiotics may be administered to prevent impending respiratory failure
D. An infusion of RSV intravenous immunoglobulin (IVIG) will hasten the patient's recovery from bronchiolitis
E. Continuous high-dose bronchodilator therapy should relieve this patient's respiratory distress

109. A 3-year-old boy has been admitted to the hospital with a history of fever, severe abdominal pain, and diarrhea. An outside CT scan of his abdomen was obtained and read as normal except for a thickening and inflammation of the pancreatic head. Further laboratory evaluation reveals an amylase of 1900 U/L and a lipase of 5000 U/L. Which of the following is an accurate statement regarding this patient's condition?

A. Blunt trauma is a common etiology
B. Amylase is always abnormal at presentation
C. Elevated amylase levels are usually diagnostic
D. Ranson's criteria can be used to predict prognosis
E. Pseudocyst development is a common complication

110. A child presents on the hospital ward with respiratory distress, exhibited by nasal flaring, intercostal retractions, grunting respirations, and cyanosis. You start oxygen by facemask, but the child is still in significant respiratory distress and becomes apneic. The best next step is:

A. Start chest compressions
B. Perform a Heimlich maneuver, as the child may have aspirated something
C. Obtain a blood gas
D. Send the child to the radiology department for a chest x-ray
E. Start bag-valve-mask ventilations with 100% oxygen

111. A newborn is found on initial exam to have a 2-cm round mass over the nasal bridge. It is soft to touch, slightly bluish in color, and darkens and swells slightly when the baby cries. An exam light transilluminates the lesion. The best next step in the management of this finding is:

A. Reassure the parents it will resolve with time
B. Obtain a biopsy
C. Inject the lesion with steroid to induce involution
D. Massage the lesion or apply a pressure bandage to induce microembolization
E. Order an MRI of the baby's head

112. A 2-year-old boy is admitted to the hospital with high fever for 5 or 6 days, swelling of the hands and feet, scarletiniform changes of the tongue, a generalized red maculopapular rash, dry red cracked lips, and scleral injection. The toddler looks miserable out of proportion to his physical findings. His initial lab work-up reveals an erythrocyte sedimentation rate (ESR) greater than 100, and thrombocytopenia with a platelet count of 60,000. A diagnosis of Kawasaki disease is made. Which of the following is the best initial treatment?

A. Cardiac catheterization and long-term follow-up by cardiology
B. IVIG 2 g/kg IV and high-dose aspirin orally
C. Aspirin 5 mg/kg by mouth (PO) daily
D. Steroid therapy
E. Avoid influenza and varicella vaccines until the child is better

The next 2 questions (items 113-114) correspond to the following vignette.

An 18-month-old girl is admitted from the ED with a chief complaint of a draining sore on her right buttock. Her grandmother reports that she first noticed an area of redness on the child's right buttock 5 days ago. Over this time period, the area enlarged and became tender and warm. Yesterday it spontaneously opened and started draining a yellow-red discharge. On physical exam, the toddler is alert and prefers to lie on her side because of the pain. Her vital signs reveal a temperature of 38.6°C and a pulse of 130. Blood pressure and respiratory rate are normal. The rest of the exam is normal except for the right buttock. There is a 6-cm area of erythema and a central 2-cm area of induration. In the center of this indurated area is a small opening through which you see the yellow-red discharge seeping out.

113. The most likely diagnosis is:

A. Osteomyelitis of the sacrum
B. Perirectal abscess
C. Irritant contact dermatitis
D. Candidal dermatitis
E. Crohn disease

114. The most appropriate next step in management would be:

A. Surgical consult for incision and drainage
B. Primary closure of the draining site with sutures
C. Oral amoxicillin for 10 days
D. Sterile dressing application and follow-up with PCP in 1 week
E. Barium enema

115. A 3300-g newborn male is born at 39 weeks' gestational age to a 25-year old mother. Prenatal labs show that the mother is rubella immune, RPR nonreactive, HIV nonreactive, hepatitis B negative, but GBS positive. The mother received IV ampicillin in adequate doses more than 4 hours before delivery. On initial exam, the baby's vital signs and physical exam are normal. He is voiding and stooling well and breastfeeding without difficulties. The most appropriate next step in management would be:

A. Lumbar puncture (LP)
B. Chest x-ray
C. Observation for 48 hours
D. CBC and blood culture
E. Empiric IV antibiotics for 72 hours

116. You are following a 2-year-old boy with septo-optic dysplasia (SOD) in the hospital for viral gastroenteritis and dehydration. Which medication needs to be adjusted during this hospitalization and illness?

A. Thyroid supplementation
B. Insulin
C. Glucocorticoid supplementation
D. Vasopressin (DDAVP)
E. Growth hormone (GH)

117. You are attending the delivery of a term infant who was born via normal spontaneous vaginal delivery with thick meconium. The baby is suctioned at the perineum and then handed to you. You notice slow irregular respirations, a heart rate of 130, limp muscle tone, grimacing, and a pale blue body throughout. What would this infant's Apgar score be at 1 minute if the exam remains unchanged?

A. 0
B. 2
C. 4
D. 5
E. 8
F. 12

118. A $2\frac{1}{2}$-week-old infant presents with a 4-day history of vomiting, decreased intake, and lethargy. The physical examination is significant for a mildly sunken fontanelle, dry mouth, and decreased activity. You notice that the scrotal sacs are hyperpigmented and small. The testes are nonpalpable and there is mild hypospadias. Electrolytes are obtained and show Na^+, 125 mmol/L; K^+, 6.4 mmol/L; Cl^- 103 mmol/L; CO_2, 15 mmol/L; and glucose, 50 mg/dL. Which of the following is accurate information to give to the family regarding this patient's illness?

A. This condition is inherited as an autosomal dominant trait
B. The most common form of the disease is 11-hydroxylase deficiency
C. Treatment includes replacement of cortisol and aldosterone
D. Ultrasound is indicated to localize the testes
E. Laboratory evaluation should include AM serum cortisol levels

119. In the delivery room, you notice that a newborn infant already has two teeth present in the lower gum. The pregnancy was uneventful without any infections and the mother received no medications other than prenatal vitamins. Which of the following is appropriate information to tell this infant's mother?

A. A deep root system is typically developed
B. Natal teeth are most commonly found in the position of the maxillary central incisors
C. A family history of natal teeth is common
D. There is no risk of aspiration
E. There is no association with cleft palate

120. A 10-month-old baby is noted to be chronically irritable. His mother, who wears a veil and gown and is a vegetarian for religious reasons, has been breastfeeding the baby exclusively. The baby's fontanelle is still open and is noted to be bulging. On physical examination you find frontal bossing, widening of the wrists, and bowed legs. Because of the irritability and bulging fontanelle, you order an MRI scan. It is reported as normal aside from showing evidence of increased intracranial pressure. An LP yields normal cerebrospinal fluid and an elevated opening pressure. The next step in the management of this patient would be to:

A. Perform serial LPs
B. Prescribe acetazolamide (Diamox)
C. Administer corticosteroids
D. Prescribe vitamin D and calcium supplements
E. Refer patient to a neurosurgeon

121. A baby seen in the newborn nursery is found to have a loud heart murmur. The baby has been feeding poorly. The chest radiograph demonstrates decreased pulmonary vascular flow and you are considering tricuspid atresia as a possible diagnosis. In preparing to tell the parents about their baby's heart defect, which of the following is most accurate?

A. In this condition, blood cannot flow from the right atrium to the right ventricle
B. In most cases, a patent ductus arteriosus (PDA) allows blood to get to the lungs
C. Most patients do not have cyanosis in the newborn period
D. The cardiogram generally shows right ventricular hypertrophy
E. The goal of medical and surgical treatment is to decrease blood flow to the lungs

122. A 3-day-old preterm infant develops intermittent apnea spells lasting greater than 20 seconds, accompanied by bradycardia. Investigation reveals no apparent infection or metabolic imbalance. These episodes seem to respond to gentle cutaneous stimulation. Which one of the following would be true for the management of this baby?

   A. The baby is too young to consider this idiopathic apnea
   B. No medication has been shown to be beneficial for frequent apnea
   C. Correction of anemia would have no effect on the frequency of apnea
   D. If the episodes are frequent, nasal continuous positive airway pressure (CPAP) might be beneficial
   E. Apnea of prematurity usually resolves at 2 months of age

123. A 4-year-old boy is seen because of increased thirst and increased urination. He was toilet trained at 2 years, but he still wets the bed every night. Your concern is that this boy could have diabetes insipidus (DI) or psychogenic water drinking. A morning urine specimen after an 8-hour fast shows a specific gravity of 1.005. His serum sodium is 140 mEq/L. What would be your next step?

   A. Administer vasopressin to see whether his urine can concentrate
   B. Administer a sodium load to see whether his kidneys can respond by increasing sodium excretion
   C. Increase the overnight fasting test to 12 to 15 hours to see whether his urine can concentrate
   D. Perform a daytime water deprivation test, measuring any changes in urine concentration and serum osmolality
   E. Because his serum sodium is normal, advise the parent that there is no need for further tests

124. An infant is born with port-wine nevus distributed and well-demarcated over the distribution of the right trigeminal area of the face. Which one of the following may apply to this syndrome?

   A. Pulsed dye laser treatments are frequently used and are quite effective for the skin lesions
   B. While seizures are common, most patients can be readily controlled with anticonvulsant therapy
   C. Medical management is the only avenue for the treatment of recalcitrant seizures
   D. Glaucoma on the affected side is always apparent in the first month of life
   E. Subsequent siblings have a 25% risk of being affected because this condition is autosomal recessive

125. You are called by the nurse to evaluate a term 3-hour-old infant who was born to a 25-year-old mother with unremarkable prenatal labs and an uncomplicated pregnancy. The baby was born via scheduled cesarean section without previous rupture of membranes secondary to a previous child born via cesarean section. On physical exam you notice a mild to moderately tachypneic infant with some coarse breath sounds bilaterally and mild intercostal retractions; the remainder of the physical exam is normal. The child is saturating 98% on room air. A chest radiograph is obtained (Figure 3-125). Your next step in management would be:

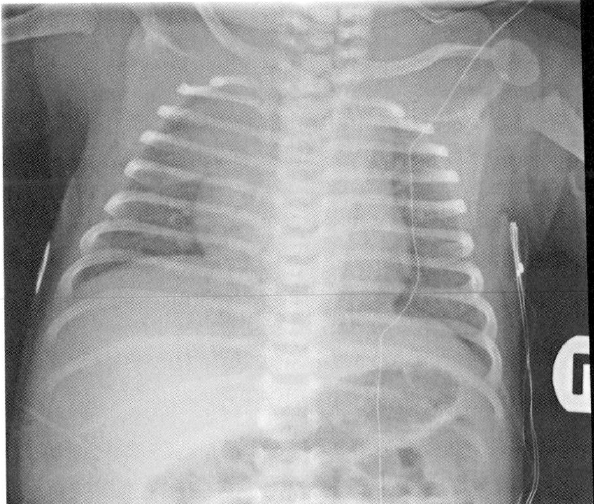

Figure 3-125 • Image Courtesy of the Department of Radiology, Phoenix Children's Hospital, Phoenix, Arizona.

   A. Place the infant on supplemental oxygen
   B. Immediately administer antibiotics
   C. Draw a CBC/blood culture and then administer antibiotics
   D. Perform an ECHO
   E. Careful observation only

126. A 7-year-old African-American girl is admitted to the hospital for the evaluation of fever with a limp. Her father has noticed low-grade fevers intermittently for the past 4 weeks. Over this time period, the girl has had progressive pain in the right knee and is now refusing to walk or bear weight on that leg. She does have sickle cell disease. On physical exam, she is febrile and irritable. The right knee is slightly swollen compared to the left. She refuses to stand unassisted. Her total serum white blood cell count and ESR are elevated. Plain radiographs of the right lower extremity reveal periosteal elevation and subperiosteal fluid collection of the medial, distal right femur. The most likely causative bacterial pathogen for this child's illness is:

A. *Pseudomonas aeruginosa*
B. *Salmonella*
C. *Brucella*
D. *Staphylococcus aureus*
E. *Candida albicans*

127. A 6-month-old child is in the PICU with pneumococcal meningitis. He weighs 5 kg. He initially presented 2 days ago. Over the last 24 hours he has received D5 0.2% normal saline IV at 20 mL/hr. Electrolytes reveal a serum sodium of 123 mEq/L, potassium of 4.5 mEq/L, chloride of 90 mEq/L, and serum CO_2 of 23 mEq/L. Heart rate is 140 beats/min, respiratory rate is 30 breaths/min, and blood pressure is 110/70 mm Hg. Urine output has been 0.8 mL/kg/hr. Urine osmolality is 800 mEq/L. What would be the best way to initially begin to correct this serum sodium?

A. Add sodium to the child's formula
B. Change the IV fluid to 0.5 normal saline
C. Fluid restriction to insensible losses
D. Administer a thiazide diuretic
E. Give 20 mL/kg normal saline bolus over 10 minutes or less

128. You are called emergently to the bedside of a 9-month-old child who appears to have stopped breathing. On your physical exam you note no active respirations and no audible heartbeat or palpable pulses. After establishment of the airway, chest compressions are best performed on an infant by:

A. Using the heel of one hand
B. Using two fingers depressing the lower half of the sternum
C. Depressing the sternum 1.5 to 2 inches
D. Depressing the chest at a rate of 90 to 100 times per minute
E. Depressing the sternum less than one third of the depth of the chest

129. A child with acute lymphoblastic leukemia has a central line placed for ease of administration of medications and blood products. His induction chemotherapy includes dexamethasone, vincristine, and asparaginase. He is in remission 7 days after the start of therapy. After 2 weeks of therapy, he develops swelling of his chest wall on the side of the central line. On physical examination, venous distention is noted around the area of swelling. His most likely diagnosis is:

A. Cellulitis of his chest wall
B. Abscess of deep structures of the chest
C. Leukemic infiltration of his skin
D. Deep venous thrombosis of his subclavian vein
E. Osteomyelitis of his ribs

130. A 14-year-old boy was hospitalized with intractable seizures of unknown cause lasting several hours. His condition is stabilized after the first 6 hours in the hospital. His vital signs are relatively normal, and his seizures are controlled. However, his urine has become brown in color, and he is becoming progressively more oliguric. Examination of the urine shows a 2+ reaction for protein, 4+ hematest, specific gravity 1.025, pH 5.5, and surprisingly few RBCs. Electrolytes reveal a mild metabolic acidosis, and are otherwise normal. His serum phosphorus is 9.0 mg/dL, calcium 8.0 mg/dL, BUN 15 mg/dL, and creatinine 0.6 mg/dL. Your immediate next course of treatment would be which one of the following:

A. Administer an intravenous bolus of normal saline 20 mL/kg, followed by maintenance-type fluids
B. Withhold IV fluids and administer furosemide IV 2 mg/kg
C. Administer a 20 mL/kg bolus of normal saline followed by mannitol 0.5 g/kg over 30 minutes, then continue with a sodium bicarbonate solution to maintain his urine pH near 7.5, watching his serum chemistries for evidence of renal failure
D. Begin maintenance fluids at a volume equal to insensible water losses plus urine output, awaiting the need to institute dialysis
E. Begin dialysis, anticipating that he will develop renal failure

131. An 8-year-old boy, who has been developmentally normal, has started to have some gait disturbance and developmental regression. His speech has become slurred, and there is a slight hand tremor bilaterally. His muscles seem tight, and there is some ataxia. Some dysarthria is also noted. Basic chemistries reveal serum sodium of 128 mEq/L, potassium 5.4 mEq/L, chloride 106 mEq/L, and CO_2 20 mEq/L. You suspect that this boy has some sort of neurodegenerative disorder. Which one of the following statements regarding neurodegenerative disorders is true?

A. Most neurodegenerative disorders are sporadic and not hereditary
B. The metabolic defect in most neurodegenerative disorders is unknown
C. Adrenal insufficiency should be a consideration in this patient
D. Adrenoleukodystrophy and metachromatic leukodystrophy are variants of the same disease
E. All the sphingolipidoses involve the storage of an abnormal lipid

132. A 3-month-old male infant is hospitalized with nonsupperative indolent infections of the skin and mouth. He also has had diarrhea for the past 4 weeks, failure to thrive, and a rather persistent respiratory infection. He was delivered at term without complications. Further pertinent history reveals that his umbilical cord did not separate until 6 weeks of age. Which one of the following tests would most likely confirm a diagnosis?

A. Test for quantitative serum immunoglobulin level
B. Test for serum complement deficiency
C. Test for leukocyte killing deficiency
D. Test for leukocyte chemotaxis
E. Test for leukocyte adhesion deficiency

133. A 3-month-old boy who was born with a large abdomen presents to the clinic. The pregnancy was characterized by oligohydramnios. The infant developed respiratory distress soon after birth, and required a ventilator for several days. There are large palpable masses bilaterally. Abdominal ultrasound shows enlarged bilateral renal masses, which are echo dense with obscured corticomedullary junctions. Serum chemistries are normal. The BUN is 10 mg/dL and the creatinine 0.5 mg/dL. A renal biopsy is performed (Figure 3-133). Counseling the parents about this child's illness would include which of the following?

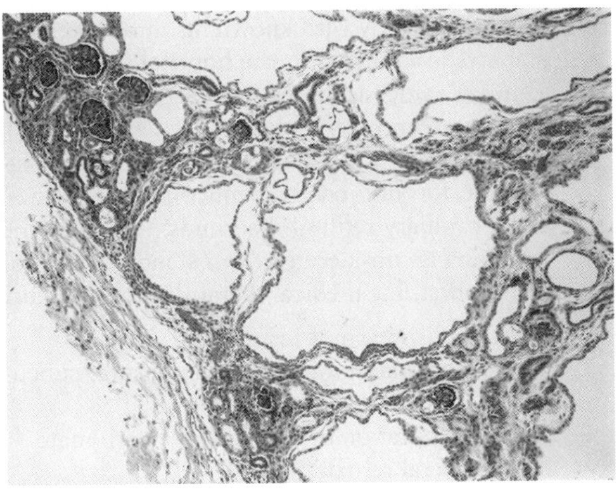

Figure 3-133 • Image Courtesy of the Department of Pathology, Phoenix Children's Hospital, Phoenix, Arizona.

A. This is an X-linked recessive disorder
B. Renal failure usually will not develop until he is an adult
C. Fifty percent of subsequent children, both male and female, will be affected
D. Large cysts of varying sizes are present early in this condition
E. Hepatic fibrosis is a common feature of this disorder

134. A newborn infant is noted to have dysmorphic features in the delivery room. The significant physical findings include hypotonia, microcephaly, wide-spaced first and second toes, simian crease, and epicanthal folds. Counseling the parents about this newborn should include:

A. Cardiac defects are seen in about 60%
B. Sterility is nearly universal in males
C. Mental retardation occurs in nearly all patients
D. Gastroschisis is commonly associated with this condition
E. Cardiac defects are seen in about 60%, and sterility is nearly universal in males
F. Cardiac defects are seen in about 60%, sterility is nearly universal in males, and mental retardation occurs in nearly all patients
G. Cardiac defects are seen in about 60%, sterility is nearly universal in males, mental retardation occurs in nearly all patients, and gastroschisis is commonly associated with this condition

135. A 4-year-old boy with known insulin-dependent diabetes is admitted to the hospital with significant lab values as follows: glucose, 650; sodium, 130; potassium, 2.5; chloride, 89; CO_2, 8; BUN, 29; and creatinine, 0.9. His physical exam is significant for dry, cracked mucous membranes, and a capillary refill of 4 seconds. Which of the following is considered to be a standard component of first-line medical therapy in this patient?

A. Administration of insulin by IV bolus
B. Administration of long-acting insulin subcutaneously
C. Administration of IV sodium bicarbonate
D. Parenteral rehydration
E. Administration of IM glucagon

136. You are called to examine a newborn infant with tachypnea. The infant's mother received no prenatal care. Vital signs are T, 37.6°C; P, 170; R, 75; BP 85/50; and saturations of 80% on room air with a physical exam significant for clear lung sounds with obvious tachypnea and no audible murmur with a normal S1 and single loud S2. A chest x-ray shows increased pulmonary markings with an egg-shaped cardiac silhouette. Which of the following would be most beneficial in the management of this infant?

A. Indomethacin
B. Captopril
C. Surfactant
D. Prostaglandin E_1
E. Propranolol

137. A 10-year-old girl who has lost significant weight over the past year is admitted to the hospital. She has been having gradually increasing difficulty swallowing solid foods, but she has been able to hold down liquids fairly well. There has been occasional vomiting, but no history of aspiration pneumonia. Her barium esophagram is shown (Figure 3-137). The most likely diagnosis is:

A. Hiatal hernia
B. Achalasia
C. Gastroesophageal reflux (GER)
D. Pyloric stenosis
E. Esophageal burn from caustic ingestion

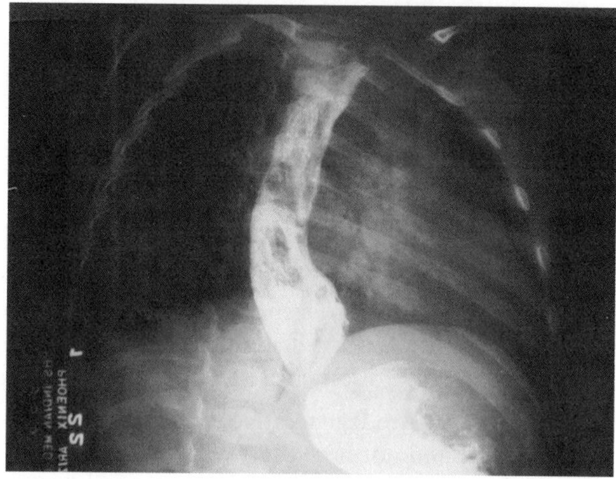

Figure 3-137 • Image Courtesy of the Department of Radiology, Phoenix Children's Hospital, Phoenix, Arizona.

138. You are admitting an 18-month-old toddler from the ED with rotavirus-positive acute gastroenteritis. She has been fluid resuscitated in the ED and is now rehydrated on physical exam. Even though maintenance IV fluids are running, she continues with frequent loose stools, but is not vomiting and acts hungry. The nurse is asking you what diet should be ordered. The most appropriate diet for this child would be:

A. NPO (nothing by mouth, IVF only)
B. BRAT diet (bananas, rice, applesauce, and toast)
C. Age-appropriate diet
D. Clear liquids only
E. Thick liquids only

139. You are called to see a newborn infant in the hospital because of feeding difficulties. The nurse reports that the child appears to be gagging with feedings and has excessive saliva. You attempt to pass an NG tube, which is unsuccessful. Which of the following is most accurate in reference to this infant's problem?

A. The least common form has the esophagus ending in a blind pouch with a distal connection between the trachea and esophagus
B. Ten percent of patients have associated anomalies such as VATER/VACTERL syndromes
C. H-type fistulas may not be detected until later in life
D. H-type fistulas are the most common type
E. Aspiration is infrequent with tracheoesophageal fistulas (TEFs)

140. A 2-month-old boy is admitted to the hospital with infantile spasms. His mother is known to have tuberous sclerosis and has normal intelligence. She is concerned that her son may also have tuberous sclerosis. Which of the following is accurate information to give to his mother?

A. Later skin manifestations of tuberous sclerosis may include shagreen patch, subungual fibromas, and café-au-lait spots
B. Mental retardation is not likely because the mother has normal intelligence
C. Tuberous sclerosis rarely affects the kidneys
D. Cataracts are common eye findings in tuberous sclerosis
E. Myxomas of the heart are common in tuberous sclerosis

141. You are called by the nurse to examine a newborn infant because of concerns over a congenital deformity. On the exam of an infant boy you observe a rather severe talipes equinovarus (clubfoot) deformity of the right foot. The parents are visibly upset and have many questions. Which of the following is appropriate information to give them?

A. Positional foot deformity must be treated like a clubfoot deformity
B. Clubfoot deformity has no genetic implications
C. Surgery is usually recommended in the newborn period for moderately severe clubfoot
D. Calf and foot atrophy frequently result in spite of adequate early treatment of clubfoot
E. The deformity in congenital clubfoot is usually limited to the foot and ankle

142. A 10-day-old premature baby in the intensive care nursery develops abdominal distension, bloody stools, and bilious vomiting. The baby has been taking a cow's milk protein-based preterm formula. An abdominal radiograph is obtained (Figure 2-142). The most appropriate management of this infant would be:

A. Switch to a protein hydrolysate formula
B. No immediate treatment is necessary; repeat radiograph in 24 hours
C. Continue to feed formula; start oral antibiotics
D. Make patient NPO, start IV antibiotics
E. Take patient to OR for bowel resection

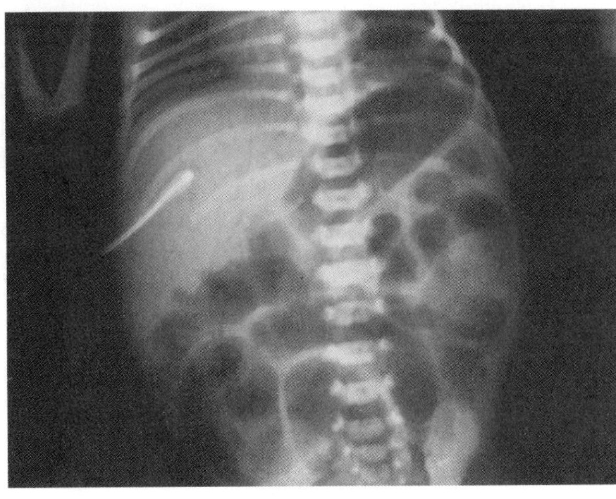

Figure 3-142 • Image Courtesy of the Department of Radiology, Phoenix Children's Hospital, Phoenix, Arizona.

143. You are called to the delivery of a full-term infant boy who was found to have the stigmata of Down syndrome. He was born to a 24-year-old primagravida mother with an unremarkable prenatal history. There is no history of the occurrence of Down syndrome in any of the family members on either the father's or the mother's side. Which one of the following statements is true?

A. The likelihood of recurrence in a subsequent offspring is about 1 in 700
B. Only 50% of Down syndrome patients result from trisomy 21
C. Almost all Down syndrome conceptions will carry to term
D. Mosaic Down syndrome results from a meiotic nondisjunction
E. Down syndrome in mothers under 30 years of age is most often a result of trisomy 21

144. You are seeing a newborn term baby in the nursery. All prenatal labs are normal as is the infant's exam. The mother reports that a cousin who visited yesterday has chicken pox. There is a history of varicella in the mother as a child. What would be the next step in the management of this newborn?

A. Acyclovir
B. Varicella-zoster immunoglobulin (VZIG)
C. Observation only
D. Cephazolin
E. Acyclovir and VZIG

145. A newborn is noted to have abdominal distension, vomiting, and failure to pass meconium in the first 48 hours of life. Abdominal radiographs show dilated loops of small bowel with air-fluid levels and a collection of "ground glass" material in the lower abdomen. The surgeon's postoperative diagnosis is meconium ileus. Which of the statements about meconium ileus would be correct information to give to the family?

A. It is commonly seen in Down syndrome
B. About 65% of infants with cystic fibrosis develop meconium ileus
C. It is less common in children whose siblings had meconium ileus
D. Rupture of the bowel wall and peritonitis are not complications of meconium ileus
E. If an enema with a hypertonic solution such as diatrizoate (Gastrografin) does not cause passage of the plug and relief of the obstruction, surgical intervention is necessary

146. A 12-year-old boy with chronic renal failure and a history of noncompliance with dialysis appointments is admitted to the floor. You are called emergently to his bedside by the nurses who fear he is in shock. An electrocardiograph reveals a chaotic rhythm with a widened QRS complex. The most effective management for this child would be:

A. Lidocaine 1 mg/kg IV bolus
B. Calcium chloride (10%), 0.2 mL/kg IV bolus
C. Magnesium sulfate, 25 mg/kg IV bolus
D. Furosemide, 5 mg/kg IV infusion
E. Mannitol, 1 g/kg IV infusion

147. A 4-year-old boy is admitted to the hospital with severe asthma. He has been admitted on two previous occasions. Oxygen saturations are 96% on 2 liters of O_2 by mask. Which one of the following arterial blood gas determinations would suggest this patient should be transferred to the ICU?

A. pH 7.35, HCO_3 20 mEq/L, pCO_2 36 mm Hg
B. pH 7.40, HCO_3 20 mEq/L, pCO_2 32 mm Hg
C. pH 7.40, HCO_3 27 mEq/L, pCO_2 45 mm Hg
D. pH 7.30, HCO_3 17.5 mEq/L, pCO_2 35 mm Hg
E. pH 7.25, HCO_3 13 mEq/L, pCO_2 30 mm Hg

148. A 6-month-old infant hospitalized for diagnostic evaluation of a congenital heart defect has echocardiographic findings consistent with tetralogy of Fallot (overriding aorta, VSD, pulmonary atresia, and right ventricular hypertrophy). You are called to see the child because he has become hypoxic and moderately cyanotic with a bout of crying. What is the first step in managing this "Tet spell?"

A. Reposition the child with knees to chest
B. Administer oxygen
C. Administer an IV fluid bolus
D. Prepare to perform cardiopulmonary resuscitation
E. Administer furosemide

The next 2 questions (items 149-150) correspond to the following vignette.

A 1-week-old baby is admitted from the ED with respiratory distress. Parents report that she has had progressive feeding and breathing difficulties since birth. Now she will only bottle feed small amounts and often will have nonprojectile regurgitation soon after feeding. Her breathing has become more rapid and includes accessory muscle use. On exam, she is

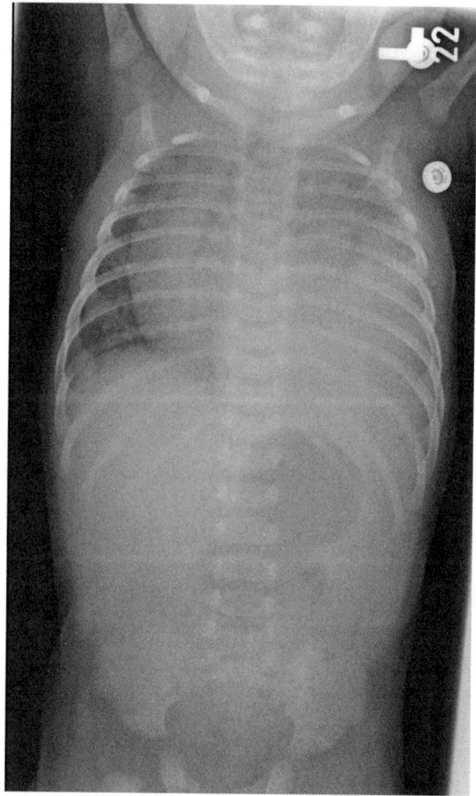

Figure 3-149 • Image Courtesy of the Department of Radiology, Phoenix Children's Hospital, Phoenix, Arizona.

afebrile with a respiratory rate of 70. She is mildly dehydrated and acts very hungry. She has mild intercostal retractions and you hear no breath sounds over the left hemithorax. Breath sounds on the right are clear. The rest of the exam is normal. CBC and basic metabolic panel (BMP) from the ED are normal. CXR taken on the way up from the ED is now available for your review (Figure 3-149).

149. The most likely diagnosis is:

A. Pyloric stenosis
B. Pneumonia with pleural effusion
C. TEF
D. Diaphragmatic hernia
E. Duodenal atresia

150. The most appropriate next step in management is:

A. NG tube decompression and surgical consultation
B. IV antibiotics
C. Chest tube insertion
D. Pyloromyotomy
E. ECHO

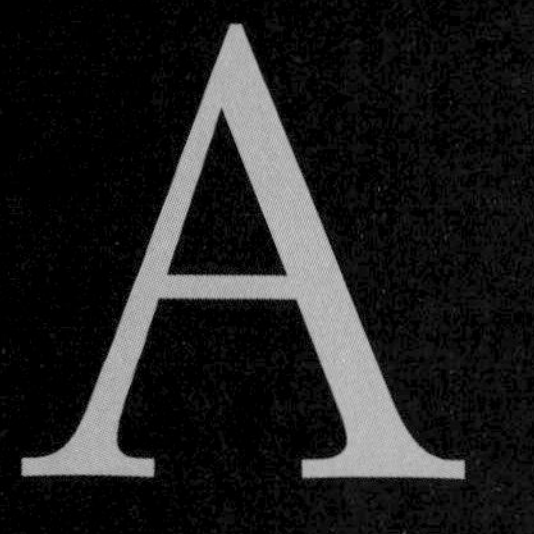

Answers and Explanations

101. D
102. D
103. A
104. C
105. C
106. A
107. A
108. B
109. A
110. E
111. E
112. B
113. B
114. A
115. C
116. C
117. C
118. C
119. C
120. D
121. A
122. D
123. D
124. A
125. E
126. D
127. C
128. B
129. D
130. C
131. C
132. E
133. E
134. F
135. D
136. D
137. B
138. C
139. C
140. A
141. D
142. D
143. E
144. C
145. E
146. B
147. C
148. A
149. D
150. A

101. D. ABO incompatibility most commonly occurs when the mother's blood type is O and the baby is either type A or B. The mother, being type O, has maternal antibodies to both A and B, which results in a hemolytic process that presents as jaundice. A blood type and direct Combs test should be obtained on all infants born to mothers who are type O.

A. Breastfeeding jaundice typically occurs in the first week of life secondary to a relative state of dehydration as a consequence of decreased breastmilk production.
B. Breastmilk jaundice usually occurs in exclusively breastfed babies in the second to third week of life. It is thought to be related to the intrinsic properties of breastmilk, which may inhibit glucuronyl transferase and the subsequent conjugation of bilirubin.
C. Biliary atresia is a disease that results in varying degrees of malformation to complete absence of the biliary tree. Although a cause of jaundice, biliary atresia typically is detected much later in life with an incidence that approximates 1 in 10,000 to 15,000.
E. By definition, any jaundice within the first 24 hours is pathological and needs further investigation. Physiologic jaundice occurs in term infants on days 2 to 4 and is believed to be related to increased red cell breakdown, increased bilirubin production, and relative immaturity of the liver's conjugation capacity.

102. D. If a positive exam is elicited in a newborn, an immediate orthopedic referral is recommended.

A. Radiographs of the pelvis and hips have limited value in the first few months of life when the femoral heads are composed mainly of cartilage. They become more reliable at approximately 4 to 6 months.
B. Although hip ultrasound is a useful exam in evaluating for DDH, treatment decisions are based on the results of the physical exam. A hip ultrasound is not recommended in the newborn with a positive exam.
C. The use of triple diapers is not recommended; they have not been shown to be effective and may even delay the onset of appropriate treatment.
E. An infant with a positive exam and concern for DDH requires fairly urgent, but not emergent, care. Simply observing and following up in 1 month is not acceptable.

103. A. The patient has a cervical lymphadenitis caused by atypical mycobacteria. The clinical history of progressing or unimproved cervical lymphadenopathy with minimal to no constitutional symptoms, a weakly positive purified protein derivative (PPD), and the lymph node biopsy showing acid fast bacilli (AFB) confirm the diagnosis. The treatment of choice is complete excision of the lymph node; incomplete excision often results in persistent drainage. Antituberculosis medications are not necessary following excision unless concern for *Myobacteria tuberculosis* cannot be ruled out.

B. IV therapy with ampicillin-sulbactam would be a good choice for the more common bacterial lymphadenitis caused by group A *Streptococcus* or *Staphylococcus aureus.*
C. There are no constitutional symptoms or other physical exam findings to suspect an oncologic process is occurring, so referral is unnecessary.
D. The use of steroids, either intralesional or systemically, is not indicated.
E. Ceftazidime and gentamycin would be appropriate choices for pseudomonal infections.

104. C. The infant in this scenario has a classic presentation of a metabolic disorder with poor feeding and vomiting without any history of fevers. The tachypnea is a result of attempted respiratory compensation for an underlying acidosis. The patient most likely has an organic acidemia, which would be revealed on urinary organic acid testing.

A. Although an ammonia level would be useful for further management, it would not solidify the final diagnosis. Organic acidemias can either present with normal or elevated ammonia levels. In evaluating an infant for inborn errors of metabolism, a key point to remember is that urea cycle defects, as well as aminoacidopathies, are expected to present *without* acidosis. In urea cycle defects, the ammonia will be elevated but normal in the aminoacidopathies.
B. Although the nonspecific signs of this child may be associated with sepsis, there is no underlying fever to suggest an infectious process.

D. Congenital adrenal hyperplasia (CAH) could present with a similar clinical picture, but laboratory evaluation should reveal hyponatremia, hyperkalemia, and possibly hypoglycemia. The elevated 17-OH-progesterone level would be expected in the most common form of CAH with a 21-hydroxylase deficiency.

E. Patients with congenital hypothyroidism would not be expected to be severely acidotic unless dehydrated—a presentation of weak cry, poor feeding, and constipation would be more suggestive.

105. **C. The physical exam and radiograph findings are consistent with a right-sided pneumothorax. After stabilization of the patient with attention to the ABCs (airway, breathing, circulation), a chest tube should be placed to evacuate pleural air. Barotrauma from mechanical ventilation is a risk factor for the development of a pneumothorax and is not uncommonly seen.**

A. Although pneumonia may predispose a patient to a pneumothorax, there is no evidence to suggest it in this patient.

B. A confirmatory left lateral decubitus radiograph is useful in determining the extent of free air seen over the liver in an abdominal process and will also aid in detecting a more subtle pneumothorax. However, the patient is in obvious respiratory distress and has a definitively diagnostic x-ray already.

D. A confirmatory ultrasound or CT has no role in this situation.

E. The use of albuterol in this scenario is not indicated.

106. **A. Extra-intestinal manifestations, such as arthritis, anemia, and erythema nodosum, are common in both forms of inflammatory bowel disease. Some of the manifestations occur only when colitis is present and some are independent of the state of the disease.**

B. Colectomy is advised in patients with ulcerative colitis when there is evidence of dysplasia on surveillance biopsies that begin around 8 years after the diagnosis.

C. Fissures and fistulas are common problems in Crohn disease.

D. Continuous involvement is typically seen in ulcerative colitis; skip lesions are commonly seen in Crohn disease.

E. Upper GI involvement is not uncommon in Crohn disease and affects perhaps 30%.

107. **A. The cause of the patient's seizures is hyponatremia. The serum sodium should be raised acutely to a level that will abort the seizure activity, typically in the range of 120 to 125 mEq/L, without being overly aggressive, which might increase the small but legitimate concern of central pontine myelinolysis caused by correcting serum sodium too rapidly. Full correction of the serum sodium acutely is therefore unnecessary. Acutely raising the sodium to 120 to 125 mEq/L in order to abort the neurologic emergency of ongoing seizure activity takes precedence over the small hypothetical risk of central pontine myelinolysis.**

B. Diuretics will not affect the serum sodium acutely enough to abort ongoing seizure activity.

C. Fluid restriction would be useful in the case of syndrome of inappropriate ADH (SIADH) but has no role in this case.

D. Acutely correcting the serum sodium to 140 mEq/L increases the theoretical risk of central pontine myelinolysis as described in the explanation for A.

E. Anticonvulsants are unlikely to be helpful in the face of seizures caused by hyponatremia, which will resolve with correction of the electrolyte abnormality.

108. **B. RSV causes inflammation of the bronchioles, which may be obstructed by edema, secretions, and cellular debris. Supportive care with oxygen, fluids, and frequent suctioning remains the mainstay of therapy for RSV.**

A. Steroids have been examined in many well-controlled studies and have never shown efficacy in the treatment of RSV, unless there is underlying asthma.

C. RSV is a virus, so antibiotics will be ineffective.

D. RSV IVIG may help reduce the severity of disease if administered to at-risk populations prior to infection, but studies have not shown efficacy in the acute treatment of active RSV infection.

E. Bronchodilators have never been shown to be effective in well-controlled studies of patients with RSV, likely because the pathophysiology of the wheezing in RSV patients is caused by bronchiole plugging with secretions, edema, and cellular debris, and not from smooth muscle bronchoconstriction.

109. **A. Blunt abdominal trauma, whether it be intentional or accidental, is a common cause of pancreatitis in the younger pediatric age group and should always be considered in the differential. Other etiologies include viral illnesses such as Epstein-Barr virus, cytomegalovirus, or coxsackie virus. Cystic fibrosis (CF), as well as a familial pancreatitis, are other known etiologies.**

B, C. Amylase can be normal in 10% to 15% of patients with acute pancreatitis. An elevated amylase level is not diagnostic of pancreatitis; elevated levels can be seen in salivary gland pathology such as parotitis, sialadenitis, or recurrent vomiting in eating disorders, as well as intestinal or esophageal perforation. Lipase is more specific for acute pancreatitis and typically remains elevated longer than amylase.

D. Ranson's criteria are factors that have been used to predict survival in adult patients; there are no prognostic factors developed for children. These criteria, used at the time of admission, include age greater than 55 years, leucocytosis greater than 16,000, hyperglycemia greater than 200 mg/dL, serum lactate dehydrogenase (LDH) greater than 400, and aspartate aminotransferase (AST) greater than 250.

E. Although pancreatic pseudocysts may be seen as a complication of pancreatitis, they are generally considered to be an uncommon sequela. They should be suspected in slowly improving cases of pancreatitis or when a palpable abdominal mass is detected following an acute episode.

110. **E. The child has stopped breathing on his own. The most important priority is to reestablish oxygenation and ventilation as suggested with 100% oxygen and bag-valve-mask.**

A. Chest compressions are not necessary unless the patient is asystolic or bradycardic with a heart rate less than 60 beats per minute (BPM). The ABCs of CPR remind one to attend to airway and breathing first.

B. You have no indication of a foreign body aspiration. Abdominal thrusts are preferable to the Heimlich maneuver in children, when indicated, to avoid rib fractures.

C. A laboratory test is not necessary to tell you the patient is not breathing, and will only waste precious time before reestablishing oxygenation and ventilation.

D. You do not want to send the child anywhere out of sight for imaging in a state of extreme respiratory distress. A portable chest x-ray should be done at the bedside *after* respirations are reestablished or the patient is intubated and ventilated.

111. **E. This lesion may be an encephalocele, because it is in the midline and swells with crying or valsalva. Neuroimaging and neurosurgical consultation are indicated.**

A. The exam findings in this newborn are descriptive of more than a simple hemangioma and deserve further investigation.

B. A biopsy would be a critical error, because the lesion could contain brain tissue.

C. The location of this lesion is suggestive that it may be much more than a hemangioma. Regardless, hemangiomas do not require steroid injection unless they are obstructing vision, the airway, or some other vital organ.

D. Massage is not helpful to either type of lesion. In addition, it is difficult to apply a pressure dressing in this location.

112. **B. Patients with Kawasaki disease are at risk of developing coronary artery dilation and aneurysms. The goal of treatment for Kawasaki disease in the acute phase is to decrease this myocardial and coronary artery (CA) wall inflammation. The use of IVIG, in conjunction with high-dose aspirin, has been shown to decrease the progression of CA dilation and aneurysms when initiated within 10 days of the onset of symptoms.**

A. Despite the initiation of treatment with IVIG and high-dose aspirin, 2% to 4% of patients will still develop CA abnormalities. ECHOs and long-term cardiology follow-up are necessary.

C. Only following the control of the acute phase is low-dose aspirin (5 mg/kg) used to prevent further CA thrombosis.

D. Steroid therapy has been shown in the past to worsen the outcome in Kawasaki disease, and is not considered standard therapy. However, in more recent literature, steroids have been reported to benefit a few patients in rare atypical cases.

E. Prolonged aspirin therapy puts the patient with Kawasaki disease at risk for Reye syndrome, especially with exposure to flu or chicken pox. Vaccines for these diseases should be given prior to hospital discharge, if not previously received.

113. B. The exam is most consistent with an area of cellulitis with overlying fluctuance and abscess formation.

A. Osteomyelitis to this degree would have a longer history than 5 days.

C, D. The two types of diaper dermatitis, candidal or contact, rarely cause such severe cellulitis.

E. Crohn disease does cause perirectal sinus tracts, but in this age group should present with symptoms such as diarrhea, poor weight gain, and poor growth.

114. A. Due to the size of this abscess, it should be incised and drained and allowed to heal secondarily. Broad-spectrum IV antibiotics that cover the common organisms (*Staphylococcus aureus, Streptococcus pyogenes*) for cellulitis, as well as those that cover anaerobes and enteric gram negatives given the location, may also be needed.

B. Simply closing up the wound with sutures would delay any further drainage.

C, D. Oral antibiotics alone or simple dressing changes with observation would not likely cure the abscess.

E. A barium enema would be painful and unnecessary in this circumstance.

115. C. Because the mother was adequately prophylaxed for GBS, according to American Academy of Pediatrics (AAP) guidelines, the baby does not need any further work-up but should be observed for at least 48 hours. The latest guidelines further allow for possible earlier discharge at 24 hours or more if the infant is 38 weeks or older and meets all other discharge criteria with reliable follow-up.

A, B, D. Babies born at a gestational age of less than 35 weeks should have a CBC and blood culture drawn and be observed for at least 48 hours. Babies of any gestational age whose GBS-positive mothers did not receive antimicrobial prophylaxis more than 4 hours before delivery should also have a CBC and blood culture drawn and be observed for at least 48 hours. A full diagnostic septic work-up, including chest x-ray and lumbar puncture, should be guided by the physical exam and further laboratory results.

E. Empiric antibiotics should not be started before obtaining relevant cultures.

116. C. SOD is a rare disorder characterized by the triad of abnormal development of the optic disc, pituitary deficiencies, and often agenesis of the septum pellucidum and/or partial or complete absence of the corpus callosum. Symptoms may include blindness in one or both eyes, pupil dilation in response to light, nystagmus, seizures, hypotonia, and deficiencies of GH, adrenocorticotropic hormone (ACTH), and TSH (panhypopituitarism). Intellectual problems vary in severity among individuals. The patient described in this vignette is on glucocorticoid replacement for ACTH deficiency. As with other patients on steroid therapy, this patient needs stress dose steroids during an acute illness such as fever above 100.5°F, nausea, vomiting, etc. Stress dosing is usually two to three times the physiologic glucocorticoid dosage of 12.5 mg/m^2/day.

A, E. Although patients with SOD may be on growth hormone and thyroid hormone therapies, these hormones are not adjusted during stress states and continuation of the same dosage will not have deleterious effects.

B. Patients with SOD and associated panhypopituitarism would not be expected to be on insulin therapy. Patients who require insulin therapy, most notably diabetics, may need to have insulin regimens adjusted during acute illnesses.

D. Patients with SOD may or may not have a central diabetes insipidus (DI) picture. In patients with DI, the adjustment of the vasopressin dosage during an acute illness depends upon the urine output and hydration status.

■ TABLE 3-117 Apgar Score Components

	0	1	2
Respirations	None	Slow, irregular	Active, crying
Heart rate	None	<100	>100
Muscle tone	Limp	Some flexion	Active movement
Reflex irritability	None	Grimace	Crying/withdrawal
Body color	Blue	Pink body, blue extremities	Entire pink body

117. **C. Respiration, heart rate, muscle tone, reflex irritability, and body color are components of the Apgar score (see Table 3-117). Each category is assigned a scale of 0 to 2, with scores at 1 and 5 minutes ranging from 0 to 10. The infant's Apgar score in the scenario is 4 from the following: respiration slow = 1, heart rate above 100 = 2, muscle tone limp throughout = 0, reflex irritability with grimace = 1, and pale, blue body color throughout = 0.**

A, B, D, E. These are all incorrect scores. See explanation for C.

118. **C. This child has the classic presentation of congenital adrenal hyperplasia (CAH), including ambiguous genitalia, hyperpigmentation, and salt wasting. The child is a genetic female with virilized genitalia. The most common form of CAH is 21-hydroxylase deficiency, which results in salt wasting and hyperkalemia. Low glucose is also common due to cortisol deficiency. These children often present with dehydration and even shock in the first 2 to 3 weeks of life. The treatment for CAH involves the essential replacement of cortisol and mineralocorticoids.**

A. CAH is inherited as an autosomal recessive trait.
B. 21-hydroxylase deficiency accounts for 90% of cases of CAH.
D. This child is a genetic female and does not have testes. This diagnosis should be considered in newborn infants with bilaterally nonpalpable testes.
E. Laboratory evaluation includes measurement of elevated 17-hydroxy-progesterone levels.

119. **C. Fifteen to twenty percent of affected children have a positive family history for natal teeth. Natal teeth are seen in about 1 in 2000 newborn infants.**

A. Natal teeth usually do not have a deep root system developed.
B. Natal teeth are typically located in the position of the mandibular central incisors.
D. There is a remote risk of aspiration should the tooth become dislodged. Elective extraction may be considered on an individual basis.
E. Natal teeth have been associated with other abnormalities such as cleft palate and Pierre Robin syndrome.

120. **D. Increased intracranial pressure with a normal MRI scan and normal cerebrospinal fluid (CSF) suggests the diagnosis of pseudotumor cerebri. The treatment of pseudotumor cerebri usually involves treating the underlying condition, in this case vitamin D-deficient rickets. Breastfed babies of women who are gowned (no sun exposure) and vegetarian may develop rickets because of a lack of vitamin D in their mother's breastmilk. Pseudotumor cerebri can be due to many diseases, including those with deranged calcium and phosphorus metabolism, as well as galactosemia, hypoparathyroidism, pseudohypoparathyroidism, hypophosphatasia, prolonged corticosteroid use, excess or deficiency of vitamin A, obesity, and pregnancy. The best treatment for this baby is to provide supplements of vitamin D and calcium.**

A. Some patients with increased intracranial pressure from pseudotumor cerebri are treated with serial lumbar taps to remove excessive CSF.
B, C. Acetazolamide and corticosteroids can also decrease intracranial pressure, but the underlying etiology should be treated first.
E. A neurosurgical consult would not be indicated in this case.

121. **A. In patients with tricuspid atresia, blood is obstructed by an atretic valve and prevents flow from the right atrium to the right ventricle.**

B. In tricuspid atresia, blood flows from the right atrium through a patent foramen ovale into the left atrium, then through the mitral valve to the left ventricle. In order to get to the lungs, some blood from the left ventricle passes through a VSD to the right ventricle. Shunting from the aorta to the pulmonary artery through a patent ductus is less common.
C. Because oxygenated and nonoxygenated blood mixes in the left atrium, patients with tricuspid atresia will have cyanosis in the newborn period.
D. The left ventricle has an increased load because of the right to left shunt that occurs; as a result left ventricular hypertrophy develops.
E. Treatment is aimed at improving pulmonary blood flow. Prostaglandins should be started immediately and balloon atrial septostomy may be needed as well. The goal of both palliative and definitive surgery is to assure better blood flow to the lungs.

122. **D. Nasal CPAP may help splint the upper airway and prevent any obstructive component of apnea that may be occurring.**

A. Generally, apnea of prematurity begins between the second and seventh day of life. Apnea on the first day, or beginning after the second week (or any time in a term infant), warrants immediate investigation.
B. Apnea of prematurity may respond to theophylline by mouth (PO), aminophylline (IV), or caffeine (PO).
C. Apnea associated with significant anemia may respond to packed RBC transfusion.
E. Apnea of prematurity generally resolves by 36 weeks postconceptional age (gestational age at birth plus postnatal age).

123. **D. The dilute urine after an 8-hour overnight water deprivation is suspicious for DI. It would be dangerous to repeat a long overnight fast if this patient has DI. Therefore, a daytime water deprivation can be done lasting 7 to 8 hours with close observation for significant rise in urine concentration and serum osmolality. After 7 to 8 hours, and no significant urine concentration or rise in serum osmolality occurs, insipidus is confirmed, and the administration of vasopressin will distinguish central from nephrogenic DI. While DI is usually accompanied by hypernatremia, patients with free access to water may retain normal serum sodium concentration.**

A. Vasopressin will result in urine concentration if the diagnosis is either psychogenic water drinking or central DI. Vasopressin can be used after an abnormal water deprivation test to distinguish between central and nephrogenic DI.
B. Sodium loading would be dangerous and offer no pertinent information.
C. Dilute urine after an 8-hour overnight water deprivation is suspicious for DI. It would be dangerous to repeat a long overnight fast if this patient has DI.
E. While DI is usually accompanied by hypernatremia, patients with free access to water may retain normal serum sodium concentration.

124. **A. This is Sturge-Weber syndrome. Pulsed dye laser is frequently effective for the skin lesions and generally avoids scarring. Such therapy can begin in infancy.**

B. Seizures are frequently unilateral on the contralateral side, and difficult to control.
C. For recalcitrant seizures, not well controlled with anticonvulsant medication, hemispherectomy or lobectomy has been effective, and may even prevent the development of mental retardation.
D. Glaucoma may develop with time, and therefore regular measurement of intraocular pressure is indicated.
E. Sturge-Weber syndrome is not hereditary, and is thought to result from anomalous development of the primordial vascular bed during the early stages of cerebral vascularization. The frequency of occurrence is 1 in 50,000.

125. **E. The infant in this scenario is experiencing transient tachypnea of the newborn (TTN). TTN represents a transient pulmonary edema resulting in delayed absorption of fetal alveolar fluid secondary to a variety of risk factors that include**

precipitous delivery, macrosomia, and operative delivery without labor, like the infant in this scenario. Most infants recover well with only supplemental oxygen, if necessary, and observation. Obtaining a chest radiograph is a logical choice in any patient showing signs of respiratory distress. The x-ray in this scenario reveals a prominent right lobe of the thymus or sail sign that may often be confused as an infiltrate of pneumonia.

A. Although the use of oxygen will most likely not harm this patient, it is unnecessary with saturations of 98% on room air.
B. Simply administering antibiotics without obtaining cultures is generally not sound medical practice unless the patient is extremely toxic appearing.
C. Further infectious work-up should be delayed, as there are no risk factors such as prematurity, fever, or prolonged rupture of membranes. If the patient continues to not improve or worsens, then a more thorough investigation would be needed.
D. With no murmur on exam, saturations of 98% on room air, and a normal-shaped heart on x-ray, performing an ECHO at this time is not necessary.

126. **D. The prolonged history of fever, limp, and radiographic findings of periosteal elevation and subperiosteal fluid collection is consistent with the diagnosis of osteomyelitis. While those affected with sickle cell anemia are more susceptible to osteomyelitis with *Salmonella*, *Staphylococcus aureus* is still the predominant pathogen of osteomyelitis.**

A. *Pseudomonas aeruginosa* infects avascular cartilaginous structures of the foot following puncture wounds.
B, C. *Salmonella* and *Brucella* tend to cause osteomyelitis of the vertebrae.
E. *Candida albicans* is not a bacterium but rather a fungus; it is an unlikely cause of osteomyelitis.

127. **C. This patient has a hypo-osmolar serum and an inappropriately concentrated urine, diagnostic of SIADH, which may be associated with bacterial meningitis. SIADH causes the retention of free water at the level of the renal collecting tubules. The initial treatment of SIADH is to restrict administration of free water and fluid.**

A. This child is probably too ill to be taking significant oral formula. However, adding additional sodium to the formula will not prevent retention of free water, and serum sodium will continue to fall.
B. Again, adding additional sodium to the IV fluids will not prevent the retention of free water caused by excess release of ADH.
D. Administration of a thiazide diuretic will result in water loss and increase sodium levels on a temporary basis, but is reserved for emergencies when sodium levels are so low that seizure activity is imminent or occurring.
E. A normal saline or hypertonic saline bolus can be helpful in patients with very severe hyponatremia (Na^+ less than 120 mEq/L) to prevent seizure activity. However, in this case fluid restriction will result in a gradual and sustained correction of the electrolytes.

128. **B. Chest compressions in infants are correctly performed using two or three fingers placed over the lower half of the sternum coordinated in a ratio of 5:1 with respirations.**

A. The heel of the hand is used in chest compressions only for a child between 1 and 8 years of age.
C. When properly performed, infant chest compressions should result in depressing the sternum to a depth of 0.5 to 1 inch.
D. The correct rate of chest compressions in an infant is *at least* 100 times per minute. The compression rate of 90 to 100 times per minute is used for children greater than 1 year of age.
E. The sternum should be compressed one third to one half of the depth of the chest in an infant, corresponding to 0.5 to 1 inch as stated in the explanation for C.

129. **D. This child has multiple risk factors for deep venous thrombosis (DVT). They include the diagnosis of cancer, the use of asparaginase, and the presence of a central line. Venous congestion and distension are more compatible with the diagnosis of a DVT.**

A. There is no erythema and/or tenderness to suggest cellulitis. Cellulitis does not typically cause venous congestion.
B. Fever and perhaps overlying erythema or fluctuance would be expected with abscess formation. In addition, abscesses do not typically cause venous congestion.

C. Because this patient is reported to be in remission, he should not have leukemic infiltration of his skin.

E. Fever and overlying bony tenderness should be seen with osteomyelitis of the ribs; there should be no associated venous distension.

130. **C. Myoglobinuria is the likely diagnosis secondary from prolonged seizure activity. The concentrated urine and normal BUN and creatinine suggest that this patient is volume depleted. It is imperative that urine flow rates be high to wash out the myoglobin, and that the urine be alkaline to expedite the myoglobin excretion. Mannitol will help the urine flow while maintaining vascular volume.**

A. The bolus is useful, but alkalinizing the urine and maintaining high urine volume is necessary in the treatment of rhabdomyolysis.

B. Diuresis and fluid restriction would be detrimental in myoglobinuria patients unless oliguric renal failure would ensue.

D. Diuresis and fluid restriction would be detrimental in myoglobinuria patients unless oliguric renal failure would ensue. Maintaining adequate hydration and urine flow rates may allay renal failure.

E. Although patients with rhabdomyolysis may develop acute renal failure, there is no need to begin dialysis in this patient unless the measures described in the explanation for C are unsuccessful.

131. **C. Addison disease occurs in about 50% of cases of adrenoleukodystrophy. When present, it generally either precedes or accompanies the onset of CNS manifestations. Occasionally Addison disease occurs without the CNS manifestations. The laboratory chemistries provided should be a clue to possible adrenal insufficiency.**

A. Most neurodegenerative disorders are autosomal recessive. The notable exception is adrenoleukodystrophy, which is inherited as an X-linked recessive disorder.

B. The metabolic defect and/or gene mutation associated with adrenoleukodystrophy has been identified in most of the neurodegenerative disorders. In adrenoleukodystrophy there is accumulation of long-chain fatty acids due to impaired degradation in the peroxizomes due to a gene mutation on the X chromosome. In metachromatic leukodystrophy there is deficiency of arylsulfatase A activity due to a gene mutation on chromosome 22.

D. While symptomatology overlaps, adrenoleukodystrophy and metachromatic leukodystrophy are distinctly different metabolic diseases. The former results from the accumulation of very long-chain fatty acids, the latter results from the accumulation of cerebroside sulfate. Also, the former is transmitted as an X-linked trait, and the latter as an autosomal recessive trait.

E. The sphingolipidoses are caused by biochemical enzyme defects that result in the accumulation of normal lipids which cannot be sufficiently degraded.

132. **E. Leukocyte adhesion deficiency is an autosomal recessive disorder causing recurrent bacterial infections with leukophilia without pus. In type 1 there is an absence of a surface adhesion glycoprotein on leukocytes. In type 2 there is a deficiency of a carbohydrate, which renders the neutrophils unable to adhere to endothelial cells. Delayed cord separation may occur (separation beyond 3 to 4 weeks of age).**

A. Quantitative serum immunoglobulin level is a measure of B-cell function, which results in a deficiency of antibody production. Delayed umbilical cord separation is not a feature. Patients with immunoglobulin deficiencies are susceptible to infections from encapsulated organisms, such as *Streptococcus pneumoniae*, *Haemophilus influenzae*, and *Neisseria meningitides*.

B. Deficiencies of various complement components are generally transmitted as an autosomal trait and produce a variety of syndromes, but delayed umbilical cord separation is not a feature. Patients are more prone to invasive bacterial infections and have a higher incidence of rheumatologic disease.

C. A test of leukocyte killing is used to test for chronic granulomatous disease in which there is inability to kill catalase-positive microbes resulting in recurrent pyogenic infections and lymphadenitis. Delayed umbilical cord separation is not a feature.

D. Test for leukocyte chemotaxis is used to test for Chediak-Higashi syndrome and other syndromes associated with defective chemotaxis. These patients generally have a partial albinism, photophobia, and nystagmus; leukopenia and recurrent pyogenic infections are seen. Delayed umbilical cord separation is not a feature.

133. **E. This patient has autosomal recessive polycystic kidney disease. Hepatic fibrosis is a common feature, and portal hypertension usually develops as patients get older. The portal hypertension and hepatomegaly may precede the renal failure. The biopsy shows diffuse cysts lined with low columnar or cuboidal epithelium representing dilated collecting ducts.**

A. This is autosomal recessive polycystic kidney disease, and is not sex linked.
B. Renal failure in patients with autosomal recessive polycystic kidney disease occurs at variable ages, but usually during childhood. Many have renal failure at birth or shortly thereafter.
C. Twenty-five percent of both male and female offspring will have this disorder. It is typically an autosomal recessive trait. The autosomal dominant polycystic kidney disease (adult form) will occur in 50% of offspring, both male and female.
D. The cysts of autosomal recessive polycystic kidney disease generally begin as small, dilated collecting ducts less than 2 mm in size. They may become larger as patient survival increases.

134. **F. Cardiac defects are seen in about 60%, sterility is nearly universal in males, and mental retardation occurs in nearly all patients. This infant is exhibiting typical features of Down syndrome including hypotonia, simian creases, epicanthal folds, widely spaced first and second toes, and microcephaly. Trisomy 21, or Down syndrome, is the most common autosomal chromosomal abnormality in humans.**

A. An ECHO is recommended for all patients with Down syndrome secondary to the high incidence of cardiac septal defects and endocardial cushion defects seen in these patients.
B. Sterility is seen in almost all males with Down syndrome. Some mosaic males may be fertile. Females with Down syndrome are fertile.
C. Mental retardation is common in trisomy 21 with an average IQ of 68.
D. Gastroschisis is not a common feature in Down syndrome, although intestinal atresia, especially duodenal atresia, is associated.
E. Cardiac defects are seen in about 60%, and sterility is nearly universal in males, but mental retardation occurs in nearly all patients, and is not mentioned in this option.
G. Cardiac defects are seen in about 60%, sterility is nearly universal in males, and mental retardation occurs in nearly all patients, but gastroschisis is not commonly associated with Down syndrome.

135. **D. Diabetic ketoacidosis (DKA) is both a very serious and a very common metabolic disturbance. It can be seen in all types of diabetes mellitus, and should be considered an emergency. Its hallmark is a metabolic acidosis caused by the build-up of ketones in the blood, and it is associated with significant dehydration. Remember the ABCs and improve circulation with volume repletion before further management. The reversal of DKA requires insulin administration and rehydration. These are typically achieved with IV insulin, given as a *continuous* infusion, and with parenteral (or oral) rehydration. In addition, blood glucose levels and blood chemistries are monitored very closely throughout the course of treatment, and replacement glucose and/or electrolytes may be provided in the rehydration solution as needed.**

A. DKA is treated with a continuous infusion of insulin. Using IV boluses of insulin contributes to eradicating glucose levels and will promote cerebral edema.
B. *Short-acting* insulin, given subcutaneously, can be used to reverse mild DKA on an outpatient basis, provided the patient has adequate social support, can tolerate oral rehydration, and has adequate follow-up with a physician. In contrast, *long-acting* subcutaneous insulin does *not* have a standard role in the acute reversal of DKA, given its late peak and longer duration of action.
C. Sodium bicarbonate administration has been demonstrated to be a risk factor for the development of cerebral edema in pediatric patients with DKA, and is therefore not recommended as a first-line therapy in these patients.
E. Glucagon administration would exacerbate DKA by stimulating glucose release.

136. **D. The infant in this scenario has clinical features consistent with transposition of the great arteries. Infants always present with cyanosis in the newborn period and a heart murmur is usually absent; a single loud S2 is often heard. Classic x-ray findings include increased pulmonary markings with an egg-shaped cardiac silhouette. Aside from attention to the ABCs with correction of an expected acidosis, prostaglandin E_1 should be initiated to promote increased oxygenation by preventing ductus arteriosus closure until surgery can be performed. The lack of prenatal care in this scenario further puts the infant at risk following delivery. A prenatal ultrasound may have been beneficial in the early detection of congenital heart disease, allowing for a planned delivery at a tertiary care center.**

A. Indomethacin would promote ductus arteriosus closure and would be contraindicated.
B. Captopril would be useful for afterload reduction or control of hypertension.
C. Surfactant would be indicated for premature infants with signs of respiratory distress syndrome.
E. Propranolol is a nonselective β-blocker that is used to control tachyarrhythmias and hypertension.

137. **B. Achalasia is a condition in which the lower esophageal sphincter fails to relax with swallowing. The cause is not clear, but pathological abnormalities of muscle fibers and ganglion cells have been seen. The average age of onset is about 10 years and many patients have problems for more than a year before being properly diagnosed. Clinically, patients have vomiting, progressive difficulty swallowing, substernal pain (esophagitis), aspiration pneumonia, and growth impairment. In patients with achalasia, the barium esophagram shows a narrowed distal esophagus with proximal esophagomegaly. The diagnosis is confirmed with esophageal manometry. Treatment involves dilatation of the sphincter or surgical (Heller) myotomy. Endoscopic injection of botulinum toxin may be effective, but it is expensive and often is effective for less than 1 year. Nifedipine (calcium channel blocker) may help on a temporary basis.**

A. The radiograph in hiatal hernia will show a portion of the stomach above the diaphragm.
C, D. In neither GER nor pyloric stenosis will the patient have a dilated esophagus.
E. Symptoms of esophagitis and esophageal stricture from a caustic ingestion would be of more acute onset. The slow progression of symptoms seen in this case is typical of achalasia.

138. **C. The AAP practice guideline for the management of acute gastroenteritis in young children states that children with diarrhea who are rehydrated should be fed age-appropriate diets.**

A. Leaving a child NPO withholds needed nutrition unnecessarily.
B. The BRAT diet is too limited and is low in energy density, protein, and fat.
D, E. Similarly, clear and thick liquids will not provide adequate nutrition.

139. **C. H-type TEFs may not be detected until later in life with recurrent pneumonias. Only 4% of TEFs are the H type. H-type TEFs have a fistula between an otherwise normal esophagus and trachea.**

A. The most common type of TEF, accounting for 85% of cases, is an esophageal atresia that ends in a blind pouch with a more distal TEF. All types of TEF, other than the H type, have an associated blind esophageal pouch that accounts for the inability to pass an NG tube to the stomach.
B. There is an increased incidence of associated anomalies with TEFs, up to 50%, such as VATER/VACTERL.
D. As in the explanation for C, only 4% of TEFs are the H type.
E. Aspiration is a great risk with TEFs and prone positioning minimizes movement of gastric contents into a distal fistula.

140. **A. Shagreen patch, subungual fibromas, and café-au-lait spots are manifestations of tuberous sclerosis. Shagreen patch is a roughened, raised, orange peel-like lesion most often seen on the thorax or lumbosacral area. Other skin lesions include adenoma sebaceum, which are angiofibromas over the nose and cheeks, which often appear between 4 and 6 years.**

B. In tuberous sclerosis the degree of mental retardation is variable, and some patients, indeed, have normal intelligence. However, severe retardation and normal intelligence can occur within the same family, and the degree of retardation in the affected parent is not predictive of the offspring's intelligence. In this case, early seizures (and other early manifestations) generally are associated with more serious mental retardation.

C. Hamartomas of the kidneys and polycystic kidneys are not uncommon in tuberous sclerosis and may result in hematuria. Kidney failure may occur but is rare.
D. Phakomas of the retina are common. Phakomas are round flat gray lesions in the region of the optic disc. Mulberry tumors of the retina also occur. Cataracts would be unusual.
E. Rhabdomyomas, not myxomas, of the heart occur in about 50% of children with tuberous sclerosis.

141. **D. Even with optimal treatment, residual abnormalities of the lower leg and foot are not unusual because there is a certain amount of deformity and atrophy to start.**

A. Positional deformity of the foot is not uncommon in the newborn and is a benign condition. It must be differentiated from true clubfoot in which there is a certain amount of rigidity, atrophy, and deformity. It requires no treatment.
B. Transmission of congenital (nonsyndromic) clubfoot deformity is considered multifactorial with a major influence by a single autosomal dominant gene.
C. Treatment of clubfoot generally starts with serial casting. Surgery is generally withheld until after 3 months if adequate correction is not obtained.
E. True congenital clubfoot is characterized by some calf atrophy, and hypoplasia of the tibia, fibula, and foot bones.

142. **D. The findings of pneumatosis intestinalis (air in the bowel wall) and gas in the portal vein are pathognomonic for neonatal necrotizing enterocolitis (NEC). NEC is a serious medical condition that primarily affects premature infants. The intestinal mucosa becomes inflamed and necrotic and the patient develops abdominal distension, bloody stools, and bilious vomiting. They may also demonstrate lethargy, apnea and bradycardia, diarrhea, acidosis, and temperature instability. NEC can be complicated by GI tract perforation, disseminated intravascular coagulation, sepsis and shock, strictures, fistulae, and abscess formation. Treatment includes cessation of all enteral feedings, placement of an NG tube for decompression, and administration of IV fluids and broad-spectrum antibiotics. Laboratory testing should include CBC, electrolytes, clotting studies, and blood and stool cultures. Frequent abdominal radiographs are obtained to monitor improvement. Patients who fail medical management or who develop bowel perforation require surgical resection of the involved intestine.**

A. In cases of suspected NEC the patient should be made NPO. Feeding intolerance following an episode of NEC is common and often necessitates the use of a protein hydrolysate formula.
B. The patient's radiograph shows evidence of NEC. It would be inappropriate to simply observe and repeat films in 24 hours.
C. As in the explanation for D, the treatment of NEC requires stopping all enteral feeds and administering IV antibiotics.
E. Although patients with NEC and free peritoneal air will require surgery, bowel resection would only be indicated in cases of bowel necrosis and/or stricture formation.

143. **E. About 9% of infants with Down syndrome born from mothers under 30 years old are a result of translocation, so the vast majority have trisomy 21. Of all Down syndrome babies, 95% are a result of trisomy 21, 5% a result of translocation, and 1% are mosaic.**

A. While the incidence of Down syndrome in all live births is 1 in 700, there is an increased risk in subsequent pregnancies even in young mothers who have had a child with trisomy 21. It may be as high as 1%. The risk goes up to 1 in 40 in mothers over 40 years old. If the Down syndrome is caused from translocation, the risk goes up to 1 in 5 live births if the mother is a balanced carrier.
B. Of all Down syndrome babies, 95% are a result of trisomy 21, 5% a result of translocation, and 1% mosaic.
C. The incidence of Down syndrome in conceptions is about twice the incidence in live births because of a high incidence of early abortions.
D. Mosaic Down syndrome results from nondisjunction in *mitosis* (cell division after meiosis). This results in two lines of cells, some with a normal chromosome complement, and some with trisomy 21. Many of these children are less severely mentally retarded.

144. C. Observation only is indicated in this scenario. Healthy term infants who are exposed to varicella postnatally are not candidates for VZIG or any other treatment. They are presumed to be carrying maternal antibody, which would be protective. The 2003 Red Book would recommend VZIG be used if the infant were less than or equal to 28 weeks. (American Academy of Pediatrics. Varicella-zoster infections. In: Pickering LK, ed. Red Book: 2003 Report of the Committee on Infectious Diseases. 26th ed. Elk Grove Village, IL: American Academy of Pediatrics, 2003:679.)

A. Acyclovir is not needed in this scenario nor is it recommended in the routine treatment of chicken pox in an immunocompetent child less than 12 years of age.

B. VZIG is not recommended in this scenario. If the mother developed chicken pox 5 days before delivery up until 2 days after delivery, the infant would be a candidate for VZIG.

D. Cephazolin can sometimes be used to treat the superinfection seen with varicella skin lesions but has no role in this scenario.

E. As in the explanations for A and B, neither acyclovir nor VZIG is indicated.

145. E. In patients with CF and meconium ileus, hypertonic enema solutions may be used in an attempt to relieve the intestinal obstruction; if unsuccessful, then surgical intervention is necessary.

A. Down syndrome can be associated with neonatal intestinal obstruction, specifically duodenal atresia. The radiographs will typically show a "double-bubble" sign and an absence of gas in the distal bowel. This is a very different appearance than is seen with meconium ileus. With meconium ileus, a contrast enema will demonstrate the sigmoid and ascending colon to have a small diameter, and the small intestine will have air-filled dilated loops of bowel. The "ground glass" appearance on abdominal radiographs is typical.

B. Approximately 10% to 20% of children with CF will develop meconium ileus. Children with meconium ileus should always be presumed to have CF until diagnostic sweat testing or genetic testing is complete.

C. A genetic predisposition for meconium ileus has been shown. Children whose siblings had meconium ileus are more likely to develop the same condition.

D. Rupture of the bowel wall and peritonitis are known complications of meconium ileus.

146. B. A child in renal failure is at risk for hyperkalemia, which may cause an acute life-threatening wide-complex arrhythmia. The progressive ECG findings seen in hyperkalemia include peaked T waves, loss of the T wave, widened QRS complexes, ST segment depression, bradycardia, and ultimately ventricular dysrhythmias or asystole leading to cardiac arrest. The acute administration of calcium, either as calcium chloride or calcium gluconate, helps to protect the heart from the arrhythmogenic effect of hyperkalemia. Other helpful acute treatments include the administration of sodium bicarbonate, insulin, and glucose, as well as an albuterol treatment. Potassium removal can be effected either by dialysis or initially with the administration of kayexelate.

A. Anti-arrhythmic agents such as lidocaine are not very effective in suppressing the arrhythmia caused by hyperkalemia.

C, D, E. Magnesium, furosemide, and mannitol are not effective in treating this acute life-threatening arrhythmia.

147. C. An asthmatic patient with severe wheezing generally will respond to his oxygen need with significant hyperventilation reducing his pCO_2, and maintaining a reasonably normal pH. Here the pCO_2 is normal, and even though his pH is near normal, this would indicate he could have impending respiratory failure and should go to intensive care. Additionally, his HCO_3 is a bit on the high side, suggesting that there has been some chronic CO_2 retention.

A. The pCO_2 is below normal, suggesting he does not have impending respiratory failure. The pH is a little low, and the HCO_3 is a little low, suggesting some metabolic compensation to the hypocapnea.

B. The pCO_2 is below normal, suggesting he does not have impending respiratory failure. The pH is normal, and the HCO_3 is a little low, suggesting complete metabolic compensation to the hypocapnea.

D. The pCO_2 is below normal, suggesting he does not have impending respiratory failure. The pH is low, and the HCO_3 is also low. There is probably some metabolic compensation, but there may also be some metabolic acidosis.

E. The pCO_2 is below normal, suggesting he does not have impending respiratory failure. However, the pH is low, as is the HCO_3. While there does not seem to be respiratory failure, there is a significant superimposed metabolic acidosis.

148. **A. Reposition the child with knees to chest. Tet spells are caused by decrease in flow through the atretic pulmonary artery, often with exercise, crying, or feeding. This causes a relative increase in the right-to-left shunting through the VSD and worsening hypoxemia with resulting cyanosis. Holding the child in a knee-to-chest position increases systemic vascular resistance, reducing the right-to-left shunt and improving oxygenation. Ideally, the parents would be able to hold the child in this position while calming and comforting him. A second appropriate management option would include a dose of morphine to relax the child and decrease respiratory drive.**

B. Oxygen would be somewhat helpful to optimize oxygenation after the right-to-left shunt is minimized, but is unlikely to be as immediately useful as the increase in systemic vascular resistance with the knee-to-chest positioning. Oxygen is, however, almost always a good idea.

C. Increased fluid volume would not address the basic problem of right-to-left shunting in the heart, and starting an IV in this child would likely increase the agitation and worsen the hypoxemia.

D. CPR is not your first choice of therapy, although a severe untreated Tet spell is life threatening.

E. The use of furosemide would be beneficial if there were signs of congestive heart failure with fluid overload, but it has no use in the management of Tet spells.

149. **D. Diaphragmatic hernias are congenital defects of the diaphragm that allow the abdominal contents to herniate into the thorax. Large defects present in the immediate neonatal period with respiratory distress. Smaller defects may present later with feeding problems and increasing respiratory distress. The x-ray shown has opacification of the left hemithorax with some evidence of bowel gas patterns and a mediastinal shift to the right suggesting a diaphragmatic hernia.**

A. Pyloric stenosis presents later, typically at age 4 to 6 weeks, with projectile vomiting and electrolyte abnormalities consisting of a hypochloremic metabolic alkalosis; a normal chest radiograph would be expected.

B. Pneumonia with pleural effusion should cause fever and an elevated WBC count.

C. TEFs present with fever, cough, and aspiration pneumonias, typically demonstrated by infiltrates in the right upper and middle lobes.

E. Duodenal atresia should present soon after delivery with bilious emesis. A classic double-bubble sign is often seen on an abdominal radiograph.

150. **A. Diaphragmatic hernias need urgent decompression and surgical correction.**

B. There is no obvious infection in this case; the use of IV antibiotics is not indicated

C. Because there is no evidence of pneumothorax or pleural effusion, inserting a chest tube is inappropriate and would cause further problems and possible bowel perforation.

D. Pyloromyotomy is the curative surgery for pyloric stenosis.

E. An ECHO would be neither diagnostic nor therapeutic.

SETTING 4: EMERGENCY DEPARTMENT

Generally, patients encountered here are seeking urgent care; most are not known to you. A full range of social services is available, including rape crisis intervention, family support, child protective services, domestic violence support, psychiatric services, and security assistance backed up by local police. Complete laboratory and radiology services are available.

151. A 7-year-old boy involved in a motor vehicle accident is transported by EMS to the ER. He has been intubated because of a Glasgow coma score (GCS) of 5 at the scene and remains unconscious in the PICU, though moves occasionally with stimulation such as suctioning. The nurse asks whether the c-collar can be removed because the c-spine films have been cleared. You answer:

    A. The patient can be removed from c-spine precautions if the films have been cleared by an attending staff radiologist
    B. The patient can remain in c-spine precautions by elevating the head of the bed but the collar can be removed
    C. The c-spine collar can be replaced by a soft collar
    D. Further studies of the c-spine (CT or MRI) would be warranted before the c-spine collar can be removed
    E. A repeat set of cervical spine films will need to be obtained first

152. When a 3-year-old presented for examination, his mother expressed concern about recent clumsiness and crossing of the eyes. He has recently been suffering from headaches and a change in his gait. The pupils were noted to be equally reactive to light, and his tracking of objects was noted to be of equal quality in each eye. Of note, the amount of crossing appeared to be less with regarding near objects than far. Which of the following would be considered the most appropriate next step in the management of this patient?

    A. Head MRI with gadolinium enhancement
    B. Lumbar puncture (LP) with opening pressure assessment
    C. Patching of the right eye
    D. Observation alone with close follow-up
    E. Tensilon testing

The following 2 questions (items 153-154) relate to the same clinical scenario.

A 10-year-old boy presents to the ED with severe headache and neck pain. He has just returned from summer camp. On exam, his temperature is 38.5°C. He resists fundoscopic exam because he says the bright light makes his headache worse. He prefers to lie still and does not want to move his neck very much. There has been no trauma. A head CT was obtained and is reported as normal.

153. The most appropriate next test for diagnosis would be:

    A. Serum drug screen
    B. Routine urinalysis
    C. MRI of the brain
    D. LP
    E. EEG

154. CSF exam reveals mild increase in WBCs with a predominance of lymphocytes. The glucose and protein levels in the CSF are normal. The Gram stain of the CSF shows no organisms. The most likely diagnosis is:

    A. Multiple sclerosis (MS)
    B. *Neisseria meningitidis* meningitis
    C. Brain tumor
    D. Migraine headaches
    E. Aseptic meningitis

End of Set

155. You arrive at a referring hospital to assist the transport of a 6-month-old with profuse watery diarrhea. The child has an HR of 200 BPM, sunken eyes, capillary refill of 5 seconds, appears gray, and has weak central pulses and absent peripheral pulses. The referring ED has tried over 12 times to get an IV started and has been unsuccessful. The most appropriate next step is:

    A. Ask for a cutdown tray to isolate the distal saphenous vein in order to provide 20 mL/kg normal saline (NS) IV ASAP
    B. Place an umbilical venous line and give 20 mL/kg IV ASAP
    C. Intubate and give 20 mL/kg NS down the endotracheal tube (ETT)
    D. Place a subclavian central venous line to give 20 mL/kg NS ASAP
    E. Place an intraosseous line and administer 20 mL/kg NS ASAP into the bone marrow cavity

156. A 6-month-old infant presents with poor feeding, fussiness, and a heart rate of 270 to 290 BPM. She is mottled, with cool extremities and capillary refill of 5 seconds. A peripheral IV is in place in the patient's antecubital space, and all medications you might wish to administer are readily available. Which of the following interventions would be the most appropriate in the treatment of this child?

A. Administration of furosemide (Lasix) 1 mg/kg rapid IV push
B. Administration of lidocaine 1 mg/kg rapid IV push
C. Administration of warm water in a plastic bag placed suddenly over the face for 15 to 20 seconds
D. Digitalizing slowly over the next 24 hours
E. Sedation and administration of synchronized cardioversion with 0.5 J/kg

157. A previously healthy, 8-week-old female infant presents with a hypoglycemic seizure and blood sugar of 14 mg/dL. On exam she is at 95% for both weight and height, well hydrated, and healthy appearing. She has been breastfeeding every 3 hours and her mother reports a normal pregnancy with good prenatal care. Aside from the hypoglycemia, a comprehensive metabolic panel is normal. Her urinalysis showed negative ketones with no reducing substances. What is the most likely diagnosis?

A. Pneumonia
B. Adrenal insufficiency
C. Glycogen storage disease
D. Galactosemia
E. Congenital hyperinsulinism (nesidioblastosis)

158. A 4-month-old infant is brought to the ED because of constipation. The mother went back to work last week and the baby was switched from breastmilk to cow's milk formula. The parents note that for the past 2 days the baby has had some difficulty sucking his bottle. On physical examination you note that the baby has no fever but is hypotonic, has a weak cry, and seems to have an expressionless face. The baby appears well hydrated and the anterior fontanelle appears normal. How would you manage this infant?

A. Switch to a soy-based formula
B. Give 4 ounces of prune juice daily for constipation
C. Obtain consultation from a speech therapist to evaluate the sucking problem
D. Obtain laboratory tests and admit the baby to the hospital
E. Observe at home; no treatment is needed

159. A 10-year-old girl comes to the ED in July because of severe right-sided ear pain that has been getting progressively worse over the last 2 days. She has had no upper respiratory symptoms or fever. When you pull on her pinna she screams out in pain. On examination, you see a whitish discharge in the ear canal. The best treatment would be:

A. Topical antibiotic/corticosteroid otic suspension
B. IM ceftriaxone
C. Benzocaine otic solution
D. Oral amoxicillin
E. Apply warm compresses to ear

160. A 10-month-old baby comes to the ER because of a fever of 40°C. Your examination reveals that the baby has an immobile, bright red, bulging eardrum. During your examination, the baby has a generalized tonic-clonic seizure. A spinal tap shows normal CSF. You suspect that the baby had a febrile convulsion. The parents are extremely anxious and have multiple questions. Which of the following is the most accurate information to give to this boy's parents?

A. Febrile convulsions commonly occur between 9 months and 5 years of age
B. Most febrile seizures last more than 15 minutes
C. Even if there is no family history of seizures, children with simple febrile convulsions are 10 times more likely to develop epilepsy than the general population
D. Children who have a simple febrile seizure require an EEG and MRI
E. Children with two or more simple febrile seizures should routinely be given prophylactic anticonvulsant medication

161. A 5-year-old boy is seen in the ED for fever and a purpuric rash on the legs and buttocks. He has been having intermittent abdominal pain and frankly bloody stools. His right knee is warm, swollen, red, and painful. Which statement regarding this patient's condition is most accurate?

A. The cause of this condition is thought to be an IgA-mediated immune vasculitis
B. The rash tends to be on the upper extremities
C. Glomerulonephritis and arthritis are quite rare
D. The platelet count is usually depressed
E. Corticosteroids should never be used in this condition

162. A 5-year-old boy presented with a history of grossly bloody urine, puffy eyes, and headache for 1 day. His diagnostic evaluation and course were consistent with the diagnosis of poststreptococcal glomerulonephritis (PSGN). The course was benign, but 10 days after the onset his urine still contained a 3+ reaction for protein and 4+ reaction for blood on a dip stick, and a microscopic examination of his urine still revealed a full field of RBCs with many RBC casts. Which one of the following can be considered normal for uncomplicated PSGN?

A. An elevated antistreptolysin O (ASO), which has normalized after 1 month
B. Low serum C3 for up to 6 weeks
C. Nephrotic syndrome within 3 months from onset
D. Gross hematuria for up to 3 months
E. Hypertension lasting 6 months or more

163. A 9-month-old infant is seen with a mild upper respiratory infection and is noted to have some pallor, slight icterus, and an enlarged spleen. The mother had a splenectomy for some unknown reason when she was about 6 years old. Which one of the following laboratory sets is compatible with the expected diagnosis?

A. Hemoglobin 10.7 g/dL, MCHC 38, reticulocyte count 1.5%
B. Hemoglobin 9.5 g/dL, MCV 80, RDW 16
C. Total bilirubin 5.0 mg/dL, MCHC 33, RDW 13
D. Total indirect bilirubin 0.5 mg/dL, MCHC 33, reticulocyte count 10%
E. Hemoglobin 9.5 mg/dL, indirect bilirubin 3.5 mg/dL, RDW 10.5

164. A 2-month-old male presents to the ED with new onset seizures. The mother states that the child "rolled from the bed a couple of days ago and has not been acting right since." After discovering biparietal subdural hematomas on exam, an ophthalmic consultation is requested as the child is awaiting further head imaging. After dilating the pupils with cycloplegic eye drops, the retina are examined. Which of the following findings would help confirm your diagnosis?

A. White-centered, dark intraretinal hemorrhages
B. Retinal detachment
C. Hemorrhages scattered throughout the posterior retina only
D. Massive bilateral eyelid ecchymoses
E. Absence of blood within the vitreous

165. A 16-year-old female is brought into the ED by her friends. She is concerned that while at a party somebody may have put something in her drink. She is particularly concerned it may have been "the date rape drug" gamma-hydroxybutyrate (GHB). Which of the following is most consistent with GHB ingestion?

A. Hypertension, tachycardia, and diaphoresis
B. Auditory and visual hallucinations
C. Nystagmus, agitation, and hyperthermia
D. Apparent coma and rapid return to consciousness when assessing a gag reflex
E. Hyponatremia seizures after attending a rave concert

The following 2 questions (items 166-167) relate to the same clinical scenario.

A 4-year-old female presents to your pediatric ED complaining of abdominal pain for the past 3 days. The pain is diffuse, intermittent, and moderate to severe at times. Sometimes her pain is so severe that she is in tears and unable to rest comfortably; sometimes it seems to go away completely and she plays normally. Her appetite has been only slightly affected. There has not been any blood in her stools, although she has not had any stool at all for the last 3 days. Review of systems is negative for fevers, vomiting, diarrhea, sore throat, respiratory symptoms, and any other complaints. Vital signs: T, 37.0°C; HR, 96; RR, 18; BP, 100/60; pulse oximetry = 100% on room air. On exam you find a soft but full abdomen; anywhere you press, she cries. Her parents are strongly opposed to the performance of a rectal exam.

166. Which of the following is an appropriate diagnostic test to order for this patient?

A. Order a kidneys/ureter/bladder radiograph (KUB) to assess for constipation
B. Abdominal ultrasound to assess for appendicitis
C. CT scan of the abdomen and pelvis to assess for appendicitis
D. Barium enema to rule out intussusception
E. Send home with reassurance that the abdominal pain will go away

167. If the diagnostic test you selected confirms your findings, what is the next step?

A. Trial of Fleet enema to see if pain resolves
B. Surgery consult for appendectomy
C. Surgery consult for manual reduction of intussusception if barium enema fails to reduce it
D. Further imaging of abdomen
E. Outpatient GI consult in 2 months

End of Set

168. A 4-year-old boy with a history of complex congenital heart disease presents with 4 days of fever, fatigue, anorexia, headache, and myalgias. On physical examination the boy is febrile and looks pale. He has a loud murmur and the spleen is enlarged. Laboratory tests reveal mild anemia and an elevated erythrocyte sedimentation rate (ESR). What is the most important next step in the management of this patient?

A. Administer digoxin and furosemide
B. Administer IV penicillin and gentamycin
C. Administer amantadine for influenza
D. Obtain blood cultures from multiple sites over the next 24 hours
E. Order an ECHO

169. A 2-year-old boy with a 1-day history of abdominal pain, bloody diarrhea, and dehydration is seen in the ED. Prior to his arrival, he had a generalized seizure in the transport ambulance. On physical examination, the patient appears pale and is found to be mildly hypertensive. Several petechiae are seen on the trunk and extremities. Laboratory tests reveal anemia, thrombocytopenia, hematuria, and elevated blood urea nitrogen (BUN). The causative organism for this condition is most commonly:

A. *Staphylococcus aureus*
B. *Streptococcus pyogenes*
C. *Shigella dysenteriae*
D. Rotavirus
E. *Escherichia coli*

170. A 12-year-old with chronic liver disease presents to the ER with hematemesis of bright red blood. Her blood pressure is 74/50 with a heart rate of 120. You suspect a recurrent bleeding esophageal or gastric varice. Which of the following should be done first for the management of her upper GI bleed?

A. Send for a CBC
B. Place two IVs and give a bolus of NS (20 mL/kg)
C. Give vitamin K
D. Endotracheal intubation
E. Start an H2 blocker

171. A pediatric intern is doing a rotation in the ER when a man enters carrying a poodle. The man is complaining of crushing chest pain and then falls to the ground dropping the dog onto the lap of a 12-year-old girl waiting for her sister and mother in another room. The dog immediately yelps and bites the 12-year-old on the right ulnar aspect of the palm. The ER physician goes to the aid of the man and sends the intern to help with the 12-year-old bite victim. The 12-year-old has no past medical history and she was given diphtheria, tetanus, acellular pertussis vaccine (DTaP) when she began school. Which of the following statements is most accurate?

A. The tetanus toxoid and diphtheria toxoid (Td) are not needed
B. Prophylactic antibiotics are indicated
C. Infections caused by dog bites are almost never the result of *Pasteurella multocida*
D. Cleaning and irrigation of the wound is the most important factor in decreasing the chance of infection
E. Wounds of the hand should be sutured after thorough cleaning

172. A 13-year-old male is seen in the ED after a minor motor vehicle accident. The patient was restrained and the right-sided impact caused him to hit his head against the window without breaking it. There is no previous medical history and no family history is available as the patient is adopted. During the examination, the physician notes marked swelling of the head and neck

and right side of the body. There is no bruising, erythema, itching, or hives noted. The patient is anxious and complaining of some abdominal pain. When swelling of the mouth was noted, the physician administered epinephrine without noticeable improvement. Which of the following is likely the cause for the problem?

A. Anaphylaxis to the powder in the examiner's gloves
B. Hereditary angioedema
C. Acute congestive heart failure secondary to pericardial tamponade
D. Acute septic shock secondary to bowel perforation
E. Infiltration of the IV

173. A 12-year-old female is brought to the ED by her friends after a house party. She is lethargic, confused, and has vomited. Her friends state that she simply "had too much to drink." Her lab work shows the following: Na^+, 140; K^+, 3.5; Cl^-, 95; CO_2, 18; BUN, 9; glucose, 120; measured osmolality, 350 mosm/kg; and ethanol, 120 mg/dL. What is the next step in managing this patient?

A. Call the child's parents to take her home
B. Obtain a toxic alcohol screen for methanol, ethylene glycol, and isopropyl alcohol
C. Administer IV thiamine
D. Administer IV fomepizole (4-MP)
E. Arrange for urgent hemodialysis

174. A 3-year-old child is seen in the ER with a history of fever, right-sided neck swelling, and dysphagia. His past medical history is negative and his shots are up to date. On physical exam you confirm right-sided cervical swelling with no tonsilar enlargement or uvula deviation without any evidence of stridor. He is saturating 98% on room air. A neck film is obtained (Figure 3-174). What would be appropriate in the management of this patient?

A. Immediate consultation with anesthesia and intubation in the OR
B. Administration of racemic epinephrine
C. Ear, nose, and throat (ENT) consultation for tonsillar drainage
D. Administration of ampicillin-sulbactam with ENT consult
E. Administration of dexamethasone

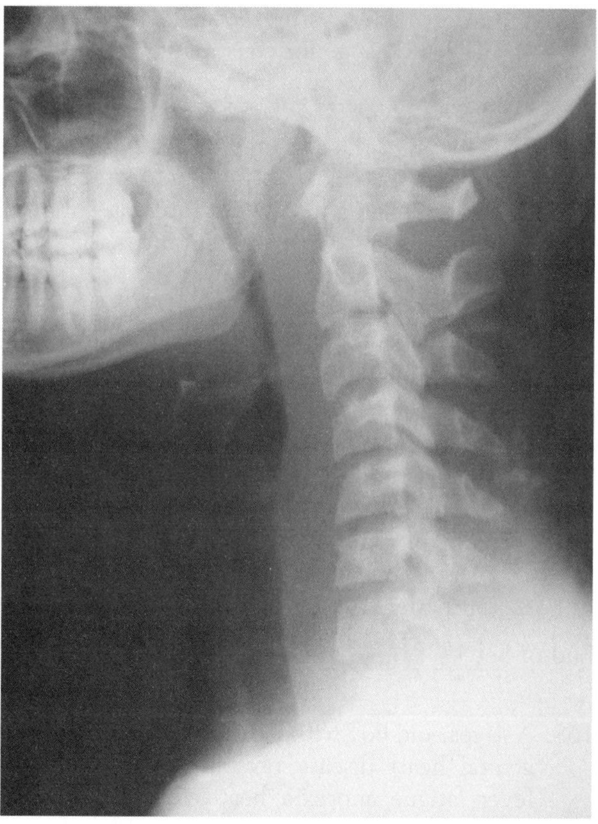

Figure 3-174 • Image Courtesy of the Department of Radiology, Phoenix Children's Hospital, Phoenix, Arizona.

175. A 5-kg infant is seen in the ED with a history of profuse diarrhea. The skin has a "doughy" texture, mucous membranes are dry, extremities are cool, and capillary refill is 4 seconds. The initial serum sodium is 170 mEq/L. Which of the following is the best immediate action?

A. Infusion of D5 (0.2%) NS plus 20 mEq/L KCl at 1.5 maintenance
B. Infusion of 10 mL/kg D10W
C. Administration of 2 mEq/kg sodium bicarbonate
D. Infusion of 20 ml/kg 0.9% NaCl
E. Administration of IV antibiotics and an LP to rule out sepsis

176. A 3-year-old boy is found playing with his older brother's D-amphetamine (Adderall) tablets that he takes for ADHD. The mother has brought him to the ED for further evaluation and treatment. Which of the following clinical features would be expected should he develop toxicity?

A. Dilated pupils (mydriasis)
B. Lethargy
C. Dry skin
D. Hyponatremia
E. Constipation

177. A 25-year-old woman at 37-weeks gestation is involved in a motor vehicle accident. En route to the ED her 2.8-kg infant is delivered. Apgar scoring is 6 at 1 minute and 9 at 5 minutes. The infant is evaluated by the trauma team and no fractures are noted. The infant is admitted to the nursery. The initial evaluation of the infant by a pediatrician reveals a healthy appearing infant with a raised area on the right posterior side of the head. There is no warmth noted and very little fluctuance. The area does not appear to cross suture lines. The most likely diagnosis is:

A. Subgaleal hemorrhage
B. Normal molding given the precipitous delivery
C. Caput succedaneum
D. Cephalohematoma
E. Infection secondary to scalp monitoring in the ER

178. A 6-year-old boy is seen in the ED because of fever, sore throat, and dyspnea. You note that he is drooling and holding his neck in a hyperextended position. The boy has had no immunizations for family religious reasons. You suspect the patient has epiglottitis. Which of the following statements about epiglottitis is true?

A. The incidence of epiglottitis has decreased dramatically since the widespread use of *Haemophilus influenzae* vaccine
B. The patient should be carefully placed in the supine position, and gently restrained so that the examiner can use a tongue blade and directly inspect the epiglottis
C. Patients with epiglottitis usually have a loud barky cough
D. The classic finding on a lateral neck radiograph is called the "steeple sign"
E. Radiographs should always be performed before endotracheal intubation or tracheostomy are considered

179. A 10-year-old boy with Ewing sarcoma presents with fever and is found to be neutropenic. After a blood culture is obtained, empiric IV antibiotics are administered. Thirty minutes later, he becomes hypotensive and unresponsive. His physical exam is remarkable for bleeding gums and petechiae. His laboratory results demonstrate a low platelet count, a prolonged partial thromboplastin time (PTT) as well as prothrombin time (PT), his d-dimers are elevated, his fibrinogen is decreased, and red blood cell fragments are noted on his blood smear. The most likely diagnosis is:

A. Disseminated intravascular coagulopathy (DIC)
B. Immune thrombocytopenia purpura (ITP)
C. Hemolytic uremic syndrome (HUS)
D. Kassabach-Merritt phenomena
E. Deep venous thrombosis (DVT)

180. A 14-year-old female presents with low-grade fever, cough, a sharp, stabbing pain over the left side of her chest extending into her left shoulder, and tachypnea. The pain is worse when she lies supine but improves with sitting upright and leaning forward. Her exam is significant for muffled heart sounds and an audible rub. A chest x-ray is obtained (Figure 3-180). Which of the following findings on exam/ECG would strengthen your diagnosis?

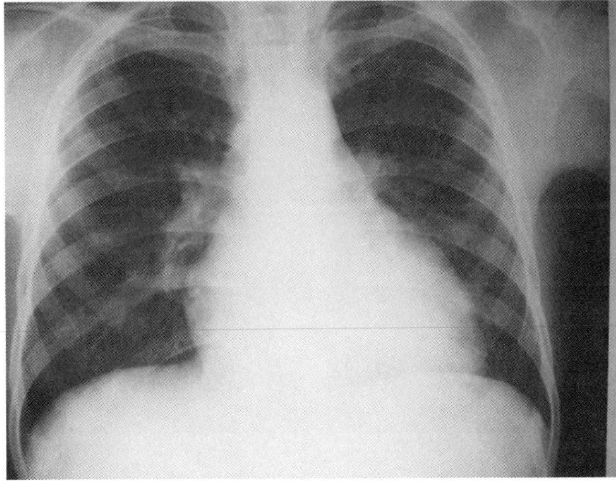

Figure 3-180 • Image Courtesy of the Department of Radiology, Phoenix Children's Hospital, Phoenix, Arizona.

A. Normal jugular venous distension in the neck
B. Wide pulses
C. Sinus bradycardia
D. Increased pulsus paradoxus
E. ST segment depression on the ECG
F. Increased QRS voltage in most leads

181. A 16-year-old girl presents to the ER with complaints of "heavy" vaginal bleeding. She had menarche at the age of 13 years. Previously her menstrual cycles were regular, lasting 28 days with 5 days of bleeding. For the past 6 months, her menstrual bleeding has lasted between 7 and 11 days. She has bled through her clothes overnight. On family history, her father required multiple cauterizations for frequent epistaxis. Laboratory evaluation revealed an isolated prolongation of the PTT. Her most likely diagnosis is:

A. Hemophilia A (factor VIII deficiency)
B. Hemophilia B (factor IX deficiency)
C. Lupus anticoagulant
D. Factor XI deficiency
E. Von Willebrand disease

182. A 13-year-old presents to the ER with a history of right leg pain that is more severe at night and relieved by ibuprofen. His physical exam is essentially normal with no limp and some mild tenderness over the lower tibial region. A radiograph is obtained (Figure 3-182a). Which of the following is the most likely diagnosis?

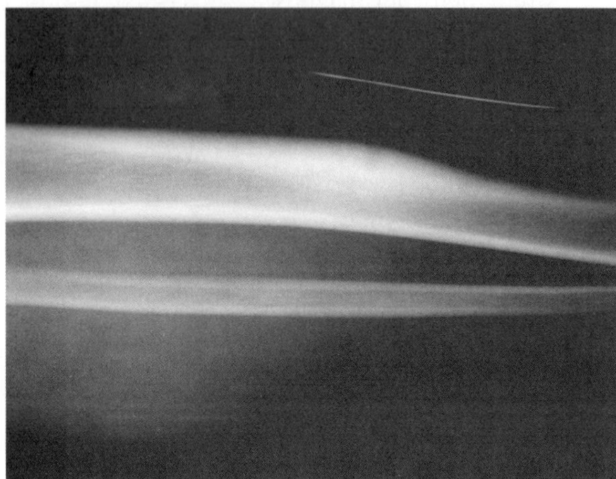

A

Figure 3-182a • Image Courtesy of the Department of Radiology, Phoenix Children's Hospital, Phoenix, Arizona.

A. Growing pains
B. Osteomyelitis
C. Osteosarcoma
D. Osteoid ostoma
E. Eosinophilic granuloma

183. A 14-year-old male has been brought into the ER following a syncopal episode. He was getting up from the toilet and reported feeling dizzy and then blacking out. His past medical and family history are unremarkable. His physical exam is completely normal, as is an ECG strip obtained during his ambulance ride over. Which of the following would be an appropriate work-up at this point?

A. Discharge home and follow-up with cardiology for a 24-hour Holter monitor
B. Admission to the ICU for inpatient monitoring
C. Stat ECHO in the ED
D. Placement of arterial line in the ED
E. Psychiatry or psychology referral

184. A 2-year-old child is brought into the ER by his mother. She reports that he was found in the bathroom with his grandmother's "iron pills" all around the floor. The mother is frantic, and to reassure her you counsel her that which of the following, once confirmed, virtually excludes the diagnosis of iron poisoning?

A. The absence of emesis 6 hours postingestion
B. Normal basic metabolic profile 1 hour postingestion
C. An alert, playful, age-appropriate child
D. The absence of leukocytosis 1 hour postingestion
E. The lack of radiolucent material on an abdominal x-ray

185. An 8-year-old male was an unrestrained front-seat passenger in an automobile accident. He was found by the paramedics in front of the car bleeding from the scalp, nose, and left lower leg. He presents with nasal flaring, intercostal retractions, and tachypnea. His pupils are reactive to light, he opens his eyes to pain, and groans with painful stimuli. His vital signs are temperature 36°C, pulse in the field 200, which has decreased to 170 with fluid, respiratory rate 60, and blood pressure 80/40. His extremities are cool, with thready pulses and capillary refill of 5 seconds. He has already received two 20 mL/kg NS infusions. He is in c-spine precautions. Which of the following interventions is most appropriate to perform first at this time?

A. Directly admit the patient to the PICU for close observation
B. Obtain an abdominal CT
C. Order a CT scan of the head
D. Repeat 20 mL/kg 0.9% NS IV
E. Placement of a femoral central venous line for central venous pressure assessment of intravascular fluid volume

186. A 4-year-old boy presents to the ED with a history of right lower quadrant abdominal pain that has been present for about 24 hours. The onset of the pain was followed by development of low-grade fever and vomiting. The patient has had no diarrhea but is not eating at all. Over the past 3 to 4 hours, the patient's pain has become more generalized and the abdomen has become distended. On physical examination the patient demonstrates generalized rebound tenderness, absent bowel sounds, and moderate dehydration. The best next step in the management of this patient is:

A. Take the patient to the OR for immediate appendectomy
B. Admit to the hospital and start oral rehydration solution
C. Start IV fluids; no antibiotics necessary
D. Start IV fluids and broad-spectrum antibiotics
E. Obtain stool specimen for microscopic examination and culture

187. A previously healthy, term 15-month-old male presents to the ER with a history of the sudden onset of rectal bleeding. The parents deny fever, vomiting, diarrhea, or abdominal pain. He has had three episodes of bright red blood per rectum. Hemodynamically, he is stable and his initial hemoglobin is 11. Which of the following tests is most likely to give you the correct diagnosis?

A. Flat plate x-ray (KUB) of the abdomen
B. Abdominal ultrasound
C. Meckel scan
D. CT of the abdomen
E. Upper GI

188. A 3-year-old girl comes to the ED because of fever, ear pain, protruding pinna, and erythematous, tender swelling in the postauricular area. There is also evidence of acute otitis media with a red, immobile, bulging tympanic membrane (TM). The patient has no signs or symptoms of meningitis. The best initial management option is:

A. Oral amoxicillin for 10 to 14 days
B. IM ceftriaxone for 3 consecutive days as an outpatient
C. Hospitalize for IV cefuroxime
D. Hospitalize for IV ampicillin-sulbactam and myringotomy
E. Arrange for otolaryngologist to perform mastoidectomy

189. A 10-month-old child is found playing with his mother's medicine bottles. There are some tablets on his shirt and some white powder around his mouth. His parents decide to take him to the ED. On arrival in the ED, the child is clearly symptomatic with a dry mouth, agitation, tachycardia, flushed skin, and hyperthermia. You would be most suspicious of which of the following medications:

A. Acetaminophen
B. Propranolol
C. Diphenhydramine (Benadryl)
D. Lithium
E. Phenytoin

190. A 16-year-old female is brought to the ER by her parents. They report that she went out with friends earlier and now has a high fever and is quite jumpy. The ER doctor examines the patient and finds her to be agitated with a heart rate of 122 and a temperature of 101°C. Her pupils are dilated, and she is diaphoretic. The patient has an infant's pacifier tied around her neck. While examining the patient, two pills with a cartoon character stamp fall out of her shirt pocket. The physician asks the parents if there has ever been a problem with illegal drug use, specifically MDMA or "ecstasy." Which of the following would be an appropriate next step for the physician?

A. Await lab analysis of the two unidentified pills
B. Administer syrup of ipecac
C. Obtain IV, and monitor airway and circulation
D. Allow patient to "detox" in the ER
E. Have emergency team locate friends for pill identification

191. A mother brings her 7-month-old baby to the ER because he has been pulling at his right ear for the last 2 to 3 weeks. The child is otherwise healthy with no symptoms of upper respiratory infection (URI), vomiting, diarrhea, or fever. On physical examination, the right TM is moderately erythematous, but no bulging or retraction is noted. Pneumatic otoscopy reveals normal mobility. The most likely diagnosis is:

A. Early acute otitis media
B. Otitis media with effusion (OME)
C. Bullous myringitis
D. Normal ears
E. Perforated TM

The following 2 questions (items 192-193) relate to the same clinical scenario.

You are evaluating an 8-year-old boy in the ED for a painful right great toe. He stubbed it playing soccer 15 days ago. Since then, he has had increasing pain, redness, and swelling of this toe. On exam, he is febrile to 38.9°C and cannot walk because of the pain in his toe. The toe is purplish-red, swollen, and the nail bed is broken.

192. The most appropriate next step in management would be:

A. MRI of the right foot
B. Whole-body bone scan
C. CBC, blood culture, and plain films of the right foot
D. Splint application and discharge for outpatient follow-up
E. IV oxacillin

193. After review of the lab and x-ray results, you note that his white count is elevated with a majority of neutrophils, and that the radiologist's dictation mentions "significant soft tissue swelling with a subperiosteal fluid collection around the base of the distal phalanx of the right great toe." The most likely diagnosis is:

A. Osteomyelitis of the right great toe
B. Cellulitis of the right foot
C. Avulsion of the right great toe nail bed
D. Right ankle sprain
E. Acute lymphoblastic leukemia (ALL)

End of Set

194. A 9-year-old girl with a known seizure disorder is brought to the ED for evaluation of prolonged hemiparesis following one of her typical focal left-sided seizures. She had been at summer camp and had neglected to take her routine medicine for seizure control. On exam, she is appropriate but drowsy. Her neurologic exam is significant for left-sided weakness and a positive Babinski reflex on the left. You suspect a diagnosis of Todd paralysis. The most appropriate next step in management is:

A. Cerebral angiogram
B. Admission to the PICU with neurosurgical consultation
C. Head MRI/MRA
D. Admission to the pediatric ward for 24-hour observation
E. LP

195. A 2-year-old girl is brought to the ED for difficulty breathing. She had been well earlier in the day. The mother states that the child had a coughing fit after she came out of her brother's room. When the mother investigated, she found the brother's piggy bank broken open on the floor. The girl has no significant past medical history. On exam, she is tachypneic and has wheezes over her right hemithorax. You suspect a foreign body aspiration. The most appropriate imaging study to confirm the diagnosis would be:

A. Contrast-enhanced CT of the chest
B. Plain films of the chest and neck
C. Modified barium swallow with speech pathology present
D. Upper GI series
E. Cervical spine x-rays

196. A 6-month-old infant is brought into the ED following a fall to a wooden floor from his mother's bed, which occurred 20 minutes ago. The child did not lose consciousness from the event and has been behaving appropriately. On physical exam you notice a mild swelling over the left parietal region, as well as significant head lag with poor truncal tone. A skull radiograph has been previously ordered by the resident and is available for your review (Figure 3-196). Your next step in the management of this patient should include:

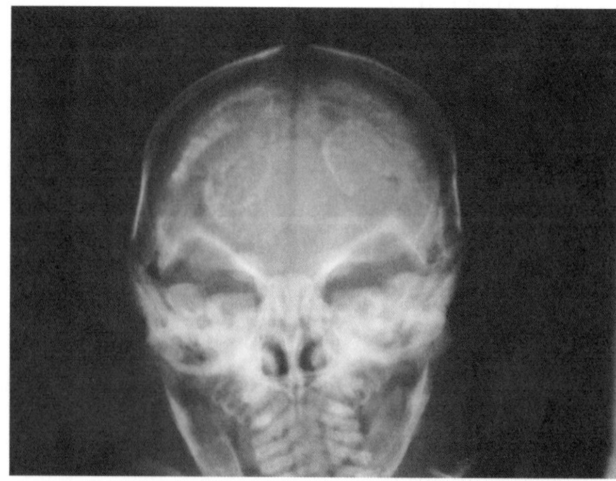

Figure 3-196 • Image Courtesy of the Department of Radiology, Phoenix Children's Hospital, Phoenix, Arizona.

A. Immediate neurosurgical consultation
B. MRI of the head
C. Discharge to the custody of child protective services
D. Admit to the hospital for overnight observation
E. Admit to the hospital for a more detailed evaluation

197. A 15-year-old male presents to the ED with a history of agitation and tachycardia. His friends say he is "on something" but refuse to say anything more. Myocardial ischemia secondary to this drug may be worsened with a β-blocker:

A. Cocaine
B. Amphetamine
C. PCP
D. Heroin
E. Codeine

The following 3 questions (items 198-200) relate to the same clinical scenario.

A 2-month-old girl is brought to the ED for evaluation after she fell out of her car seat off a table and landed on a concrete floor. She cried immediately, but over the next 4 hours got progressively drowsy and was not interested in feeding. On exam her vital signs are all within normal limits; however, she does have a 2-cm oval raised hematoma over her left parietal bone. The rest of the exam is normal.

198. The best next step in management would be:

A. Skull radiography
B. Head CT
C. Head MRI
D. Bone scan
E. Head ultrasound

199. The appropriate imaging study reviewed by yourself and the housestaff reveals a linear, non-depressed skull fracture. The best next step in management would be:

A. Discharge to a teenage relative while the parents are at work
B. Discharge to the parents who can observe the baby at home
C. Admission to the hospital for 24-hour observation
D. Neurosurgical consultation
E. Rapid sequence intubation and hyperventilation

200. You are beginning to write up the appropriate paperwork for your child when the radiologist calls with his interpretation of the study: "A depressed skull fracture of 6-mm depth over the left parietal bone with no obvious intracranial injury." Following this information, the best next step in management would be:

A. Discharge to a teenage relative while the parents are at work
B. Discharge to the parents who can observe the baby at home
C. Admission to the hospital for 24-hour observation
D. Neurosurgical consultation
E. Rapid sequence intubation and hyperventilation

End of Set

A Answers and Explanations

151. D
152. A
153. D
154. E
155. E
156. E
157. E
158. D
159. A
160. A
161. A
162. B
163. B
164. A
165. D
166. A
167. A
168. D
169. E
170. B
171. D
172. B
173. B
174. D
175. D
176. A
177. D
178. A
179. A
180. D
181. E
182. D
183. A
184. A
185. D
186. D
187. C
188. D
189. C
190. C
191. D
192. C
193. A
194. D
195. B
196. E
197. A
198. B
199. C
200. D

151. D. A child can have spinal cord injury without radiologic abnormality (SCIWORA), where the spinal cord has been damaged but the cervical vertebrae appear normal by x-ray. Therefore, a pediatric patient's c-spine should only be cleared when both the c-spine radiographs are normal *and* a clinical exam of the neck and spine can be reliably performed. If such a clinical exam cannot be performed, then further evaluation of the cervical spinal cord, such as with CT or MRI, would need to be performed to rule out the possibility of SCIWORA.

A, B, C, E. See explanation for D.

152. A. Elevated intracranial pressure is quite likely in this case. Crossing of the eyes, which is worse with distant gaze than near gaze, typifies a sixth nerve palsy. Active abduction is needed to maintain the straightness of the eyes at a distance, but not at closeness. The symptoms of possible ataxia with a history of recent clumsiness are concerning for a posterior fossa mass and warrant further investigation with a head MRI.

B. Prior to sampling the cerebral spinal pressure, the possibility of herniation from the pressure drop should be eliminated by cranial imaging.

C. Patching is indicated for the treatment of amblyopia, commonly associated with strabismus. In such cases, the unaffected eye is patched to force or stimulate the use of the amblyopic eye.

D. Given the constellation of symptoms in this patient, observation alone would not be appropriate.

E. Tensilon testing for myasthenia gravis is unnecessary, as it is not a likely source of this set of symptoms. Myasthenia is quite unusual in this age group, and while it often presents with strabismus, gait issues are quite unusual as well.

153. D. This boy presents with signs of meningitis, which include nuchal rigidity and/or pain, photophobia, and an associated fever; an LP would be the appropriate next step in management.

A, B, E. A serum drug screen, routine urinalysis, and EEG would not reveal any information about his CSF or meninges.

C. MRI of the brain, after a normal head CT scan, would be costly, delay appropriate treatment, and not provide any useful, additional information.

154. E. This is the typical pediatric presentation of aseptic meningitis in late summer: headache, neck pain/stiffness, photophobia, and CSF findings showing an increased WBC count with a predominance of lymphocytes with a normal CSF glucose and protein.

A. MS is a slowly progressive neurologic disease with insidious onset, not acute as in this case.

B. If *Neisseria meningitidis* were the cause of his illness, the patient would be expected to be sicker and have CSF findings more consistent with a bacterial process: increased WBC count with a predominance of neutrophils and increased protein with a decreased glucose.

C. A brain tumor should have been seen on the head CT and would not be expected to present with fever and neck pain.

D. Migraine headaches would not be expected to produce fever and the CSF findings seen in this patient, although associated photophobia and neck pain may occasionally be seen.

155. E. The child presented is in significant shock, manifested by gray color, prolonged capillary refill, absent peripheral pulses, and weak central pulses. This child needs vascular access immediately before bradycardia and irreversible cardiac arrest occurs. If IV access cannot be readily and *immediately* obtained, a needle should be inserted into the bone marrow cavity and rapid fluid resuscitation initiated. The usual location for intraosseous access is the proximal tibia, just below the tibial tuberosity, but any bone marrow access can be utilized in such an emergency (such as the humerus, anterior or posterior ileac crest, etc.). Fluid resuscitation can be ongoing through this site while attempts at securing further vascular access via a cutdown, central line, or peripheral vein ensue.

A. A cutdown procedure to isolate the saphenous vein may be necessary if no other IV access can be obtained. However, an intraosseous (IO) line is much easier to place and allows much more rapid treatment for this gravely ill child.

B. An umbilical venous line can be used in premature infants and neonates, but would not be possible in a 6-month-old child.
C. The primary problem in this patient is circulatory shock, not respiratory compromise. With proper fluid resuscitation, intubation and ventilation may be avoided.
D. Placement of a subclavian line is not the first choice in a 6-month-old infant. Intraosseous line placement is the appropriate first step.

156. E. The scenario presented above describes a child with supraventricular tachycardia (SVT) who is *unstable* and in shock. The shock is manifested by cool extremities, mottled skin color, and prolonged capillary refill. Synchronized cardioversion is the first-line treatment of SVT in an unstable patient with hypotension.

A. Furosemide (Lasix) would be an effective treatment for a patient with evidence of congestive heart failure and fluid overload with pulmonary edema. It has no role for the initial treatment of SVT.
B. Lidocaine is a group-1B antiarrhythmic drug that is indicated for the treatment of acute ventricular arrhythmias, most commonly that of ventricular fibrillation. Adenosine is considered the drug of choice when treating SVT.
C. Administration of ice and water increases vagal tone, which will also slow conduction in the atrioventricular (AV) node and can result in rapid conversion of SVT. The use of warm water would have the opposite intended effect of tachycardia.
D. Digitalizing slowly over 24 hours is not an appropriate choice for someone who is unstable and in shock because it does not correct the dysrhythmia rapidly enough. Once the child has been converted to a stable rhythm, digitalization can be started to reduce the risk of subsequent events.

157. E. This patient has a ketone-negative hypoglycemia without failure to thrive. Congenital hyperinsulinism is the most likely diagnosis. An uninterrupted flow of glucose in the blood is essential for normal brain metabolism. Categories of hypoglycemia include abnormalities in hormonal regulation; inborn errors of glucose, fat, or protein metabolism; prematurity; drugs; organ failures; and certain neoplasms. Hormonal conditions include deficiencies in the growth hormonal axis, adrenal hormonal axis, thyroid hormonal axis, or insulin hormone excess.

The algorithm below can be useful in helping to diagnose hypoglycemic disorders:

Ketotic
- **High lactate**
  - **→ Inborn errors of glucose metabolism**
- **Normal lactate**
  - **→ Glycogen storage diseases, hormonal deficiency, ketotic hypoglycemia**

Nonketotic
- **Reducing substances**
  - **→ Hereditary fructose intolerance, galactosemia**
- **No reducing substances**
  - **→ Hyperinsulinism, fatty acid oxidation defect, drugs**

A. The patient is not noted to have tachypnea, cough, or fever, and thus pneumonia is unlikely.
B. Adrenal insufficiency should present with electrolyte abnormalities, most notably hyponatremia and hyperkalemia, as well as ketonuria if hypoglycemic.
C. Patients with glycogen storage disease often present with hepatomegaly and failure to thrive, and would be expected to be able to produce ketones.
D. Galactosemia is a disorder of carbohydrate, specifically galactose, metabolism. Infants often present with jaundice, failure to thrive, hepatomegaly, and hypoglycemia. Negative ketones, but positive reducing substances, would be expected on a urinalysis.

158. D. This is a classic case of infant botulism. Babies with this condition are listless and hypotonic and may have a weak cry, poor head control, feeding difficulties, and constipation. As in this case, there is often a recent change in feeding practice. Additionally, honey has been implicated as a cause in several cases. In adult cases of botulism, the patient swallows the toxin from improperly prepared foods, but infants become infected by ingesting *Clostridium botulinum* spores that colonize the baby's colon. Because paralysis of the respiratory muscles can cause respiratory failure, these babies must be admitted to the hospital for careful supportive care, which may include endotracheal intubation. Antibiotics are not helpful. Stools should be tested for botulinum toxin.

A. Cow's milk allergy or intolerance generally causes diarrhea, not constipation, and would not account for difficulties in suck and hypotonia.
B. The natural sugars in prune juice can act to draw water into the gut lumen and help hydrate and soften stools. In this case of botulism, the constipation is toxin mediated and stool softeners would not be effective.
C. This baby may be too ill for a speech therapy evaluation at this time. The gag, suck, and swallowing reflexes begin to return to normal after approximately 1 to 3 weeks. At that time, the speech therapist can be helpful with decisions regarding resumption of oral feedings.
E. Infant botulism can be fatal. When the condition is recognized early and babies get adequate supportive care and proper airway management in the hospital, the mortality rate is less than 5%.

159. **A. During the summer, many children who go swimming develop external otitis, also known as "swimmer's ear." This condition is due to maceration of the ear canal epithelium caused by moisture or chemical irritation. The pain can be intense, especially with manipulation of the pinna or pressure on the tragus. Unlike acute otitis media, most cases are not associated with signs or symptoms of an upper respiratory condition. Secondary bacterial infection is common with external otitis. The best treatment for most cases is a topical combination antibiotic-steroid suspension that is instilled into the ear canal for about 7 to 10 days. For prevention, the ear canals should always be dried well after swimming. Some experts also suggest acetic acid (vinegar) for prophylaxis.**

B. Systemic antibiotics, such as ceftriaxone, are not necessary for external otitis.
C. Drops containing benzocaine can be effective in reducing pain, but will not help with the infection or inflammation seen in external otitis.
D. Topical treatment is adequate. Oral agents such amoxicillin can be associated with unnecessary systemic side effects, such as diarrhea or rash.
E. Because the pain originates from the ear canal, warm compresses to the external ear would not help.

160. **A. It is true that most febrile seizures occur between 9 months and 5 years of age.**

B. Febrile convulsions are considered "atypical" if they last longer than 15 minutes, occur multiple times in the same day, or are associated with focal seizure activity or focal neurologic findings. If a child has "atypical" seizures, a family history of epilepsy, seizure onset before 9 months, delayed development, or preexisting neurologic disease, there will be greater risk for developing epilepsy later.
C. Children with a typical simple febrile convulsion without risk factors are not significantly more likely to develop epilepsy than the general population.
D. While it is extremely important to rule out meningitis, an extensive diagnostic work-up with serum electrolytes, toxicology screening, an EEG, or neuroimaging is not recommended in children with a simple febrile seizure.
E. Prolonged anticonvulsant prophylaxis is not recommended for simple febrile seizures. Some experts feel diazepam (Valium) may be given at the onset of a febrile illness to children with a history of very frequent recurrences of simple febrile seizures.

161. **A. The case history is a typical presentation of Henoch-Schönlein purpura (HSP). Most cases are preceded by a viral infection and the symptoms are secondary to an immune-mediated vasculitis involving IgA antibodies and complexes.**

B. The rash tends to be crops of palpable purpuric lesions that have a predilection for the buttocks and lower extremities.
C. In addition to the rash, arthritis, glomerulonephritis, hypertension, and abdominal pain are common.
D. As opposed to idiopathic thrombocytopenic purpura, the platelet count in HSP is normal or elevated.
E. The abdominal pain is sometimes associated with intussusception, which should be considered whenever the abdominal pain is severe or if the stools are grossly bloody (currant jelly stools). Many patients with HSP have a mild illness and do not require hospitalization. Severe abdominal pain, renal disease, and hypertension are criteria for admission. Corticosteroids may help abdominal pain due to intestinal vasculitis. Their use may also prevent serious chronic renal disease.

162. B. The C3 is low early in the course of PSGN, but in all cases returns to normal in 6 to 8 weeks. A persistently low C3 suggests a different type of hypocomplementemic glomerulonephritis.

A. ASO is usually elevated early and frequently remains high for 3 to 6 months. When PSGN is secondary to skin infection the anti-DNAase B is often more strongly positive.
C. Diminishing significant proteinuria can last as long as 3 months, but heavy proteinuria with or without nephritic syndrome suggests a complicated course and warrants reevaluation.
D. While gross hematuria is a common initial finding, this should gradually disappear in 2 to 3 weeks.
E. Hypertension is common during the acute phase of PSGN, but it should not persist as the urine clears and the other symptoms abate.

163. B The diagnosis is most likely hereditary spherocytosis. The findings of anemia, normal MCV, and high RDW are all compatible with the diagnosis of hereditary spherocytosis.

A. The diagnosis is most likely hereditary spherocytosis. The findings of anemia and high MCHC are compatible with the diagnosis of hereditary spherocytosis, but the absence of reticulocytosis would be unusual in a hemolytic process.
C. The diagnosis is most likely hereditary spherocytosis. The anemia is hemolytic, and the finding of both a high MCHC (above 35) and a high RDW (over 14.5) is almost pathognomonic of this disease. Anemia, reticulocytosis, and an elevated indirect bilirubin are the rule. Therefore this selection, which includes a normal MCHC and RDW, is not compatible with the diagnosis of hereditary spherocytosis.
D. A normal direct bilirubin and high reticulocyte count both occur in hereditary spherocytosis. However, you would expect the *indirect* bilirubin to be elevated. The normal MCHC is also expected and is not of any clinical assistance in making the diagnosis.
E. The diagnosis is most likely hereditary spherocytosis. The findings of anemia and high indirect bilirubin both support the diagnosis of hemolytic anemia. However, the RDW should be high in hemolytic anemia.

164. A. The delay in treatment and suspicious story of a 2-month-old being unattended and rolling off a bed are highly suggestive of abuse. The infant in this scenario should have a thorough physical exam for abuse as well as diagnostic studies to include a head CT, skeletal survey, and retinal exam. Shaken baby syndrome, which manifests as subdural hematomas and retinal hemorrhages, is a concern in this case. After several days, the yellow centers of intraretinal hemorrhages, so typical of shaken baby syndrome, begin to turn white or gray.

B. Retinoschisis, a splitting of the layers of the retina, rather than detachment, is only rarely seen spontaneously.
C. Shaken baby syndrome is typified by hemorrhages of multiple layers of the retina, and multiple areas from posterior to anterior.
D. Shaken baby syndrome is typified by a normal examination of the external eye, and internal eye hemorrhaging.
E. Bridging retinal vessels and subarachnoid sources can produce marked vitreal bleeding in shaken baby syndrome.

165. D. GHB is a concern for potential abuse as a date rape drug. Although the mechanism of action of GHB is not clearly understood, GHB appears to influence dopaminergic activity, probably by GHB receptors. A clue to the diagnosis of GHB is an apparent coma with a rapid return to consciousness when stimulated (usually when attempting to intubate).

A. Hypertension, tachycardia, and diaphoresis may be seen following the ingestion of sympathomimetic drugs such as cocaine or methamphetamine.
B. Auditory and visual hallucinations would be more consistent with phencyclidine (PCP).
C. Nystagmus, agitation, and hyperthermia may be seen following excessive diphenhydramine (Benadryl) ingestion.
E. Ecstasy ingestion would be more typical with a presentation of hyponatremic seizures after a rave concert, most likely secondary to the excessive drinking of water in an effort to stay hydrated from prolonged dancing.

166. A. The patient's clinical presentation is consistent with constipation-induced abdominal pain, which is a common mimic for appendicitis in the

pediatric age range. Factors suggesting against appendicitis in this case are:

- No fevers despite 4 days of symptoms
- Intermittent pain that sometimes is severe, and at other times goes away completely
- No significant change in appetite
- No vomiting

If a rectal exam had been performed that confirmed the presence of a large amount of stool in the vault, a KUB would not be necessary before a therapeutic trial of an enema. However, in this case, it is quite justifiable to obtain a KUB to confirm the presence of increased fecal material.

B, C. The above-listed factors argue against appendicitis and the need for a CT scan or an ultrasound.

D. Intussusception would certainly be high in the differential if this patient were between 6 months and 2 years of age. Although it can occur in older children, it is much less common. In this patient with no blood in her stools, it would be more reasonable to exclude constipation first before embarking upon a more extensive work-up.

E. Simple reassurance would not be appropriate in this patient.

167. A. Typically, when a Fleet enema is given and a large stool results, the patient who was previously writhing in pain now becomes quite happy and comfortable and no further work-up or consultation is needed. However, if such a patient stools after an enema but still has significant abdominal pain, further work-up is necessary, as the presence of constipation does not rule out more serious etiologies of abdominal pain.

B, C. A surgical consult would not be necessary in this patient with constipation.

D. Further imaging of the abdomen would most likely not be necessary unless severe pain persists as described in the explanation for A.

E. Although patients with a chronic history of constipation may need further GI involvement, it would be inappropriate to refer a patient to subspecialty care without initial interventions of dietary change and the use of stool softeners and/or laxatives. It is unlikely that the patient in this scenario, who has no significant past medical history, will need subspecialty involvement in the near future.

168. D. A presumptive diagnosis of infective endocarditis is made whenever a patient with underlying heart disease has an unexplained fever for several days' duration associated with typical clinical findings. Patients may have a new murmur or an increased intensity of an existing murmur. There may be petechiae of the skin, mucous membranes, or conjunctiva, but the classic Osler nodes, Janeway lesions, and splinter hemorrhages are rare. Embolic complications include pulmonary emboli, hematuria and renal failure, and seizures or hemiparesis. Patients generally require treatment with at least 4 to 6 weeks of IV antibiotics. *Streptococcus viridans, Staphylococcus aureus,* and group D streptococcus (enterococcus) are responsible for 90% of cases of infectious endocarditis. The diagnosis is generally made by isolation of these organisms from blood culture. The timing of the blood cultures is not important because the bacteremia is constant.

A. This patient is not in cardiac failure and does not require digoxin or furosemide.

B. Antibiotic pretreatment significantly decreases the chance of isolating the organism, so antibiotics should not be given prior to obtaining cultures.

C. While some of the symptoms are similar to those seen in influenza, this patient's history, physical exam, and lab results are more typical of infectious endocarditis. Amantadine would not be beneficial.

E. An ECHO may show the vegetation, but a normal ECHO does not rule out the possibility of endocarditis. Small vegetations early in the course of the disease may not be detected.

169. E. This patient's clinical presentation is typical of hemolytic-uremic syndrome (HUS). Many cases follow ingestion of poorly cooked hamburger meat that contains a toxin produced by *E. coli* O157:H7. The syndrome consists of microangopathic hemolytic anemia, thrombocytopenia, and acute renal failure. Patients may develop toxic megacolon, bowel wall necrosis, intussusception, and/or bowel perforation. Many patients have CNS findings such as irritability, lethargy, coma, seizures, or hallucinations. Thrombotic or hemorrhagic stroke may occur. Chronic renal insufficiency occurs in 5% to 10% of patients. The blood smear in HUS shows fragmented red blood cells or schistocytes. Historically, 10% to 20% of patients with *E. coli* O157:H7 infection

develop HUS. Recently, it has been shown that administration of antibiotics to patients with *E. coli* infection can actually increase the chance of developing HUS. Treatment includes supportive care to manage fluid and electrolyte imbalance, hypertension, anemia, and bleeding. Renal dialysis is necessary in 30% to 50% of patients.

A. *Staphylococcus aureus* can produce a clinical picture consistent with food poisoning, but is typically not associated with HUS. *S. aureus* is further associated as a causative organism in toxic shock syndrome, scalded skin syndrome, pneumonia, osteomyelitis, arthritis, cellulitis, and other localized skin infections.
B. *Streptococcus pyogenes* is responsible for causing cellulitis and other localized skin infections, as well as arthritis, osteomyelitis, and, less commonly, toxic shock syndrome.
C. *Shigella dysenteriae* infection can result in HUS, but less commonly than *E. coli*. Patients with *S. dysenteriae* typically present with bloody diarrhea and systemic symptoms of fever, vomiting, and abdominal pain. Treatment with a third-generation cephalosporin is recommended and shortens the duration of illness.
D. Rotavirus is a common cause of diarrhea in the pediatric population and often produces diffuse, foul-smelling, water loss stools. It does not commonly cause bloody diarrhea and/or HUS.

170. **B. In any unstable patient with an upper GI bleed, the first step is to place two IVs and give volume resuscitation.**

A. Following the establishment of IV access, attempts are made to type and screen/cross blood for transfusion and perform further diagnostic testing.
C. Vitamin K may be helpful in patients with a known elevated prothrombin time (PT) but the effect is not immediate.
D. Endotracheal intubation is needed infrequently and only in those patients who develop as altered level of consciousness due to rapid blood loss.
E. The use of an H2 blocker while the patient remains with nothing by mouth (NPO) or for the treatment of suspected ulcer may be useful, but it is not the first step in management of the patient with an upper GI bleed.

171. **D. Irrigation and cleaning is the mainstay of wound management.**

A. In this case Td is indicated given that more than 5 years have passed since vaccination.
B. Prophylactic antibiotics are not necessary. The wound should be monitored for further signs of infection and antibiotics prescribed if then necessary.
C. Early infections are often caused by *Pasteurella multocida* in both cat and dog bites.
E. Suturing of the hand, particularly following a dog bite, should be avoided if at all possible given the higher chance of infection.

172. **B. Hereditary angioedema is an autosomal dominant defect in the complement system. Angioedema that does not respond to epinephrine and is not associated with hives should be the clue to the health care provider. Often there is a family history of edema associated with minor trauma and/or stress. The differential would include anaphylaxis, but one should see some resolution with epinephrine in that case.**

A. Anaphylaxis to the gloves' powder would be expected to be more generalized and should respond to epinephrine.
C. There is no history of blunt chest trauma or signs on physical exam, such as muffled heart sounds, jugular venous distension, or hypotension, that would be consistent with pericardial tamponade.
D. There are no peritoneal signs or other acute physical findings to suggest bowel perforation and septic shock.
E. IV infiltration is a local reaction that occurs at the catheter site and would not explain these symptoms.

173. **B. This patient's elevated anion and osmolal gap indicate that she may have ingested a toxic amount of alcohol in addition to the ethanol; therefore she requires supportive care while the levels are obtained.**

A. This child has a very elevated ethanol level for her age and is not stable to go home. In addition, the metabolites of methanol, ethylene glycol, and isopropyl alcohol can be extremely toxic and dangerous. Fortunately, the coingestion of ethanol will result in the preferential inhibition of alcohol dehydrogenase, preventing metabolism of the toxic ethanols and acting as an antidote.
C. IV thiamine is important to replace with chronic alcoholism but would not be indicated in this patient.

D. Fomepizole is a potent inhibitor of alcohol dehydrogenase and can be used in the treatment of ethylene glycol or methanol ingestion. This is an expensive therapy that has not yet been widely used in children.
E. Hemodialysis is an effective and rapid technique to remove ethylene glycol and methanol and their toxic metabolites. Indications for hemodialysis would include severe metabolic acidosis, renal failure, or high levels of ethylene glycol or methanol.

174. **D. The patient in this scenario is presenting with a retropharyngeal abscess. Classic symptoms include fever, dysphagia, neck swelling or pain, a muffled voice, drooling, or stridor. The lateral neck film reveals a widening of the retropharyngeal soft tissue (prevertebral) space as defined by more than one half of a vertebral body below C3. The diagnosis should be confirmed by CT scan to further evaluate the extent of the infection. Appropriate management consists of controlling the airway, use of parenteral antibiotics such as ampicillin-sulbactam, and drainage in a majority of patients.**

A. Immediate consultation with anesthesia and intubation in the OR would be indicated if epiglottitis were suspected, unlikely in a case of a child with current vaccines and no evidence of stridor or respiratory distress. The classic x-ray finding is a swollen or thumbprint-like epiglottis.
B. The use of racemic epinephrine would be indicated in a scenario of croup.
C. Peritonsillar abscesses are more common in the adolescent population and rare in younger patients. The exam of the oropharynx should demonstrate unilateral tonsillar fullness with possible uvula deviation.
E. The use of dexamethasone would be indicated in cases where the abscess may cause upper airway inflammation significant enough to cause symptoms such stridor; it would also be indicated in the treatment of croup.

175. **D. The clinical description of dry mucous membranes, cool extremities, prolonged capillary refill, doughy skin texture, and hypernatremia describes a child in hypovolemic shock. The treatment is intravascular volume expansion with isotonic fluid, such as 0.9% sodium chloride, 20 mL/kg per infusion, pushed IV followed by immediate reevaluation and repetition as needed to correct the clinical condition of shock.**

A. Infusion of D5 (0.2%) NS plus 20 mEq/L at 1.5 maintenance may be appropriate after the initial phase of shock has passed and the patient has been stabilized.
B. Infusion of 10 mL/kg of D10W is the treatment for hypoglycemia.
C. Administration of 2 mEq/kg sodium bicarbonate would be appropriate to correct a severe metabolic acidosis after the initial phase of fluid replacement has occurred.
E. Administration of IV antibiotics and an LP to rule out sepsis is not the initial management choice for a patient suffering from hypovolemic shock probably as a result of diarrhea.

176. **A. D-Amphetamine is a sympathomimetic agent. Dilated pupils, diaphoresis, agitation, hyperthermia, and seizures would all be expected symptoms associated with toxicity from D-Amphetamine or any other amphetamine-related product.**

B. Agitation, rather than lethargy, would be an expected result of the ingestion of a sympathomimetic agent.
C. Diaphoresis, rather than dry skin, would be an expected side effect of D-amphetamine.
D. Hyponatremia would not be a likely result in this case.
E. GI symptoms may include nausea, vomiting, or diarrhea. Constipation would not be expected.

177. **D. Cephalohematomas are a common occurrence in newborns. They do not cross suture lines of the skull, present as a fluctuant mass, and are the result of a subperiosteal hemorrhage. They can be rarely associated with skull fractures.**

A. Subgaleal hemorrhages are rare conditions that must be diagnosed quickly, as a relatively large amount of blood can collect and shock can occur. They are often associated with vacuum deliveries.
B. Molding is a normal finding in newborns. Commonly it is seen after prolonged delivery.
C. Caput succedaneum is swelling that is noted after birth and crosses the suture lines.
E. Scalp monitoring is used for prolonged labor. As this baby was delivered quickly en route to the ED, there was no opportunity for scalp monitor placement.

178. **A. Since the release of the Haemophilus vaccine, the incidence of epiglottitis due to this organism has dropped greatly. Other agents, such as *Streptococcus pyogenes, S. pneumoniae,* and *Staphylococcus aureus,* now represent a larger proportion of pediatric cases of epiglottitis.**

B. Anxiety-provoking interventions should always be avoided in patients with epiglottitis. Phlebotomy, IV line placement, placing the child supine, or direct visualization of the oral cavity should be delayed until the airway is secure.

C. Patients with epiglottitis do not show the typical barky cough seen in viral croup. Stridor is a late finding and may not be present until the airway is nearly completely obstructed. Epiglottitis is a potentially lethal condition in which a child may develop air hunger, restlessness, cyanosis, and coma in just hours.

D. The classic finding on lateral neck radiographs is the "thumb sign" consistent with the large, swollen, cherry-red epiglottis seen on laryngoscopy. The "steeple" sign results from subglottic edema and is seen in viral croup, not epiglottitis.

E. Patients suspected of having epiglottitis should never be taken to the radiology department until after endotracheal intubation (or tracheostomy if necessary) is performed to prevent complete airway obstruction, regardless of the degree of respiratory distress.

179. **A. This boy has the classic picture of DIC with widespread activation of the coagulation system, usually resulting from some form of shock, in this case septic shock.**

B. There are no abnormalities of the PT or PTT in ITP.

C. Children with HUS present with renal insufficiency and a microangiopathic hemolytic anemia.

D. A Kassabach-Merritt phenomenon is associated with large hemangiomas that consume both platelets and clotting factors.

E. Elevated levels of d-dimer can be seen in deep venous thrombosis; however, microangiopathic changes of the red cells are rarely seen.

180. **D. The patient in this scenario is presenting with pericarditis with impending cardiac tamponade. The chest x-ray shows evidence of an enlarged heart with increased pulmonary marking. Pulsus paradoxus is caused by the normal slight decrease in systolic arterial pressure during inspiration. With cardiac tamponade, this is exaggerated because of decreased filling of the left side of the heart. To hear the first Korotkoff sound, use a manometer while the patient takes a normal inspiration, and then listen to when the first Korotkoff sound is heard continuously. The difference between the two points is the pulsus paradoxus. If it is greater than 20 in a child with pericarditis, it is indicative of cardiac tamponade.**

A, B, C. The impaired filling of the heart leads to distended jugular veins, narrow pulses, and a compensatory tachycardia.

E, F. An ECHO is the most sensitive technique for evaluating the pericardial effusion and looking for evidence of tamponade, but an ECG typically reveals widespread low-voltage QRS complexes with mild ST segment elevation and T wave inversion. Electrical alternans can be seen with a variable QRS complex amplitude.

181. **E. Hemophilia A, hemophilia B, lupus anticoagulant, factor XI deficiency, and Von Willebrand disease can all cause an isolated prolongation of the PTT. Von Willebrand disease is the most common inherited bleeding disorder, affecting 1% to 2% of the population. It is inherited in either an autosomal dominant or recessive manner. It typically presents with recurrent epistaxis or prolonged menstruation.**

A, B. Factor VIII and IX deficiency are inherited in an X-linked pattern. Therefore, females are carriers and only extremely rarely affected.

C. Lupus anticoagulant is associated with thrombosis, not bleeding.

D. Factor XI deficiency is an autosomal recessive trait, though much more rare than Von Willebrand disease.

182. **D. The classic history of nighttime pain relieved by nonsteroidal anti-inflammatory drugs (NSAIDs), coupled with the radiographic findings of a sclerotic bone surrounding a radiolucent area, is consistent with the diagnosis of an osteoid osteoma. This is a benign bone tumor that may require resection if pain becomes intolerable.**

A. Growing pains are worse at night and are relieved by NSAIDS, but they are typically bilateral and accompanied by a normal physical exam and normal radiographs.

B. There is no history of fever, limp, or systemic illness that would suggest osteomyelitis.

C. Although osteosarcomas are often diagnosed during adolescence and periods of rapid bone growth, the typical radiographic appearance is one of severely sclerotic bone with overlying new bone formation (Figure 3-182b).

E. The classic radiograph findings of eosinophilic granuloma are more lytic, punched out-type lesions. Patients often present in early childhood and have systemic or skin involvement in a large proportion of cases.

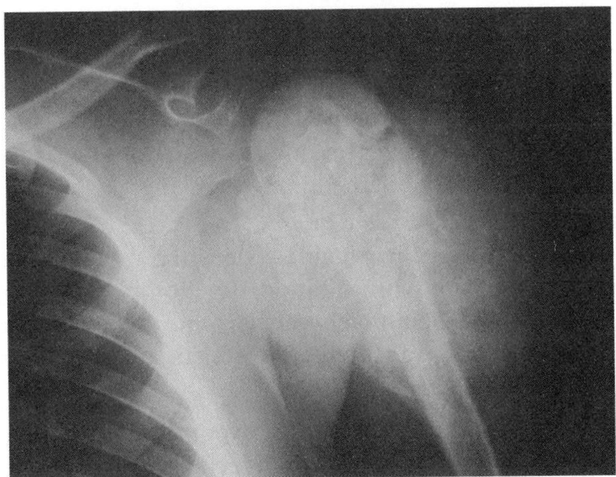

B

Figure 3-182b • Image Courtesy of the Department of Radiology, Phoenix Children's Hospital, Phoenix, Arizona.

183. **A. Many would argue that follow-up is not even necessary for a single suspected vasovagal episode. Of all the options listed, discharge home and follow-up with cardiology for a 24-hour Holter monitor is the only option that is appropriate.**

B. This patient clearly does not need ICU monitoring because the etiology is most likely a vasovagal syncope.

C. An ECHO would not be helpful in this scenario given the normal physical exam and past medical history.

D. An arterial line would be invasive and useless in a patient with a normal blood pressure.

E. Referral to psychology/psychiatry would only be appropriate if the patient was willfully fainting as can be seen following hyperventilation—something unlikely in this case.

184. **A. Emesis occurring prior to 6 hours after ingestion implies significant iron ingestion. The absence of emesis 6 hours postingestion virtually excludes the diagnosis of iron poisoning.**

B, D, E. Laboratory parameters and radiographs are not usually helpful with the exception of a confirmatory iron level. It is important to understand that iron poisoning is a clinical diagnosis and iron levels or other laboratory values do not dictate treatment.

C. Iron exerts its initial toxic effect on the gastric mucosa by direct irritation. Nausea, vomiting, and diarrhea may occur with accompanying electrolyte abnormalities. However, aside from the associated vomiting and diarrhea, a child may appear alert and playful without any other signs following iron ingestion.

185. **D. The patient presents with signs of decompensated hypotensive shock after major trauma. He is tachycardic, hypotensive, and poorly perfused. Aggressive stabilization with attention to ensuring a stable airway, adequate oxygenation and ventilation, and improved circulation is mandatory. Of the answers provided, only repeat immediate volume expansion with an additional rapid infusion of 20 mL/kg isotonic crystalloid is immediately appropriate.**

A. Although this patient will need to be admitted to the PICU, it is important to continue his initial resuscitation and attempt further stabilization of his circulation.

B. The possibility that the patient suffered a head injury following this accident needs to be considered, but further stabilization needs to occur before being sent for a CT scan.

C. Blunt abdominal trauma is common and an abdominal CT would be warranted after stabilization.

E. Placement of a femoral central line would be a useful form of IV access to supply more fluids, but not simply to monitor or assess central venous pressure.

186. **D. This patient has the clinical picture that is typical of a perforated acute appendicitis. Perforation is much more common in very young children. When perforation occurs, patients require IV fluid resuscitation and broad-spectrum antibiotics (ampicillin, gentamycin, clindamycin) for treatment of peritonitis for several hours prior to appendectomy. Antibiotics should provide coverage for *E. coli, Klebsiella, Pseudomonas,* and anaerobes. The patient should be placed on NG suction and be given nothing to eat or drink by mouth. Following the appendectomy, patients with perforation may develop paralytic ileus and**

bowel obstruction, persistent fever, abdominal abscess, wound infection, and/or sepsis.

A. Although this patient will eventually require surgical intervention, it is important to first stabilize the patient with particular attention to the ABCs (airway, breathing, circulation), while providing adequate antibiotic therapy to control the further progression of disease.
B. The patient has evidence of an acute surgical abdomen and should not be given anything by mouth.
C. As in the explanation for D, broad-spectrum antibiotics should be initiated to control the further progression of disease.
E. There is no need for a microscopic examination or culture of the stool in this case. Such tests may be valuable in suspected infectious gastroenteritis. In gastroenteritis, diarrhea is common, and the vomiting and fever usually precede the abdominal pain.

187. **C. Painless rectal bleeding in this age group without any signs of intestinal obstruction is most likely due to a Meckel diverticulum. Hemorrhage is the result of peptic ulceration and is typically bright red or maroon and painless. A Meckel scan uses technetium, which is excreted by the gastric mucosa and will demonstrate increased intake at the site of the diverticulum.**

A. In this patient, a flat plate of the abdomen will typically show nonspecific findings.
B. Abdominal ultrasound is not specific for diagnosing Meckel diverticulum and is not the study of choice for GI bleeding.
D. CT of the abdomen may be helpful if the Meckel scan is normal and a colonoscopy does not reveal the source of the lower GI blood loss. It would not be the study of choice in a patient with GI bleeding unless there was a history of trauma or an abdominal mass.
E. An upper GI will not demonstrate a diverticulum near the level of the ileum.

188. **D. The patient presented in the case scenario has typical findings of acute mastoiditis. Acute mastoiditis is caused by extension of infection from otitis media into the mastoid air cells. The presentation usually includes fever, ear pain, postauricular swelling and erythema, and a protruding pinna. The common causative organisms are *Streptococcus pneumoniae, Streptococcus pyogenes,* and *Staphylococcus aureus*. The initial treatment should combine IV, broad-spectrum antibiotic administration with drainage of the middle ear (myringotomy).**

A. Oral amoxicillin does not provide adequate coverage for the common causative organisms.
B. While ceftriaxone may provide adequate antibiotic coverage, most patients should be hospitalized and observed for complications such as meningitis, sepsis, brain abscess, venous sinus thrombosis, osteomyelitis, labyrinthitis, or Bezold (deep neck) abscess.
C. Cefuroxime alone without drainage of the middle ear is not considered optimal treatment.
E. Mastoidectomy is usually reserved for cases in which antibiotics and drainage do not result in marked improvement in 48 hours.

189. **C. Diphenhydramine (Benadryl) toxicity is associated with agitation, dry mouth, dry axilla, flushed skin, tachycardia, and hyperthermia due to its anticholinergic effects.**

A. Acetaminophen toxicity is most likely to present with nausea, vomiting, abdominal pain, and anorexia, which may progress to jaundice and liver failure.
B. Propranolol ingestion is likely to produce bradycardia, hypotension, lightheadedness, fatigue, nausea, and vomiting.
D. Lithium overdosage may result in nausea, vomiting, tremor, drowsiness, and lack of muscle coordination.
E. Phenytoin may cause nystagmus, tremor, ataxia, and dysarthria. Severe overdose may result in respiratory and circulatory depression.

190. **C. Unfortunately, the use of amphetamines and derivatives is quite common in the United States. Substances such as methamphetamine and MDMA are actually becoming more of a problem in recent years. While the above presentation could indeed be the result of these substances, it is important to complete a thorough examination with appropriate lab evaluation. The ABCs are the important priorities.**

A. Often, street drugs have more than one active substance whether the buyer knows this or not. Lab analysis of the pills is important but often is a later source of information.

B. Ipecac is not appropriate in this setting as emesis can cause more problems in an altered level of consciousness. Activated charcoal is more likely to be of benefit in unknown ingestions.

D. It is necessary to proceed with the ABCs and provide supportive care rather than simple observation.

E. Further identification of the pills will not immediately help in the management of this patient.

191. **D. Erythema of the TM alone is rarely indicative of acute otitis media. Normal eardrum position and normal mobility with pneumatic otoscopy should be interpreted as normal. Many babies without ear pathology pull at or play with their ears.**

A. The most important diagnostic features of acute otitis media are a bulging TM and decreased mobility when positive and negative pressure are applied into the ear canal with a rubber bulb attached to the otoscope (pneumatic otoscopy). There is often pain. Fever is present in only about 50% of cases, but almost all ear infections are preceded by URI symptoms.

B. Otitis media with effusion, previously known as serous otitis media, is caused by a blocked eustachian tube. The TM is usually in the retracted position secondary to a negative middle ear pressure. Fluid levels and air bubbles are often seen through the TM. Most patients do not have pain, but temporary conductive hearing loss is common.

C. The eardrum in bullous myringitis has hemorrhagic or serous bubble-like blisters on the TM. This condition is caused by the same organisms that cause acute otitis media. The patient usually has a great deal of ear pain.

E. When the eardrum perforates in acute otitis media, the ear canal generally becomes filled with purulent material and the TM is not visible. A more chronic perforation may appear as a dark hole in the TM. Pneumatic otoscopy will be abnormal with decreased or absent mobility.

192. **C. The most appropriate next step would involve obtaining a complete blood count, blood culture, and plain radiographs of the foot.**

A, B. Obtaining plain films before going straight to a bone scan or MRI is preferable. The suspected injury and inoculation occurred approximately 15 days ago. Radiographic findings of a fracture or osteomyelitis should be evident on plain films. If further suspicion is still high and plain radiographs are negative, an MRI or bone scan may then be indicated.

D. Simply applying a splint without first determining the extent of injury would be inappropriate.

E. Obtaining a blood culture before giving antibiotics is a good general principle.

193. **A. Osteomyelitis causes soft tissue swelling around the infected bone and subperiosteal fluid collections and reaction. This diagnosis also makes sense given the mechanism and timing of the injury and physical findings.**

B, C, D. Simple cellulitis, nail bed avulsion, or a right ankle sprain would not cause the bony changes seen on radiograph.

E. ALL should show a majority of lymphoblasts on the CBC and bony changes, if any, should be in the marrow. Occasionally leukemic infiltrates can present as destructive, sclerotic-type lesions seen on plain films.

194. **D. Todd paralysis is temporary hemiparesis following a focal seizure and may be confused with a stroke. The symptoms should completely resolve within 24 hours of the seizure. Observation is likely warranted in the hospital given the weakness and risk of falling at home.**

A, C. A cerebral angiogram and head MRI/MRA are used in the evaluation for stroke and are unnecessary in this case of Todd paralysis.

B. PICU admission is unnecessary if the patient is hemodynamically and neurologically stable; neurosurgical consultation is not indicated.

E. An LP and CSF analysis are not useful or necessary for cases of simple Todd paralysis.

195. **B. Plain films of the chest and neck are indicated to look for radio-opaque foreign bodies and to assess for the presence of any hyperinflation of the involved hemithorax.**

A. CT is too costly and may require sedation in a young child.

C, D. A modified barium swallow and upper GI series are used to assess for swallowing dysfunction and gastroesophageal reflux disease, not acute lung pathology.

E. Cervical spine x-rays are used to assess for bony injuries after trauma and are not indicated in this scenario.

196. E. This child's skull radiograph shows evidence of periventricular calcifications consistent with a possible diagnosis of congenital CMV. The child's developmental delay would also be consistent with the diagnosis. Congenital infection occurs in 1% of all newborns and may manifest itself in the immediate newborn period as sepsis with hepatosplenomegaly and growth retardation. Another 10% to 20% of infants may be asymptomatic at birth but progress to sequelae consisting of developmental delay, seizures, retinitis, and deafness. Although this child's work-up may be completed as an outpatient, the most appropriate choice listed is admission to the hospital.

A. Neurosurgical consultation is not indicated at this time.

B. A head CT would be useful in the continued management of this patient and probably would have been preferred over simple radiograph for better visualization of intracranial injury/hemorrhage following the fall; an MRI is not as useful in detecting calcifications.

C. There is no reason to suspect abuse in this patient; there is no delay in treatment nor is the injury inconsistent with the mother's story.

D. The child has developmental delay and periventricular calcifications that need further evaluation.

197. A. β-blockers may lead to unopposed α blockade that may cause hypertension and worsening ischemia in the setting of cocaine abuse. In general, β-blockers are not indicated in toxin-induced tachycardia.

B, C. Although amphetamine and PCP abuse is expected to result in agitation and tachycardia, myocardial ischemia secondary to either of these drugs has not been definitively shown to be worsened with a β-blocker. However, as in the explanation for A, β-blockers are generally not indicated in toxin-induced tachycardia.

D, E. Heroin and codeine would not be expected to result in significant tachycardia. The expected toxic side effects would be bradycardia and respiratory depression.

198. B. Head CT is the most appropriate choice of imaging study.

A. According to the AAP practice guideline, *The Management of Minor Closed Head Injury in Children*, a skull radiograph is not sensitive enough to pick up intracranial injuries. (Committee on Quality Improvement, American Academy of Pediatrics, Commission on Clinical Policies and Research, and American Academy of Family Physicians. The management of minor closed head injury in children. Pediatrics 1999;104:1407–1415.)

C. Head MRI has no added benefit than head CT and costs more.

D. Bone scans would not show intracranial injuries.

E. Head ultrasounds are not sensitive enough to detect skull fractures.

199. C. Given the baby's drowsiness and poor feeding, in-hospital observation is warranted.

A, B. Home observation would be risky, even with a responsible adult.

D. Neurosurgical consultation is warranted with depressed skull fractures, but not generally for a simple, nondepressed fracture without any intracranial injury.

E. Rapid sequence intubation and hyperventilation are used in the intensive care setting for severe head injuries showing signs of increased intracranial pressure.

200. D. Depressed skull fractures must be treated surgically if a neurologic deficit is present, if a compound wound is present, or if the depression is greater than 3 to 5 mm.

A, B. Given the new diagnosis, home observation would be wholly inappropriate, even with a responsible adult.

C. Simple admission to the hospital for observation without neurosurgical involvement is not appropriate.

E. Rapid sequence intubation and hyperventilation are used in the intensive care setting for severe head injuries showing signs of increased intracranial pressure. In this case, the child has no obvious intracranial injuries or clinical exam that would necessitate intubation at this time.

Section

4 Psychiatry

SETTING 1: COMMUNITY-BASED HEALTH CENTER

You work at a community-based health facility where patients seeking both routine and urgent care are encountered. Many patients are members of low-income groups; many are ethnic minorities. Several industrial parks and local businesses send their employees to the health center for treatment of on-the-job injuries and employee health screening. There is a facility that provides x-ray films, but CT and MRI scans must be arranged at other facilities. Laboratory services are available.

1. A 54-year-old divorced Hispanic man is being evaluated at the community clinic for daytime sleepiness. His 20-year-old daughter is concerned that her father might have narcolepsy. Symptoms of narcolepsy include which one of the following?

   A. Absence-like seizures
   B. Cataplexy
   C. Catalepsy
   D. Snoring
   E. Continued tiredness even after napping

2. A 33-year-old divorced mother of three being seen in the community clinic is diagnosed with the rapid-cycling variant of bipolar disorder. Her liver function and renal functions are normal. Which of the following options would be the best initial treatment?

   A. Sertraline
   B. Paroxetine
   C. Lithium
   D. Valproic acid
   E. Outpatient observation only

3. A 28-year-old waitress is brought to the clinic's urgent care service by her boyfriend after she ingested 10 diazepam tablets. Which of the following medications is the benzodiazepine antagonist used as a possible treatment for benzodiazepine toxicity?

   A. Narcan
   B. *N*-acetyl-cysteine
   C. Flumazenil
   D. Methadone
   E. Temezepam

4. A 32-year-old tile setter with a history of frequent insomnia presents to the clinic's urgent care service with the complaint of a persistent, painful penile erection for the last 5 hours. He is diagnosed with priapism and treated accordingly. Which of the following medications is most likely to have caused this side effect?

   A. Bupropion
   B. Trazodone
   C. Nortriptyline
   D. Haloperidol
   E. Divalproex sodium

The next two questions (items 5 and 6) correspond to the following vignette.

An 83-year-old retired janitor with a history of hypertension and mild heart failure has been referred by his family physician. Over the past 5 years, the patient has experienced a declining memory and the presumed diagnosis has been senile dementia, Alzheimer's type (SDAT). The patient's PCP initially prescribed donepezile, but was required to stop it due to side effects. A trial of rivastigmine was better tolerated and proved helpful until the past 3 months. Increased doses have not made a difference. Presently, the patient's Mini-Mental Status Examination (MMSE) score is 19.

5. In regard to the patient's pharmacologic treatment, which one of the following options is the best step to take next?

   A. Stop the rivastigmine and start galantamine
   B. Add galantamine to the rivastigmine
   C. Add risperidone to the rivastigmine
   D. Add memantine to the rivastigmine
   E. Stop the rivastigmine and start memantine

6. What is the primary mechanism of action of the new medication prescribed to this patient?

   A. Specifically inhibits acetylcholinesterase but not butyrlcholinesterase
   B. Reversibly inhibits actylcholinesterase and butyrlcholinesterase
   C. Acts as an N-methyl-D-aspartate (NMDA) receptor antagonist
   D. Has agonistic effects at the $5HT_3$ receptor
   E Inhibits acetylcholinesterase and modulates nicotine receptors

End of Set

7. A 16-year-old high school honors student is being seen in the community clinic's walk-in service for agitation, combativeness, and paranoid thoughts. His speech is rapid, and on exam he has tachycardia with pupillary dilation. His presentation is consistent with which type of substance intoxication?

   A. Heroin
   B. Methamphetamine
   C. Inhalants
   D. Marijuana
   E. Alcohol

8. A 13-year-old gang member with a history of truancy and petty theft is brought to the clinic's urgent care service by police after being arrested for vandalism. He is aggressive and disoriented. Physical exam reveals slurred speech, ataxia, poor motor coordination, and silver stains around his lips. What is the most likely diagnosis?

   A. Bipolar disorder
   B. Conduct disorder
   C. Cocaine intoxication
   D. Acute alcohol ingestion
   E. Inhalant intoxication

9. A 23-year-old law student has been under considerable stress lately while preparing for her final exams. She is brought into the community clinic by her parents because she "can't stop talking." According to her friends, the patient has been extremely hyperactive and productive for the last 5 days. Upon examination, she is smiling, friendly, and talking rapidly. She states that she has been "painting nonstop" without sleep for almost a week because God has chosen her to be the "world's greatest artist!" The triage nurse informs you that the patient's urine drug screen is negative. What is the most likely diagnosis for this patient?

   A. Schizophrenia
   B. Delusional disorder, grandiose type
   C. Bipolar disorder, manic phase
   D. Bipolar disorder, mixed phase
   E. Dissociative identity disorder

The next two questions (items 10 and 11) correspond to the following vignette.

A 33-year-old seriously mentally ill man presents to the clinic's urgent care clinic with urinary retention, tachycardia, mydriasis, and dry skin.

10. Which of the following psychiatric medications is most likely causing this syndrome?

    A. Fluoxetine
    B. Paroxetine
    C. Valproic acid
    D. Alprazolam
    E. Clozapine

11. Which of the following medications is used to reverse the syndrome?

    A. Lorazepam
    B. Physostigmine
    C. Atropine
    D. Thioridazine
    E. Valproic acid

End of Set

12. An 18-year-old high school senior and body builder is brought to the clinic by his family for "bizarre behavior." Upon examination, the patient is physically agitated and restless, stating that he needs to buy a gun because he believes people are following him. On physical exam, he is noted to be diaphoretic and tachycardic, and has dilated pupils. The patient is guarded and distrustful for most of the interview. His parents state that their son's behavior has become increasingly erratic and distrustful over the last few weeks since he began hanging out with a "bad group of kids." What would be the most appropriate next step in this case?

A. Admit the patient to the psychiatric unit for observation
B. Order a CT scan of the brain
C. Order a urine drug screen
D. Give the patient 2 mg of intramuscular lorazepam to calm him down
E. Discharge the patient home if he can contract for safety

13. A 45-year-old special-education teacher with a past history of episodic alcohol abuse complains of being depressed. During an interview, the patient states that for the last 2 years she has felt sad "throughout the day" almost every day, with feelings of low energy, low self-esteem, poor concentration, and decreased appetite. The patient denies any current or past thoughts of harming herself. What is the most likely diagnosis for this patient?

A. Major depressive disorder, single episode
B. Major depressive disorder, recurrent
C. Dysthymic disorder
D. Cyclothymic disorder
E. Bipolar disorder, depressed phase

14. A 45-year-old recently separated accountant with two children presents to the clinic with the complaint that he "can't stop worrying." He reports that his work has suffered over the last few weeks because he constantly has to check to make sure he has done everything "just right." The patient admits that his behavior may be excessive, but he is unable to control it. He also complains of several unpleasant, intrusive thoughts of an aggressive nature that he cannot make go away. The patient reports that he stopped driving a car about a week ago because he had to constantly stop and make sure he had not "run anybody over." What is this patient's most likely diagnosis?

A. Generalized anxiety disorder
B. Schizophrenia
C. Delusional disorder
D. Obsessive-compulsive disorder
E. Panic disorder

15. A mother brings her 8-year-old son to the clinic because she is concerned about his "bad behavior." For the last year, the child has had problems both at home and at school because of his failure to complete chores and homework. His teachers say that he is unable to sit still or pay attention in class, is easily distracted, and is unable to follow instructions. When asked, his mother responds that her son has never gotten into a fight at school, nor has he been truant or deceitful. The child fidgets in his chair throughout the entire interview. When asked what he thinks is wrong, he replies, "I just get bored real easy." What is this child's most likely diagnosis?

A. Conduct disorder
B. Attention deficit hyperactivity disorder
C. General anxiety disorder
D. Adjustment disorder with disturbance of conduct
E. Malingering

16. A 28-year-old single grocery store cashier followed at the community clinic for her bipolar disorder is concerned that she is pregnant and worried about possible birth defects caused by her medication. You tell her that the use of lithium during the first trimester of pregnancy is associated with which teratogenetic effect?

A. Neural tube defect
B. Ebstein's anomaly
C. Craniofacial defects
D. Fingernail hypoplasia
E. Acromegaly

17. The nurse practitioners at the clinic ask you, the only psychiatrist on staff, to give them an in-service presentation on prescribing psychotropic medications to older patients. Which of the following effects do you tell them is associated with pharmacokinetics and aging?

A. Volume of distribution increases for lipid-soluble drugs
B. Volume of distribution increases for water-soluble drugs
C. Decreased metabolism causes decreased half-lives
D. Unbound percentage of albumin-bound drugs decreases
E. Total body weight increases

The following three questions (items 18, 19, and 20) relate to the same clinical scenario.

A 34-year-old public defender presents to his primary care physician's office at the clinic with a complaint of increased stress. He appears to be having difficulty getting to work on time in the morning and reports that he is frequently showing up 2 to 3 hours late despite waking up earlier each day. Increasing time is spent on his morning routine, and he is beginning to recognize it as being excessive. Upon further questioning, the patient remarks that he has been spending most of his morning time trying to avoid contaminating germs. He is neatly dressed but his hands are raw with cracked, dry skin. Otherwise, the physical examination is normal.

18. What is the most likely diagnosis?

 A. Generalized anxiety disorder (GAD)
 B. Paranoid schizophrenia
 C. Delusional disorder
 D. Obsessive-compulsive disorder (OCD)
 E. Hypochondriasis

19. What medication and dosage range would be most effective for this patient over the long term?

 A. Fluoxetine, low dose
 B. Fluoxetine, high dose
 C. Olanzapine, low dose
 D. Olanzapine, high dose
 E. Venlafaxine, low dose

20. The appropriate medication and dosage has been prescribed. When would a clinical response to the medication be expected?

 A. Immediately
 B. Within 3 days
 C. Within 1 to 2 weeks
 D. Within 2 to 4 weeks
 E. Within 6 to 8 weeks

End of Set

The next two questions (items 21 and 22) correspond to the following vignette.

A 40-year-old home health provider is referred by her primary care physician at the clinic for psychiatric consultation. She complains of depression and insists that her husband has been cheating on her. She also thinks that several months ago the front door of her home was painted while she was away. There were paint drops on the floor, and she assumed that her husband's "mistress" had been in the home. The patient has had periods of depression in the past but no hospitalizations. When she is not depressed, she does not have suspicions of her husband's fidelity. She denies auditory or visual hallucinations. The patient works full-time in addition to managing her home. She denies use of illicit drugs or alcohol, and she cannot identify any recent acute stressors. Her MMSE score is 30/30.

21. What is this patient's most likely diagnosis?

 A. Major depressive disorder with psychotic features
 B. Schizophrenia, paranoid type
 C. Adjustment disorder not otherwise specified
 D. Schizoaffective disorder
 E. Alzheimer's disease

22. The patient has no active medical issues but does admit to a history of binging and purging. What is a possible effective treatment strategy for her current illness?

 A. Sertraline and diazepam
 B. Fluoxetine
 C. Valproic acid
 D. SSRI and an antipsychotic
 E. Bupropion

End of Set

23. A 28-year-old art student with a history of sickle cell anemia presents to her community clinic for the first time complaining of "spells" lasting several minutes and leaving her confused. Which of the following symptoms is most typically associated with partial complex seizures?

 A. Hemiballism
 B. Lacunar states
 C. Dissociative phenomena
 D. Scanning speech
 E. Akathisia

24. A young couple have brought their 6-year-old child to the clinic quite concerned that the youngster has been wetting the bed while asleep at night. Bed-wetting is most typically associated with which of the following characteristics?

 A. Girls
 B. Pathological at age 3
 C. Higher socioeconomic status
 D. Genetic factors
 E. Psychosis

25. After their 8-year-old son refused to go to school 6 days in a row, a perplexed and frustrated couple bring the boy to the community clinic. School phobia is most likely associated with which of the following conditions?

A. Fire setting
B. Depression
C. Enuresis
D. Learning disabilities
E. Separation anxiety

26. As the faculty psychiatrist at the community clinic, you have been asked to give the next group of second-year medical students a talk about relaxation therapy. Which one of the following is a specific type of relaxation therapy?

A. Confrontation
B. Interpretation
C. Guided imagery
D. Self-revelation
E. Silence

27. Your next talk to the medical students rotating through the clinic will cover the epidemiology of psychiatric illness. Which of the following psychiatric disorders has an equal lifetime prevalence for men and women?

A. Depression
B. Seasonal affective disorder (SAD)
C. Panic disorder
D. Alcohol dependence
E. Bipolar disorder

28. The community clinic's advisory board has decided to create a discrete Women's Health Program. The clinic pharmacists have requested that you speak with them about how this development might affect their stocking medications. Which of the following has an essentially equal effect between men and women in terms of the pharmacokinetics of medications?

A. Hepatic metabolism
B. Drug absorption
C. Protein binding
D. Middle age
E. Milligram per kilogram (mg per kg) dosing

29. The Women's Health Program has asked that you provide psychiatric consultations to its gynecologic clinic related to premenstrual dysphoric disorder (PMDD). Which of the following is considered the greatest risk factor for PMDD?

A. Clinical depression
B. Postpartum blues
C. OCD
D. Oral contraceptives
E. Panic disorder

30. A 26-year-old woman on parole for shoplifting is seeking pediatric care at the community clinic for her 18-month-old daughter. The mother is concerned about her daughter's development and is worried that her alcohol use during the pregnancy might have damaged the child. Which one of the following is a feature of fetal alcohol syndrome (FAS)?

A. Hypertonia
B. Attention deficit disorder
C. Normal intelligence
D. Growth acceleration
E. Incidence of 1 to 2 cases per 100,000 live births

31. The community clinic has partnered with a nearby halfway house for recovering alcoholics. You are asked to see a 28-year-old woman with a history of hepatitis to establish a primary caregiver relationship with her. Which of the following gender-specific differences related to alcoholism is true?

A. Alcohol dehydrogenase is more active in women
B. Men have relatively higher mortality rates from alcoholism
C. Alcoholism is far less common in young women than in young men
D. Risk factors for alcoholism in women include sexual abuse
E. Alcoholism tends to precede depression in women

32. A 46-year-old divorcee with a history of marijuana use has been prescribed lorazepam through the community clinic routinely for 3 years. Lately she has been asking for more than is called for by her usual dosage schedule. The treatment team members would like to help this patient develop alternative strategies for stress management and wean her off the medication, but are concerned about managing the side effects of withdrawal. Which one of the following statements is true regarding withdrawal from benzodiazepines?

A. Hyperpyrexia, seizures, psychosis, and death can occur in severe withdrawal.
B. Bradycardia, decreased blood pressure, and hypersomnia occur in moderate withdrawal.
C. Withdrawal symptoms typically occur several weeks after discontinuation.
D. Withdrawal typically continues for 3 to 4 days.
E. A reasonable dose reduction rate is 25% per week for patients treated with alprazolam for longer than 2 to 3 months, if discontinuation of the medication is desired.

33. The community mental health clinic has decided to establish a program for patients with panic disorder and agoraphobia that will include educational groups and medication management. Which of the following drugs has been shown to have the best efficacy and tolerance in treating panic disorder?

A. Selective serotonin reuptake inhibitors (SSRIs)
B. Tricyclic antidepressants (TCAs)
C. Beta blockers
D. Antiarrhythmics
E. Dilantin

34. Faced with increasing budget constraints, the community mental health center's residential alcohol detoxification program is shifting its resources and clientele to the outpatient clinic. To ensure that medications are stocked appropriately, you need to know that which one of the following is a medication used during the recovery phase to help maintain sobriety?

A. Disulfiram
B. Thiamine
C. Folate
D. Lorazepam
E. Chlordiazepoxide

35. During her first postpartum follow-up appointment at the clinic, a 26-year-old woman's husband relates that she has developed symptoms of agitation, labile mood, auditory hallucinations, and paranoia over the 2 weeks following delivery of a healthy baby boy. Which one of the following statements is most accurate regarding postpartum psychosis?

A. There is no increased incidence with a family history of psychiatric illness.
B. There is no increased incidence with a history of previous postpartum psychiatric illness.
C. The incidence is greatest with a history of postpartum blues.
D. Most episodes occur within 1 to 2 weeks after delivery.
E. Overall incidence is 5% to 10% of all deliveries.

36 A 63-year-old widow presents to her primary care physician at the clinic with symptoms of crying, insomnia, and trouble concentrating since the death of her husband 4 weeks earlier. Which one of the following characteristics is most reflective of a normal grieving process?

A. Survivor guilt
B. Usually resolves in 2 to 3 months
C. Is similar throughout all cultures
D. Decreased vulnerability to physical illness
E. Is not affected by preparation for the loss

37. The clinic's walk-in substance abuse treatment program continues to be busy. The most popular drugs in the neighborhood lately have been stimulants and alcohol. Which of the following symptoms is associated with amphetamine intoxication?

A. Depression
B. Indifference
C. Grandiosity
D. Lethargy
E. Constricted pupils

The next four questions (items 38–41) correspond to the following vignette.

A 33-year-old female presents to her primary care physician's office at the clinic with a chief complaint of a 13-year history of unstable mood and difficulty controlling her anger. Her medical history is unremarkable. Social history is significant for three divorces, a history of alcohol and methamphetamine abuse currently in remission, and difficulty holding the same job for longer than 3 months. Physical exam is significant for multiple lengthwise scars on her wrists. She is dressed in darkly colored, baggy clothing, makes minimal eye contact, and becomes tearful when talking about her symptoms.

38. Which of the following personality disorders does this patient most likely have?

A. Antisocial personality disorder
B. Obsessive-compulsive personality disorder
C. Borderline personality disorder
D. Schizoid personality disorder
E. Histrionic personality disorder

39. Considering the patient's presentation, what would be the most important area of inquiry at this appointment?

    A. Depressive symptoms
    B. Family history
    C. Alcohol use
    D. Developmental history
    E. Suicidal ideation

40. Over the course of the patient's treatment, which primitive defense mechanism would this patient most likely exhibit?

    A. Undoing
    B. Splitting
    C. Intellectualization
    D. Altruism
    E. Humor

41. Assuming her diagnosis is correct, what is the preferred method of treatment for this patient's personality disorder?

    A. Medication management only
    B. Long-term psychotherapy with medication management
    C. Short-term therapy only
    D. Electroconvulsive therapy (ECT) with medication management
    E. There is no appropriate treatment for this condition

End of Set

42. A 23-year-old African American graduate student with a history of sarcoidosis presents to the walk-in service of the clinic complaining of "nervousness" for 6 weeks. Upon further examination, she relates a 20-pound weight loss despite a good appetite. On physical examination, her pulse is 130 beats per minute. Which of the following psychiatric symptoms is typically seen in patients with severe hyperthyroidism?

    A. Indifference
    B. Slowed speech
    C. Psychosis
    D. Compulsions
    E. Neologisms

43. The community clinic has a large number of patients with dual diagnoses, often including both schizophrenia and substance abuse. Today, a 43-year-old homemaker is seen in consultation after being referred by her internist, who is concerned about the patient's alcohol consumption and wishes to start her on benzodiazepines to aid in withdrawal. The patient has been diagnosed with paranoid schizophrenia for 15 years. Which of the following statements is true regarding benzodiazepines?

    A. Benzodiazepines provide adequate coverage for heroin withdrawal.
    B. Benzodiazepines function via dopaminergic receptors to cause influx of chloride ions into a cell.
    C. Benzodiazepines are useful in the treatment of catatonia.
    D. Lorazepam and chlordiazepoxide are seldom used for alcohol withdrawal states.
    E. Benzodiazepines may decrease clozapine levels.

44. A 16-year-old high school honors student is reluctantly brought to the clinic by her parents, who are very concerned with their daughter's weight loss, moodiness, and fixation on getting good grades. Which of the following symptoms is typically seen in patients with anorexia nervosa?

    A. Disinterest in food
    B. Binge eating
    C. Premenstrual dysphoria
    D. Diminished appetite
    E. Hypersexuality

45. A 21-year-old liberal arts major was recently hospitalized for her first manic episode. Her hospitalization was complicated by a suicide attempt and a urinary tract infection. She has been referred to the clinic for follow-up care as she tries to finish her last semester of college. She has several poignant questions about potential problems if she continues taking the prescribed lithium. Which of the following is a side effect of lithium?

    A. Weight loss
    B. Leukopenia
    C. Acne
    D. Decreased urine output
    E. Hyperthyroidism

The next three questions (items 46, 47, and 48) correspond to the following vignette.

A 53-year-old woman presents to the clinic's walk-in service with tachycardia, tremor, anxiety, psychomotor agitation, and insomnia.

46. This constellation of symptoms is most closely associated with which of the following conditions?

    A. Alcohol intoxication
    B. Barbiturate intoxication
    C. Barbiturate withdrawal
    D. Benzodiazepine intoxication
    E. Chloral hydrate intoxication

47. What is the standard initial dose for a pentobarbital challenge test?

    A. Pentobarbital 50 mg
    B. Pentobarbital 200 mg
    C. Pentobarbital 400 mg
    D. Pentobarbital 800 mg
    E. Pentobarbital 1000 mg

48. What is the usual daily decrease of the barbiturate dosage to facilitate an uncomplicated withdrawal?

    A. 10% decrease per day
    B. 20% decrease per day
    C. 30% decrease per day
    D. 40% decrease per day
    E. 50% decrease per day

End of Set

The next two questions (items 49 and 50) correspond to the following vignette.

A 50-year-old mother of three supported by government disability presents to the clinic with a 15-year history of schizoaffective disorder, bipolar type. She has a history of syncope and has been recently diagnosed with long QT syndrome. She is currently taking the five medications listed in question 49, A–E.

49. Which medication should be stopped?

    A. Sodium divalproex
    B. Clonazepam
    C. Thioridazine
    D. Gabapentin
    E. Diphenhydramine

50. The inappropriate medication has been discontinued. Considering this fact, which medication would be best to start her on?

    A. Lithium carbonate
    B. Risperidone
    C. Benztropine
    D. Nortiptyline
    E. Carbamazepine

End of Set

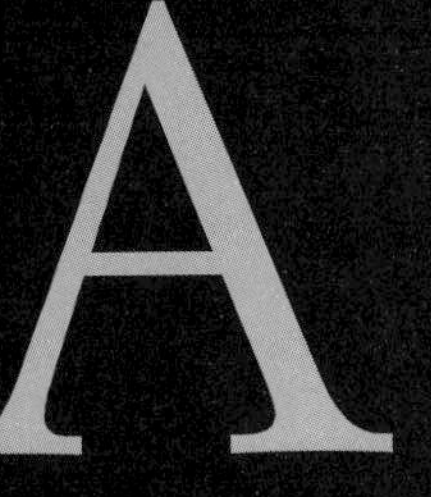

Answers and Explanations

1. B
2. D
3. C
4. B
5. D
6. C
7. B
8. E
9. C
10. E
11. B
12. C
13. C
14. D
15. B
16. B
17. A
18. D
19. B
20. E
21. A
22. D
23. C
24. D
25. E
26. C
27. E
28. E
29. A
30. B
31. D
32. A
33. A
34. A
35. D
36. A
37. C
38. C
39. E
40. B
41. B
42. C
43. C
44. B
45. C
46. C
47. B
48. A
49. C
50. B

1. **B. Cataplexy is an abrupt paralysis or paresis of skeletal muscles that typically follows awakening, highly emotional experiences (such as anger, surprise, or laughter), and physical exercise. It may be generalized, resulting in collapse, or it may remain isolated to a particular muscle group, resulting in transient loss of function. Duration typically lasts a few minutes, and the patient remains awake during the episode. Afterward, the patient usually regains full function without any impairment. Although cataplexy is the pathognomonic symptom of narcolepsy, it can be elicited in only approximately half of all narcoleptics. Other symptoms of narcolepsy include daytime sleepiness; hypnagogic (just before sleep), hypnopompic (prior to complete awakening) hallucinations; restless sleep; and sleep paralysis.**

   A. Seizures are not associated with narcolepsy.
   C. Cataplexy should not be confused with catalepsy, the waxy flexibility that may be seen in the catatonic type of schizophrenia.
   D. Snoring is often a sign of obstructive sleep apnea, rather than narcolepsy.
   E. Narcoleptics typically awaken from naps feeling refreshed.

2. **D. Valproic acid is a mood-stabilizing medication.**

   A. Antidepressants such as sertraline would not be used alone in bipolar disorder because they can precipitate a manic episode.
   B. Monotherapy with an antidepressant such as paroxetine is not appropriate treatment for bipolar disorder.
   C. Although lithium is one of the mainstays of treatment for bipolar disorder, valproic acid appears to be more effective at stabilizing rapid-cycling bipolar disorder. Rapid-cycling mood disorder is diagnosed when an individual with bipolar disorder experiences frequent cycles, defined as four or more mood disturbances per year.
   E. It is important to treat these individuals with medication and hospitalization as needed, as the suicide rate in rapid cyclers may be higher than that in non-rapid cyclers.

3. **C. Flumazenil is a benzodiazepine antagonist approved for the treatment of benzodiazepine overdose and the reversal of benzodiazepine oversedation. This drug binds competitively and reversibly to the GABA-benzodiazepine receptor complex and inhibits the effects of benzodiazepines. Flumazenil may not fully reverse benzodiazepines' inhibitory effects on the hypoxic respiratory drive. Continued monitoring of respiration is necessary. Flumazenil also has a short duration of action and may need to be repeatedly administered to antagonize long-acting benzodiazepines. The drug may induce seizures in patients who are prone to seizures. Caution must also be used due to the risk of causing a seizure from benzodiazepine withdrawal in patients who take benzodiazepines chronically.**

   A. Narcan is given for opioid toxicity.
   B. *N*-acetyl-cysteine is given for acetaminophen overdose.
   D. Methadone is given for long-term maintenance treatment of heroin dependence.
   E. Temezepam is a benzodiazepine used primarily as a hypnotic agent.

4. **B. A number of cases of priapism have been reported in patients taking the antidepressant trazodone.**

   A. Bupropion, an antidepressant, is not associated with priapism.
   C. Nortriptyline, a tricyclic antidepressant, is not associated with priapism.
   D. Haloperidol, a typical antipsychotic, is not associated with priapism.
   E. Divalproex sodium, or valproic acid, is an anticonvulsant with mood-stabilizing properties. It is not associated with priapism.

5. **D. Adding memantine to the rivastigmine regimen is the best next step because the two drugs have different mechanisms of action and are usually tolerated together. Memantine is helpful for patients with moderate to severe SDAT, which is indicated by this patient's MMSE score of 19 out of a possible 30.**

   A, B. Galantamine would not likely be more helpful in combination with rivastigmine or alone for a patient with moderately severe SDAT.
   C. Risperidone is an antipsychotic. There is no specific indication for prescribing such a medication to the patient described.
   E. Because rivastigmine and memantine have different mechanisms of action, an additive effect should be pursued rather than administration of memantine alone.

6. **C. Memantine's primary mechanism of action is as a moderate-affinity NMDA receptor antagonist.**
   - A. Donepezil specifically inhibits acetylcholinesterase.
   - B. Rivastigmine inhibits acetylcholinesterase and butyrlcholinesterase.
   - D. Memantine has antagonistic effects at the $5HT_3$ receptor.
   - E. Galantamine inhibits acetylcholinesterase and modulates nicotine receptors.

7. **B. Methamphetamine is a stimulant. As such, it commonly produces agitation, paranoia, rapid speech, tachycardia, diaphoresis, muscle twitching, and dilated pupils.**
   - A. Heroin intoxication should not cause agitation or combativeness. Intoxication will cause pupillary constriction and sedation. While withdrawal from heroin might have a presentation similar to that seen in this patient, paranoia is not commonly associated with heroin withdrawal or intoxication.
   - C. Inhalants such as glue or paint thinner may produce aggression, impulsivity, and occasionally psychosis, but usually will not cause pupillary dilation.
   - D. Marijuana intoxication occasionally will cause paranoia and anxiety, but would not account for pupillary dilation or combativeness.
   - E. Patients intoxicated with alcohol can display rapid shifts from agitation to mood lability, but they are unlikely to have dilated pupils or paranoid thoughts.

8. **E. Aromatic hydrocarbons found in products such as gasoline, glue, and paint can be abused through inhalation. In addition to the symptoms observed in this patient, signs of intoxication can include grandiosity, euphoria, and visual disturbances. The silver stains are likely from inhaling spray paint.**
   - A. Bipolar disorder would not account for the physical exam findings in this patient.
   - B. Conduct disorder would not account for the physical findings in this patient.
   - C. Cocaine intoxication might cause impulsivity and aggression, but would not cause slurred speech or ataxia.
   - D. Alcohol can cause mood lability, irritability, slurred speech, ataxia, and motor incoordination, but would not account for the silver stains around this patient's mouth.

9. **C. This patient is exhibiting symptoms of an acute manic episode of a bipolar disorder: acute hyperactivity, pressured speech, psychomotor agitation with goal-oriented activity, decreased need for sleep, and mood elevation to the point of developing a delusion of grandeur. Her negative drug screen helps eliminate the possibility of substance-induced mania or psychotic behavior.**
   - A. The patient does not exhibit enough symptoms consistent with a diagnosis of schizophrenia (e.g., auditory or visual hallucinations, ideas of reference, thought blocking, thought insertion, avolition, catatonia).
   - B. Although the patient does indeed have a grandiose delusion, the diagnosis of delusional disorder would not explain her other symptoms such as pressured speech and increased psychomotor activity.
   - D. The patient is neither complaining nor exhibiting any symptoms of depression; therefore this is likely not a mixed phase of mania.
   - E. No evidence indicates that this patient's symptoms are due to dissociative states or multiple personalities.

10. **E. Clozapine is an antipsychotic medication with potent anticholinergic effects. It is typically reserved for use in seriously mentally ill patients with chronic persistent symptoms.**
    - A. Fluoxetine has essentially no anticholinergic properties.
    - B. Paroxetine has minimal anticholinergic properties.
    - C. Valproic acid has no anticholinergic properties.
    - D. Alprazolam has no anticholinergic properties.

11. **B. Physostigmine reverses the syndrome by inhibiting acetylcholinesterase, the enzyme that breaks down acetylcholine.**
    - A. Lorazepam and other benzodiazepines may calm the agitated patient but will not reverse the condition.
    - C. Atropine, as an anticholinergic agent, would worsen the condition.
    - D. Thioridazine and other typical antipsychotics have anticholinergic effects.
    - E. Valproic acid is an anticonvulsant with mood-stabilizing properties but would not be helpful in this patient.

12. **C. It would be extremely helpful at this time to determine what is causing the patient's symptoms, whether a primary psychiatric condition (schizophrenia) or an organic condition (substance-induced psychosis). The patient's physical exam findings and his parents' information suggest that this is likely a stimulant-induced psychotic episode.**

    A. Admitting the patient is not the best option at this time. He currently needs a more thorough medical evaluation (i.e., urine drug screen, possible head CT). If this is indeed a substance-induced psychosis, his symptoms may diminish after a period of detoxification.
    B. Ordering a CT scan is not the most appropriate step at this time. It would be more prudent to await the results of the urine drug screen before ordering additional tests. If the drug screen is negative, then a CT of the brain may be warranted, especially if the patient has a history of recent head trauma.
    D. The patient is restless and agitated but is not currently threatening or combative. Lorazepam can be given at any time if needed.
    E. It would be inappropriate to discharge this patient until a diagnosis has been made and a thorough risk assessment of his suicidal and homicidal status has been performed. Currently, this patient is paranoid and is talking about buying a gun. His symptoms may improve over a short time course if this is a substance-induced disorder, but discharge at this time is premature. It is likely that he will require admission.

13. **C. The chronology and intensity of the patient's symptoms are consistent with the diagnostic criteria for dysthymic disorder (feeling depressed most of the day, more days than not, for a period of at least 2 years).**

    A, B. Although the symptoms of depressed mood, low energy, low self-esteem, poor appetite, and decreased sleep are found in both major depressive disorder and dysthymic disorder, the consistency and length of this patient's symptoms are more diagnostic of dysthymic disorder than a major depressive disorder, single or recurrent. No evidence suggests a recurrent or episodic condition.
    D. The patient has not exhibited any current or past symptoms of hypomania, which would be required for a diagnosis of cyclothymic disorder.
    E. A history of mania would be required to make a diagnosis of bipolar disorder.

14. **D. Obsessive-compulsive disorder is the correct answer. The patient has both obsessions and compulsions that he recognizes are excessive and are causing him marked distress.**

    A. The patient is not complaining of constant anxiety over numerous life events, which would be necessary to make a diagnosis of GAD.
    B. This patient does not have hallucinations, delusions, disorganized speech, catatonic behavior, or any of the other major symptoms typical of schizophrenia.
    C. This patient is not really delusional, seemingly appreciating an irrationality to his excessive worrying and unusual behavior.
    E. This patient does not describe a history of panic attacks, which would be required to make a diagnosis of panic disorder.

15. **B. This child has attention deficit hyperactivity disorder (ADHD). He has had problems for more than 6 months in two different settings with regard to paying attention, sitting still, being easily distracted, following instructions, and demonstrating hyperactivity. These symptoms are severe enough to have caused him impaired functioning both at home and in school.**

    A The patient does not have a history of truancy from school, fighting, or deceitfulness, so a diagnosis of conduct disorder is inappropriate.
    C. The patient complains of boredom and his symptoms are marked by distractibility and hyperactivity, not anxiety.
    D. No identifiable stressor has occurred within the last 3 months that would account for the child's behavior. Also, the patient's symptoms have been present for longer than 1 year.
    E. There are no external incentives or secondary gains to explain this child's behavior.

16. **B. Ebstein's anomaly is a serious cardiac defect involving the tricuspid valve. First-trimester use of lithium increases the risk to 1/1000 from 1/20,000 in the general population.**

A. Neural tube defects are associated with valproic acid and carbamazepine exposure during pregnancy.
C. Craniofacial defects are associated with valproic acid and carbamazepine exposure during pregnancy.
D. Fingernail hypoplasia is associated with valproic acid and carbamazepine exposure during pregnancy.
E. Acromegaly is a condition associated with pituitary tumors and excessive levels of growth hormone.

17. **A. There is an increase in total body fat with aging, especially in women.**

B. The volume of distribution for water-soluble drugs decreases with aging.
C. The decreases in renal blood flow and hepatic enzyme activity associated with aging result in decreased metabolism rates and, therefore, longer half-lives for medications.
D. Albumin decreases with aging, so the unbound percentage increases.
E. Typically the elderly experience a decrease in total body weight, which affects milligram per kilogram prescribing.

18. **D. OCD is characterized by obsessions, compulsions, or both. This patient engages in compulsive hand washing and cleaning rituals to avoid contamination. The diagnosis of OCD also requires that he recognize the symptoms as being excessive, and that they produce noticeable interference with his usual functioning.**

A. GAD might be a consideration, but the presence of specific obsessions and compulsions is better explained by OCD.
B. This patient does not exhibit any symptoms of psychosis, which makes a diagnosis of schizophrenia unlikely.
C. Delusional disorder is unlikely because the patient is not psychotic.
E. Patients with hypochondriasis usually do not try to resist their thoughts of contamination, nor do they think them unreasonable.

19. **B. The most effective medications for OCD are SSRIs such as fluoxetine, and higher doses are typically required.**

A. The lower dose of fluoxetine might be started, but the dosage goal would be approximately 60 to 80 mg per day.
C, D. There is no evidence supporting the use of the atypical antipsychotic olanzapine at any dose for OCD.
E. A mixed serotonin/norepinephrine reuptake inhibitor such as venlafaxine might be efficacious for OCD (although it is not approved for this use), but the goal would likely be a higher dose to achieve a sufficient serotonin effect.

20. **E. The bulk of scientific evidence on treating OCD with SSRIs supports the notion that a delayed response is the rule. A response would be expected in 6 to 8 weeks at the earliest, but it might take several months to achieve clinical improvement. When used to treat depression, SSRIs typically produce improvements in 3 to 5 weeks. An earlier response might be seen in either illness, but it is no more likely than with placebo.**

A, B, C, D. An expected time frame for a medication response for OCD is not less than 6 to 8 weeks.

21. **A. The patient most likely has a major depressive disorder with psychosis.**

B. The significant mood component and the fact that she does not exhibit a typical picture of schizophrenia (e.g., early age of onset and chronic deteriorating clinical course) make schizophrenia an unlikely diagnosis in this patient.
C. There is no identifiable acute stressor that would lead to an adjustment disorder.
D. To make a diagnosis of schizoaffective disorder, there would have to be a significant period during which psychotic symptoms existed in the absence of mood symptoms.
E. The patient's age makes dementia unlikely. Furthermore, she shows no evidence of cognitive decline.

22. **D. The patient requires an antidepressant, most likely an SSRI, for her mood disorder, as well as an antipsychotic for her delusional perceptions.**

A. Sertraline and the anxiolytic diazepam would not likely sufficiently treat her psychosis.
B. Fluoxetine alone would not likely treat her psychosis adequately.
C. Valproic acid is a mood stabilizer that is effective in treating bipolar disorder and may also be effective in treating schizoaffective disorder. It would not be effective in treating this patient's depression or depression-related psychosis.
E. The patient should not be prescribed bupropion due to her history of an eating disorder and the increased risk of seizures in such individuals who take bupropion.

23. **C. Partial complex seizures may cause prolonged dissociative states resembling catatonia.**

A. Hemiballism involves unilateral involuntary movement typical of chorea.
B. Lacunar states are the pathological findings in the brain associated with atherosclerosis.
D. Scanning speech is a nonspecific abnormality associated with conditions such as multiple sclerosis.
E. Akathisia is a subjective experience of jitteriness and difficulty remaining still that is typically seen as a side effect of antipsychotic medications.

24. **D. Bed-wetting runs in families, typically in fathers and sons.**

A. Bed-wetting, or enuresis, is much more common in boys.
B. Bed-wetting is pathological if it occurs repeatedly in someone at least 5 years old and is not caused by a physical condition or medication.
C. For reasons that remain unclear, but perhaps are related to stress, bed-wetting is more common in institutionalized children and children of lower socioeconomic status.
E. Psychosis itself is not associated with bed-wetting. Psychological stresses such as birth of a sibling, moving, and parents divorcing may exacerbate bed-wetting.

25. **E. Children with separation anxiety fear that something bad will happen to them or their caretakers while they are at school.**

A. Fire setting, or pyromania, can be seen in school-aged children but is not associated with school phobia.
B. Depression reduces energy and motivation and may dampen a desire to attend school, but it is not the condition most commonly associated with school phobia.
C. Enuresis may cause embarrassment in school so that children want to stay away, but it is not the condition most commonly associated with school phobia.
D. Learning disabilities often bring ridicule from other students and prompt children to want to stay away from school, but they are less common than separation anxiety as an associated condition.

26. **C. Guided imagery is a specific relaxation-inducing technique. The patient is coached to visually imagine a relaxing, serene setting as a strategy to reduce stress and anxiety.**

A. Confrontation is an aspect of psychotherapy that helps in the interview process by breaking through the defense of denial.
B. Interpretation is an aspect of psychotherapy that helps clarify conflicts.
D. Self-revelation is an aspect of psychotherapy that may help unmask a patient's hidden concerns.
E. Silence fosters contemplation but also tends to create anxiety for the patient.

27. **E. Bipolar disorder is essentially equally prevalent in men (7%) and women (9%). This holds true for bipolar types I and II.**

A. The lifetime prevalence of depression in men and women is 12% versus 20%, respectively.
B. The lifetime prevalence of SAD in men and women is 1% versus 6%, respectively.
C. The lifetime prevalence of panic disorder in men and women is 2% versus 5%, respectively.
D. The lifetime prevalence of alcohol dependence in men and women is 20% versus 6%, respectively.

28. **E. Despite the various possible pharmacokinetic gender-related differences between men and women, a standardized mg per kg dosing approach serves either sex well.**

A. Estrogen has an inhibitory effect on some hepatic enzymes.
B. Progesterone can delay gastric emptying and subsequently absorption.

C. Both estrogen and progesterone are protein bound and may compete with medications for binding sites.
D. Case reports suggest that hormonal fluctuations associated with menopause affect medication levels as well.

29. **A. Clinical depression is highly correlated with PMDD. Although no single cause of PMDD has been established, fluctuations of normal levels of reproductive hormones appear to promote psychological symptoms in susceptible women. Specific symptoms seen in PMDD include depression, anxiety, emotional lability, trouble concentrating, and lethargy.**

B. Postpartum blues are not associated with PMDD.
C. OCD has no direct causative relationship to PMDD.
D. Oral contraceptives, especially when continued through the menstrual cycle, may alleviate PMDD.
E. Panic disorder itself does not cause PMDD, but panic episodes may be more frequent premenstrually.

30. **B. Attention deficit disorder, with or without hyperactivity, is often manifested in childhood as a feature of FAS.**

A. Hypotonia is often present at birth in babies with FAS.
C. Cognitive deficits, including intellectual deficiencies and other learning disabilities, are associated with FAS.
D. FAS is associated with growth retardation.
E. FAS is a relatively common occurrence; even occasional consumption of alcohol may result in fetal defects. The incidence is 1 to 2 cases per 1000 live births.

31. **D. Sexual abuse is a risk factor for alcoholism.**

A. Alcohol dehydrogenase, the enzyme that breaks down alcohol, is less active in women and likely causes women to more readily become intoxicated.
B. Alcohol-related medical complications occur more quickly in women.
C. Although the overall prevalence of alcoholism among women is much less than among men, this discrepancy is becoming less pronounced in the younger age groups.
E. Mood disorders frequently precede alcoholism in women.

32. **A. Hyperpyrexia, seizures, psychosis, and even death can be seen in benzodiazepine withdrawal.**

B. Tachycardia, increased blood pressure, and insomnia occur in moderate withdrawal from benzodiazepines.
C. Withdrawal symptoms can occur as soon as the day after discontinuation of benzodiazepines.
D. Withdrawal symptoms can continue for weeks to months after stopping a benzodiazepine.
E. For patients treated with benzodiazepines for longer than 2 to 3 months, a typical dose reduction rate would be 5% to 10% per week. The faster the benzodiazepine's onset of action, the slower the taper should be.

33. **A. SSRIs are the most efficacious and well-tolerated agents for the long-term treatment of panic disorder.**

B. TCAs are useful in the long-term treatment of panic disorder but are not as well tolerated as SSRIs.
C. Beta blockers have shown limited efficacy in the acute treatment of panic disorder but are not as efficacious as SSRIs for long-term treatment.
D. Antiarrhythmics are not used to treat panic disorder.
E. Although some anticonvulsants have shown efficacy in the treatment of panic disorder, dilantin is not one of them.

34. **A. Disulfiram promotes sobriety by accumulating acetaldehyde and producing very unpleasant physical effects when combined with alcohol.**

B. Thiamine deficiency can occur in chronic alcohol abuse, resulting in Wernicke's encephalopathy. Thiamine is prescribed during the withdrawal phase of treatment.
C. Folate deficiency is common in chronic alcohol abuse, resulting in neurologic symptoms if left untreated. Folate does not help with sobriety.
D. Lorazepam is a short-acting benzodiazepine used to minimize withdrawal symptoms and seizures.
E. Chlordiazepoxide is a longer-acting benzodiazepine used to minimize withdrawal symptoms and seizures.

35. D. Most postpartum psychotic episodes occur relatively soon after delivery.

A. Inquiring about a family history of psychiatric illness with special consideration being paid to incidence of bipolar disorder and postpartum psychosis may identify a higher risk.
B. A patient with a previous history of postpartum psychiatric illness should be educated and monitored for a recurrence.
C. All affective disorders, but bipolar disorder in particular, may be manifested for the first time postpartum.
E. Postpartum psychosis is a relatively rare disorder and occurs after 0.1% to 0.2% of all pregnancies.

36. A. Blaming oneself for how the deceased was treated is common in normal grieving.

B. Normal grieving is self-limited, but commonly persists for 6 to 12 months.
C. Grieving is manifested differently from culture to culture, so the clinician must be mindful of what is appropriate for the patient.
D. The increased vulnerability to physical illness should be monitored and may allow for follow-up visits for supportive therapy.
E. The course of grieving is affected by the abruptness of the loss.

37. C. Grandiosity is a behavioral effect associated with amphetamine intoxication.

A. Depression, fatigue, and hypersomnia are characteristic of amphetamine withdrawal, rather than intoxication.
B. Hypervigilance, rather than indifference, is a behavioral effect associated with amphetamine intoxication.
D. Agitation, rather than lethargy, is a behavioral effect associated with amphetamine intoxication.
E. Dilated pupils, tachycardia, and hypertension are physical effects caused by amphetamines.

38. C. The diagnostic traits of borderline personality disorder seen in this patient include a pattern of unstable relationships, impulsivity (substance abuse), chronic self-destructive behavior, affective instability, and intense anger.

A. The patient does not show the pattern of disregard for the law and lack of remorse seen in antisocial personality disorder.
B. There is no evidence of perfectionism, preoccupation with rules, or moral inflexibility as would be seen in obsessive-compulsive personality disorder.
D. Schizoid personality disorder is unlikely because the patient does not report engagement in solitary activities, emotional detachment, or flattened affect. On the contrary, she reports excessive mood reactivity, and her desire to have close relationships is evidenced by her multiple divorces.
E. If this patient had histrionic personality disorder, she would likely be using her appearance to draw attention to herself or to appear seductive.

39. E. Suicidal ideation. Long-term data on borderline personality disorder indicate a lifetime suicide rate exceeding 5%. The scars on this patient's wrists indicate prior self-mutilation or suicide attempts.

A, B, C, D. While it would be helpful to inquire about depressive symptoms, family history, current alcohol use, and developmental history, the single most important thing to assess in this patient would be dangerousness to herself or to others.

40. B. Examples of primitive defenses include splitting, denial, projection, dissociation, and acting out. The personality disorders—particularly borderline personality disorder—are characterized by use of these more primitive defense mechanisms. Splitting can be described as black-and-white thinking, such as treating someone as if that person were all evil or all good. This consideration is relevant here because this patient may eventually come to view her physician, nurse, or other office staff as all good or all evil.

A. Undoing is considered a "neurotic defense" and might be seen in patients with an anxiety disorder.
C. Intellectualization is another "neurotic defense."
D. Altruism is a mature defense mechanism commonly observed in a psychologically healthy person.
E. Humor is a mature defense mechanism.

41. B. The standard of care for a patient with borderline personality disorder is long-term psychotherapy with adjunctive use of medications for treatment of co-morbid Axis I disorders.

A. Medication management alone may be helpful to some degree, but more significant gains would be expected with concomitant psychotherapy.
C. Personality disorders may initially respond to short-term therapy, but longstanding dysfunctional patterns are likely to return after therapy ends.
D. While ECT may treat an underlying severe mood or persistent psychotic disorder, it is generally not indicated for the treatment of personality disorders.
E. Although often challenging, psychotherapy and prudent use of medications as the borderline patient matures can produce rewarding results.

42. C. More severe hyperthyroidism can result in psychotic symptoms of hallucinations and delusions.

A. Irritability, rather than passivity or indifference, is one of the many mood and personality changes experienced with hyperthyroidism.
B. Hyperthyroidism may be manifested as an energy disorder with rapid speech, racing thoughts, and increased activity.
D. Compulsions are not psychiatric symptoms typically associated with hyperthyroidism, although generalized anxiety is commonly experienced.
E. Neologisms involve the creation of novel words, a behavior sometimes manifested by patients with schizophrenia.

43. C. Benzodiazepines are often used to treat catatonia.

A. Benzodiazepines do not provide adequate coverage for opioid withdrawal. Agents like methadone are more appropriate.
B. Benzodiazepine receptors are closely linked with the GABA receptor. Activity at the benzodiazepine receptor potentiates the action of GABA. This major inhibitory neurotransmitter causes chloride channels to open, allowing influx of chloride into the cell to occur.
D. For a patient in alcohol withdrawal, lorazepam is sometimes preferred to chlordiazepoxide if the patient has liver disease or is elderly, due to the former agent's brief half-life. Both drugs are efficacious, however.
E. Benzodiazepines must be used with caution in patients on clozapine, as they may cause clozapine levels to rise.

44. B. Individuals with anorexia typically eat secretively and often binge.

A. Patients with anorexia nervosa have a preoccupation with food.
C. Starvation commonly produces menstrual irregularities leading to amenorrhea.
D. Despite the use of the term "anorexia," diminished appetite is not the rule in these patients.
E. Loss of sexual interest, decreased alertness, and social withdrawal may occur in conjunction with the starvation of anorexia nervosa.

45. C. Dermatologic side effects from lithium include acne and hair loss.

A. Presumably related to carbohydrate craving and lowered metabolism, lithium frequently causes weight gain.
B. Lithium commonly produces leukocytosis rather than leukopenia.
D. Increased thirst and decreased ability to concentrate follow from lithium-related polyuria.
E. Hypothyroidism is a potential side effect of lithium and is more often seen in women taking lithium than in men.

46. C. Barbiturate and similarly acting sedative, hypnotic, anxiolytic, and alcohol withdrawal syndromes present with similar symptoms. Nausea, vomiting, hallucinations, illusions, and seizures may also develop.

A, B, D, E. Intoxication with alcohol, barbiturates, benzodiazepines, and sedative-hypnotics such as chloral hydrate would result in slurred speech, incoordination, nystagmus, and stupor.

47. B. Pentobarbital 200 mg is given orally, and the patient is observed for intoxication after 1 hour. If not intoxicated, the patient is given another 100 mg every 2 hours, up to a maximum of 500 mg over 6 hours.

A, C, D, E. These are incorrect dosages.

48. **A. A decrease of approximately 10% per day typically allows for an uncomplicated withdrawal, but the rate must be adjusted if the patient shows signs of intoxication or withdrawal.**

    B, C, D, E. Decreasing barbiturate doses more than 10% per day could result in a medically dangerous withdrawal state characterized by seizures, psychosis, and even death.

49. **C. Thioridazine is an antipsychotic that has been found to cause significant increases in the corrected QT interval. It is absolutely contraindicated in patients with long QT syndrome.**

    A. Sodium divalproex is not known to cause increases in the QTc.
    B. Clonazepam is not known to cause increases in the QTc.
    D. Gabapentin is not known to cause increases in the QTc.
    E. Diphenhydramine is not known to cause increases in the QTc.

50. **B. As an antipsychotic medication, risperidone would be an appropriate replacement for thioridazine. It is not known to cause significant alterations in EKG parameters.**

    A. Lithium carbonate should not be used in a patient with arrhythmias, and it would not be an effective replacement for an antipsychotic.
    C. Benztropine is an anticholinergic medication commonly used to treat extrapyramidal side effects of antipsychotics. It would not be an effective replacement for an antipsychotic.
    D. Nortriptyline is a tricyclic antidepressant that may cause tachycardia; it would be contraindicated in a patient with bipolar disorder.
    E. Carbamazepine is an anticonvulsant that may be used adjunctively as a mood stabilizer. It would not be an effective replacement for an antipsychotic.

SETTING 2: OFFICE

Your office is in a primary care generalist group practice located in a physician office suite adjoining a suburban community hospital. Patients are usually seen by appointment. Most of the patients you see are from your own practice and are appearing for regular scheduled return visits, with some new patients as well. As in most group practices, you will often encounter a patient whose primary care is managed by one of your associates; reference may be made to the patient's medical records. You may do some telephone management, and you may have to respond to questions about articles in magazines and on television that will require interpretation. Complete laboratory and radiology services are available.

The next three questions (items 51, 52, and 53) correspond to the following vignette.

An 83-year-old widow is accompanied to your office by her daughter, with whom she lives. On examination, the patient is pleasant and attentive, and she denies any specific psychiatric symptoms except for some trouble with her memory. Her Mini-Mental State Examination (MMSE) score is 23.

51. Which of the following medications would be the most appropriate choice for this patient?

    A. Lorazepam
    B. Risperidone
    C. Buspirone
    D. Donepezil
    E. Sertraline

52. Over the course of 2 months, the patient's MMSE score improves to 26, then it plateaus. You increase the donepezil dose, but she soon complains that the side effects are intolerable. What should be your next step?

    A. Reduce the donepezil to the earlier dose
    B. Switch to rivastagmine
    C. Add risperidone
    D. Add sertraline
    E. Inform the patient and her daughter that nothing more can be done

53. Over the course of time, your patient's Alzheimer's disease (AD) progresses such that she becomes increasingly paranoid and is experiencing auditory hallucinations. Which of the following statements about antipsychotic medication usage by elderly patients such as this woman is true?

    A. Elderly patients are at increased risk for developing extrapyramidal symptoms (EPS).
    B. Olanzepine does not cause diabetes in the elderly.
    C. Quetiapine does not cause triglyceride elevations in the elderly.
    D. Weight gain is not seen when using atypical antipsychotics in the elderly.
    E. Elderly patients are at less risk for developing anticholinergic side effects.

End of Set

54. A patient referred to your outpatient office has been self-medicating with herbs and vitamins and asks for your advice on any possible drug interactions. Of the following, which complementary or alternative medicine is most appropriate for a patient with rapid-cycling bipolar disorder?

    A. Kava
    B. Fish oils containing omega 3 fatty acids
    C. Valerian
    D. St. John's wort
    E. Gingko biloba

55. A 68-year-old retired teacher with hypertension is followed in your office. He is otherwise in good health but expresses concern about his sexual performance. You counsel him that which of the following statements is most correct regarding sexuality and normal aging?

    A. Libido generally decreases with age for men and women.
    B. In men, decreased levels of testosterone and follicle-stimulating hormone (FSH) affect libido.
    C. In women, decreased estrogen levels and increased testosterone levels reduce libido.
    D. Few people older than 65 years have a chronic disease that may affect sexual function.
    E. Most men in their seventies report erectile dysfunction.

The next two questions (items 56 and 57) correspond to the following vignette.

A 16-year-old high school student is referred to your outpatient practice. When you ask her to describe her problems, she relates that she breaks into a cold sweat at supermarket checkout counters and most any other casual social activity. You diagnose her with social anxiety disorder (SAD).

56. Which of the following statements regarding SAD is true?

    A. SAD often begins early in life.
    B. Males are affected more often than females.
    C. SAD is an uncommon disorder.
    D. The majority of individuals with SAD suffer from the nongeneralized type.
    E. Recovery without treatment is common.

57. Which of the following pharmacologic treatments may be helpful for this patient's SAD?

    A. Sertraline
    B. Amitriptyline
    C. Imipramine
    D. Nortriptyline
    E. Desipramine

End of Set

58. A 73-year-old retired printer with a history of depression, a movement disorder, and progressive dementia is being followed in your outpatient office practice. Which of the following statements is most true about dementia?

    A. Dementia with Lewy bodies (DLB) accounts for one-fifth of all dementias.
    B. Few patients with DLB experience extrapyramidal symptoms.
    C. Neuroimaging is not helpful to differentiate the various forms of dementia.
    D. Few patients with Parkinson's disease (PD) experience cognitive impairment.
    E. The prevalence of Alzheimer's disease decreases after age 80.

59. A well-groomed, attractive, 38-year-old Hispanic female comes to your outpatient office. She is complaining of stress related to the break-up of her 15-year relationship with the father of her two children. Three months ago her boyfriend went to Mexico, and when he returned he announced that he had married a woman whom he had met just 9 days earlier. Since receiving this news, the patient has experienced initial insomnia, poor energy, and depressed mood for most of the day nearly every day. She has been unable to concentrate in the classes she is taking to become a beautician. However, she continues to enjoy spending time with her two children. The patient denies feelings of guilt, any thoughts of death, or wanting to hurt herself or others. She is anxious about how she will support herself and her children. She has no previous psychiatric history. The patient visits her primary care physician for annual check-ups and has no history of physical illness. She remains composed until the end of the interview, when she becomes tearful and asks, "Doctor, do you think he ever loved me?" Which of the following is her most likely diagnosis?

    A. Major depressive disorder, first episode
    B. Dysthymia
    C. Adjustment disorder, chronic type, with depressed mood
    D. Adjustment disorder, acute type, with mixed anxiety and depressed mood
    E. Post-traumatic stress disorder

The next two questions (items 60 and 61) correspond to the following vignette.

A 33-year-old woman presents to your office with signs and symptoms of a major depressive episode, recurrent, and without psychotic features. You plan to prescribe an antidepressant medication.

60. Which of the labeled dose-response curves in Figure 4-60 demonstrates a "therapeutic window" effect for antidepressant medication?

    A. Curve A
    B. Curve B
    C. Curve C
    D. Curve D

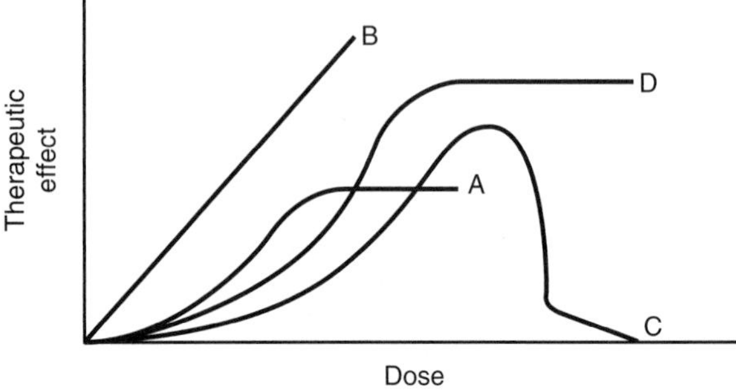

Figure 4-60 •

61. A "therapeutic window" dose-response curve is most typically associated with which of the following antidepressants?
    A. Desipramine
    B. Nortriptyline
    C. Fluoxetine
    D. Paroxetine
    E. Risperidone

End of Set

62. A 30-year-old receptionist with a history of premenstrual dysphoric disorder (PMDD) and lupus survives a serious car accident without any physical injuries. In the week immediately following the accident, she is seen for follow-up care at your office. She has developed feelings of detachment, does not remember details about the accident, and appears to be in a daze. She tells you that she is having nightmares about cars and has been unable to go to work for 1 week. What is her most likely diagnosis?
    A. Post-traumatic stress disorder (PTSD)
    B. Depersonalization disorder
    C. Malingering
    D. Generalized anxiety disorder
    E. Acute stress disorder

63. A 36-year-old flight attendant is referred to your outpatient office practice for assessment and treatment of her refractory depression. Her PCP has prescribed a variety of SSRIs with only moderate success. Which of the following antidepressant combinations or potentiators is most appropriate?
    A. Fluoxetine plus sertraline
    B. Sertraline plus bupropion
    C. Sertraline plus nardil
    D. Imipramine plus nardil
    E. Lithium plus nardil

The next two questions (items 64 and 65) correspond to the following vignette.

A PCP has asked you to assess his 36-year-old male patient for depression in your outpatient office. The patient's symptoms include fatigue, depressed mood, irritability, sleep disturbance, and poor concentration. To rule out possible medical causes of his symptoms, you pay close attention to the symptoms review portion of the history.

64. Which of the following statements is most likely correct?
    A. Inquiring about endocrinologic review of systems is irrelevant.
    B. Inquiring about hematologic review of systems is irrelevant.
    C. Inquiring about neurologic review of systems is irrelevant.
    D. Inquiring about dermatologic review of systems is irrelevant.
    E. Inquiring about infectious disease review of systems is irrelevant.

65. Thorough history and exam are performed on the patient to rule out physical causes for his symptoms, and you correctly diagnose him with major depressive disorder. You decide to initiate treatment with paroxetine, as he had taken another SSRI in the past. You carefully educate the patient about which side effect that is especially associated with this medication?
    A. Dry mouth
    B. Rapid discontinuation syndrome
    C. Nausea
    D. Headache
    E. Delayed ejaculation

End of Set

The next two questions (items 66 and 67) correspond to the following vignette.

A 35-year-old hotel concierge presents to your outpatient office. He has a longstanding history of HIV infection and is concerned about new psychiatric symptoms.

66. Which of the following statements regarding the psychiatric manifestations of HIV infection is true?
    A. Short-term memory is almost always more affected than long-term memory.
    B. Hallucinations are symptoms of a separate primary psychiatric disorder.
    C. Opportunistic infections will not cause new psychiatric symptoms.
    D. Antiretroviral drug side effects are not a likely cause of new psychiatric symptoms.
    E. Neuropsychological testing is unnecessary.

67. During your evaluation of the patient, he admits to hearing voices recently. You suspect auditory hallucinations and recognize the importance of following up on this symptom. Which is the most appropriate follow-up question?

    A. Is the voice male or female?
    B. Are the voices telling you to do anything?
    C. How does that make you feel?
    D. Would you allow me to refer you to a psychiatrist?
    E. Are you remembering to take your medications?

End of Set

68. A 49-year-old man followed in your outpatient practice relates that he "hates himself" because he has been secretly dressing in women's underwear for years. The patient adds that he has successfully concealed this practice from everyone, including his wife and children. He finds this behavior "disgusting" and has tried to stop it, but cannot resist the sexual arousal associated with it. Which of the following interventions is the most appropriate for this patient?

    A. Discuss the possibility of sexual reassignment surgery
    B. Initiate treatment with medroxyprogesterone
    C. Have the patient explore the reasons why he finds the behavior disgusting
    D. Tell the patient that many men participate in this behavior
    E. Suggest that the patient disclose his behavior to his wife and begin marital counseling

69. A 12-year-old boy with a history of truancy is referred by his pediatrician for consideration of antidepressant treatment. The boy is accompanied to your office by his mother and stepfather. Which of the following statements is true regarding mood disorders in children and adolescents?

    A. The prevalence of depression in children approaches 1 in 10.
    B. The prevalence of depression in adolescents decreases as they approach adulthood.
    C. The male to female ratio for depression is 1:1 in childhood.
    D. Tricyclics are the antidepressants of choice for younger patients.
    E. Antidepressant dosage should be halved upon achieving symptom control in younger patients.

The next three questions (items 70, 71, and 72) correspond to the following vignette.

A 68-year-old retired physician has been referred for outpatient consultation by his neurologist. The patient experienced a stroke 3 months ago but except for daytime somnolence and fatigue has no significant sequelae. The patient's neurologist wonders whether he is depressed, but you discern no specific symptoms to warrant that diagnosis.

70. Which of the following medications is best indicated?

    A. Sertraline
    B. Ziprasidone
    C. Modafinil
    D. Carbamazepine
    E. Rivastigmine

71. The patient's spouse, who is a retired nurse, asks you how modafinil works. What is the best description of its mechanism of action?

    A. It is a selective serotonin reuptake inhibitor (SSRI)
    B. It is a dopamine receptor-blocking agent
    C. It prevents reuptake of dopamine
    D. It enhances release of GABA
    E. It stabilizes neuronal membranes

72. The patient's spouse also questions you about side effects associated with modafinil. Which of the following statements is correct?

    A. Symptoms of withdrawal are common after several weeks of use.
    B. Extra caution is not necessary while driving.
    C. Modafinil can precipitate symptoms of depression.
    D. Modafinil does not affect levels of other medications metabolized by the liver.
    E. The patient's blood pressure should be monitored.

End of Set

The next two questions (items 73 and 74) relate to the following vignette.

A 48-year-old house painter is referred to you by his family practitioner for complaints of anxiety related to "kidney problems." Despite a thorough evaluation and his PCP's reassurance that there is no evidence of disease, the patient is convinced he is "going to die in the next 10 years" from kidney disease. A typical episode of anxiety begins when he starts to feel warm when he is working, followed by shortness of breath. He starts to worry about his blood pressure rising and his kidneys malfunctioning, leading to a build-up of toxins. His PCP prescribed citalopram initially, but the patient believed that it made his "breathing" worse so he discontinued it. His PCP then prescribed clonazepam, which helps his anxiety. The patient admits that he sometimes takes an extra afternoon and evening dose to deal with a particularly stressful day. At one point he discusses the possibility that his brain may be causing some of his symptoms, but later in conversation refers again to his imminent "kidney failure." The patient reveals that his brother died 18 months ago from pancreatic cancer. The patient has a history of alcohol abuse 5 years ago.

73. What is the patient's most likely diagnosis?

    A. Adjustment disorder
    B. Somatization disorder
    C. Hypochondriasis
    D. Somatoform disorder
    E. Pain disorder

74. What should be your next step in management?

    A. Admit him to the psychiatric inpatient unit because of his poorly controlled panic attacks and his abuse of clonazepam
    B. Explain to the patient why you would like him to taper the clonazepam and start him on an SSRI and communicate your plan to his PCP
    C. Continue the clonazepam and introduce cognitive behavioral therapy into the treatment regimen
    D. Discontinue the scheduled clonazepam and start lorazepam as needed for anxiety in addition to cognitive-behavioral therapy
    E. Continue the clonazepam and start a noradrenergic antidepressant like bupropion or venlafaxine

End of Set

75. Your upcoming geriatric community outpatient office rotation will be at a facility known as "Threepoints" because it is situated among three different ethnic-minority neighborhoods. In preparation for this assignment, you review a current textbook about cultural variables in clinical psychiatry. Which one of the following statements is correctly associated with ethnic-minority elderly groups?

    A. Elderly Japanese are expressive about revealing symptoms of depression.
    B. Schizophrenia is underdiagnosed in elderly African Americans.
    C. Elderly Hispanic individuals are high utilizers of mental health care.
    D. Elderly immigrants assimilate more readily than younger immigrants.
    E. Elderly immigrants are more likely to manifest culture-bound syndromes.

The next two questions (items 76 and 77) correspond to the following vignette.

A 27-year-old sexually active postal carrier is being evaluated in your office with signs and symptoms of a moderately severe major depressive disorder. As you begin to discuss the merits of medication treatment, he makes a point to interject that he does not want to take a medication that might interfere with his sex life.

76. Which of the following neurotransmitters is most closely linked to sex drive?

    A. Nitric oxide
    B. Acetylcholine
    C. Dopamine
    D. Serotonin
    E. Norepinephrine

77. Which of the following antidepressants is most likely to maintain this patient's sexual functioning?

    A. Bupropion
    B. Fluoxetine
    C. Paroxetine
    D. Sertraline
    E. Amitriptyline

End of Set

78. A 46-year-old Gulf War veteran presents to your outpatient office with symptoms of rage attacks, hyperarousal, insomnia, and nightmares of his combat experience. You decide to treat his PTSD with SSRIs, as they have proven beneficial in the treatment of which of the following symptoms of PTSD?

A. Autonomic hyperarousal
B. Insomnia
C. Suspiciousness
D. Rage attacks
E. Nightmares

79. A 32-year-old male with a history of localized head injury is visiting his primary care physician's office with his sister. She does not know exactly where he was injured but is able to provide a history of his recent unusual behavior. His sister describes the patient as not acting like himself anymore. Since the accident, he has been impulsive, irresponsible, and without motivation, and he now seems to be a poor decision maker. While in the office, the patient makes inappropriate jokes and frequently uses profanity. On neurological exam, the motor and sensory exams are normal and visual fields are intact. As shown in Figure 4-79, which area of the patient's brain was most likely affected by the injury?

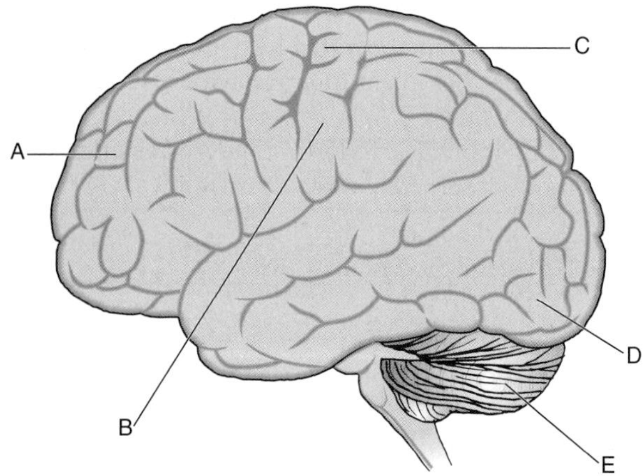

Figure 4-79 •

A. A
B. B
C. C
D. D
E. E

The next four questions (items 80–83) correspond to the following vignette.

A 23-year-old single receptionist has been referred by her gynecologist for psychiatric assessment. She is 8 weeks pregnant and is considering an elective abortion.

80. Which of the following statements is most accurate regarding the psychological effects of an elective abortion?

A. Most women experience significant psychological sequelae after an elective abortion.
B. The strongest predictor of poor post-abortion psychological outcome is a history of depression.
C. Medical or genetic indications for an abortion decrease the likelihood of negative emotional experiences.
D. A first-trimester decision to abort has the most negative psychological impact.
E. The rate of PTSD in women who undergo first-trimester abortion is higher than the rate in the general population.

81. An interview of the patient reveals that she has had a significant mood disorder for at least 5 years. She is presently taking valproic acid to control her symptoms. Regarding the special concerns of treating women with bipolar disorder, which of the following statements is true?

A. Symptoms may recur or worsen premenstrually.
B. Carbamazepine does not affect contraceptives.
C. Women with bipolar disorder are at no higher risk for postpartum psychosis.
D. Valproic acid is not associated with higher rates of fetal anomalies.
E. Medication levels remain stable across the menstrual cycle.

82. Which one of the following, if true, would be a risk factor for postpartum blues in this patient?

A. Family history of bipolar disorder
B. History of PMDD
C. History of bipolar disorder
D. Previous postpartum psychosis
E. Primiparity

83. The patient decides to continue her pregnancy but stop her mood-stabilizing medication. She does well over the remainder of her pregnancy. Following delivery, which would be the best step to take next in her treatment?

A. Start an antidepressant
B. Electroconvulsive therapy (ECT)
C. Start an antipsychotic
D. Start a mood stabilizer
E. Do nothing

End of Set

84. A 38-year-old married administrative assistant is referred by her gynecologist. The patient and her husband have been trying to become pregnant since she stopped using a diaphragm 18 months ago. Which of the following statements is best associated with the psychological factors of infertility?

A. Women tend to be more emotionally affected than their male partners but this effect is short-lived.
B. The demands for sexual performance for men during the fertile portion of the menstrual cycle have few negative effects.
C. Infertile couples typically feel socially supported by their families and peers.
D. Guilt and anger because of past decisions to postpone conception are common problems.
E. It is better to see the two partners individually rather than as a couple.

85. A 53-year-old janitor in your office building is referred for outpatient assessment by her supervisor, who suspects that the patient is a victim of violence. Which of the following statements about female victims of violence is true?

A. Most female victims of sexual assault seek professional help.
B. Rates of sexual abuse are lower in African American women than in the general population.
C. Older women are more likely to be sexually assaulted by strangers.
D. The initial therapeutic approach should be couple, rather than individual, therapy.
E. Female patients presenting with ambiguous physical findings should be evaluated for physical abuse.

86. A 52-year-old single attorney with a history of myocardial infarction and bipolar disorder is seen for her first office visit for lithium maintenance. The patient refuses to tell her primary care physician and cardiologist about her diagnosis of bipolar disorder because she fears the "stigma" of psychiatric illness and is "scared to death" of losing her license to practice law. What would be the best course of action?

A. Tell her that in keeping her safety in mind, you would be unwilling to treat her unless she allows you to relay her medication list to her other physicians; you would also educate her that legally you are permitted to do so without her consent
B. Inform the other physicians without the patient's consent, as it is in her best interests, without her knowing that you have done so and have them maintain secrecy on this issue
C. Encourage the patient to tell her physicians, but reassure her that you would not contact them without her written consent, as it would be illegal and unethical
D. Enlist a member of her family to disclose the information to her other physicians
E. Inform her at the end of the interview that because this is an initial consultation, you are not bound by rules of confidentiality and you feel it is necessary to inform her physicians of what she has just disclosed

87. During your primary care treatment team's weekly staff meeting, a nurse practitioner expresses concern that many of the clinic's depressed patients stop taking their prescribed antidepressant medication prematurely. You recently read a research article on this topic. What is the most important variable to accomplish higher adherence to long-term antidepressant therapy?

A. Planful coping skills training
B. Favorable attitudes toward antidepressant medication
C. Involvement in pleasant activities
D. Increased socialization
E. Monitoring depressive symptoms

The next five questions (items 88–92) correspond to the following vignette.

A single mother of an 8-year-old boy accompanies her son to your outpatient office. The pair has been referred by the boy's second-grade teacher for assessment of possible attention deficit disorder. During your interview, the boy sits quietly and answers your questions to him succinctly; the mother does most of the talking.

88. Which of the following statements regarding attention deficit hyperactivity disorder (ADHD) is true?

A. ADHD is limited to childhood years.
B. The effects of stimulants on ADHD are recently discovered phenomena.
C. Little scientific literature supports the use of stimulants to treat ADHD.
D. The use of stimulants to treat children with ADHD is no longer controversial.
E. There has been a steady increase in the rate of diagnosis of ADHD.

89. After taking a detailed medical and psychiatric history and listening to the mother's observations, it seems the boy may well have ADHD with prominent inattentive symptoms. Which of the following is the best next step?

A. Prescribe methylphenidate twice a day and schedule a follow-up appointment in 3 months
B. Prescribe dextroamphetamine three times a day and instruct the child to keep the mid-day dose in his lunch box to take during recess
C. Prescribe a long-acting stimulant and instruct the mother to not inform the school so there will be no stigma from his teachers
D. Engage the boy's teacher
E. Do nothing and schedule a follow-up visit in 6 months

90. One month later, after baseline ratings of symptoms in the school setting have been made, there is general agreement that a stimulant trial is indicated. Which of the following statements regarding the prescription of stimulants is true?

A. A history of drug abuse is a contraindication to prescribe stimulants.
B. Treated glaucoma is a contraindication to prescribe stimulants.
C. Any cardiovascular disease is a contraindication to prescribe stimulants.
D. Hyperthyroidism is a contraindication to prescribe stimulants.
E. Hypertension is a contraindication to prescribe stimulants.

91. The boy's mother also inquires about the role of play therapy to treat ADHD. Which of the following techniques is most closely associated with play therapy?

A. Emotional catharsis
B. Positive reinforcement
C. Response cost
D. Time-out
E. Token economy

92. Which of the following is the best example of the behavioral technique called "response cost"?

A. Child completes homework and is permitted to play with his or her friends
B. Child pushes classmate on playground and is required to sit alone for 5 minutes
C. Child loses time playing video games for not finishing homework
D. Spanking
E. Child earns stars for completing household chores and can cash them in at the end of the week for a toy

End of Set

93. **A 76-year-old Navajo man is referred by his daughter, who is concerned that her father is depressed. His wife died 6 months ago, and he seldom leaves the house. Which of the following is most appropriate first step in the therapy of Native American patients?**

A. Indoctrinate the patient to traditional psychotherapy techniques
B. Limit involvement of others
C. Maintain direct eye contact
D. Clarify expectations
E. Minimize genetic influence in regard to psychopharmacology because the patient is elderly

The next two questions (items 94 and 95) correspond to the following vignette.

A 36-year-old computer program analyst is required to travel by air frequently. She is seeking outpatient consultation for her fear of flying.

94. Regarding the pharmacokinetics of benzodiazepines, which of the following statements is true?

A. A benzodiazepine's elimination half-life determines how long it accumulates in the body.
B. Benzodiazepine steady-state concentrations are usually achieved over 2 to 3 half-lives of dosing.
C. Benzodiazepines with longer elimination half-lives result in more severe withdrawal symptoms upon discontinuation.
D. Benzodiazepines initially oxidized by hepatic microsomal enzymes have shortened elimination half-lives in the elderly.
E. Benzodiazepines initially conjugated by hepatic microsomal enzymes have prolonged elimination half-lives.

95. Which of the following benzodiazepines is the best to prescribe for this patient for an upcoming cross-country airplane trip for business?
    A. Chlordiazepoxide
    B. Clonazepam
    C. Diazepam
    D. Clorazepate
    E. Lorazepam

End of Set

96. A 38-year-old legal assistant is self-referred with symptoms of anxiety, insomnia, and thoughts of suicide. She associates the onset of her symptoms with the termination of a romantic relationship with her employer 2 weeks ago. When you ask her about the relationship, she will only provide evasive answers, implying she fears there could be a breach in confidentiality if she is forthright. Regarding confidentiality in the psychiatrist–patient relationship, what do you tell her?
    A. The duty to maintain confidentiality is absolute
    B. Confidentiality ends upon the patient's death
    C. Consent to disclose revealing information is not necessary for scientific reports
    D. Revelation of a past crime warrants breaching confidentiality to law-enforcement authorities
    E. A psychiatrist may release confidential information under legal compulsion

97. A 33-year-old woman and her 4-year-old son are referred by the son's pediatrician. When you ask the mother about her son, she says, "He never speaks to me . . . he only looks away . . . he either rocks or flaps his hands . . . he stares at lights . . . when I call his name there is no response . . . if I drop a book he shudders . . ." Your initial diagnosis is autism. Which of the following statements regarding autism is correct?
    A. Autism is associated with *Streptococcus* infection.
    B. Core clinical characteristics include social withdrawal, inflexibility, and impairment in communication.
    C. This disorder is limited to children of parents with higher educational and occupational success.
    D. Higher rates of developmental and psychiatric disabilities are not observed in family members of autism patients.
    E. Few children with autism develop seizures.

98. A 23-year-old single dog groomer is referred for consultation by her psychologist. The patient has been engaged in cognitive-behavioral therapy (CBT) for symptoms of depression, panic disorder, compulsive cleaning, and bulimia for the past 18 months but with limited success. Which of the following medications is the best choice to treat this patient's constellation of symptoms?
    A. Nortriptyline
    B. Phenelzine
    C. Sertraline
    D. Bupropion
    E. Imipramine

The next two questions (items 99 and 100) relate to the following vignette.

A 53-year-old divorced school teacher is referred for outpatient consultation by another psychiatrist. She has a 20-year history of dysthymic disorder and recurrent depressions with only a limited response to a variety of antidepressants at seemingly adequate doses. When you ask her how she tolerated each of the antidepressants prescribed over the past two decades, she recalls that one in particular made her very sleepy, constipated, and light-headed.

99. Which of the following antidepressants most likely caused these side effects?
    A. Bupropion
    B. Citalopram
    C. Paroxetine
    D. Amitriptyline
    E. Venlafaxine

100. After further discussion, the patient recalls that she has been treated with amitriptyline, citalopram, paroxetine, and desipramine with little help. Which one of the following antidepressants would be the next logical one to prescribe this patient?
    A. Fluoxetine
    B. Bupropion
    C. Doxepin
    D. Imipramine
    E. Sertraline

End of Set

A Answers and Explanations

51. D
52. B
53. A
54. B
55. A
56. A
57. A
58. A
59. D
60. C
61. B
62. E
63. B
64. D
65. B
66. A
67. B
68. C
69. C
70. C
71. C
72. E
73. C
74. B
75. E
76. C
77. A
78. D
79. A
80. B
81. A
82. B
83. D
84. D
85. E
86. A
87. B
88. E
89. D
90. E
91. A
92. C
93. D
94. A
95. E
96. E
97. B
98. C
99. D
100. B

51. **D. Donepezil is one of several cholinesterase inhibitors that may be effective in treating the early memory impairment experienced with Alzheimer's disease (AD).**

A. Lorazepam, a benzodiazepine anxiolytic, may worsen the memory problems.
B. Risperidone, an antipsychotic, may be helpful in reducing the agitation and psychotic symptoms experienced with dementia but is not presently necessary for this patient.
C. Buspirone, a non-benzodiazepine anxiolytic, may have some efficacy for the anxious patient with dementia, but this patient is not experiencing such symptoms.
E. Sertraline is an SSRI antidepressant. Depression may be manifested as a pseudo-dementia but the MMSE score would likely be higher.

52. **B. Rivastigmine, a cholinesterase inhibitor, is helpful in improving the early cognitive and memory deficits experienced with AD. Due to the up-regulation effects of donepezil, its efficacy may diminish; another cholinesterase inhibitor may recapture the positive effect before the disease progresses noticeably.**

A. A lower dose of the same medication would not be efficacious.
C. Because the patient does not have any reported psychotic symptoms, risperidone is not necessary.
D. Because the patient does not have any reported depressive symptoms, sertraline is not necessary.
E. Active treatment of cognitive and memory deficits, especially early in the course of AD, can be very helpful to lengthen the patient's period of self-sufficiency.

53. **A. Older patients are at increased risk for both EPS and tardive dyskinesia when taking antipsychotic medications. These side effects are less common with atypical antipsychotic agents.**

B. Olanzepine is associated with the development of diabetes in all age groups.
C. Quetiapine can cause triglyceride elevation in the elderly.
D. Weight gain can occur in all age groups taking atypical antipsychotic medications.
E. Elderly patients are at increased risk for anticholinergic side effects. The more-sedating typical antipsychotics, such as chlorpromazine and thioridazine, are especially problematic.

54. **B. Several controlled trials have suggested that fish oils may be an effective adjunct treatment for bipolar disorder. This supplement might be of benefit to the patient in this case.**

A. Some anecdotal evidence suggests that kava may have some anxiolytic properties, but this supplement is not known to affect mood. Reports of hepatotoxicity have caused kava to be banned in some European countries.
C. Valerian has been used as both a sleep agent and an anxiolytic, although currently no objective clinical evidence supports its use. There is no evidence of toxicity or effects on mood with valerian.
D. In randomized, double-blind, placebo-controlled trials, St. John's wort has been shown to have some antidepressant activity and is thus contraindicated in a patient with bipolar disorder. The primary concerns would be elevating the patient's mood into mania or increasing the rate of cycling.
E. Gingko biloba has been reported as being beneficial to memory, although most placebo-controlled trials have failed to show a significant effect. It is not associated with antidepressant or antimanic activity.

55. **A. Libido does tend to decrease with age for both men and women.**

B. Decreased testosterone levels and increased FSH levels affect men's libido as they age.
C. Decreased estrogen and testosterone levels reduce women's libido.
D. Approximately 80% of all individuals older than 65 years have at least one illness that may affect sexual function.
E. Approximately 25% of men in their seventies and 55% of men older than 80 years report sexual dysfunction.

56. **A. SAD often begins early in life with a mean onset at age 15; 35% of the time SAD occurs before age 10.**

B. Females are affected with SAD more often than males are.
C. SAD has a lifetime prevalence of 13%, making it the third most common psychiatric disorder after depression and alcohol abuse.
D. The majority of people with SAD suffer from generalized SAD, implying that they fear and avoid most all social interaction.
E. Recovery without treatment for SAD is rare.

57. **A. SSRIs such as sertraline can be helpful in treating generalized SAD.**

B, C, D, E. TCAs such as amitriptyline, imipramine, nortriptyline, and desipramine are not helpful for SAD.

58. **A. DLB does account for 15% to 20% of all dementias.**

B. Approximately 75% of patients with DLB experience extrapyramidal symptoms.
C. Neuroimaging technologies such as MRI, SPECT, and PET may be useful to differentiate the dementias.
D. Approximately 60% of patients with PD experience minimal cognitive impairment and dementia.
E. The prevalence of AD is 10% for those older than 65 years and 32% for those older than 85 years.

59. **D. This patient likely has adjustment disorder, acute type, with mixed anxiety and depressed mood. Adjustment disorder is the development of significant emotional or behavioral symptoms due to an identifiable stressor, occurring within 3 months of the stress. An increased risk of suicide is associated with adjustment disorders. Treatment of adjustment disorders typically involves psychotherapy, but treatment with antidepressants is warranted in severe cases.**

A. Although the patient is anxious and depressed, the full clinical picture of a major depressive disorder or an anxiety disorder (such as generalized anxiety disorder) is not present.
B. Dysthymia is chronic, low mood that lasts for at least 2 years. This patient has had symptoms for only 3 months.
C. Adjustment disorder is considered chronic if the disturbance lasts for 6 months or longer.
E. In PTSD, a patient exhibits avoidance behaviors, reexperiences the traumatic event, and has symptoms of increased arousal. These symptoms are not indicated in this patient's history.

60. **C. Curve C illustrates a curvilinear dose response with a therapeutic window; both low and high doses are less effective than midrange doses.**

A. Curve A illustrates a curvilinear dose response but no loss of efficacy at higher doses.
B. Curve B illustrates a linear response.
D. Curve D illustrates a curvilinear dose response with no loss of efficacy at higher doses.

61. **B. Nortriptyline, a tricyclic antidepressant, is most typically associated with a "therapeutic window" dose-response curve.**

A. Desipramine, a tricyclic antidepressant, is more typically associated with a linear dose-response curve.
C. SSRI antidepressant medications such as fluoxetine typically do not have established dose-response curves.
D. SSRIs such as paroxetine do not have established dose-response curves.
E. Risperidone is an antipsychotic, not an antidepressant.

62. **E. Given that her symptoms developed within 4 weeks of the traumatic event, this patient's symptoms are most consistent with acute stress disorder.**

A. If the patient's symptoms persist for longer than 1 month, then her diagnosis will become PTSD.
B. She does not have symptoms of anxiety and depersonalization.
C. There is no indication of the purposeful exaggeration of symptoms or a secondary gain, such as financial reward, that is typical of malingering.
D. Generalized anxiety disorder is a prolonged syndrome of persistent anxiety lasting for more than 6 months.

63. **B. An SSRI such as sertraline plus the dopaminergic antidepressant bupropion may provide broader neurotransmitter activation and be a relatively safe combination.**

A. Fluoxetine and sertraline are both SSRIs and would have limited potentiating effects.
C. The combination of an SSRI, such as sertraline, and an MAOI is always contraindicated. When such agents are used together, a life-threatening serotonergic syndrome can develop.
D. A TCA such as imipramine used cautiously in combination with an MAOI can be a potent antidepressant regimen but is not the safest combination proposed.

E. Lithium can be a valuable potentiator for most all antidepressants but must be used cautiously. Lithium plus the MAOI nardil is not the safest combination proposed.

64. **D. Diseases that are dermatologic in origin are very rarely associated with the neurovegetative symptoms of depression. Dry skin may be a sign of hypothyroidism, but it would more appropriately fall under the category of endocrine review of symptoms.**

A. Common causes of depressive symptoms include hypothyroidism, panhypopituitarism, and adrenal dysfunction. It is important to elicit other signs of these diseases before diagnosing depression.
B. Anemia can be associated with symptoms that mimic depression. Ruling out anemia and other blood diseases is important in the screening process for depression.
C. Patients with neurological diseases such as multiple sclerosis and stroke can appear to be depressed.
E. It is always important to consider infections such as Epstein-Barr virus and HIV before treating someone for depression.

65. **B. Rapid discontinuation of paroxetine has been associated with a syndrome characterized by paresthesias, headache, nausea, flu-like symptoms, and photophobia.**

A. Dry mouth can occur with paroxetine treatment but can also be a side effect of other SSRIs and TCAs.
C. Nausea can be a side effect of paroxetine treatment but is not unique to this medication.
D. Headache is a side effect common to many SSRIs.
E. Delayed ejaculation and decreased libido are side effects common to many SSRIs.

66. **A. Short-term memory usually shows a steeper decline and is affected before long-term memory with HIV infection. In particular, attention and learning can be impaired.**

B. Psychosis can occur as a result of HIV infection and may signify direct viral effects on the CNS, medication side effects, delirium, opportunistic infection, or a primary psychiatric condition.
C. New psychiatric symptoms may be due to opportunistic CNS infection with fungi, parasites, viruses, or bacteria.
D. Antiretroviral medication side effects can include psychosis, depression, mania, restlessness, agitation, or irritability.
E. Neuropsychological testing of this patient could be beneficial to objectively evaluate the extent of his dysfunction.

67. **B. Asking the patient if the voices are telling him to do anything is the single most important follow-up question. Command auditory hallucinations can be very disturbing to patients. If the patient is hearing commands, then inquiring whether he feels compelled to follow the commands would be the next question to ask with regard to the patient's immediate safety.**

A. Asking whether the voice is male or female may help elicit discussion, but assessing the patient's immediate safety is much more important.
C. Inquiring about the patient's feelings may elicit further discussion, but it less important than asking about command hallucinations.
D. Referral to a mental health professional may be appropriate in this case, but determining the patient's immediate dangerousness to himself or to others is the primary concern.
E. While medication compliance may be questionable in a patient with new-onset hallucinations, assessment of his safety should be the primary concern.

68. **C. This patient's symptoms are suggestive of a transvestic fetishism. The most appropriate step is to explore the reasons he finds his behavior disturbing. The self-loathing typically found with this disorder usually will respond to psychotherapy.**

A. Sexual reassignment surgery is sometimes used in the treatment of gender identity disorder, not transvestic fetishism.
B. Exogenous progesterone may be used to treat some paraphilias but would probably not be appropriate to treat someone with transvestic fetishism, as libido and other areas of sexual function are likely to be affected as well.

D. The prevalence of this disorder is unknown. It would be dishonest and misleading to try to comfort the patient by trying to tell him that "many men" participate in this behavior.
E. Disclosing this behavior to his spouse may or may not improve his self-image or may just cause interpersonal conflict. The more immediate concern here is to address why the patient feels disgusted by his behavior.

69. **C. The male to female ratio for depression is 1:1 in childhood but during adolescence approaches the 1:2 ratio associated with adulthood.**

A. The prevalence of depression is approximately 2% in children.
B. The prevalence of depression in adolescents ranges from 4% to 8%, approaching the higher prevalence rate as the age group approaches adulthood.
D. SSRIs are the antidepressants of choice for children and adolescents. Despite their widespread use, relatively few controlled studies have examined the effects of these drugs in younger patients.
E. As in adults, antidepressants should be continued in children at the same dose to maintain remission unless significant dose-related side effects arise. Treatment should continue at the successful dose for at least 6 to 12 months.

70. **C. Modafinil is indicated to improve wakefulness in patients with excessive daytime sleepiness.**

A. Sertraline is an antidepressant. Because there are no symptoms except low energy to indicate a depression in this case, it would not be indicated in this patient.
B. Ziprasidone is an atypical antipsychotic. Because there are no symptoms of psychosis in this case, it would not be indicated in this patient.
D. Carbamazepine is an anticonvulsant also used as a mood stabilizer in bipolar disorder. Because there are neither seizures nor mood symptoms in this case, it would not be indicated in this patient.
E. Rivastigmine is an acetylcholinesterase inhibitor used in patients with dementia.

71. **C. Modafinil binds to dopamine reuptake sites, causing an increase in extracellular dopamine but not an increase in its release.**

A. Modafinil does not block serotonin reuptake; this effect occurs with SSRI antidepressants.
B. Modafinil does not block dopamine receptors; this effect occurs with antipsychotics.
D. Modafinil does not affect GABA; this effect occurs with anxiolytics.
E. Modafinil does not stabilize neuronal membranes; this effect occurs with anticonvulsants.

72. **E. Modafinil can cause both hypertension and hypotension.**

A. No specific symptoms of withdrawal are typically observed upon stopping modafinil, although it is likely that the patient's sleepiness will return.
B. Caution should be used when prescribing any medication that affects the CNS.
C. As a stimulant, modafinil can precipitate symptoms of mania, psychosis, and anxiety but is not expected to produce depression.
D. Modafinil can both induce and suppress various cytochrome P-450 isoenzymes.

73. **C. This patient meets the criteria for a diagnosis of hypochondriasis, a specific type of somatoform disorder in which there is a preoccupation with the idea that one has a serious disease based on one's misinterpretation of bodily symptoms. The preoccupation persists despite appropriate medical evaluation and reassurance. The belief does not have a delusional intensity (as in delusional disorder, somatic type). The duration of the disturbance is at least 6 months. With this patient's history, it is apparent that the preoccupation with his health is the cause of the panic attacks and depressive symptoms. The likelihood of an underlying or secondary depression or anxiety disorder should always be considered with hypochondriasis. Physical disease must be excluded as well.**

A. Although the patient suffered from the loss of his brother 18 months ago, an adjustment disorder as defined in DSM-IV occurs within 3 months of a traumatic or stressful event and resolves within 6 months of the onset of the stressor (assuming that the stressor and its consequences have ended).

B. This patient does not meet the criteria for a diagnosis of somatization disorder, which requires that a person have four distinct complaints of pain, two non-pain gastrointestinal symptoms, and one pseudo-neurological symptom, all beginning before age 30 and occurring over a period of several years; these symptoms must not be fully explained by a medical condition after appropriate investigation to warrant this diagnosis.
D. Enough information is presented for the diagnosis of a specific type of somatoform disorder, hypochondriasis, which causes anxiety due to the preoccupation with disease that is present most of the time.
E. Pain is not this patient's main complaint. What seems to be of most concern to him is the anxiety related to the fear of having serious disease.

74. **B. Treatment is most effective when there is collaboration between a PCP who continues regular appointments and a consulting psychiatrist who focuses on coping skills and treats symptoms of anxiety, depression, or psychosocial distress. First-line treatment for hypochondriasis is an SSRI, which would target both depression and anxiety. Because some SSRIs can worsen anxiety early in treatment, it is important to start with the smallest possible dose and increase the dose slowly. Most likely, the dose will have to be increased to the higher range to adequately treat the patient's panic attacks. Some studies have shown that individuals with a history of alcohol abuse are more vulnerable to abusing benzodiazepines, as in this patient.**

A. Although the patient does have recurrent thoughts of death, he does not currently have active suicidal thoughts and is not in imminent danger of hurting himself or others. Thus hospitalization is not warranted.
C. It is best to discontinue the benzodiazepine, clonazepam, because of the patient's higher risk of substance abuse.
D. Lorazepam would not be recommended for the same reason as given in the explanation for C. However, CBT can be helpful for treatment of hypochondriasis and to decrease the frequency of panic attacks.
E. SSRIs are first-line therapies because hypochondriasis appears to respond best to a serotonergic agent. If the SSRI is ineffective when administered alone, another medication (e.g., an antidepressant that has a noradrenergic component) can be added as an adjunct therapy. Noradrenergic medications can also be useful for a patient who experiences sexual dysfunction as a side effect of taking an SSRI.

75. **E. Elderly individuals more often manifest culture-bound syndromes, which complicates making an accurate diagnosis.**

A. Japanese are socialized to behave in a deferential manner, which may result in inhibition about revealing emotional symptoms to an authority figure such as a psychiatrist.
B. Both schizophrenia and dementia are overdiagnosed in elderly African Americans.
C. Both Hispanic and Asian elderly persons underuse mental health services.
D. Migration at a later stage of life is often marked by more difficulty acculturating.

76. **C. Sex drive, or libido, is the first stage of sexual response. This dopaminergic function is mediated by the mesolimbic region of the brain.**

A. Nitric oxide is a chemical messenger that controls erections in the penis, which is a major component of the second stage of the sexual response cycle.
B. Acetylcholine is an autonomic parasympathetic neurotransmitter also involved in the second stage of the sexual response cycle, resulting in erections for men and lubrication and swelling for women.
D. Serotonin exerts inhibitory actions on orgasm, the third stage of the sexual response cycle.
E. Norepinephrine is a noradrenergic sympathetic neurotransmitter facilitating ejaculation and orgasm in the third stage of sexual response.

77. **A. Bupropion is a dopaminergic antidepressant. Not only is it least likely to interfere with this patient's sexual functioning, but it may actually enhance it.**

B. Fluoxetine, an SSRI, may result in inhibitory actions on orgasm.
C. Paroxetine, an SSRI, may result in inhibitory actions on orgasm.

D. Sertraline, an SSRI, may result in inhibitory actions on orgasm.
E. Amitryptyline, a TCA, has both serotonergic and anticholinergic properties, potentially causing inhibition of both orgasm and erection.

78. **D. Rage, impulsivity, suicidality, depressed mood, panic symptoms, and obsessional thinking associated with PTSD may be helped by SSRIs.**

A. Autonomic hyperarousal may be helped by beta blockers and benzodiazepines, which should be used cautiously in patients with PTSD because of the frequent concomitant alcohol and substance abuse.
B. Insomnia may also be helped by benzodiazepines, other sedative-hypnotics, and clonidine.
C. Antipsychotics are not routinely used for PTSD, but may prove helpful in low doses for paranoia and suspiciousness.
E. Clonidine, a presynaptic a-adrenergic agonist, may be helpful for traumatic nightmares.

79. **A. The presentation is similar to the case of Phineas Gage, a laborer whose left frontal lobe was impaled by an iron bar after an accidental explosion. The classic frontal lobe syndrome is characterized by poor judgment, disinhibition, irresponsibility, and social inappropriateness.**

B. The postcentral gyrus is associated with sensory function; an injury to this area would result in abnormal sensory findings on exam. If the motor sensory cortices had been affected, then abnormal neurological findings would be present.
C. The precentral gyrus is associated with motor function; an injury to this area would result in abnormal motor findings on exam.
D. The patient's visual fields are intact, indicating that the occipital lobe is unaffected.
E. A lesion in the cerebellum would cause difficulty with balance and coordination.

80. **B. A history of depression is the strongest predictor of poor post-abortion psychological outcome.**

A. Of course, some women experience significant distress after an elective abortion, but most do not.
C. Medical or genetic indications for an abortion increase the likelihood of negative emotional experiences.
D. Mid-trimester abortion increases the likelihood of negative emotional experiences.
E. The rate of PTSD in first-trimester post-abortion women is lower than the rate in a general age-related female population.

81. **A. Mood symptoms frequently recur or worsen premenstrually.**

B. Carbamazepine, an anticonvulsant used as a mood stabilizer for bipolar patients, may render oral contraceptives ineffective.
C. Women with bipolar disorder are at higher risk for postpartum psychosis.
D. Mood-stabilizing agents such as carbamazepine, valproic acid, and lithium, especially if taken in the first trimester of pregnancy, are associated with higher rates of fetal anomalies.
E. Medication levels fluctuate across the menstrual cycle.

82. **B. PMDD is associated with a higher risk for postpartum blues.**

A. A family history of bipolar disorder is a risk factor for postpartum psychosis but not postpartum blues.
C. A history of bipolar disorder confers a 35% risk for postpartum psychosis.
D. A previous postpartum psychosis is associated with a 30% risk of recurrence following delivery.
E. Primaparity increases the risk of postpartum psychosis but not necessarily postpartum blues.

83. **D. This patient is at significant risk for postpartum psychosis. Initiation of a mood-stabilizing agent in her third trimester or immediately after delivery can reduce the rate of relapse.**

A. An antidepressant alone would be contraindicated in a bipolar patient because it may cause rapid mood cycling or mania.
B. ECT is used as an alternative for patients who do not respond to medications.
C. The patient is not presently psychotic, so an antipsychotic is not indicated.
E. Considering the patient's history, prophylactic pharmacologic treatment is indicated. Patients with postpartum psychosis are at risk for child abuse, infanticide, and suicide.

84. D. It is not uncommon for women who have purposely postponed childbearing to experience guilt and anger for being unsuccessful at achieving pregnancy.

A. Women tend to be more emotionally affected by infertility than men, and this condition persists after years of treatment.
B. Sexual performance for men during fertile periods can become an issue, especially if they have anxious personalities.
C. Infertile couples typically become socially isolated from their families and friends to avoid painful questions and preoccupations with child rearing.
E. Even if one member of the infertile couple is more psychiatrically distressed, it is more helpful to see both partners as a couple for several sessions.

85. E. Female patients with ambiguous physical findings should be queried privately about sexual and physical abuse.

A. Only 1 in 10 female victims of sexual assault seeks treatment.
B. Approximately 20% of all women, 15% of female college students, and 12% of adolescent girls have experienced sexual abuse or assault. These rates are higher for African American women.
C. Although sexual assault affects women of all ages, older women are more likely to be sexually assaulted by marital or ex-marital partners.
D. Individual therapy is indicated first in suspected sexual or physical abuse, as couple therapy is likely to cause defensive behaviors.

86. A. Confidentiality can be waived within the clinical treatment circle. Therefore, one does not need to obtain specific consent to discuss information with other members treating the patient, or with supervisors or consultants. This is true even under the new HIPAA regulations. The patient should be told that treatment cannot continue if she is not agreeable to you communicating critical health data to her other treating physicians.

B. This plan does not fall under beneficence, disregards patient autonomy, and would be unethical.
C. On the contrary, not informing her other physicians could be extremely dangerous for the patient's health. Other examples that would not require written consent would be in emergencies, when treating a minor, or if the patient is incompetent.
D. The patient's consent is needed to share information with his or her family, with similar exceptions as stated above.
E. A consultant doing an initial evaluation does not have a relationship with the patient and would be able to relay relevant findings and history to the physician who requested the consultation. The patient should be informed of this possibility at the beginning of the consultation. In this instance, the patient was not first educated about this fact.

87. B. Long-term adherence to antidepressant therapy is a frequent problem in a primary care practice. Active intervention by the treatment team has consistently been found to be helpful. More recent studies have found that instillation of a favorable attitude toward antidepressant treatment by the professional staff, as well as confidence in the management of side-effects are the most significant variables to promote adherence.

A. Planful coping does not affect medication adherence.
C. Involvement in pleasant activities does not significantly affect medication adherence.
D. Increased socialization does not significantly affect medication adherence.
E. The self-management activities of checking for depressive symptoms do not significantly improve medication adherence.

88. E. Over the past two decades, there has been a steady increase in the diagnosis of ADHD.

A. ADHD is now known to persist into adolescence and adulthood, and adults are increasingly being treated for this disorder.
B. The effects of stimulants on the disruptive behavior of ADHD were discovered in 1937.
C. Studies of the short-term benefits of stimulants on the symptoms of ADHD constitute perhaps the largest body of scientific literature for any childhood psychiatric disorder.
D. The use of stimulants to treat children remains controversial, particularly among the lay media.

89. **D. Teacher ratings of ADHD symptoms using age and sex-normed instruments should be obtained at baseline and after treatment has begun.**

A. Although a stimulant such as methylphenidate may well be indicated eventually, baseline target symptoms in school should be identified first.
B. Baseline target symptoms in the school setting should be identified and arrangements made for school personnel to provide supervision for in-school doses of medications.
C. Engagement of appropriate school staff (e.g., teachers, nurses, coaches) is in the best interest of the child.
E. Minimally, formal assessment of the child's symptoms in school should be documented and monitored.

90. **E. Untreated hypertension, concomitant use of MAOIs, and active psychosis are contraindications to stimulant use.**

A. Stimulants are not contraindicated but should be used cautiously if there is a history of drug abuse. If a member of the household has a history of stimulant abuse, steps should be taken to ensure that the medications are not abused.
B. Untreated glaucoma is a contraindication to stimulant use.
C. Untreated cardiovascular disease is a contraindication to stimulant use.
D. Untreated hyperthyroidism is a contraindication to stimulant use.

91. **A. Play therapy is a psychological intervention designed to evaluate and change a child's emotional status through catharsis. It has little documented efficacy in the treatment of ADHD.**

B. Positive reinforcement provides rewards contingent on the child's performance; it is more closely associated with behavior therapy.
C. Response cost includes withdrawing rewards or privileges contingent on the performance of problem behavior; it is more closely associated with behavior therapy.
D. Time-out involves removing access to positive reinforcement contingent on problem behavior.
E. Token economy includes earning rewards that may be cashed in; it is associated with behavior therapy.

92. **C. Losing playtime for not finishing homework is an example of the behavioral technique known as response cost.**

A. Being allowed to play after completing homework is an example of positive reinforcement.
B. Having to sit alone after pushing is an example of the time-out technique.
D. Spanking, although in the realm of response cost, is more appropriately termed aversive conditioning.
E. Earning tokens for a grander reward is an example of a token economy.

93. **D. As with all cultural subgroups, some Native American patients do not know what is expected of them when seeing a mental health professional.**

A. The therapist must be mindful to be sensitive and flexible to the cultural influences that a Native American patient brings to the therapy situation.
B. Consultation with resources such as the tribe, Indian Health Services, family members, and traditional healers can all be of assistance.
C. Direct eye contact may be seen as a sign of disrespect by some Native Americans and may generate anxiety.
E. As with other ethnic groups, there may be variations in the response to the dosages of psychotropic medications compared to the standard doses prescribed to Caucasians. The patient's age also affects medication prescribing.

94. **A. A benzodiazepine's elimination half-life determines how long it accumulates in the blood and brain.**

B. Benzodiazepine steady-state concentrations are usually achieved over 4 to 5 half-lives of dosing.
C. Benzodiazepines with longer elimination half-lives result in less severe withdrawal symptoms upon discontinuation.
D. Benzodiazepines metabolized by oxidation have longer elimination half-lives, so they should be prescribed cautiously in the elderly and patients with liver disease.
E. Benzodiazepines metabolized by conjugation have shorter elimination half-lives.

95. E. The duration of a benzodiazepine's effect following a single dose is primarily related to its distribution half-life rather than its elimination half-life. A short-acting benzodiazepine such as lorazepam would be the best choice from this list because of its relatively intermediate onset (1 to 6 hours) and distribution times, and its short elimination half-life (10 to 20 hours).

A. Chlordiazepoxide has a slow distribution time and long elimination half-life (30 to 200 hours).
B. Clonazepam has a longer elimination half-life (18 to 50 hours).
C. Diazepam has very fast onset (0.5 to 2 hours) and distribution times, but a long elimination half-life (30 to 200 hours).
D. Chlorazepate has fast onset and distribution times, but a long elimination half-life (30 to 200 hours).

96. E. Proper legal compulsion and patient authorization are the two mainstays of disclosing confidential information.

A. The duty to maintain confidentiality is not absolute. Exceptions to confidentiality include the duty to warn and evidence of child abuse.
B. Ethically, confidences survive the patient's death.
C. If a patient's identity cannot be disguised, consent must be obtained before publication.
D. Typically, revelation of a past crime does not warrant breaching confidentiality unless it is recent, particularly heinous, and likely to be repeated.

97. B. Social withdrawal, inflexibility, and communication impairment are core clinical characteristics of autism.

A. *Streptococcus* infection is associated with the abrupt onset of tics in children.
C. There is no special social class issue that distinguishes parents of children with autism.
D. Genetic research of autism shows associations with other developmental and psychiatric disabilities in family members.
E. As many as 25% of persons with autism develop seizures.

98. C. The SSRI sertraline is the best choice among the medications listed because SSRIs are efficacious in treating depression, panic disorder, OCD, and bulimia.

A. The TCA nortriptyline is not helpful in treating OCD.
B. The MAOI phenelzine is not helpful in treating OCD.
D. The antidepressant bupropion is not helpful in treating panic disorder, OCD, or bulimia.
E. The TCA imipramine is not helpful in treating OCD.

99. D. Amitriptyline is a TCA. Its potency for blocking histamine, acetylcholine, and α-adrenergic receptors, resulting in sedation, constipation, and light-headedness, respectively, is very high.

A. Bupropion has essentially no histamine-, acetylcholine-, and α-adrenergic-blocking properties.
B. Citalopram has minimal histamine-blocking properties and no effect on acetylcholine or adrenergic neurotransmitters.
C. Paroxetine has minimal anticholinergic properties but no histamine- or α-adrenergic-blocking properties.
E. Venlafaxine has no histamine-, acetylcholine-, or α-adrenergic-blocking properties.

100. B. Bupropion, a dopamine-enhancing antidepressant, would be the next logical choice from this group. The patient reports a poor response to serotonergic and noradrenergic antidepressants in the past.

A. Fluoxetine is an SSRI, as are citalopram and paroxetine, which have not helped the patient in the past.
C. Doxepin is a TCA much like amitriptyline with serotonergic and noradrenergic properties that have not particularly helped the patient in the past. It also has a higher propensity for histamine, acetylcholine, and α-adrenergic blocking—properties that were problems for this patient in her earlier treatment.
D. Imipramine is another TCA similar to amitriptyline and doxepin in efficacy and side effects.
E. Sertraline is an SSRI similar to citalopram and paroxetine, which evidently were not helpful to the patient in the past.

SETTING 3: INPATIENT FACILITIES

You have general admitting privileges to the hospital. You may see patients in the critical care unit, the pediatrics unit, the maternity unit, or recovery room. You may also be called to see patients in the psychiatric unit. A short-stay unit serves patients who are undergoing same-day operations or who are being held for observation. There are adjacent nursing home/extended-care facilities and a detoxification unit where you may see patients.

101. An 83-year-old female with a history of aortic valve stenosis and hypertension was admitted to the hospital 2 weeks ago for worsening dyspnea. Her outpatient medications included citalopram and alprazolam. She denied any alcohol use. She has never abused her anxiolytic medication and has been on the same dose for the past 14 years. Her alprazolam was ordered at half her usual outpatient dose on admission. For the past 10 days she has been "seeing people" around her bed at night. She is also very anxious about the aortic valve replacement scheduled later in the week. The patient has a nearly perfect score on her MMSE and has no previous diagnosis of dementia. She has not shown any confusion or any change in her sleep-wake cycle. Which of the following is most likely the source of her visual hallucinations?

    A. Dementia of the Alzheimer's type
    B. Schizophrenia
    C. Schizoaffective disorder
    D. Delirium secondary to general medical condition
    E. Benzodiazepine withdrawal

102. A 51-year-old female with a history of coronary artery disease and previous myocardial infarction is admitted for chest pain. Her cardiologist requests that she be evaluated by the consultation service for complaints of chronic chest pain, pain in both of her lower extremities, migraine headaches, and abdominal pain. The abdominal pain is accompanied by nausea and vomiting. On admission she also expresses concern about new-onset "seizures.". Her cardiologist, who reveals that this is her tenth admission in the past year, states that an EEG was normal. During these episodes she has tremors in all four extremities, remains conscious for the duration of the episode, and does not have postictal confusion. She had a hysterectomy for "excessive bleeding" when she was 28 years old. Her cardiologist asks for advice about "setting rules" due to the fact that every week she either calls him at home complaining of "10 out of 10 chest pain," or drops by his office unexpectedly for an emergency visit. What is her most likely diagnosis?

    A. Pain disorder
    B. Undifferentiated somatoform disorder
    C. Somatization disorder
    D. Hypochondriasis
    E. Conversion disorder

103. A 19-year-old Asian honors college student is admitted to the inpatient psychiatric service. She exhibits pressured speech, admits to having racing thoughts, and appears unable to sit still. Her family relates that she has not slept for more than 2 or 3 hours each night since she came home 1 week ago for spring break. Despite being difficult to direct during interview, she is fairly compliant with staff requests but is suspicious of the other patients. When one male patient walks by, she states that she can "feel evil" emanating from him. She also believes that she has special healing powers. Her family reveals that she was started on isoniazid 2 weeks ago for having a positive skin test for tuberculosis. Her urine drug screen is negative, and the patient has no family history of bipolar disorder. What is her most likely diagnosis?

    A. Major depressive disorder
    B. Bipolar disorder, type I
    C. Substance-induced mood disorder
    D. Schizophrenia
    E. Hypomania

104. A consultation is requested for a surgery patient for a "change in mental status." The patient is a 77-year-old female who is 2 days status post surgery for hip fracture repair. Her chart indicates no prior psychiatric history. The patient's vital signs are as follows: temperature 101.8°F, heart rate 97, respiratory rate 26, blood pressure 156/97. Her current medications include Colace, glucophage, lisinopril, propranolol, and IV meperidine for pain. Upon examination, the patient is disoriented to location, day, date, and year. She is agitated, pulling at soft restraints and yelling, "They're all out to get me! I can see them standing in the shadows!" What is the most likely diagnosis for this patient?

A. Schizophrenia
B. Delusional disorder
C. Delirium
D. Dementia
E. Brief psychotic disorder

The next two questions (items 105 and 106) correspond to the following vignette.

A disheveled, middle-aged man has been admitted to the inpatient teaching service for assessment of suicidal ideation to jump in front of a bus. He has a very strong odor of alcohol and various neurological signs on physical exam, including ophthalmoplegia, weakness, confusion, and a staggering gait.

105. This history and findings are most likely related to which of the following vitamin deficiencies?

A. Vitamin B_{12}
B. Vitamin A
C. Ascorbic acid
D. Niacin
E. Thiamine

106. The ophthalmoplegia associated with this patient's Wernicke's encephalopathy is related to which of the following?

A. External strabismus
B. Conjugate gaze
C. Ptosis
D. Sixth cranial nerve palsy
E. Seventh cranial nerve palsy

End of Set

107. As a member of the hospital's professional staff, you are asked to participate on the pharmacy committee. Which of the following medications is a nonstimulant medication approved by the FDA to treat ADHD?

A. Citalopram
B. Amitriptyline
C. Atomoxetine
D. Methylphenidate
E. Dextroamphetamine

The next two questions (items 108 and 109) correspond to the following vignette.

A 36-year-old graduate student is hospitalized for a recurrence of his bipolar disorder. This is his fourth hospitalization for manic symptoms during the past 10 months.

108. Which of the following statements is true about the symptom phenomenology of bipolar disorder?

A. Bipolar patients are symptomatically ill approximately 10% of the time.
B. Approximately 80% of bipolar patients relapse within 5 years.
C. Bipolar patients do best with pharmacologic treatment alone.
D. Manic symptoms typically initiate rapid cycling.
E. Duration of episodes is approximately 1.5 months for depression and 3 months for mania.

109. Regarding the socioeconomic costs of bipolar disorder, which of the following statements is true?

A. Bipolar disorder is among the top 10 disabling disorders as measured by disability-adjusted life-years.
B. Hospitalization costs outweigh bipolar disorder's indirect costs to society and families.
C. Subsyndromal symptoms cause less social disruption than acute phases.
D. Despite the nature of their illness, bipolar patients tend to remain married.
E. There is little correlation between relapse and psychosocial functioning.

End of Set

The next three questions (items 110, 111, and 112) correspond to the following vignette.

A 23-year-old single college student was very distraught over her break-up with her boyfriend of 2 weeks. She was admitted to the hospital because she was cutting her forearms and threatening to overdose on her prescribed medications. Her symptoms have now stabilized, and the treatment team is developing a plan for her follow-up care.

110. Which of the following is the most appropriate antidepressant to prescribe to this patient?

A. Fluoxetine
B. Phenelzine
C. Parnate
D. Amitriptyline
E. Imipramine

111. The team's faculty supervisor suggests a treatment trial with venlafaxine. Before prescribing venlafaxine, which particular vital sign should be assessed and documented?

A. Weight
B. Blood pressure
C. Temperature
D. Respiration
E. Pulse

112. Which of the following types of psychotherapy is best indicated in a patient with a borderline personality disorder (BPD) and the symptoms described for this patient?

A. Psychoanalysis
B. Psychodynamic psychotherapy
C. Cognitive therapy
D. Behavioral therapy
E. Dialectical behavior therapy (DBT)

End of Set

113. A 20-year-old Caucasian male with a history of gang involvement and imprisonment for aggravated assault is transferred from the jail psychiatric inpatient unit for evaluation of suicidal ideation. When asked about his history of violence, he states that he cannot remember the details of the assault. He recounts other similar episodes of "blanking out" and being unable to recall past events. He admits that he was out "partying" with friends immediately before the assault took place. Which of the following conditions should be considered in the DSM IV Axis II differential diagnosis?

A. Antisocial personality disorder
B. Seizure disorder
C. Substance abuse
D. Dissociative amnesia
E. Malingering

114. A 56-year-old man with chronic alcoholism was admitted to the hospital for pneumonia. Several days into the hospitalization, he developed signs and symptoms of Wernicke's encephalopathy. Although he has since improved, concern remains that he may progress to Korsakoff's syndrome. Which of the following is associated with Korsakoff's syndrome?

A. Reversible short-term memory impairment
B. Impaired sensorium
C. Confabulation
D. Heavy alcohol intake for weeks
E. Structural lesions in the amygdala

115. A 20-year-old homeless man has been admitted directly to the inpatient psychiatric unit. He claims that he cannot remember who he is. He says that he found himself in New York City, but that he cannot recall where he comes from, the circumstances of his trip, or any other information. The only identification he has is a bus ticket from Chicago. Which of the following is the most likely diagnosis?

A. Dissociative amnesia
B. Depersonalization disorder
C. Dissociative identity disorder
D. Dissociative fugue
E. Substance-induced amnestic disorder

The next five questions (items 116–120) correspond to the following vignette.

A 26-year-old woman is admitted through the emergency department to the inpatient psychiatric unit. On examination, she demonstrates rapid speech, extreme irritability, and flight of ideas. Although she is too distractible to provide a coherent history, her boyfriend relates that she stopped taking her usual medications nearly 2 months ago.

116. What are the average noncompliance rates among patients with bipolar disorder?

A. 20% to 30%
B. 30% to 40%
C. 40% to 50%
D. 50% to 60%
E. 60% to 70%

117. The patient's boyfriend adds that she stopped taking her medication because she did not like the side effects. Which of the following side effects linked to lithium is most commonly associated with noncompliance?

A. Cognitive dysfunction
B. Tremor
C. Weight gain
D. Acne
E. Hair loss

118. The patient's boyfriend, a third-year medical student, also relates that she experienced amenorrhea, galactorrhea, and gynecomastia. Which of the following best describes the physiologic mechanism underlying this patient's antipsychotic-induced hyperprolactinemia?

A. Dopamine-2 (D_2) blockade in the tuberoinfundibular pathway of the brain
B. D_2 blockade in the mesolimbic area of the brain
C. D_2 blockade in the mesocortical area of the brain
D. D_2 blockade in the nigrastriatal pathway
E. $5HT_{2C}$ receptor affinity

119. After presenting the history of this complicated patient to your faculty supervisor, he quizzes you about the variety of medication-related side effects. Which of the following antipsychotics is most likely to cause hyperprolactinemia in this patient?

A. Risperidone
B. Quetiapine
C. Olanzapine
D. Ziprasidone
E. Haloperidol

120. The patient is also obese. Which of the following atypical antipsychotics is least likely to cause weight gain?

A. Risperidone
B. Quetiapine
C. Olanzapine
D. Ziprasidone
E. Haloperidol

End of Set

121. A 28-year-old male with a history of paranoid delusions is brought to the hospital wearing leg shackles and handcuffs. He is accompanied by two armed guards. During a brief break from the examination, one of the guards asks you if you have ever participated in a prisoner execution. Which of the following statements about the involvement of physicians in executions is most consistent with the profession's code of ethics?

A. A physician may assist in an execution by selecting injection sites and starting intravenous lines.
B. A physician may supervise lethal injection personnel.
C. A physician may testify as to medical diagnoses as they relate to the legal assessment of competence for execution.
D. A physician may declare the executed person dead.
E. A physician may witness an execution in a professional capacity.

122. A 32-year-old male is admitted to the inpatient unit for depression with suicidal ideation. He has had two previous trials of antidepressants. The patient says that he has heard about bupropion and is interested in trying it. You counsel him that which of the following statements is true regarding this medication?

A. Its major mechanism of action involves serotonin.
B. The advantage of the sustained-release (SR) formulation is that it is effective when taken once a day and is better tolerated.
C. It is safe for individuals with a history of anorexia but not those with bulimia.
D. The immediate-release formulation can be prescribed for a maximum dose of 300 mg daily.
E. If sexual side effects are a concern, this medication may be better tolerated than an antidepressant that is selective for serotonin.

123. A 53-year-old physician is admitted to the inpatient service with symptoms of weight loss, frequent familiar songs in his head, and visions of friends he knows are not really present. In which region of the brain depicted in Figure 4-123 (A–E) would you expect a tumor to be present?

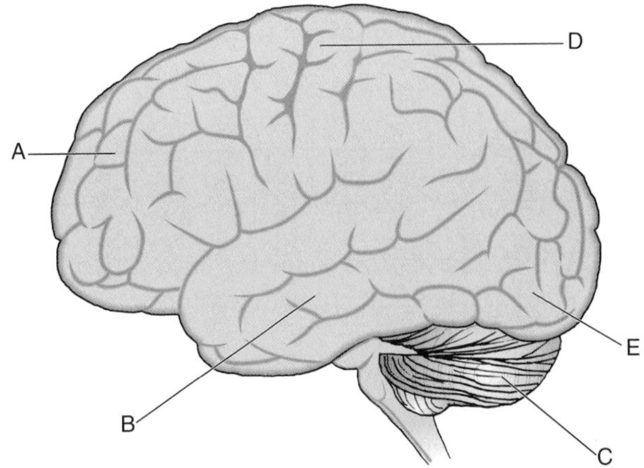

Figure 4-123 •

A. A
B. B
C. C
D. D
E. E

The next three questions (items 124, 125, and 126) correspond to the following vignette.

You have admitted a 22-year-old male with schizophrenia to the inpatient psychiatric unit. He has been started on haloperidol for management of his illness. After taking several doses of the medication, the patient complains of stiffness in his neck and jaw muscles. On exam, cogwheel rigidity is noted in his arms.

124. The patient's symptoms are consistent with a drug effect in which area of the brain depicted in Figure 4-124 (A–E)?

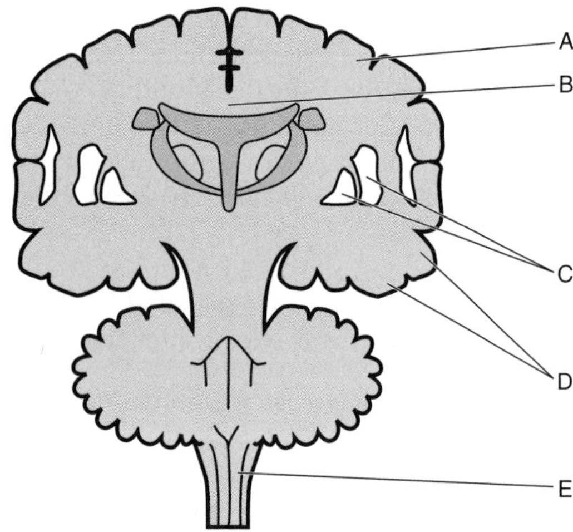

Figure 4-124 •

A. A
B. B
C. C
D. D
E. E

125. Which one of the following medications will provide rapid relief of his symptoms?

A. Benztropine
B. L-Dopa
C. Quetiapine
D. Phenytoin
E. Metoprolol

126. You treat the patient accordingly, and then educate him on the risk of which serious long-term neurological condition associated with haloperidol?

A. Extrapyramidal symptoms (EPS)
B. Parkinson's disease
C. Tardive dyskinesia
D. Huntington's disease
E. Akathisia

End of Set

127. A 49-year-old Caucasian male with a history of bipolar disorder, alcohol dependence, and hepatitis C infection is admitted to the medical floor for upper gastrointestinal bleeding, sepsis, and hyponatremia. The patient reports having a depressed mood for the past 9 months after his 20-year-old son committed suicide. Most recently he was on lithium and citalopram, which he stopped taking 3 months ago. He admits to poor sleep, poor appetite, and an increase in crying spells. He denies suicidal ideation but states, "I need to get back on my meds." His labs include the following results: BUN 46, creatinine 1.4, sodium 128, potassium 3.1, AST 138, and ALT 69. Which of the following would be the best step in management regarding his psychiatric medications?

A. Start lithium to prevent a manic episode from occurring
B. Start citalopram due to his depressive symptoms
C. Start lithium and citalopram concurrently to get the patient back on therapeutic doses of his medication as soon as possible
D. Continue to hold his psychiatric medications
E. Start the patient on another mood stabilizer such as valproic acid because the previous medications did not seem to be effective

128. A 29-year-old obese female graduate student is admitted to the inpatient psychiatric unit after an overdose. Her liver enzymes are trending down, and she no longer complains of nausea. She endorses having depression with accompanying anxiety, manifested by restlessness, primary insomnia, and irritability. She meets the criteria for the diagnosis of a recurrent major depression. Although the patient is agreeable to starting a selective serotonin reuptake inhibitor

(SSRI), she admits to being wary about antidepressants because she is concerned about their side effects. You counsel her that which of the following statements is true regarding the various medications in this antidepressant class?

A. Paroxetine would be ideal because of its low risk of weight gain.
B. Fluoxetine can be started at 20 mg/day with little risk of increasing her anxiety.
C. Sertraline may cause diarrhea initially, with a decrease in this side effect typically by the second or third week of dosing.
D. Citalopram is purported to have fewer side effects than escitalopram.
E. Sexual dysfunction is a possible side effect of SSRIs but is primarily seen in males and is manifested as erectile and ejaculatory dysfunction.

129. A 33-year-old woman remains in the hospital several days after the cesarean section delivery of a healthy infant boy. You are asked to evaluate the mother because she is experiencing mood lability, tearfulness, and anxiety. Which of the following is her most likely diagnosis?

A. Postpartum psychosis
B. Postpartum depression
C. Postpartum panic disorder
D. Postpartum blues
E. Postpartum obsessive-compulsive disorder (OCD)

130. A 36-year-old married man has been admitted from the emergency center to the inpatient psychiatric unit. Over the past several weeks he has experienced a new onset of psychotic symptoms. On examination, the patient demonstrates choreic movements, dysarthria, and a supranuclear gaze palsy. What is his most likely diagnosis?

A. Parkinson's disease
B. Rett's syndrome
C. Tardive dyskinesia
D. Syndenham's chorea
E. Huntington's disease

131. A 68-year-old widower with a history of hypertension and hypothyroidism is being seen in consultation on the inpatient rehabilitation service. He suffered a stroke 2 weeks ago with resultant right-sided hemiplegia and dysarthria. Which of the following statements is true about the psychiatric manifestations of stroke?

A. Depression occurs in 60% to 80% of stroke patients within 2 years of the initial event.
B. Stroke lesions producing depression are more commonly found in the right frontal lobe than in the left frontal lobe.
C. PET reveals bilateral frontal hypometabolism in stroke patients with depression.
D. Poststroke depression does not typically respond to antidepressant medications.
E. Mania occurs almost exclusively with lesions of the left hemisphere.

132. A 13-year-old girl with a long-standing history of seizures, excessive nail biting, and recent onset of menses has been admitted to the neurology service. A psychiatric consultation has been requested. Which of the following is true about the risk factors for the development of psychosis in epilepsy?

A. Seizure focus tends to be right-sided
B. More frequent in males
C. Age of onset during latency
D. Seizure type is often complex-partial
E. Seizure frequency is increased

The next two questions (items 133 and 134) correspond to the following vignette.

A 29-year-old Marine has been admitted through the emergency center to the inpatient unit with symptoms of severe abdominal pain with nausea and vomiting but a soft abdomen, psychosis, and third cranial nerve palsy.

133. What is this patient's most likely diagnosis?

A. Acute intermittent porphyria
B. Narcolepsy
C. Paget's disease
D. Amaurosis fugax
E. Pavor nocturnus

134. Which of the following medications might have precipitated the attack described in this vignette?

A. Aspirin
B. Digoxin
C. Penicillin
D. Chloroquinone
E. Tetracycline

End of Set

135. A 43-year-old married woman with multiple sclerosis (MS) has been admitted to the psychiatric inpatient unit with symptoms of insomnia, trouble concentrating, sadness, and vague thoughts of suicide. Which of the following statements is true about MS?

A. The incidence of MS decreases with latitude.
B. Risk for the development of MS correlates with the latitude at which one lived before age 15.
C. Men are more commonly affected than women.
D. Blacks are more commonly affected than whites.
E. CT scans are more sensitive than MRI for detecting MS plaques.

136. A 26-year-old graduate student with a history of depression has been admitted to the neurology inpatient service for evaluation of persistent headaches. You have been asked to see the patient to evaluate him for mental status changes. The neurologic assessment included an EEG with continuous, focal, polymorphic delta activity with depressed ipsilateral background rhythms. These EEG findings are most consistent with which one of the following diagnoses?

A. Epilepsy
B. Focal brain lesion
C. Early encephalopathy
D. Coma
E. Hepatic encephalopathy

137. A 14-year-old adolescent girl has been admitted to the adolescent psychiatric inpatient unit for evaluation and treatment of anorexia nervosa. The treatment team decides that family therapy is indicated. Which of the following characterizations best describes structural family therapy?

A. Focuses on both the hierarchy of family relationships and the rules of relating that define boundaries within the family
B. Strives to change the repetitive and maladaptive interactional patterns within the family through paradoxical techniques
C. A brief therapy approach that is entirely present-centered
D. Focuses on the understanding of emotions and transference phenomena within the family
E. Relies primarily on object-relations theories

138. A 43-year-old man with a long-standing history of schizophrenia has been hospitalized for the past 10 days after an acute exacerbation of psychotic symptoms and suicidal ideation. The treatment team is meeting to discuss a discharge plan. Which of the following statements about suicide and schizophrenia is true?

A. Approximately 40% of patients with schizophrenia complete suicide.
B. Suicide is more common during middle age.
C. Females with schizophrenia are at higher risk for suicide than are males.
D. Patients with schizophrenia are more likely to complete suicide when their psychosis is under control.
E. Higher education decreases the risk of suicide.

139. A 36-year-old African American male with a history of schizophrenia is admitted to the hospital for pneumonia. He says that he no longer hears voices because he has been stable on clozapine for the past 3 years. Which of the following statements is true regarding this medication?

A. Clozapine differs from other atypical antipsychotics in that it has little effect on the serotonergic system.
B. Because of the 1% to 2% risk for the development of agranulocytosis, monthly monitoring of their white cell counts is mandatory for all individuals taking this medication.
C. Common side effects of clozapine are sedation, excessive salivation, hypotension, hyperthermia, sexual dysfunction, tachycardia, and enuresis.
D. Clozapine is more effective in treating the positive symptoms of schizophrenia than the "typical" antipsychotics such as haloperidol.
E. Clozapine is associated with significant extrapyramidal side effects, including the development of tardive dyskinesia.

140. A 49-year-old married teacher has been admitted to the inpatient psychiatric unit for evaluation and treatment of manic symptoms. Although she has suffered bouts of depression in the past, this occasion is her first psychiatric hospitalization. After treating her with olanzapine and lorazepam for 2 days, the treatment team decides to start her on lithium. Which of the following side effects is most commonly associated with lithium's long-term systemic effects?

A. Weight loss
B. Elevated risk of renal concentrating ability
C. Hyperthyroidism
D. Memory loss
E. Psoriasis

141. A 26-year-old single beautician has been admitted to the inpatient psychiatric unit for treatment of an acute manic episode. Her symptoms include irritability, increased energy, racing thoughts, and rapid speech. She is started on valproic acid and the benzodiazepine clonazepam. Which of the following statements about benzodiazepine treatment is most accurate?

A. High-potency benzodiazepines with short half-lives are less likely to cause physiologic dependence.
B. Low-potency benzodiazepines are associated with treatment-emergent depression.
C. Memory impairment is more commonly associated with high-potency benzodiazepines.
D. The water solubility of benzodiazepines is associated with their effects on memory.
E. The active metabolite of clonazepam is the therapeutic agent.

142. After morning report on the adult inpatient service, the attending psychiatrist asks the first-year residents about the prevalence of psychosis on the unit. Which of the following is the most accurate description of prevalence?

A. The chance of having a negative finding given that no disease is present
B. The proportion of people with a finding or disease in a given population at a given time
C. The chance of having a positive finding given that a disease is present
D. A person without the target condition who has a negative finding
E. The number of new cases of a condition occurring in the population over a specified period of time

The next two questions (items 143 and 144) correspond to the following vignette.

A 33-year-old unemployed computer analyst has been readmitted to the inpatient psychiatric unit for treatment of an acute exacerbation of paranoid schizophrenia.

143. Which of the following statements is true about schizophrenia?

A. The onset of symptoms typically occurs earlier in life for women than for men.
B. One in 100 people will develop schizophrenia in their lifetime.
C. Outcome is worse in people with an acute onset of symptoms.
D. Negative symptoms are easier to treat than positive symptoms.
E. The average age of onset of symptoms is 18 years of age.

144. Which of the following is an accurate statement about the evidence-based management of schizophrenia?

A. Chlorpromazine does not improve symptoms any better than placebo.
B. Considerable evidence indicates that polyunsaturated fatty acids reduce the subsequent need for antipsychotic medication in the treatment of schizophrenia.
C. Continuing antipsychotic medication for at least 6 months after an acute episode significantly reduces relapse rates.
D. Social skills training does not reduce relapse rates.
E. Family therapy is likely to improve adherence with antipsychotic medication.

End of Set

145. A 27-year-old graduate student has been referred for inpatient assessment by his student health center counselor. The student has revealed to his counselor that he has been stalking another student. Which one of the following, if present, would best predict stalking violence in this patient?

A. A major mental disorder
B. Prior sexual intimacy
C. Sobriety
D. Citizenship
E. Threats

The next two questions (items 146 and 147) correspond to the following vignette.

A 46-year-old separated pilot was admitted to the ICU after attempting suicide by overdose with his estranged spouse's medications. His presenting symptoms included hyperreflexia, myoclonus, tremors, confusion, diaphoresis, agitation, and hyperthermia.

146. The patient's symptoms are most consistent with which of the following syndromes?

A. Neuroleptic malignant syndrome (NMS)
B. Lethal catatonia
C. Anticholinergic toxicity
D. Serotonin syndrome
E. Malignant hyperthermia

147. Which of the following medications is most likely causing this patient's syndrome?

A. Chlorpromazine
B. Amitriptyline
C. Haloperidol
D. Alprazolam
E. Paroxetine

End of Set

148. A 26-year-old lawyer has been admitted to the inpatient substance abuse program for treatment of his cocaine addiction. Which one of the following medications is most likely to dampen his cocaine euphoria?

A. Bupropion
B. Naltrexone
C. Fluoxetine
D. Lorazepam
E. Methylphenidate

149. A 16-year-old high school junior has been admitted to the inpatient substance abuse program. Which of the following statements about alcohol use disorders (AUDs) in adolescents is true?

A. Binge drinking in adolescents usually progresses to alcohol dependence in adulthood.
B. Concurrent use of many substances is the exception rather than the rule.
C. Environmental factors account for a significant amount of AUDs in adolescents.
D. There is less psychiatric co-morbidity in adolescents with AUDs than in adults.
E. Adolescents with early-onset alcoholism are less likely to have familial alcoholism.

150. An 83-year-old retired schoolteacher has been admitted to the inpatient psychiatric unit for evaluation and treatment of her recurrent mood disorder. She also suffers from hypertension, mild congestive heart failure, and emphysema. Which of the following statements about combined drug therapy in the elderly is true?

A. A combination of nefazadone and digoxin increases digoxin serum concentrations.
B. Phenelzine combined with nadolol results in tachycardia.
C. Lithium combined with angiotensin-converting enzyme (ACE) inhibitors lowers lithium levels.
D. Nortriptyline combined with lithium is contraindicated in the elderly.
E. Fluvoxamine combined with theophylline may decrease theophylline plasma concentrations.

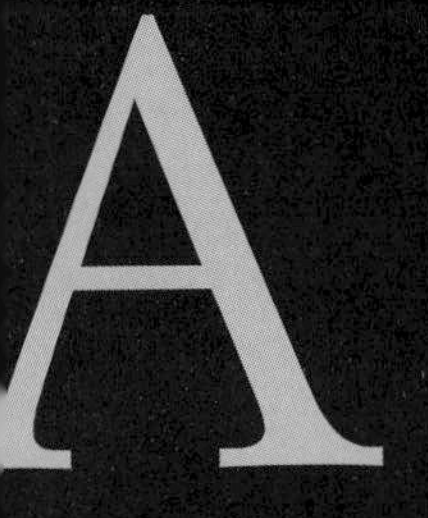

Answers and Explanations

101. E
102. C
103. C
104. C
105. E
106. D
107. C
108. B
109. A
110. A
111. B
112. E
113. A
114. C
115. D
116. E
117. C
118. A
119. E
120. B
121. C
122. E
123. B
124. C
125. A
126. C
127. D
128. C
129. D
130. E
131. C
132. D
133. A
134. D
135. B
136. B
137. A
138. D
139. C
140. B
141. C
142. B
143. B
144. C
145. B
146. D
147. E
148. B
149. C
150. A

101. E. Physical dependence may occur when benzodiazepines are taken in higher than usual dosages or for prolonged periods of time. Other manifestations of anxiolytic withdrawal include autonomic hyperactivity, tremor, insomnia, nausea, anxiety, and even seizures.

A. Although patients with Alzheimer's dementia can experience hallucinations, this patient's presentation with a nearly perfect score on her MMSE is not indicative of dementia.
B. New-onset schizophrenia is highly unlikely in an 83-year-old.
C. New-onset schizoaffective disorder is unlikely at this patient's age.
D. In a hospitalized elderly individual, delirium should always be considered as part of the differential diagnosis. However, this patient does not show other signs of delirium, such as a change in her sleep-wake cycle, a fluctuating level of consciousness, or agitated confusion.

102. C. This patient meets the criteria for a type of somatoform disorder called somatization disorder. A person must have pain in four different body sites or involving four different body functions, two gastrointestinal symptoms (other than pain), one pseudo-neurological symptom (other than pain), and one symptom related to a reproductive organ (other than pain) to be diagnosed with somatization disorder. Some of these symptoms have to be present before age 30 and have persisted for several years. As in this individual, there is often a history of medical and surgical treatments that actually lead to iatrogenic complications. Furthermore, true illness may occur concurrently with somatization disorder, making diagnosis and treatment more complicated.

A, B, D, E. Pain disorder, hypochondriasis, and conversion disorder are types of somatoform disorders. Given the information in this case, the more specific diagnosis of somatization disorder can be made.

103. C. This patient has a substance-induced mood disorder, related to isoniazid. Other mental side effects associated with isoniazid include memory impairment and confusion.

A. The patient is not exhibiting symptoms typical of a major depression except diminished sleep.
B. While she meets the criteria for a manic episode with symptoms lasting at least 1 week or requiring hospitalization, the fact that this patient was recently started on isoniazid requires the consideration of a substance-induced mood disorder, as this medication can induce euphoria, agitation, grandiosity, and psychosis.
D. In this young adult, one might consider the possibility of psychotic symptoms related to the onset of schizophrenia, but manic symptoms would generally not be present. Also, her symptoms have not been present for 6 months or longer, which would be necessary to meet the criteria for schizophrenia.
E. The patient's symptoms are typical of mania, not hypomania, and are seemingly caused by exposure to a substance.

104. C. This is a classic example of delirium. The diagnosis of an elderly patient with no prior psychiatric history, status post a recent operation, with a sudden change in mental status usually is delirium until proven otherwise. This patient is also febrile and is on an IV narcotic, meperidine, which can cause visual hallucinations, especially in the elderly. The primary treatment of delirium is to correct the underlying organic cause.

A. This patient has no prior psychiatric history, and it is unlikely that she would develop schizophrenia at age 77. Her multiple medical issues make delirium a much more logical choice.
B. The patient is disoriented to location, day, date, and year and having visual hallucinations, none of which would likely occur in a pure delusional disorder.
D. Dementia is a slow, insidious change in cognition and mental status seen over a period of weeks, months, or years. This patient's change in mental status occurred within the last few days, status post an operation, making delirium a more accurate diagnosis.
E. The patient's symptoms are more accurately accounted for by her recent medical history and current medical condition rather than by a nonspecific diagnosis such as a brief psychotic disorder, especially given her advanced age and no prior history of psychiatric illness.

105. E. Thiamine deficiency is associated with alcoholism and causes Wernicke's encephalopathy.

A. Vitamin B_{12} deficiency results in pernicious anemia, amblyopia, paresthesias, lower motor weakness, and memory impairment.
B. Vitamin A deficiency results in night blindness, xerophthalmia, and keratomalacia.
C. Ascorbic acid (vitamin C) deficiency results in scurvy. Symptoms of scurvy include lassitude, weakness, irritability, and vague arthralgias.
D. Niacin deficiency results in pellagra. Signs and symptoms of pellagra include glossitis, diarrhea, dermatitis, and mental status changes.

106. D. A sixth cranial nerve palsy causes the ophthalmoplegia associated with Wernicke's encephalopathy.

A. A sixth cranial nerve palsy causes internal strabismus.
B. A sixth cranial nerve palsy causes dysconjugate gaze.
C. A third cranial nerve lesion causes ptosis.
E. A seventh cranial nerve palsy causes facial muscle paralysis and loss of taste on the anterior portion of the tongue.

107. C. Atomoxetine is a clinically effective, FDA-approved nonstimulant useful in treating ADHD. It is a potent inhibitor of presynaptic norepinephrine transporters in the brain.

A. Citalopram is a serotonergic antidepressant; it is not used for the treatment of ADHD.
B. Amitriptyline is a tricyclic antidepressant; it is not used for the treatment of ADHD.
D. Methylphenidate is an FDA-approved stimulant treatment for ADHD.
E. Dextroamphetamine is an FDA-approved stimulant treatment for ADHD.

108. B. Bipolar disorder is both a chronic and a recurrent illness. More than 80% of patients will have a recurrence of depression or mania within 5 years.

A. Bipolar patients are symptomatic 50% of the time, mostly in a depressed phase.
C. Bipolar patients do best with a combination of pharmacologic and psychosocial treatments.
D. Depressed symptoms more typically initiate rapid cycling.
E. Manias tend to be shorter in duration than depressive episodes.

109. A. Along with heart disease, cancer, and AIDS, bipolar disorder is a leading disabling illness.

B. Indirect costs such as missed days at work and burden on caregivers far outweigh the costs for direct medical care.
C. Patients with prolonged subsyndromal symptoms have a worse socioeconomic outcome than simple acute-episode counting.
D. Patients with bipolar disorder have a high rate of divorce.
E. Impaired psychosocial functioning causes more stressful events such as the loss of family supports and financial difficulties, which can exacerbate relapses.

110. A. Fluoxetine is an SSRI antidepressant that can be helpful in relieving symptoms of anger, depression, and aggressive behavior. It is much safer when overdosed than an MAOI or TCA.

B. Phenelzine is an MAOI; although it is an efficacious antidepressant, it would be contraindicated in this patient because of its high lethality upon overdosing.
C. Parnate, an MAOI, would also be contraindicated.
D. Amitriptyline, a TCA, can be lethal on overdose.
E. Imipramine, a TCA, can be lethal on overdose.

111. B. Venlafaxine has a particular side effect of frequently elevating the patient's blood pressure in the range of 5 mm Hg, but sometimes produces even higher pressures. This could be problematic in the borderline hypertensive patient.

A. Although there is a potential for weight gain with many psychotropic medications, venlafaxine is not particularly associated with such effects.
C. Temperature elevation is not an expected side effect from venlafaxine.
D. Respiratory changes are not expected side effects from venlafaxine.
E. Any serotonergic agent has the potential to decrease a patient's pulse rate; the nonspecific noradrenergic property of venlafaxine may elevate the heart rate.

112. E. DBT is a psychotherapeutic strategy specifically helpful for individuals with BPD to decrease suicidal behaviors and mitigate symptomatology.

A. The uncovering process and ambiguities of psychoanalysis tend to promote regression in the BPD patient, which may result in immature behaviors.
B. Although more directive than psychoanalysis, psychodynamic psychotherapy has a similar theoretical base and tends to be reserved for the higher-functioning BPD patient.
C. Cognitive therapy is merely one element of DBT; both employ collaborative problem solving and a focus on the present.
D. Behavioral therapy is another element of DBT; both use direct reinforcement of behavior.

113. A. Antisocial personality disorder (like all of the personality disorders) is listed on Axis II. The other listed diagnoses are included in Axis I or III in the DSM IV format.

B. A differential diagnosis of dissociative symptoms may include seizure disorder, particularly complex partial seizures (especially those originating in the temporal lobe); head injury; sequelae of electroconvulsive therapy or anesthesia; delirium; or dementia.
C. Substance abuse and withdrawal should always be considered when a patient presents with complaints of memory loss. This is particularly true for this young male, who would be at high risk for alcohol and street drug use.
D. Dissociative amnesia is characterized by an inability to recall important personal data beyond what could be explained by ordinary forgetfulness. It is typically precipitated by an intense psychological trauma or stressor, some threat of harm or death, an intolerable or inescapable life situation, or a morally unacceptable impulse or act.
E. A psychological differential diagnosis of the dissociative disorders includes malingering, particularly if a patient in legal difficulties stands to gain by withholding incriminating information.

114. C. Korsakoff's syndrome is associated with filling in memory deficits with false information, a condition called confabulation.

A. Only 20% of patients with Korsakoff's syndrome make a significant recovery.
B. Remarkably, a clear sensorium is typically present.
D. Chronic alcohol abuse for years and nutritional deficiencies cause the syndrome.
E. Postmortem brain studies reveal bilateral lesions in the mamillary bodies rather than in the amygdala.

115. D. Amnesia, unexplained travel, and identity confusion are classic symptoms of dissociative fugue. The treatment approach for dissociative fugue and amnesia includes an adaptational approach in a safe and stable environment. A phasic process with paced retrieval of dissociated information typically works best.

A. Dissociative amnesia is associated with the inability to recall emotionally charged memories; it would not explain this patient's broad symptoms.
B. Depersonalization disorder deals with a sense of detachment from one's body. It would not explain this patient's recent travel, amnesia, or identity confusion.
C. This patient gives no evidence of having multiple personalities, which would be required for a diagnosis of dissociative identity disorder.
E. There is no evidence presented that this patient has abused alcohol or drugs, nor would that explain his recent travel.

116. E. Noncompliance rates among bipolar patients run between 60% and 70%.

A, B, C, D. The 20% to 50% rates are too low in regard to noncompliance among patients with bipolar disorder. After an acute episode resolves, users of lithium take their medication an average of 38% of the days it is prescribed. Only 8% of these patients take the lithium 90% of the days it is prescribed.

117. C. Weight gain is the side effect most commonly related to medication discontinuation.

A. Cognitive dysfunction, including short-term memory and lessened creativity, can occur even with lower or therapeutic lithium levels.
B. Tremor can occur at lower lithium levels but tends to be dose dependent.

D. Acne can occur with lithium use at any age, but especially in adolescent and younger-adult age groups.
E. Hair loss can occur at any lithium level; zinc sometimes helps with this side effect.

118. **A. Dopamine-2 (D_2) blockade in the tuberoinfundibular pathway results in loss of normal suppression of prolactin by dopamine.**
B. D_2 blockade in the mesolimbic area reduces psychosis.
C. D_2 blockade in the mesocortical area reduces psychosis.
D. D_2 blockade in the nigrastriatal pathway causes extrapyramidal symptoms.
E. $5HT_{2C}$ receptor affinity results in weight gain.

119. **E. Haloperidol elevates prolactin levels the most significantly.**
A. Risperidone elevates prolactin levels above the normal range but not as severely as haloperidol.
B. Only quetiapine and clozapine are truly prolactin-sparing antipsychotics.
C. Olanzapine produces transient increases in prolactin levels that usually diminish in weeks.
D. Ziprasidone also produces transient increases in prolactin levels.

120. **B. Quetiapine has the lowest affinity of all the atypical antipsychotics for $5HT_{2C}$ receptors; $5HT_{2C}$ blockade is associated with weight gain.**
A. Risperidone's affinity for $5HT_{2C}$ receptors is much greater than that of quetiapine but less than that of olanzapine and ziprasidone.
C. Olanzapine's affinity for $5HT_{2C}$ receptors is between that of risperidone and ziprasidone.
D. Ziprasidone has the greatest affinity for $5HT_{2C}$ receptors of the medications listed.
E. Haloperidol is not an atypical antipsychotic. Its affinity for $5HT_{2C}$ receptors is the least of the medications listed.

121. **C. According to the AMA code of ethics, a physician should not be part of a legally authorized execution. A physician may testify regarding medical history, diagnoses of mental state as they relate to competence to stand trial, or competence for execution.**
A, B. The prohibitions against involvement in a legally authorized execution include selecting injection sites, starting intravenous lines, and prescribing, administering, or supervising the injection of lethal drugs.
D. A physician may certify death provided that the executed person has been declared dead by someone else.
E. A physician can observe an execution only in a nonprofessional capacity.

122. **E. Bupropion is not commonly associated with sexual side effects; in fact, it is sometimes added to SSRIs to decrease sexual side effects.**
A. Bupropion's major mechanism of action is inhibition of norepinephrine and dopamine reuptake.
B. The immediate-release formulation of bupropion may be started at 100 mg twice a day and increased after 3 days to a standard dosing of 100 mg three times a day. The sustained-release formulation of bupropion has allowed the dosing frequency to be decreased to only twice daily. Bupropion SR also has increased tolerability, especially in terms of possibly reducing the frequency of seizures associated with the immediate-release formulation. A third preparation of bupropion (extended release) allows once-daily dosing.
C. A careful eating-disorder history should be obtained before starting a patient on bupropion, as studies have shown an increased risk of seizures in these individuals.
D. The maximum recommended dose of immediate-release bupropion is 150 mg three times daily, for a total of 450 mg/day. Sustained-release bupropion has a maximum recommended dose of 400 mg/day. The risk of seizures is increased significantly when higher dosages are used.

123. **B. A patient with temporal lobe tumors may have auditory and visual hallucinations. The hallucinations may recall a previous experience.**
A. Frontal lobe tumors typically result in memory disturbance and social inappropriateness.
C. A tumor in the cerebellum would likely cause a problem with balance.
D. A tumor in the somesthetic postcentral gyrus region would cause numbness.
E. A tumor in the occipital lobe would result in a visual deficiency.

124. **C. The globus pallidus and putamen are areas of the basal ganglia that receive dopaminergic innervation from the substantia nigra. In combination, these areas are thought to play an important role in movement disorders associated with dopamine-blocking medications.**

A. The motor cortex is associated with voluntary movements but not directly with medication-induced movement disorders.

B. The corpus callosum contains fibers that communicate between the right and left hemispheres.

D. Lesions in the temporal lobe may cause behavioral and emotional changes.

E. Lesions in the spinal cord may cause paralysis and paresthesias, but this region is not directly associated with the medication side effects described here.

125. **A. This patient is having a dystonic reaction to the haloperidol, also called extrapyramidal symptoms (EPS). Benztropine is an anticholinergic medication that is the best treatment for an acute dystonia. Diphenhydramine is another anticholinergic medication that is typically used for this condition. Both medications may be administered orally or intramuscularly if the patient is having difficulty swallowing.**

B. L-Dopa is an accepted treatment for Parkinson's disease, but is not an effective treatment for acute dystonia. Haloperidol is a strong antagonist to the dopamine receptor, and L-Dopa is unlikely to displace the tightly bound haloperidol.

C. Quetiapine is an atypical antipsychotic medication that has a low incidence of EPS, but it would not be an effective acute treatment for a dystonic reaction.

D. Phenytoin is an anticonvulsant that is not an effective treatment for acute dystonias.

E. Metoprolol is a beta blocker that is not an effective treatment for acute dystonias.

126. **C. Tardive dyskinesia (TD) is a potentially irreversible involuntary movement disorder associated with the use of dopamine-blocking drugs such as haloperidol. The risk of developing TD and the potential severity are thought to increase with length of treatment and amount of drug exposure. The risk of TD is also thought to be increased in patients who experience dystonic reactions and other EPS, as in this case.**

A. EPS can include dystonias, akathisia, and cogwheel rigidity. These symptoms may occur during the course of drug exposure, but almost always resolve after the drug is discontinued. While EPS may be a medication side effect, this is not the best answer.

B. EPS can mimic certain features of Parkinson's disease, but these are distinct entities. Development of Parkinson's disease is not associated with use of antipsychotic medications.

D. EPS can mimic certain features of Huntington's disease, but these are distinct entities. Development of Huntington's disease is not associated with use of antipsychotic medications. Patients with Huntington's disease may, over the natural course of their illness, eventually develop psychosis.

E. Akathisia, which is best described as motor restlessness, may cause voluntary movements such as pacing or leg movements. While it may be a side effect experienced during the course of antipsychotic use, it is not the best answer for this question.

127. **D. In this patient who has hyponatremia and hypokalemia, it would not be prudent to start lithium, as this medication could further disrupt the patient's electrolyte status. His BUN:creatinine ratio is greater than 20:1, indicating that the patient is dehydrated. Lithium, even within the recommended therapeutic range, can cause diabetes insipidus and worsen the dehydration. There is no urgent need to restart the medication. An antidepressant such as citalopram should not be started until the patient is on a therapeutic dose of a mood stabilizer to decrease the risk of precipitating a manic episode. Furthermore, any SSRI can cause (or, in this case, worsen) hyponatremia. The patient should be reassessed periodically during his hospital stay and medications restarted pending resolution of his acute medical problems.**

A, B, C. As in the explanation for D, holding this patient's medications is the prudent approach.

E. Valproic acid, which is metabolized in the liver, would not be a good choice in this patient with hepatitis and elevated liver enzymes. Stabilization of the acute physical issues supercedes the need to restart his psychiatric medication.

128. **C. Like many SSRIs, sertraline can cause gastrointestinal disturbance such as diarrhea, constipation, or abdominal pain. The diarrhea may be quite significant and inconvenient. Patients should be informed that this side effect typically lessens in severity the longer one takes the medication.**

A. Paroxetine has been known to cause significant weight gain. In a patient who is already overweight, this agent may not be the SSRI of choice.
B. In a patient who has significant agitation and anxiety in addition to depressed mood, it is a good idea to start fluoxetine at 10 mg/day for several days, then increase the dose to 20 mg/day. Fluoxetine may have an "activating" effect during initial dosing, so starting with a low dose will decrease the risk of increasing the patient's subjective feelings of anxiety and restlessness.
D. Escitalopram is the enantiomer of citalopram and is often better tolerated than the older citalopram.
E. Patients of both genders should be educated about the possible risk of sexual dysfunction with SSRIs, which some studies show to be as high as 70%. This side effect can be manifested as decreased libido, erectile dysfunction, or difficulty with orgasm and ejaculation. Particularly in an individual such as this patient, who views starting medication with some trepidation, it would be prudent to reassure her that many options are available to decrease the severity of this side effect. Some examples would be lowering the dose or adding an adjunct agent such as buspirone or bupropion.

129. **D. As many as 85% of new mothers experience postpartum blues, which is a temporary condition usually beginning 2 to 4 days after delivery and relenting within 2 weeks.**

A. Postpartum psychosis is a serious but relatively rare illness. It is characterized by extreme mood lability, agitation, hallucinations, and delusions.
B. Postpartum depression shows the hallmarks of a major depressive episode and has a prevalence of approximately 10%.
C. Postpartum panic disorder is manifested in much the same way as typical panic disorder and can also occur with or without agoraphobia.
E. Postpartum OCD has gained increased recognition and would be manifested with the expected obsessional and/or compulsive symptoms, none of which are described in this patient.

130. **E. Huntington's disease is the most likely diagnosis considering the constellation of symptoms.**

A. Parkinson's disease is manifested by bradykinesia rather than chorea.
B. Rett's syndrome is manifested by autism, ataxia, and stereotypical hand movements in girls.
C. Tardive dyskinesia is also a choreiform disorder but generally occurs when there has been chronic exposure to dopamine-blocking agents such as the typical antipsychotics. TD would be unlikely in a patient with new-onset psychosis.
D. Syndeham's chorea follows group A streptococcal infections. It can be accompanied by irritability and obsessive-compulsive symptoms rather than psychosis. Psychosis is present in 5% to 15% of patients with Huntington's disease.

131. **C. PET reveals bilateral frontal hypometabolism in stroke patients with depression.**

A. Depression occurs in 30% to 50% of stroke patients. Major depression is not correlated with the severity of disability, whereas minor depression is more closely correlated with the severity of disability.
B. Stroke lesions producing depression are more commonly found in the left frontal lobe.
D. Poststroke depression commonly responds to conventional antidepressants.
E. Mania occurs almost exclusively with lesions of the right hemisphere.

132. **D. Psychosis is more likely to occur in individuals with a history of complex-partial seizures.**

A. The seizure focus tends to be left-sided in those developing psychosis.
B. Psychosis is more frequent in females with seizures.
C. Psychotic symptoms usually start during puberty when they are associated with seizures.
E. Psychosis is associated with a diminished frequency of seizures.

133. **A. The porphyrias are rare disorders of heme biosynthesis with neurologic, psychiatric, cutaneous, and other organ manifestations. They are caused by autosomal dominant enzyme defects of heme biosynthesis.**

B. Narcolepsy is a sleep disorder characterized by excessive daytime somnolence, sleep attacks, cataplexy, and sleep paralysis.
C. Paget's disease is a disorder of local bone remodeling, resulting in pain. It usually develops after age 40.
D. Amaurosis fugax is the symptom of partial or complete transient monocular blindness caused by a transient ischemic attack of the retinal vasculature.
E. Pavor nocturnes, also known as sleep terrors, occurs almost exclusively in children.

134. **D. Chloroquine is one of many drugs that may precipitate an attack of acute intermittent porphyria. These drugs activate heme biosynthesis.**

A, B, C, E. Aspirin, digoxin, penicillin, and tetracycline do not exacerbate acute intermittent porphyria.

135. **B. The risk for the development of MS is correlated with the latitude at which one lived before age 15.**

A. The incidence of MS increases with latitude.
C. Women are more commonly affected by MS than are men.
D. Whites are more commonly affected by MS than are blacks.
E. MRI is more sensitive than CT scan for detecting MS plaques.

136. **B. Continuous, focal, polymorphic delta activity strongly suggests a focal lesion.**

A. Spikes, sharp waves, or spike-wave complexes suggest epilepsy.
C. Early encephalopathy typically causes α-rhythm slowing and generalized theta activity on the EEG.
D. The EEG findings of a coma include lack of normal background and reactivity with continuous, generalized, polymorphic delta activity.
E. Hepatic and other metabolic encephalopathies result in periodic triphasic waves on the EEG.

137. **A. Structural family therapy focuses on the hierarchy of family relationships and the rules of relating that define the boundaries between the subsystems of the family.**

B. Strategic family therapy utilizes paradoxical strategies to change repetitive and maladaptive patterns within the family.
C. Solution-focused family therapy is a brief therapy model focusing only on the present.
D. Psychodynamically-oriented family therapy focuses on the understanding of emotions and transference phenomena.
E. Object-relations therapy is a form of psychodynamically-oriented therapy emphasizing the importance of projection and projective identification in family relationships.

138. **D. Patients with schizophrenia are more likely to complete suicide when the psychosis is under control, coincidental with a depressive recovery phase of the illness.**

A. Approximately 10% of patients with schizophrenia complete suicide.
B. The majority of suicides in patients with schizophrenia occur in younger patients.
C. Males with schizophrenia—especially younger males—are at a higher risk for suicide.
E. Higher education is associated with increased suicide risk in patients with schizophrenia, perhaps related to a heightened awareness that their lives have become different.

139. **C. All of these are common side effects of clozapine. Among the atypical antipsychotics, clozapine has very strong anticholinergic effects, compared to quetiapine, risperidone, and olanzapine, which have only mild anticholinergic effects.**

A. Clozapine, like other atypical antipsychotics such as olanzapine, risperidone, and quetiapine, has a relatively weak D_2 binding effect combined with a relatively potent serotonergic effect, which accounts for its side-effect profile.
B. Clozapine is a very effective antipsychotic. However, due to its 1% to 2% risk of causing agranulocytosis, a weekly check of the white blood cell count is a must for patients who take this medication; they are often enrolled in "clozapine clinics" for this reason. Sometimes the white cell count can be done every 2 weeks instead of weekly. The risk of agranulocytosis is the main reason why

clozapine is used only in treatment-resistant psychosis—that is, after an individual has failed previous trials of antipsychotics.

D. Like other atypical agents, clozapine is more effective at treating the negative, as well as the positive, symptoms of schizophrenia as compared to the typical antipsychotics such as haloperidol.

E. Clozapine appears to carry no risk of TD and is not associated with significant EPS. Researchers propose that atypical agents such as clozapine bind more strongly to D_3, D_4, and D_5 receptors than older antipsychotics such as haloperidol and chlorpromazine. These more recently discovered dopamine receptors are found in the frontal cortex and limbic areas rather than in the striatum, which may account for the decreased risk of EPS and TD.

140. **B. The long-term effect of lithium on the kidneys is controversial, but the balance of literature suggests an increased risk of impaired renal concentrating ability.**

A. As many as 50% of lithium recipients will experience a 5% to 10% weight gain; weight loss is practically unheard of.

C. Hypothyroidism, rather than hyperthyroidism, occurs in lithium recipients at rates of 5% to 35%. This effect is much more common in women.

D. Memory loss—in particular, recall or retrieval—is a dose-related, rather than long-term, effect of lithium.

E. Psoriasis is a rare dermatologic effect of lithium use.

141. **C. Memory impairment is more commonly associated with high-potency benzodiazepines such as triazolam and lorazepam.**

A. High-potency benzodiazepines with short half-lives are more likely to cause physiologic dependence.

B. Treatment-emergent depression is more commonly associated with high-potency benzodiazepines.

D. The lipid solubility, rather than water solubility, of benzodiazepines is associated with impact on memory. Clonazepam has low lipid solubility.

E. There is no active metabolite of clonazepam.

142. **B. Prevalence is the proportion of people with a finding or disease in a given population at a given time.**

A. Specificity is the chance of having a negative finding given that no disease is present.

C. Sensitivity is the chance of having a positive finding given that a disease is present.

D. True negative refers to a person without the target condition who has a negative finding.

E. Incidence is the number of new cases of a condition occurring in a population over a specified period of time.

143. **B. Schizophrenia is a relatively common illness; one in 100 people will develop schizophrenia in their lifetime.**

A. The onset of symptoms for schizophrenia is typically earlier in life for men than for women.

C. Outcome is better in people with an acute onset of schizophrenia symptoms. An insidious onset is generally associated with a worse prognosis.

D. Positive symptoms such as hallucinations, delusions, and ideas of reference are easier to treat than the negative symptoms of apathy, self-neglect, and reduced emotion.

E. The average age of onset for schizophrenia is 25 years.

144. **C. Continuing antipsychotic medication for at least 6 months after an acute episode reduces relapse rates.**

A. Chlorpromazine, the prototypical classic antipsychotic agent, does improve symptoms of schizophrenia better than placebos but has many unpleasant side effects such as sedation, orthostatic hypotension, dry mouth, and EPS at higher doses.

B. Little evidence indicates that polyunsaturated fatty acids reduce the need for antipsychotic medications in schizophrenia.

D. Social skills training compared to medication management alone does reduce relapse rates.

E. Family therapy beyond education is unlikely to improve compliance with antipsychotic medication.

145. **B. A strong correlation exists between sexual intimacy and stalker violence. This holds true for both male and female stalkers.**

A. A major mental illness such as schizophrenia does not positively correlate with stalking violence. Stalkers who are psychotic tend to stalk public figures, whereas those who are not psychotic tend to stalk private individuals.
C. Drug and alcohol abuse are predictors of physical injury during stalking.
D. Several studies found prior criminal convictions to be a predictor of stalker violence, but there is no established correlation with citizenship.
E. Only a moderate predictive relationship exists between threats and stalking violence. This correlation tends to be stronger with stalking private individuals versus public individuals.

146. D. The symptoms of hyperreflexia, myoclonus, tremors, confusion, diaphoresis, agitation, and hyperthermia are most consistent with a serotonin syndrome.

A. NMS is typically manifested by severe muscular rigidity, EPS, tachycardia, and hyperthermia.
B. Lethal catatonia has many similarities to NMS.
C. Anticholinergic toxicity results in hot, dry skin, mydriasis, tachycardia, urinary retention, delirium, muscular relaxation, and hyperthermia.
E. Malignant hyperthermia is an inherited disorder whose onset occurs after exposure to specific anesthetic agents that block the neuromuscular junction.

147. E. Paroxetine is an SSRI antidepressant. An overdose with any SSRI could result in a serotonin syndrome.

A. Chlorpromazine is a dopamine receptor-blocking antipsychotic. An overdose with this medication could result in NMS.
B. Amitriptyline is a highly anticholinergic TCA. An overdose with this medication could result in anticholinergic toxicity.
C. An overdose with the antipsychotic haloperidol could result in NMS.
D. Alprazolam is a potent benzodiazepine. An overdose with benzodiazepines results in sedation.

148. B. Naltrexone is an opioid receptor antagonist that might attenuate cocaine euphoria by blocking the endorphins released by cocaine.

A. Bupropion, a dopaminergic antidepressant, could accentuate the effects of cocaine.
C. Fluoxetine, a serotonergic antidepressant, has limited direct effect on cocaine-induced euphoria.
D. Lorazepam, a benzodiazepine, has limited direct effect on cocaine-induced euphoria.
E. Methylphenidate, a dopaminergic stimulant, would enhance the effects of cocaine.

149. C. Environmental factors account for approximately 40% of AUDs in adolescents. They include peer pressure, product advertising, and self-medication for anxiety, depression, and ADHD.

A. Binge drinking in adolescents usually does not progress to alcohol dependence.
B. Concurrent use of many substances such as opiates, marijuana, and cocaine is the rule in adolescents with AUDs.
D. There is more psychiatric co-morbidity in adolescents with AUDs than in adults.
E. Adolescents with early-onset alcoholism are more likely to have familial alcoholism.

150. A. Digoxin combined with the antidepressant nefazodone increases digoxin levels by approximately 25%.

B. The beta blocker nadolol combined with the MAOI antidepressant phenelzine results in bradycardia.
C. Lithium combined with ACE inhibitors increases lithium levels.
D. Lithium combined with the TCA nortriptyline can improve response in major depression but should be used cautiously in the elderly.
E. Fluvoxamine, an SSRI antidepressant, inhibits cytochrome P-450 1A2 and, as a result, can increase theophylline concentrations when the two agents are combined.

SETTING 4: EMERGENCY DEPARTMENT

Generally, patients encountered here are seeking urgent care; most are not known to you. A full range of social services is available, including rape crisis intervention, family support, child protective services, domestic violence support, psychiatric services, and security assistance backed up by local police. Complete laboratory and radiology services are available.

The next four questions (items 151–154) relate to the following vignette.

A 36-year-old Hispanic woman was grocery shopping with her nephew when she experienced a rapid onset of chest pain, diaphoresis, hot flashes, and shortness of breath. She stated that she felt like she was dying. An ambulance was called and transported her to the emergency department (ED), where she was found to be diaphoretic, mildly tachycardic (pulse 106), and hypertensive (142/94). Otherwise, the physical exam was normal. Further testing revealed normal CBC, CMP, cardiac enzymes, and ECG. Urine drug screen was negative. Pregnancy testing was also negative. Within 15 minutes of her arrival to the ED, the patient's vitals had normalized. The patient revealed that she has had several similar but less severe episodes in the past 6 months.

151. What is the most likely diagnosis for this patient?

A. Delusional disorder, somatic type
B. Post-traumatic stress disorder (PTSD)
C. Obsessive-compulsive disorder (OCD)
D. Panic disorder
E. Generalized anxiety disorder (GAD)

152. Which of the following specific phobias is strongly associated with this woman's diagnosis?

A. Apiphobia
B. Agoraphobia
C. Claustrophobia
D. Gynophobia
E. Hydrophobia

153. Which other lab test is routinely performed on patients with these symptoms and is important for accurate diagnosis?

A. Thyroid function test
B. Fasting plasma glucose
C. Plasma cortisol
D. Testosterone level
E. Arterial blood gases

154. Which of the following pharmacologic treatments would most benefit the patient in her acute situation?

A. Sertraline
B. Zolpidem
C. Bupropion
D. Paroxetine
E. Lorazepam

End of Set

155. A 68-year-old male with a longstanding history of bipolar disorder was recently discharged from the hospital. Tonight he is brought to the ED with gait problems, shoulder shaking, elbow rigidity, and tremor. Which of the following combinations of medications is most likely producing these symptoms?

A. Fluphenazine and lithium
B. Risperidone and lithium
C. Risperidone and carbamazepine
D. Risperidone and valproate
E. Fluphenazine and benztropine

156. A 26-year-old graduate student presents to the university hospital ED complaining of insomnia for the past 2 weeks. She is quite distraught because finals are approaching and her poor sleep is making it hard to concentrate. After performing a careful history and examination, you are unable to identify any other problems, so you proceed to instruct her about good sleep hygiene. Which of the following tactics is consistent with that approach?

A. Sleeping-in on the weekends
B. Frequent naps
C. Wind-down time between work and sleep
D. Exercise just before bedtime
E. Later dinner meals

The next three questions (items 157, 158, and 159) correspond to the following vignette.

A 20-year-old college sophomore is brought to the ED by her two roommates. She is tachycardic, hypertensive, and sweating, and she has dilated pupils. Her roommates inform the triage nurse that they were all at a rave dance club several hours before the patient became agitated and incoherent.

157. What is this patient's most likely diagnosis?

A. Acute alcohol intoxication
B. Acute alcohol withdrawal
C. Ecstasy intoxication
D. Marijuana inhalation
E. LSD ingestion

158. What is the correct chemical name for the substance that this patient has taken?

A. Ketanserin
B. Olanzapine
C. 3,4-Methylene dioxymethamphetamine
D. D-lysergic acid
E. Citalopram

159. Which of the following is an expected acute effect from intoxication with the substance that this patient has taken?

A. A sense of distance or aloofness toward others
B. Muscle relaxation
C. Increased appetite
D. Sleepiness
E. Decreased libido

End of Set

160. A 26-year-old separated mother of two infant children has been brought to the emergency center by her older sister. The patient has bruises about her eyes, shoulders, and forearms. She is weeping profusely. In regard to the negative family consequences of substance abuse, which of the following statements is correct?

A. Serious neglect is present in few families with substance abuse.
B. Few male child abusers are substance abusers.
C. Most female child abusers are substance abusers.
D. Nearly half of the women treated for domestic violence drink alcohol heavily.
E. Few male domestic violence assailants drink heavily.

The next three questions (items 161, 162, and 163) correspond to the following vignette.

A 33-year-old man embarking on a cross-country trip was hospitalized at a rural facility for religious grandiosity and extreme verbosity. He is transferred to the university hospital emergency center for further mental status changes, muscular rigidity, elevated temperature, and irregular heartbeats.

161. What is this patient's most likely diagnosis?

A. Manic delirium
B. Akathisia
C. Neuroleptic malignant syndrome
D. Pseudo-parkinsonism
E. Oculogyric crisis

162. Which of the following options is indicated in the management of this patient?

A. Dantrolene
B. Broad-spectrum antibiotics
C. Risperidone
D. Thioridazine
E. Fluid restriction

163. What of the following statements is true regarding this patient's diagnosis?

A. It is an uncommon but potentially fatal condition.
B. It is a common and potentially fatal condition.
C. It is a common and relatively benign condition.
D. It is an uncommon and relatively benign condition.
E. It is seen more frequently with atypical antipsychotic medications than with typical antipsychotic medications.

End of Set

164. A 29-year-old Hispanic homemaker is persuaded to go to the emergency room by a girlfriend who is concerned that she has not left her home in the past 3 weeks. The patient admits that she typically avoids crowded places because she has a fear that she will accidentally urinate in public. This has never happened, but her anxiety about the possibility of this scenario has gotten so severe that she has had to rely on friends to do all of her errands, including grocery shopping. The patient has no history of urinary incontinence, nor any condition that would make this a likely event. When she is at home, she realizes that the likelihood of this event ever happening is close to nil. She denies any episodes of rapid-onset, severe anxiety accompanied by chest pain, shortness of breath, or fears of losing control. What is her most likely diagnosis?

A. Social phobia
B. Agoraphobia without history of panic disorder
C. Panic disorder with agoraphobia
D. Generalized anxiety disorder
E. Delusional disorder

The next two questions (items 165 and 166) correspond to the following vignette.

An 8-year-old girl is brought to the ED by her parents. The parents are bewildered because their daughter has been mute for the past 3 days. The girl's physical exam is normal.

165. What is the most likely diagnosis in this patient?

 A. Catatonia
 B. Stroke
 C. Infection
 D. Drugs
 E. Elective mutism

166. Which of the following is the best approach in the management of an adult patient with mutism?

 A. Prolonged interviewing
 B. Elaborate mental status examination
 C. Empathetic concern
 D. Persistent and close-at-hand observation
 E. Sedative-hypnotic medication

End of Set

167. A 19-year-old college student returns to the emergency room 10 days after being sexually assaulted. Since the assault, she has had recurrent thoughts about the event. She finds it distressing to be in physical proximity to male strangers, even on a crowded street in broad daylight. She has experienced feelings of numbness and "being outside" her body. The patient makes an effort to avoid television shows involving crime and violence. She finds it difficult to sleep at night. Family and friends have remarked to her that she is much more irritable and "jumpy." Because of these symptoms, she has been unable to attend classes and avoids meeting friends at night. This individual meets the criteria for which of the following?

 A. Post-traumatic stress disorder
 B. Acute stress disorder
 C. Adjustment disorder with a mixture of depressed and anxious features
 D. Major depressive disorder
 E. Anxiety disorder not-otherwise-specified

The next two questions (items 168 and 169) correspond to the following vignette.

A 23-year-old woman is brought to the ED by her boyfriend. She is hyperreflexic, hallucinating, and practically insensitive to pain. Her boyfriend admits that both smoked a joint laced with phencyclidine (PCP) only hours before.

168. The proper management of PCP intoxication should include which of the following steps?

 A. Enhanced sensory stimulation
 B. Risperidone
 C. Fluoxetine
 D. Alkalinize urine
 E. Outpatient care

169. Which of the following is a common street name for PCP?

 A. Black beauties
 B. Angel dust
 C. Crack
 D. Horse
 E. Mother's little helpers

End of Set

170. A man brings his wife to the emergency room complaining that she is "out of control." Her behavior changed when she stayed up several nights in a row trying to meet a deadline for her editor. Her sleep has been poor for the past 10 days. The patient is extremely talkative and jumps from topic to topic. She states loudly her plan to author the "greatest novel ever written" and sell it to the largest publishing houses. She has completely disrobed and is attempting to seduce her male nurse. She is very restless and shows extreme affective instability, with laughter often dissolving into crying. In the past year, her husband recalls two episodes lasting approximately 3 to 4 weeks at a time when the patient complained of overwhelming sadness and hopelessness. She seemed uninterested in everything and lost weight due to her poor appetite. During these episodes, she was unable to function at work or at home. In between these depressive episodes there was a period that lasted about 3 or 4 days when the patient talked faster than usual, finished several chapters of her book, and slept for only a few hours at night. In the emergency room, a urine drug screen is negative. Physical exam and routine laboratory results, including TSH level, are normal. The patient has no history of medical problems and is not on any medications. Which of the following statements is true regarding this patient?

A. For a diagnosis of bipolar disorder, type I, to be made, an individual must have at least one manic episode lasting longer than 1 week and one depressive episode lasting at least 2 weeks.
B. Major depressive disorder would have a higher rate of transmission than would bipolar disorder if this couple requested counseling regarding the likelihood of their children having psychiatric illness.
C. This patient meets the criteria for bipolar disorder, type I, with rapid cycling.
D. Prognosis for bipolar disorder is usually better than in major depressive disorder, as patients tend to "burn out" as they age.
E. If this patient had significant hallucinations and delusions, she may have met the criteria for an official diagnosis of schizophrenia and bipolar disorder.

The next three questions (items 171, 172, and 173) correspond to the following vignette.

A 28-year-old part-time carpet cleaner is brought to the ED by the police. He had been picked up outside a nearby convenience market where he was screaming obscenities at customers as they entered the store. On exam he is disheveled, unkempt, agitated, and wild-eyed.

171. Which of the following would constitute an improper reason for using restraints on this patient?

A. Prevention of imminent harm
B. For the convenience of staff
C. Decreasing stimulation
D. Prevention of disruption to the treatment setting
E. As a contingency in behavioral therapy

172. The best practice of subduing a patient by restraints includes which of the following?

A. Including only staff unfamiliar to the patient
B. A three-member restraining team
C. Debriefing
D. Limiting staff involvement to unit personnel
E. Oral medication

173. The means of restraining a pre-adolescent child typically includes which of the following?

A. A five-point restraining technique
B. Negotiation
C. Employing a holding technique
D. Surreptitiously placing medication in the patient's food beforehand
E. Asking involvement from the patient's peers

End of Set

174. A 51-year-old retired postal worker is brought to the emergency room by a close friend for complaints of gross blood in the urine. He is diagnosed by the internist as having hypertrophy of the prostate, and follow-up is scheduled up with a urologist. A psychiatric consultation is requested because the friend who accompanied the patient is worried about the patient's belief that the CIA is spying on him. The patient believes that his house is bugged and that the CIA has started to monitor his movements in his home by flying helicopters over his property at night. He denies having auditory or visual hallucinations, and his friend denies that the patient has shown any bizarre behavior. You diagnose him with delusional disorder. Which of the following statements is true regarding this patient's diagnosis?

A. For this diagnosis to be made, symptoms must be present for at least 1 month.
B. In delusional disorder, the delusional thinking is pervasive, affecting many aspects of the patient's life.
C. The subtype of delusional disorder in this man is best described as grandiose.
D. Even in delusional disorder with a significant depressive component, sole treatment with an antipsychotic for the major symptom of delusional thinking results in a better outcome than a more complicated regimen combining an antipsychotic with an antidepressant.
E. This disorder is mainly distinguishable from schizophrenia, paranoid type, by the time course of the symptoms.

175. A man is brought into the emergency room by the police for treatment of various cuts and abrasions after he was assaulted by a neighbor for spying on the neighbor's wife as she undressed. The patient has had two previous brief incarcerations for similar infractions in the past 12 months. Which of the following statements is true regarding this patient's diagnosis of paraphilia?

A. One paraphilia is mutually exclusive of another paraphilia, making it inadvisable to ask about other possible behaviors.
B. Affected individuals typically are comfortable with self-disclosure of details regarding their behavior.
C. In paraphiliacs whose behavior harms others, cognitive therapy may play a role in treatment.
D. Paraphiliac fantasies are equivalent to paraphiliac disorders.
E. This patient exhibits a type of paraphilia known as frotteurism.

The next four questions (items 176–179) correspond to the following vignette.

A 26-year-old obese, part-time student with a long-standing history of paranoia is brought to the ED by his sister. She is concerned that her brother will act on his threats to harm their neighbor.

176. Which of the following court cases refers to duty to warn?

A. *Rennie vs. Klein*
B. *Stone vs. Proctor*
C. *Blanchard vs. Levine*
D. *Tarasoff vs. Regents of University of California*
E. *Clifford vs. United States*

177. Regarding violent patients, which of the following statements is most correct?

A. Standards for assessment of risk factors do not exist.
B. Standards of care for the prediction of violent behavior do exist.
C. The clinician should assess the risk of violence frequently.
D. A risk-benefit assessment should be conducted after discharge.
E. The potential for violence is independent of the patient's mental state at any given time.

178. The "four D's" of malpractice include which of the following?

A. Data
B. Deviation
C. Debenture
D. Drugs
E. Decree

179. Which of the more common allegations of psychiatric malpractice is claimed most frequently?

A. Undue familiarity
B. Incorrect treatment
C. Suicide
D. Incorrect diagnosis
E. Medication error

End of Set

The next three questions (items 180, 181, and 182) correspond to the following vignette.

A 46-year-old homeless man was brought to the ED by paramedics. He was found lying face down and mumbling to himself at a nearby city park. As he is being placed on a gurney, one of the nurses relates, "I know this patient . . . his name is Bill . . . last time he was here he went into DTs . . . "

180. Which of the following characterizations of delirium tremens (DTs) is correct?

A. Occurs in the majority of chronic alcoholics
B. Usually begins 24 to 36 hours after the last drink
C. Usually occurs in those who have been drinking heavily for 1 to 3 years
D. May last 1 to 5 days
E. If untreated, mortality is the rule

181. Which of the following diets is the best option in the treatment of this patient with impending DTs?

A. Low-fat diet
B. Low-calorie diet
C. Salt-restricted diet
D. High-calorie, high-carbohydrate diet
E. High-protein, low-calorie diet

182. A complication of alcohol withdrawal is Wernicke-Korsakoff syndrome. Which of the following supplements is indicated to help prevent the syndrome from developing in this patient?

A. Folate
B. Multivitamins
C. Vitamin B_{12}
D. Magnesium
E. Thiamine

End of Set

The next two questions (items 183 and 184) correspond to the following vignette.

A 32-year-old former professional boxer is brought to the ED by paramedics. He was found obtunded in the alley next to a nearby convenience store. On examination, he has pinpoint pupils, bradycardia, depressed respiration, and hypothermia.

183. What is this patient's most likely diagnosis?

  A. Cocaine intoxication
  B. Alcohol intoxication
  C. Phencyclidine intoxication
  D. Benzodiazepine intoxication
  E. Opioid intoxication

184. Which pharmacologic intervention is indicated for the treatment of this patient's intoxication?

  A. Diazepam
  B. Flurazepam
  C. Naloxone
  D. Haloperidol
  E. Thiamine

End of Set

185. A 32-year-old single woman comes into the emergency room complaining of fever that has persisted despite multiple trials of oral antibiotics. Her medical record reveals that she has an extensive history of hospitalizations and procedures. One of the residents who treated the patient during the past hospital stay confides that there has been previous suspicion that the woman is inducing these fevers by covert means for the sole purpose of obtaining medical attention. Which of the following statements is true regarding this patient's suspected diagnosis of factitious disorder?

  A. Munchausen's syndrome is a less severe form of factitious disorder.
  B. The patient benefits from or has external incentives for the production of signs or symptoms.
  C. The symptoms in factitious disorder are unconsciously produced.
  D. Patients with this diagnosis often have a background in a medically related field, and are typically educated, intelligent young women of a higher socioeconomic class.
  E. Coexisting medical disease is, by definition, not a possibility with this diagnosis.

186. A 19-year-old soldier is triaged from the field for emergency treatment. He cannot remember the events of a skirmish in which most members of his squad were killed. Which of the following statements is true regarding this patient's diagnosis of dissociative amnesia?

  A. It is more common in males than in females.
  B. Its incidence is thought to increase during disasters.
  C. This disorder is consciously motivated.
  D. Substance abuse is rarely the cause of amnestic episodes.
  E. Psychotropic medications are frequently useful in these episodes.

The next two questions (items 187 and 188) correspond to the following vignette.

A 32-year-old woman comes into the emergency room accompanied by her husband. She has recurrent thoughts and images of drowning her 3-week-old baby in the bathtub. The patient denies having auditory hallucinations commanding her to take this step, and is very distressed by these thoughts. Because of these thoughts and images, she excessively checks on her baby "to make sure he is safe." She denies having poor energy, tearfulness, irritability, periods of sadness, or mood lability. Physical examination reveals a healthy-appearing female who is clean and well groomed. The remainder of the exam and routine labs are unremarkable.

187. What is this patient's most likely diagnosis?

  A. Postpartum blues
  B. Postpartum depression
  C. Puerperal psychosis
  D. Adjustment disorder
  E. Obsessive-compulsive disorder

188. Which of the following medications would be considered first-line treatment of the patient in the preceding clinical scenario?

  A. Sertraline
  B. Risperidone
  C. Haloperidol
  D. Lithium carbonate
  E. Valproic acid

End of Set

189. A 19-year-old, HIV-positive waitress is brought to the emergency center by paramedics after she abruptly "passed out" at work. This is the fourth such episode in less than 3 months. Which of the following signs and symptoms is more likely in seizures than pseudo-seizures and will help confirm your diagnosis?

A. Aura
B. Secondary gain
C. Affected by suggestion
D. Asynchronous body movements
E. Normal EEG

190. A 29-year-old man presents to the emergency center complaining of muscle aches, nausea, and vomiting. Physical exam reveals a fever of 101.4°C, diaphoresis, dilated pupils, and rhinorrhea. Which of the following abused substances is most likely responsible for this presentation?

A. Alcohol
B. Cocaine
C. Amphetamines
D. Heroin
E. Phencyclidine (PCP)

The next two questions (items 191 and 192) correspond to the following vignette.

A 25-year-old homemaker accompanied by her husband is seen in the emergency room complaining of sudden loss of vision. Earlier that day she witnessed her son being hit by a car outside her home. During her neurological exam, she blinks when presented with visual threat. The remainder of her physical and neurological exam is normal. The patient's son sustained only minor fractures. Surprisingly, the patient denies any current anxiety and appears to be quite unconcerned by her loss of vision.

191. What is her most likely diagnosis?

A. Post-traumatic stress disorder
B. Conversion disorder
C. Acute stress disorder
D. Somatization disorder
E. Histrionic personality disorder

192. Which of the following statements is true regarding treatment of this patient's disorder?

A. Studies have shown that confronting the patient results in the most rapid resolution of symptoms.
B. The presence of histrionic personality disorder, "la belle indifference," and secondary gain are sufficient to support a diagnosis of this disorder.
C. Estimates for prevalence of this disorder's symptoms are that it is very rare for patients admitted to a general medical setting.
D. Approximately one in five patients initially diagnosed with this disorder is later diagnosed with somatization disorder.
E. The deficit or symptom in this disorder is intentionally produced, as it is in malingering and factitious disorder.

End of Set

193. A 33-year-old schoolteacher is brought to the emergency center after taking an overdose of her psychiatric medications. She is very irritable, complaining of diarrhea and on examination demonstrating myoclonus, elevated blood pressure, tachycardia, hyperpyrexia, and diaphoresis. Which of the following medications did she most likely take an overdose of?

A. Bupropion
B. Fluoxetine
C. Clozapine
D. Alprazolam
E. Diazepam

The next two questions (items 194 and 195) correspond to the following vignette.

A 16-year-old girl is accompanied to the emergency center by her mother and stepfather. She is acting oddly and responding as if someone not visible to you is in the examination room. She is also grabbing her abdomen as if she is in pain. On physical exam, you are struck by her physical immaturity and a tremor. Screening labs are normal except for an anemia.

194. Which of the following metabolic diseases is the likely diagnosis?

A. Hypothyroidism
B. Wilson's disease
C. Hyperthyroidism
D. Hyperparathyroidism
E. Hypoparathyroidism

195. Which element is associated with the disease described in this vignette?

A. Calcium
B. Phosphorus
C. Copper
D. Iron
E. Sodium

End of Set

196. A 53-year-old attorney with a history of episodic alcohol abuse presents to the emergency center with ataxia and confusion. His clothes smell of urine. He vomits, and then has a tonic clonic seizure and becomes unresponsive. His wife is present and thinks he may have overdosed on his medication. Which medication would be most likely to cause his symptoms?

A. Gabapentin
B. Valproic acid
C. Fluphenazine
D. Lithium carbonate
E. Clonazepam

197. A 68-year-old widower with severe rheumatoid arthritis and hypertension has been transported by the paramedics to the emergency center. His neighbors found him sitting on his front porch, mumbling and disoriented. Which of the following symptoms, if exhibited, would be considered the hallmark for a diagnosis of delirium?

A. Fluctuating mental status
B. Visual hallucinations
C. Illusions
D. Disorientation
E. Affective symptoms

The next two questions (items 198 and 199) correspond to the following vignette.

A 22-year-old Asian student is brought to the university hospital emergency center by her parents. The patient is very distressed, believing both her parents are imposters and involved in a complicated scheme to control the young woman's life. The remainder of the mental status examination is normal, and a urine drug screen is negative.

198. What is this patient's most likely diagnosis?

A. Folie á deux
B. Capgras syndrome
C. Schizophrenia, paranoid type
D. Depersonalization disorder
E. Dissociative identity disorder (DID)

199. The medical student accompanying you during the examination asks you to tell her more about DID. Which of the following characterizations is correct regarding DID?

A. The number of reported cases has been decreasing
B. Often presents after age 40
C. Is frequently associated with substance abuse
D. Cannot be helped with hypnosis
E. Is frequently helped by medications

End of Set

200. A 53-year-old airport security guard is brought to the emergency center by her spouse. You are asked to provide psychiatric consultation because she is irritable, paranoid, and depressed. During your examination of the patient, you are struck by her dry skin, Parkinsonian-like faces, and cogwheel rigidity of her arms. Which of the following endocrine disorders should be included in your differential diagnosis?

A. Addison's disease
B. Cushing's syndrome
C. Hyperparathyroidism
D. Hypoparathyroidism
E. Hyperthyroidism

A

Answers and Explanations

151. D
152. B
153. A
154. E
155. A
156. C
157. C
158. C
159. C
160. D
161. C
162. A
163. A
164. B
165. E
166. C
167. B
168. B
169. B
170. C
171. B
172. C
173. C
174. A
175. C
176. D
177. C
178. B
179. B
180. D
181. D
182. E
183. E
184. C
185. D
186. B
187. E
188. A
189. A
190. D
191. B
192. D
193. B
194. B
195. C
196. D
197. A
198. B
199. C
200. D

151. **D. Chest pain, diaphoresis, hot flashes, shortness of breath, and fear of dying can all be symptoms of panic disorder. Other symptoms of panic may include palpitations, tremulousness, choking, nausea, dizziness, numbness or tingling, chills, feelings of unreality and depersonalization, and fear of going crazy. The rapid onset and short duration are also consistent with a panic attack.**

A. Somatic delusions typically involve concern about parasites, an altered self-image, or fears of giving off a foul body odor. These symptoms must be present consistently for 1 month to make a diagnosis.
B. PTSD is incorrect. There is no evidence that the patient's symptoms are a result of trauma.
C. Although anxiety is also a central feature in OCD, no evidence indicates that the patient had been experiencing recurrent or persistent obsessional thoughts or compulsive behaviors.
E. The patient's symptoms follow a time frame more consistent with a panic disorder in that they are acute, relatively brief, and episodic, unlike the persistent, long-term symptoms of GAD.

152. **B. Agoraphobia, or fear of open spaces, is most closely associated with panic disorder. The other four phobias can be found in persons with panic disorder but are not as prevalent.**

A. Apiphobia is the fear of bees.
C. Claustrophobia is the fear of enclosed spaces.
D. Gynophobia is the fear of women.
E. Hydrophobia is the fear of water.

153. **A. Thyroid function testing is routinely used to rule out hyperthyroidism. Patients with hyperthyroidism can present with symptoms similar to panic disorder.**

B. Fasting glucose is not a routine test in the work-up of panic disorder, although hypoglycemia may cause similar symptoms.
C. Plasma cortisol is not a routine test in the work-up of panic disorder.
D. Testing of testosterone levels is not indicated in the work-up of panic disorder.
E. Arterial blood gases are not routinely measured in the evaluation of panic disorder. If the patient's symptoms persisted or there was evidence of a cardiac or pulmonary condition, such tests could be pursued.

154. **E. Lorazepam is a fast-acting benzodiazepine that is most appropriate for patients for acute management of panic symptoms.**

A. Sertraline, a selective serotonin reuptake inhibitor (SSRI), is useful in the long-term management of panic disorder but will have no immediate beneficial effects for patients.
B. Zolpidem, a non-benzodiazepine hypnotic, is used for the short-term management of insomnia.
C. Bupropion, a selective dopamine reuptake inhibitor (SDRI), is not typically used for first-line treatment of panic disorder.
D. Paroxetine, an SSRI, is useful in the long-term management of panic disorder but will have no immediate beneficial effects for patients.

155. **A. Typical, or first-generation, antipsychotics such as fluphenazine in combination with lithium frequently cause extrapyramidal symptoms (EPS). Their synergistic therapeutic effect likely also causes this side effect, which is more common in elderly patients.**

B. The atypical antipsychotic risperidone combined with lithium is generally well tolerated.
C. Risperidone plus carbamazepine is often well tolerated, although discontinuation of the carbamazepine may elevate the risperidone level and produce EPS.
D. Risperidone combined with valproate is well tolerated.
E. Presumably, the anticholinergic agent benztropine combined with fluphenazine would prevent EPS.

156. **C. Allowing some wind-down time is important before going to bed.**

A. Sleep hygiene includes maintaining a consistent bedtime and wake-up schedule, even on weekends.
B. Good sleep hygiene includes avoiding naps or at least keeping them short.
D. Exercise, but not within 3 hours of going to bed, is considered important to promote good sleep.
E. Good sleep hygiene includes avoiding heavy eating, as well as consumption of tobacco, alcohol, and caffeine near bedtime.

157. **C. Ecstasy is an increasingly popular "club drug" that is often used at all-night dance parties and clubs. The patient's clinical presentation resembles amphetamine toxicity.**

A. Alcohol intoxication would not result in tachycardia and dilated pupils, but more likely vomiting and a strong odor of alcohol.
B. Alcohol withdrawal typically takes many hours after the last drink in a chronically dependent person and is unlikely to cause dilated pupils.
D. Marijuana ingestion is unlikely to result in such a severe physiologic response.
E. LSD, another "club drug," tends not to result in such severe physiologic changes.

158. **C. 3,4-Methylene dioxymethamphetamine (MDMA) is the chemical name for the club drug Ecstasy. As its name implies, Ecstasy is an amphetamine derivative.**

A. Ketanserin is a serotonin antagonist, which, if given before exposure to Ecstasy, can attenuate the response.
B. Olanzapine is an atypical antipsychotic with serotonin- and dopamine-blocking properties.
D. D-lysergic acid is a hallucinogen, better known as LSD.
E. Citalopram is a serotonergic antidepressant that may attenuate some of the psychological effects of Ecstasy.

159. **C. During acute intoxication from Ecstasy, an increased appetite is common but anorexia may follow.**

A. Reported positive effects from Ecstasy include decreased defensiveness and a decreased sense of alienation rather than increased distance or aloofness.
B. Trismus, or jaw clenching, as well as teeth grinding occur with Ecstasy use.
D. Sleepiness, as well as decreased motivation and fatigue, are not experienced during acute intoxication with Ecstasy but rather are after-effects experienced the next day or later.
E. Sexual arousal and increased libido are sought-after positive effects from Ecstasy.

160. **D. Approximately 50% of women treated for domestic violence drink heavily.**

A. Serious neglect is present in more than 40% of drug-abusing families.
B. More than 40% of male child abusers are substance abusers.
C. Approximately 30% of female child abusers are substance abusers.
E. Nearly 90% of male domestic violence assailants drink heavily.

161. **C. Neuroleptic malignant syndrome (NMS) is the likely diagnosis. The clinical history suggests an acute manic episode, necessitating hospitalization in the rural setting and likely exposure to antipsychotic medications as an acute intervention.**

A. It is quite possible that the mania remains, but the physical abnormalities are consistent with NMS.
B. Akathisia is a subjective sense of jitteriness experienced with antipsychotic medications.
D. Pseudo-parkinsonism or EPS would not have the constellation of findings, including rigidity, hyperthermia, and arrhythmia, associated with NMS.
E. Oculogyric crisis is a specific acute dystonia associated with antipsychotic medications.

162. **A. Dantrolene, a skeletal muscle relaxant, can lessen the rigidity and hyperthermia of NMS.**

B. An underlying or concurrent infection is not uncommon in the pathogenesis of NMS, but a specific organism should be identified first as fever is part of the syndrome as well.
C. Risperidone and all other antipsychotics are contraindicated in the management of NMS.
D. Thioridazine, an antipsychotic, is contraindicated in the management of NMS.
E. The hyperthermia, elevated CPK associated with muscular rigidity, and other symptoms all warrant aggressive fluid management.

163. **A. NMS is an uncommon but potentially fatal illness. Approximately 0.2% of patients exposed to typical antipsychotics develop NMS of varying severity. Nearly 40% of patients with NMS develop significant physical complications, and as many as 20% die.**

B, C, D. See the explanation for A.
E. NMS was much more common with the typical antipsychotic medications such as the phenothiazines and haloperidol.

164. B. The diagnosis is agoraphobia without history of panic disorder. This patient has markedly restricted her normal activities due to a fear that she will develop urinary incontinence in public. Agoraphobia is the fear of being in situations from which escape might be difficult if the person develops an embarrassing or incapacitating symptom. More rarely, there is no history of panic disorder, and the fear relates to developing some specific symptoms such as urinary incontinence, vomiting, or cardiac distress.

A. Social phobia is a persistent fear of a situation in which a person is exposed to possible scrutiny by others. In this disorder, the individual is trying to accomplish a voluntary activity (e.g., speaking, writing, eating, urinating) and fears that this activity will be impaired by signs of anxiety (e.g., stuttering, being tremorous while writing, being too self-conscious to urinate). By contrast, in agoraphobia without a history of panic disorder, the individual is afraid of suddenly developing a symptom that is unrelated to the activity he or she is attempting to accomplish.

C. Usually agoraphobia is diagnosed as a qualifier of panic disorder, in which a person avoids certain situations that are associated with having panic symptoms. In this patient, there is no history of symptoms indicating the occurrence of unprovoked panic attacks.

D. This patient has a very specific anxiety, whereas generalized anxiety disorder is characterized by excessive worry about everyday things, more than the average person.

E. A delusion is a fixed, false belief. In contrast, when this individual is not in a public place she has the insight to acknowledge that her thinking is not logical. Insight is typically poor in a person with delusional disorder.

165. E. In children, mutism is more often than not elective. In young adults, it may arise from a multitude of conditions including psychiatric conditions. In older patients, a top concern would be a neurologic condition.

A. Catatonia associated with schizophrenia and mood disorders can be manifested as mutism. Although not the most likely diagnoses in an 8-year-old, these possibilities would be included in the differential diagnosis.

B. A neurologic condition such as stroke would be unusual in a child, especially without other physical findings.

C. A CNS infection could cause mutism but other symptoms would be expected as well.

D. Sedating agents can cause mutism as well as a variety of abused drugs such as hallucinogens. This diagnosis would be less likely in a child.

166. C. Empathetic nursing staff who are with the patient for extensive periods may gain more information.

A. Frequent but brief contacts are more useful than a prolonged interview.

B. Simple, concrete questions are more likely to evoke responses.

D. Surreptitious observation may reveal a malingering aspect or other odd behavior.

E. Often there is an underlying psychosis, so antipsychotic medications are the preferred treatment.

167. B. Acute stress disorder lasts between 2 days and 4 weeks. This patient shows a reexperiencing symptom ("recurrent thoughts about the event"), avoidance symptoms (violent television shows and meeting friends at night), and hyperarousal symptoms (being jumpy and finding it difficult to sleep at night) with onset after a traumatic event.

A. A time period of at least 4 weeks is required for a diagnosis of PTSD, as well as at least one reexperiencing symptom, three avoidance symptoms, and two hyperarousal symptoms.

C. The time course of adjustment disorder involves symptoms that appear within 3 months of a significant event, but then resolve by 6 months after the event. In adjustment disorder, the event that caused the change in mood must be something that may be experienced by the average person during his or her lifetime, such as the loss of a job or the end of a relationship. A violent assault does not fit into this category.

D. Although this patient does have some depressive symptoms, the fact that a traumatic episode that could have led to severe bodily harm or even death precipitated the symptoms is more indicative of an acute stress disorder. Another clue that would eliminate a diagnosis of clinical depression is the time course of 10 days; the time course for major depression is at least 2 weeks.

E. Acute stress disorder is a type of anxiety disorder, but enough details are presented in the history to allow for a more accurate diagnosis of acute stress disorder.

168. **B. Psychotic symptoms should be actively treated with an antipsychotic medication such as risperidone.**

A. Sensory stimulation should be minimized; attempts to reassure the patient may aggravate the situation.
C. An antidepressant such as fluoxetine is not indicated in the treatment of PCP intoxication.
D. The urine should be acidified with ascorbic acid or ammonium chloride to increase excretion.
E. The patient should be monitored closely because large ingestions may result in seizures, coma, and death. Hospitalization is usually indicated.

169. **B. Although relying on street jargon to correctly discern which drugs have been ingested is precarious, the nickname "angel dust" is commonly associated with PCP.**

A. "Black beauties" typically refers to stimulants.
C. "Crack" refers to cocaine.
D. "Horse" refers to heroin.
E. "Mother's little helpers" commonly refers to sedative-hypnotics and benzodiazepines.

170. **C. According to the husband's history, in the past year the patient has had a depressed episode, a hypomanic episode, another depressed episode, and now a full-blown manic episode. Thus the patient meets the requirement for four or more mood cycles in a 1-year period to warrant the qualifier "with rapid cycling." Rapid cycling usually involves one or more manic or hypomanic episodes, but is also diagnosed if all the episodes are depressed, manic, or hypomanic as long as they are separated by periods of remission (or switches to the opposite pole). This qualifier is of clinical relevance, as patients with rapid-cycling bipolar disorder have high rates of nonresponse to lithium. Outcomes may be more successful if the disorder is treated with anticonvulsants, such as carbamazepine or valproic acid.**

A. This patient shows rapid speech, decreased need for sleep, grandiosity, hyperactivity, hypersexuality, and a suggestion of loose associations and flight of ideas. A single manic episode is sufficient for a diagnosis of bipolar disorder, type I.
B. Studies have shown that bipolar disorder has a higher rate of genetic transmission than both major depressive disorder and schizophrenia. In fact, the risk of bipolar disorder transmission is 60% for people with two parents with bipolar disorder, 20% for first-degree relatives of patients with bipolar disorder, and 1% for the general population.
D. Bipolar disorder tends to carry a worse prognosis than major depressive disorder, with episodes of depression or mania occurring closer in time as a person ages.
E. When patients or well-meaning family members give a confusing history of multiple diagnoses, including schizophrenia and bipolar disorder in the same individual, it indicates a lack of communication and education by the patient's treating professional. It may also result from different diagnoses being made by different individuals at different times in the person's life. Interestingly, although no ethnic differences have been found in the occurrence of bipolar disorder, in African American and Hispanic patients of low socioeconomic class, bipolar disorders are often misdiagnosed as schizophrenia. A mixture of mood and psychotic symptoms should be explored in depth to differentiate among a possibility of diagnoses; some examples would be major depressive disorder, severe with psychotic features, or schizoaffective disorder, bipolar subtype. Until clarification can be made, it is best to assign a diagnosis of psychosis not-otherwise-specified or mood disorder not-otherwise-specified to avoid further confusion.

171. **B. Restraints are improperly used for the convenience of the staff or to punish a patient. The expectation is to provide care in the least restrictive environment.**

A. Restraining for the prevention of imminent harm to the patient or staff is indicated if other means such as medication or verbal interventions are ineffective.

C. The agitated, labile patient may require restraints until he or she can be placed in a less stimulating environment than the ED.
D. Restraints are indicated to prevent substantial damage or disruption to the setting. The confined space of an ED may require such measures.
E. Restraining a patient may serve as a contingency to help eliminate disruptive or dangerous behavior.

172. **C. The team, ideally with input from an observer, should critique the intervention with debriefing. This is instructional for the staff, as well as helping them work through antecedent distress on their part.**

A. Including a staff member familiar with the patient may be more comforting to the patient.
B. A five-member team is more appropriate to restrain a patient—one person for each limb and a team leader who also manages the patient's head.
D. Back-up resources—perhaps hospital security—as a show of force can be helpful in encouraging the patient to comply with the intervention.
E. More often than not, once the patient is securely in restraints, providing injectable medication is necessary and should be quickly available to help diminish the inappropriate behavior, agitation, psychosis, or other troublesome symptoms. Oral medications may be offered once the patient becomes cooperative and is able to swallow safely.

173. **C. Pre-adolescent children are not generally restrained in the same manner as larger teenagers or adults. A firm hugging of the child from behind as the patient's arms are held securely to each side may suffice.**

A. The five-member team approach is reserved for larger or markedly agitated younger patients.
B. Once the decision to restrain a patient is made, negotiation may merely lead to further escalation.
D. Medications should not be given to patients surreptitiously.
E. Patient peer involvement is contraindicated.

174. **A. Delusional disorder, formerly termed "paranoia," is a type of psychotic disorder characterized by a nonbizarre, fixed delusional system of at least 1 month's duration. The delusion is nonbizarre, meaning that it involves a situation that can occur in real life, such as being followed, infected, loved at a distance, and so forth. Although the phenomenon that is purported to occur is not real or likely, it is nevertheless possible.**

B. The delusional thinking is circumscribed, not affecting other aspects of the patient's life. Although these patients may appear odd, eccentric, or reclusive, they usually remain outside of hospital settings because they may experience little impairment. Contact with professionals may be more likely related to litigation or general medical problems, as these individuals actively oppose psychiatric treatment and often have poor insight into their illness.
C. The subtypes of delusional disorder are erotomanic, grandiose, jealous, persecutory, somatic, and mixed. A delusion of the grandiose type focuses on possessing inflated worth, power, knowledge, identity, or a special relationship to a deity or famous person. This patient's delusion is best described as persecutory, in which the central theme is that the individual (or someone to whom the individual is close) is being attacked, harassed, cheated, persecuted, or conspired against.
D. Studies indicate that treatment of both the psychotic and the mood symptoms results in an improved outcome. This would also be true in other disorders, such as major depressive disorder with psychotic features.
E. While the time course for delusional disorder (at least 4 weeks) does differ from schizophrenia (at least 6 months), these two conditions are also distinguishable in another way—in delusional disorder there is an absence of bizarre delusions, hallucinations, or disorganized speech and behavior.

175. **C. Paraphiliacs may engage in a variety of distortions to assuage the guilt they feel about the behavior, such as blaming the victim ("he/she made me do it"), or denying the effects on the victim ("I could tell he/she enjoyed it"). Challenging belief systems may involve treatment programs that utilize testimony written by the victim or videos presented from the victim's standpoint.**

A. Paraphilias are characterized by the preferential use of unusual objects of sexual desire or engagement in unusual sexual activity over a period of at least 6 months, causing impairment in occupational or social functioning. Some types of paraphilias are fetishism, frotteurism, pedophilia, and exhibitionism. Multiple paraphilias may be present in the same individual. Thus, when one paraphilia is known, one should screen for other paraphilias.
B. A clinician should never rely solely on report of symptoms by the patient, particularly when the behavior may inflict harm on others. An attempt to obtain corroborative information is necessary in any case of paraphilia.
D. Unless they are recurrent or intense, paraphilic fantasies are not paraphilias but simply normal components of human sexuality.
E. This individual exhibits a disorder called voyeurism, in which a person obtains sexual pleasure from secretly watching people (often with binoculars) undressing or engaging in sexual activity. In contrast, frotteurism is diagnosed when a person has recurrent urges over a 6-month period to rub against or touch a nonconsenting individual, for the purpose of sexual excitation, and either is distressed by these urges or has acted on them.

176. D. *Tarasoff vs. Regents of University of California* and related cases resulted in a ruling in most jurisdictions that a physician has the duty to warn or protect potential victims.

A. *Rennie vs. Klein* dealt with a patient's right to refuse treatment.
B. *Stone vs. Proctor* dealt with standards of care.
C. *Blanchard vs. Levine* dealt with failure to evaluate a patient before administrating medications.
E. *Clifford vs. United States* dealt with the expectation to monitor patients receiving psychotropic medications.

177. C. The clinician should assess the risk for violence frequently and during critical junctures for treatment (e.g., granting of passes, discharge).

A. Professional standards do exist for the assessment of risk factors.
B. There is no standard of care (care is not the same as assessment) for predicting violent behavior.
D. A risk-benefit assessment should be conducted and documented *before* discharge.
E. The potential for violence is dependent on the patient's mental state and concurrent situational factors.

178. B. The "four D's" of malpractice include duty, deviation, damage, and direct causation.

A, C, D, E. See the explanation for B.

179. B. Incorrect treatment is claimed most frequently, accounting for 33% of psychiatric malpractice cases.

A. Allegations of undue familiarity account for approximately 3% of psychiatric malpractice claims.
C. Suicide and attempted suicide claims account for 20% of psychiatric malpractice cases.
D. Incorrect diagnosis is claimed in 11% of psychiatric malpractice cases.
E. Medication error and drug reactions are claimed in 7% of psychiatric malpractice cases.

180. D. DTs may last 1 to 5 days.

A. DTs occur in fewer than 5% of chronic alcoholics.
B. DTs usually begin 48 to 96 hours after cessation or decrease in alcohol intake.
C. DTs usually occur in those who have been drinking heavily for 5 to 15 years.
E. Left untreated, DTs may have a mortality rate as high as 20%.

181. D. The patient with impending DTs should be placed on a high-calorie, high-carbohydrate diet.

A, B, C, E. These are not the best diets in the treatment of impending DTs.

182. E. Thiamine deficiency is thought to be the cause of Wernicke's encephalopathy.

A. Folate deficiency is common in chronic alcoholics, but is not the cause of Wernicke's encephalopathy.
B. Vitamin deficiencies in general are common in chronic alcoholics.
C. Vitamin B_{12} deficiency does not cause Wernicke's encephalopathy.
D. Magnesium is sometimes used to ward off seizures, but does not treat Wernicke's encephalopathy.

183. E. Opioids include opium, morphine, heroin, meperidine, methadone, pentazocine, and propoxyphene. The pinpoint pupils are unresponsive to light.

A. Cocaine and other stimulant intoxication results in restlessness, tachycardia, and dilated reactive pupils.
B. Alcohol intoxication typically causes tachycardia, not bradycardia.
C. Phencyclidine intoxication causes tachycardia and nystagmus.
D. Benzodiazepine intoxication does not alter pupillary response; rather, it resembles alcohol intoxication.

184. C. Naloxone 0.4 to 2.0 mg IV every 2 to 3 minutes until respirations are stable is the antidote for opioid intoxication.

A. Diazepam, as a benzodiazepine, may worsen the patient's respiratory status.
B. Flurazepam, a benzodiazepine, is primarily used to promote sleep.
D. Haloperidol, as an antipsychotic, is not indicated and may complicate this patient's physical status.
E. Thiamine is used in alcohol withdrawal states.

185. D. Having a background in a medically related field allows these individuals to feign symptoms that are initially plausible. Affected persons are typically educated, intelligent individuals.

A. Munchausen's syndrome is a severe form of factitious disorder in which the person tends to wander from hospital to hospital and to change health care practitioners frequently to escape detection of the feigned illness.
B. Unlike malingering patients, the patient with factitious disorder does not benefit from or have external incentives for the production of signs or symptoms. The main goal is to assume the sick role.
C. The symptoms in factitious disorder are consciously produced, but the motivations for the clinical presentation are unconscious and should be addressed in therapy in this manner.
E. True illness may very well be present in a person with factitious disorder, particularly given that these individuals are often the recipients of well-intentioned diagnostic procedures that may result in complications (for example, the formation of adhesions after exploratory surgery). A thorough physical exam and lab work-up should always be done, but reservation should be used when considering invasive diagnostic procedures.

186. B. The incidence of dissociative amnesia is believed to rise during disasters, and this condition may affect as many as 5% to 8% of combat soldiers during wartime.

A. Dissociative amnesia is most common in adolescent and young adult females; it is most rare in the elderly.
C. The psychoanalytic model describes dissociative amnesia as unconsciously motivated. A memory may be so traumatic or laden with conflict that conscious awareness of it would be accompanied by insupportable anxiety. Therefore, the mind activates defense mechanisms such as repression and dissociation to keep the memory from entering conscious awareness.
D. Alcohol and hallucinogen abuse (as well as withdrawal syndromes) must be ruled out when confronted with memory disturbance in an individual. The "alcoholic blackout" is the classic substance-induced amnesia.
E. Psychotropic medications are rarely useful in the treatment of dissociative amnesia. Therapy relies on two principles: (1) removing the patient from the threatening circumstances by hospitalization if needed, and (2) addressing the emotional distress through psychotherapy.

187. E. Obsessive-compulsive disorder (OCD) is a type of anxiety disorder. Patients experience recurrent intrusive, unwanted feelings, thoughts, and images (obsessions) that cause marked anxiety and are to some extent relieved by performing repetitive actions (compulsions). The postpartum period may represent a time of increased risk for the development of OCD.

A. Although this patient is postpartum with the onset of symptoms within 4 weeks after delivery, she does not meet the criteria for postpartum blues, in which women experience mild depressive symptoms during the first week after delivery. This patient denies depressive symptoms other than the distress caused by the recurrent ego dystonic thoughts. Symptoms indicative of "the blues" include dysphoria, mood lability, irritability, tearfulness, anxiety, and insomnia.

B. Postpartum depression is a diagnosis made when a patient meets the criteria for major depressive disorder, with onset of the depressive episode occurring within 4 weeks postpartum.

C. Puerperal psychosis is the most severe form of postpartum psychiatric illness. Puerperal psychosis is rare, affecting approximately 1 to 2 women per 1000 mothers postpartum. Psychotic symptoms and disorganized behavior are observable and cause significant dysfunction. The psychosis is often sudden, appearing within 2 to 4 weeks after delivery, and may include auditory hallucinations or delusions that the child is somehow defective. An affective psychosis is often present.

D. Although having a child is certainly a significant life stressor, the prominent obsessional thoughts make the diagnosis of OCD more appropriate in this case.

188. **A. SSRIs are considered first-line agents for the treatment of OCD. Other options besides sertraline are fluoxetine, paroxetine, citalopram, escitalopram, and fluvoxamine. Clomipramine, a mixed-action agent with potent serotonergic effects, was the first medication found to have an effect on OCD. It is now considered second-line therapy, because the dose titration needed to achieve a therapeutic effect often results in intolerable drowsiness and weight gain.**

B. Risperidone, an antipsychotic, should not routinely be used to treat OCD.

C. Haloperidol, an antipsychotic, is not indicated for OCD.

D. Lithium carbonate, a mood stabilizer, is primarily used to treat bipolar disorder but not OCD.

E. Valproic acid, an anticonvulsant with mood-stabilizing properties, is not routinely used for OCD.

189. **A. Auras are common in organic seizures but not in pseudo-seizures. The pseudo-seizure patient has some conscious control over mimicking the signs and symptoms of a seizure.**

B. Secondary gain should arouse suspicion for pseudo-seizures.

C. Suggestibility should arouse suspicion for pseudo-seizures.

D. Asynchronous body movements should arouse suspicion for pseudo-seizures.

E. A normal EEG should arouse suspicion for pseudo-seizures.

190. **D. Withdrawal from opioids such as heroin will present clinically with nausea, muscle aches, rhinorrhea, pupillary dilation, sweating, fever, and diarrhea. Treatment options include symptomatic stabilization with tapering doses of methadone.**

A. Patients with alcohol withdrawal usually present with agitation, tremors, and elevated vital signs. Alcohol withdrawal would not explain this patient's dilated pupils or rhinorrhea.

B, C. Stimulants such as cocaine or amphetamines would cause agitation and elevated vital signs during intoxication, but usually cause the patient to develop somnolence and dysphoria upon withdrawal. Neither stimulant would explain all of this patient's symptoms. This patient's clinical presentation is more consistent with opioid withdrawal than with either stimulant intoxication or withdrawal.

E. Patients suffering from PCP intoxication typically are agitated, are combative, may demonstrate psychotic symptoms, and have a decreased sensitivity to pain. These symptoms are not consistent with this patient's clinical presentation.

191. **B. This individual suffers from conversion disorder, in which there is an abrupt, dramatic loss of motor or sensory function suggestive of a neurological or medical condition. However, psychological factors are deemed the cause of the illness, as the loss of function is typically preceded by a particular stressor and may have symbolic significance.**

A. To meet criteria A in DSM-IV for PTSD, an individual must have been exposed to a traumatic event. Further diagnostic criteria require a "1-3-2" symptom cluster (referring to criteria B, C, and D in DSM-IV): one reexperiencing symptom, three avoidance symptoms, and two hyperarousal symptoms. PTSD is categorized as an anxiety disorder. This patient denies any anxiety symptoms that would fit criteria B, C, or D for PTSD and, in fact, displays "la belle indifference" that is typical of conversion disorder. The time course for diagnosis of PTSD is greater than 4 weeks.

C. In acute stress disorder, the criteria are essentially the same as those in PTSD except that the time course lasts from 2 days to 4 weeks. Another contrast between acute stress disorder and PTSD is that only a "1-1-1" symptom cluster is required: at least one reexperiencing symptom, one avoidance symptom, and one hyperarousal symptom.
D. Diagnosis of somatization disorder requires a "4-2-1-1" symptom cluster: four gastrointestinal symptoms, two non-gastrointestinal pain symptoms, one pseudo-sexual symptom, and one pseudo-neurological symptom.
E. This patient is not exhibiting any of the symptoms of histrionic personality disorder.

192. D. When a symptom occurs in isolation, it is appropriate to make the diagnosis of conversion disorder. However, conversion symptoms may also occur as a component of other major syndromes, including somatization disorder, schizophrenia, depression, and even general medical or neurological disease.

A. Confrontation is not considered beneficial. Rather, suggestion of cure typically results in eventual resolution of the symptom or deficit.
B. Several traditional clinical features previously associated with conversion, such as secondary gain, histrionic personality, and "la belle indifference," have been shown to have little diagnostic significance. These are considered "soft signs" assisting in a possible diagnosis but having no concrete diagnostic validity. The diagnosis of conversion must ultimately rest on positive clinical findings clearly demonstrating that the etiology of the symptom is not physical disease.
C. Conversion symptoms are actually relatively common in medical practice, especially among patients admitted to a general medical setting.
E. The deficit or symptom in conversion disorder is not intentionally produced or feigned, in contrast to malingering and factitious disorder.

193. B. Fluoxetine is a serotonergic antidepressant. This patient's signs and symptoms of irritability; diarrhea; elevated blood pressure, pulse, and temperature; and diaphoresis are typical of a serotonin syndrome.

A. An overdose with the dopaminergic antidepressant bupropion would cause nausea, vomiting, dry mouth, and possibly seizures.
C. An overdose of the antipsychotic clozaril would likely cause postural hypotension, sedation, hypersalivation, constipation, and possibly seizures.
D. An overdose of the benzodiazepine alprazolam would likely cause drowsiness, ataxia, hypotension, bradycardia, and respiratory depression.
E. An overdose of the benzodiazepine diazepam would have much the same effects as described in the explanation for D.

194. B. Wilson's disease, or hepatolenticular degeneration, can present with a variety of psychiatric symptoms, including psychosis, as well as the physical sequelae associated with impaired hepatic function.

A. Hypothyroidism can also occur in adolescence. The psychiatric symptoms can be those seen in other endocrine or metabolic diseases but the physical findings are quite different, including dry, cold skin and bradycardia.
C. Hyperthyroidism usually occurs later in life (e.g., the fourth or fifth decade) and has different physical findings such as tachycardia; warm, moist skin; and tremor.
D. Hyperparathyroidism typically occurs in the 50- to 60-year-old age group and has physical symptoms expected with hypercalcemia.
E. Hypoparathyroidism can occur at any age. It has similar psychiatric symptoms but different physical findings than those associated with hypocalcemia.

195. C. Copper excess is associated with Wilson's disease.

A. Calcium is associated with parathyroid disease.
B. Phosphorus is also associated with parathyroid disease.
D. Iron deficiency is associated with anemia.
E. Sodium is associated with inappropriate antidiuretic syndrome as well as many other conditions.

196. D. The hallmarks of lithium toxicity include ataxia, tremor, confusion, vomiting, and urinary incontinence. Overdose with lithium carbonate can also lead to coma and seizures.

A. Gabapentin, an anticonvulsant with mood-stabilizing properties, may cause confusion and ataxia in overdose, but would not cause urinary incontinence or seizures.
B. Valproic acid is an anticonvulsant with mood-stabilizing properties; the symptoms experienced with its toxicity or overdose are similar to those observed with gabapentin overdose.
C. Fluphenazine, a phenothiazine antipsychotic, may cause sedation and convulsions in overdose, but its anticholinergic effects would cause urinary retention.
E. Benzodiazepines, such as clonazepam, have anticonvulsant properties, so overdose would not cause seizures.

197. A. Fluctuating mental status is the hallmark of delirium.

B. Visual hallucinations can occur in every psychotic syndrome but suggest an organic etiology and are a common form of hallucinations in delirium.
C. Illusions are associated with the sensory misperception experienced in delirium but are not specific to that syndrome.
D. Disorientation is frequently seen in patients with delirium as well as in dementia, head injury, mental retardation, and other conditions.
E. Affective symptoms such as depression, irritability, and mania are seen in delirium but are not very specific to the condition.

198. B. Capgras syndrome is a nonspecific delusion implying that the patient believes family members have been replaced by imposters. It can exist independent of more extensive psychiatric illness, or can be a component of schizophrenia, dementia, and other syndromes with psychotic symptoms.

A. Folie á deux is a delusion shared between two people.
C. Schizophrenia is too broad a diagnosis for this patient because the patient lacks other specific symptoms typical of that illness.
D. Depersonalization is the experience of detachment from oneself; a true disorder implies persistent symptoms.
E. DID is also known as multiple personality disorder.

199. C. DID is frequently associated with substance abuse.

A. There has been a rise in reported cases of DID, perhaps related to mental health professionals' increased awareness of the disorder.
B. DID typically emerges between adolescence and the twenties; it can occur in childhood but rarely presents as a new disorder after age 40.
D. Hypnosis can be helpful in facilitating access to associated personalities.
E. No evidence indicates that any medication is particularly therapeutic for the dissociative process manifested by patients with DID.

200. D. Hypoparathyroidism can be manifested as dry skin, EPS, diarrhea, tetany, and heart failure.

A. Addison's disease (adrenal cortical insufficiency) is associated with hyperpigmentation and hypotension.
B. Cushing's syndrome (hyperadrenalism) produces symptoms of central obesity, hypertension, diabetes, and acne.
C. Hyperparathyroidism can be very similar to hypoparathyroidism in regard to psychiatric symptoms, but the physical symptoms would be different. They include weakness, anorexia, nausea, constipation, polyuria, and thirst.
E. Hyperthyroidism would likely result in warm and moist skin.

Section

5 Surgery

SETTING 1: COMMUNITY-BASED HEALTH CENTER

You work at a community-based health facility where patients seeking both routine and urgent care are encountered. Many patients are members of low-income groups; many are ethnic minorities. Several industrial parks and local businesses send their employees to the health center for treatment of on-the-job injuries and employee health screening. There is a facility that provides x-ray films, but CT and MRI scans must be arranged at other facilities. Laboratory services are available.

The next three questions (items 1–3) correspond to the following vignette.

A 33-year-old female is seen at your clinic complaining of a 2-month history of diarrhea and intermittent abdominal pain. Prior to her current problem, she was healthy without any medications or prior surgeries. Review of symptoms reveals a recent 25-pound weight loss and recurrent mouth sores. On physical exam, the patient is cachectic with a soft, nontender abdomen. A colonoscopy with biopsy is scheduled for the next day.

1. Which of the following is characteristic of this clinical setting?

   A. Sclerosing cholangitis
   B. Rectal involvement
   C. Treatment via ileoanal pouch procedure
   D. Linear ulcers
   E. Rectal bleeding

2. Your suspicion is confirmed with the biopsies obtained, and medical management is initiated. One year later, the patient is admitted to the hospital due to nausea and vomiting with abdominal pain and distention. An abdominal CT is obtained (Figure 5-2a). Treatment with bowel rest, nasogastric decompression, and IV fluids is instituted. What is the most likely diagnosis?

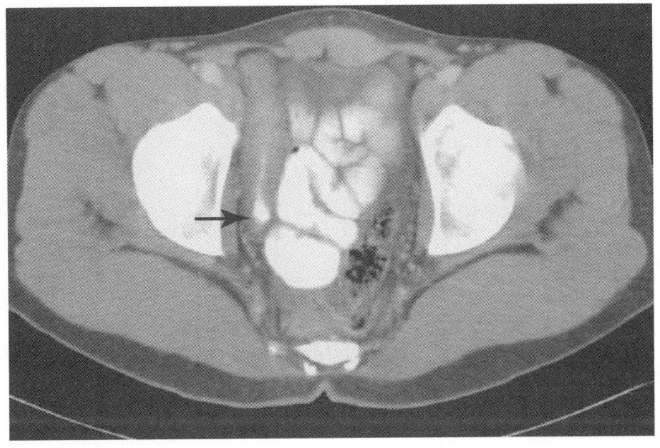

A

Figure 5-2A • Image Courtesy of the University of Utah School of Medicine, Salt Lake City, Utah.

   A. Adhesions
   B. Stricture
   C. Volvulus
   D. Femoral hernia
   E. Pelvic abscess

3. Which of the following is an extra-intestinal manifestation of IBD?

   A. Abdominal pain
   B. Risk of carcinoma
   C. Thickened bowel wall
   D. Sclerosing cholangitis
   E. Lymphoid aggregation

End of Set

The next two questions (items 4 and 5) correspond to the following vignette.

A 50-year-old male with known ulcerative colitis visits your clinic. The patient complains of abdominal pain, pruritis, malaise, fever, and a recent 15-pound weight loss. History includes a total colectomy more than 10 years ago. On physical exam, the patient has mild scleral icterus and is tender in the right upper quadrant.

4. What is the most appropriate next step in this patient's management?

   A. Exploratory laparotomy
   B. CT scan of abdomen
   C. ERCP
   D. MRI of the abdomen
   E. Colonoscopy

5. As this disease progresses, it will most likely result in the need for which surgery?

   A. Laparoscopic cholecystectomy
   B. Liver transplant
   C. Choledochojejunostomy
   D. Open cholecystectomy
   E. Whipple procedure

End of Set

The next two questions (items 6 and 7) correspond to the following vignette.

A 67-year-old male comes to your clinic complaining of a 2-day history of persistent nausea and vomiting, without relief from use of over-the-counter medications. The last time this patient saw a doctor was 2 years ago. He reports to you that he has not had any previous medical problems, takes no medications, and has had a remote appendectomy. On physical exam, the patient appears acutely ill and is tachycardic, with a benign abdominal exam. The following labs are obtained: Na, 147 mmol/L; K, 4 mmol/L; Cl, 110 mmol/L; BUN, 25 mg/dL; Cr, 1.0 mg/dL; glucose, 120 mg/dL; Ca, 13.5 mg/dL.

6. What is the most appropriate first step in management of this patient?

   A. PTH levels
   B. Furosemide administration
   C. Sestamibi scan
   D. IV hydration
   E. Plicamycin

7. This patient's disorder will cause which of the following lab values?

   A. Increased PTH, decreased serum calcium, increased serum phosphate
   B. Increased PTH, increased serum calcium, decreased serum phosphate
   C. Decreased PTH, increased serum calcium, increased serum phosphate
   D. Decreased PTH, decreased serum calcium, increased serum phosphate
   E. Normal PTH, normal serum calcium, normal serum phosphate

End of Set

The next two questions (items 8 and 9) correspond to the following vignette.

A 63-year-old male with a 55-pack-per-year history of smoking and a 35-pound weight loss over the last 4 months presents to your community-based health center with the complaint of blood in his urine for the last 3 weeks. You obtain a urinalysis and confirm the presence of hematuria. You are concerned for the possibility of bladder cancer.

8. Which of the following is the most accurate means of confirming your diagnosis?

   A. Urine culture
   B. Intravenous pyelogram
   C. Cystoscopy with directed and random biopsies
   D. Bladder washings for cytology
   E. MRI of the abdomen and pelvis

9. The patient is diagnosed with a transitional cell cancer of the bladder. A transurethral resection of the bladder tumor (TURBT) is performed through the cystoscope. The tumor is found to be superficial on pathology, with no evidence of invasive or metastatic disease. Regarding bladder cancer, what can generally be stated about treatment, cell type, or the degree of invasiveness?

   A. Most bladder tumors are transitional cell and superficial in depth.
   B. Most bladder tumors are transitional cell and invasive beyond the lamina propria.
   C. Most bladder tumors are metastatic when diagnosed.
   D. Most bladder tumors are high grade, aneuploid when diagnosed.
   E. Most bladder tumors require chemotherapy.

End of Set

The next three questions (items 10–12) correspond to the following vignette.

A 67-year-old male presents to your community-based health center with a history of weight loss, chronic cough, and hemoptysis. The patient has a 65-pack-per-year smoking history. You obtain a chest x-ray, which shows a mass near the hilum of the lung. A CT scan (Figure 5-10) confirms the presence of a centrally located 3 cm mass (indicated by arrow).

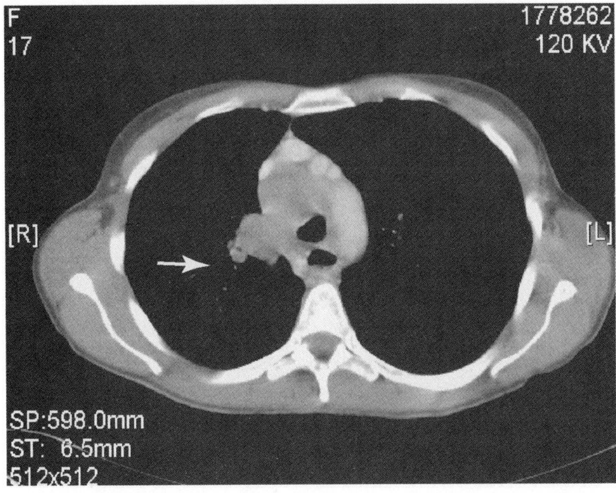

Figure 5-10 • Image Courtesy of the University of Utah School of Medicine, Salt Lake City, Utah.

10. What is the most appropriate next step in management?

    A. Repeat the CT scan in 6 months to look for advancement of the tumor
    B. CT-guided biopsy of the mass
    C. Bronchoscopy with transbronchial biopsy
    D. Mediastinoscopy
    E. Thoracoscopy with biopsy

11. When you receive the pathology report of your biopsy 5 days later, you determine the mass to be unresectable based solely on the biopsy results. Which of the following tumor histologies has the most aggressive natural history?

    A. Squamous cell carcinoma
    B. Adenocarcinoma
    C. Small cell carcinoma
    D. Large cell carcinoma
    E. Hodgkin's disease

12. If the pathology report on this patient showed the tumor to be a squamous cell carcinoma, which paraneoplastic syndrome would he be at most risk for developing?

    A. SIADH
    B. Eaton-Lambert syndrome
    C. PTH-like peptide syndrome
    D. Cushing's syndrome
    E. Ectopic acromegaly

End of Set

The next two questions (items 13 and 14) correspond to the following vignette.

You see a 64-year-old homeless Caucasian male in the outreach clinic who is complaining of abdominal distention. The patient was diagnosed with cirrhosis of the liver secondary to hepatitis C infection more than 10 years ago. He has not seen a physician in more than 5 years.

13. Which of the following is used in determining this patient's Child's classification?

    A. Age
    B. History of smoking
    C. Encephalopathy
    D. Hepatocellular enzyme elevation (ALT, AST)
    E. PTT

14. You determine that the patient fits the definition of Child's class B. The patient also gives a history concerning for diabetes, coronary artery disease, and a 45-pack-per-year history of smoking. What is the best option for intervention for this patient with esophageal varices?

    A. Mesocaval shunt "H" graft
    B. Transjugular intrahepatic portosystemic shunt
    C. Warren distal splenorenal shunt
    D. End-to-side portal caval shunt
    E. Emergent liver transplant

End of Set

15. A 6-week-old male infant is brought to your clinic because of a 2-week history of emesis. The mother describes the emesis as non-bilious and reports it has become projectile over the last 48 hours. On physical exam, the infant's abdomen is soft and a palpable mass is detected in the right upper quadrant. A contrast study is obtained (Figures 5-15A and 5-15B). What is this child's most likely diagnosis?

    A. Duodenal atresia
    B. Cholangiocarcinoma
    C. Hirschsprung disease
    D. Hypertrophic pyloric stenosis
    E. Intestinal malrotation

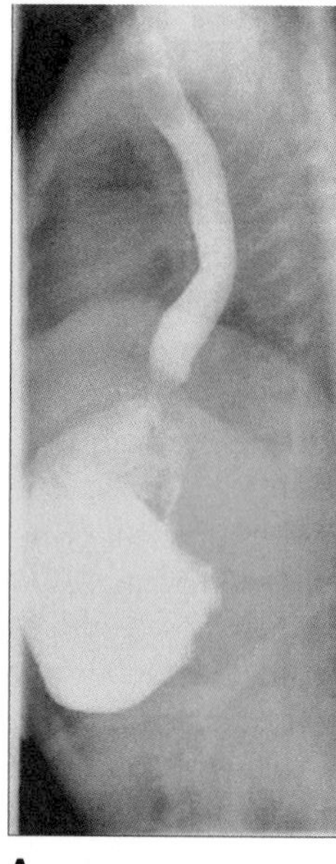
A

Figure 5-15A • Image Courtesy of the University of Utah School of Medicine, Salt Lake City, Utah.

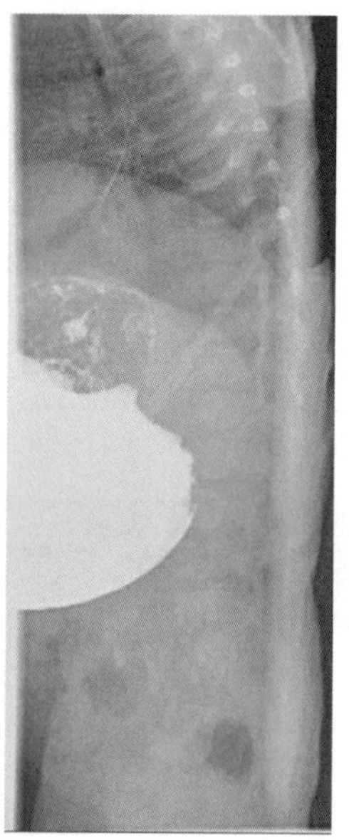
B

Figure 5-15B • Image Courtesy of the University of Utah School of Medicine, Salt Lake City, Utah.

16. A 60-year-old male comes to your clinic with a large mass in his groin that he believes is a hernia. The patient has had this mass for the last 6 months, and it had been easily reducible until this morning. The mass has become increasingly more painful, and the patient is experiencing nausea and vomiting. On exam, the mass is tender to palpation and the hernia appears incarcerated. After giving the patient some midazolam and morphine sulfate in the clinic procedure room, you are still unable to reduce the hernia. What is the next step in management of this patient?

    A. Have the patient return in 12 hours for reevaluation
    B. Ultrasound of the mass
    C. CT scan of the abdomen and pelvis
    D. Upper GI imaging with small bowel follow-through
    E. Emergency surgery

The next two questions (items 17 and 18) correspond to the following vignette.

A 72-year-old male comes to your clinic complaining of a 2-day history of urinary hesitancy, frequent urination, and discomfort upon urinating. A urinalysis demonstrates bacteria, more than 75 WBC, and the presence of leukocyte esterase and nitrites. The patient has non-insulin-dependent diabetes and suffers from arthritis. Currently the patient is not taking any medications. Surgical history includes an appendectomy, cholecystectomy, and cataract surgery. Vital signs are normal. On physical exam, the patient is thin, but otherwise well developed. There is no urethral discharge, and his testicles are nontender to examination. A rectal exam reveals a large, smooth prostate. The remainder of his exam is unremarkable.

17. What is the most likely etiology of these symptoms?

    A. Gonorrhea
    B. Prostate cancer
    C. Kidney stone
    D. Hydronephrosis
    E. Bladder outlet obstruction
    F. Rectal cancer

18. After initial medical management, the patient returns to your clinic 2 months later to report that the symptoms initially improved, but later returned and recently have become significantly worse. You recommend a transurethral resection of the prostate. What should you tell the patient regarding risks if the proposed procedure reveals prostatic cancer?

A. Prostate cancer is rarely fatal
B. Caucasians are the most likely to develop cancer
C. Risk factors include a high-fat diet and tobacco consumption
D. Prostate cancers are universally indolent
E. The majority of patients have locally advanced or metastatic disease when diagnosed

End of Set

19. An 18-month-old male is referred to your clinic by his pediatrician for evaluation of right cryptorchidism. On exam, you are unable to palpate his right testicle and note that his left testicle has descended properly into the scrotum. What is the most appropriate management of this child's cryptorchidism?

    A. Ultrasound
    B. CT scan of the abdomen and pelvis
    C. Orchiectomy
    D. Surgical exploration and scrotal placement of the testicle
    E. Wait until age 4 before operating to allow time for descent of the testicle

The next two questions (items 20 and 21) correspond to the following vignette.

A 38-year-old African American patient with diabetes comes to your outreach clinic complaining of rectal pain and fevers up to 103.1°C. On exam the patient reports that the onset of pain was approximately 5 days ago; it has gotten progressively worse since that time. Fevers started 2 days ago and subside somewhat with acetaminophen administration, but they return as the medication wears off. The only abnormal lab is the WBC, which is 14,800. You perform a rectal exam and find a fluctuant mass on the anterior rectal wall.

20. What is the best initial treatment for this patient's problem?

    A. Admission and IV antibiotics
    B. Referral to radiology for needle drainage
    C. Localization via CT
    D. Evaluation via endorectal ultrasound (ERU)
    E. Surgical drainage

21. Which of the following is a relatively common sequelae of this condition?

    A. Anal incontinence
    B. Colovesical fistula
    C. Anal stricture
    D. Fistula in ano
    E. Anal fissure

End of Set

22. A 42-year-old female visits your clinic for her annual mammogram and breast exam. Upon examination, both her breasts appear normal and there are no palpable masses. The radiology report for the mammogram states there is an area concerning for ductal carcinoma in situ (DCIS). DCIS is a precursor lesion to invasive ductal carcinoma and is treated with surgical resection. Which of the following statements is true of DCIS?

    A. DCIS is usually found on physical exam.
    B. Microcalcifications are usually seen on mammogram in DCIS.
    C. Lumpectomy with axillary dissection is the surgery of choice.
    D. Radiation therapy has no role in the treatment of DCIS.
    E. There is a high risk of lymph node involvement in DCIS.

The next two questions (items 23 and 24) correspond to the following vignette.

A 29-year-old Hispanic male with a 3-week history of vague abdominal pain is referred to your clinic. The patient has been living in the United States for the past 4 months, and he has no prior history of medical illness or surgery. In addition to the pain, the patient complains of some fever and chills, and he has no desire to eat. Vital signs are as follows: T 38.1°C, HR 85, BP 132/65, RR 12, SaO_2 95% on room air. On your exam, the patient is ill appearing, and has fullness in the right upper quadrant associated with pain upon palpation. You observe the following CT scan (Figure 5-23A).

23. Which of the following tests is most likely to aid in the diagnosis of this patient's disease?

    A. Liver function test
    B. Indirect hemagglutination titer
    C. Complete blood count
    D. Indirect Coomb's test
    E. Chemistry panel

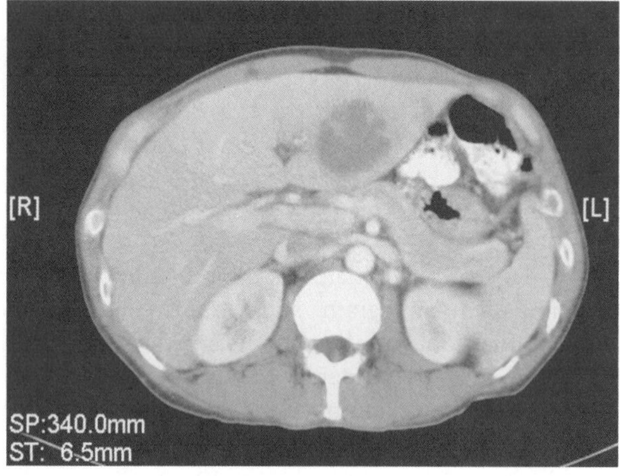

A

Figure 5-23A • Image Courtesy of the University of Utah School of Medicine, Salt Lake City, Utah.

24. What is the most appropriate initial management of this disease?
    A. Oral metronidazole with percutaneous drainage
    B. Operative drainage
    C. Oral metronidazole
    D. IV gentamicin /ampicillin/metronidazole with percutaneous drainage
    E. IV gentamicin /ampicillin/metronidazole

End of Set

The next three questions (items 25–27) correspond to the following vignette.

A 37-year-old female is referred to clinic due to a hepatic mass found on CT scan. The patient denies current right upper quadrant pain and is otherwise healthy. A thorough investigation for cancer by her primary care physician revealed nothing. Patient history does not include any prior abdominal surgery or recent travel outside the United States, but she is allergic to penicillin and takes NSAIDs for occasional headaches. The patient is afebrile and hemodynamically stable, and her labs are within normal limits. You observe the following CT scan (Figure 5-25A).

25. What is the most likely diagnosis?
    A. Hepatic hemangioma
    B. Hamartoma
    C. Hepatocellular carcinoma
    D. Bacterial abscess
    E. Hydatid cyst

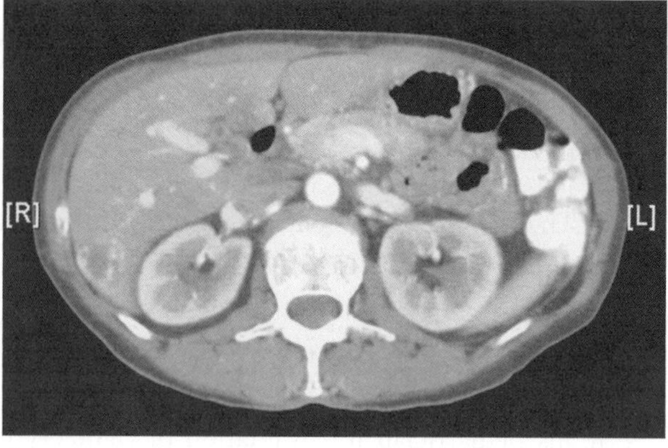

A

Figure 5-25A • Image Courtesy of the University of Utah School of Medicine, Salt Lake City, Utah.

26. Which of the following is the best initial treatment?
    A. Hepatic wedge resection
    B. Percutaneous drainage
    C. Hepatic lobectomy
    D. Observation
    E. Sclerotherapy

27. Which of the following is the most common worldwide cause of hepatocellular carcinoma?
    A. Polyvinyl chloride
    B. Hepatitis B
    C. Hepatitis A
    D. Cirrhosis
    E. Aflatoxins

End of Set

The next three questions (items 28–30) correspond to the following vignette.

A 21-year-old male presents to the emergency department with a 15-hour history of abdominal pain associated with vomiting and a fever. The pain localizes to the right lower quadrant and the WBC count approaches 13,000. The patient undergoes a laparoscopic appendectomy without incident and is discharged from the hospital the next day. The appendectomy pathology report shows a 3 cm mass at the base of the appendix.

28. What is the correct treatment at this point?
    A. Right hemicolectomy
    B. Radiation therapy
    C. Hepatic wedge resection
    D. Observation alone
    E. Trastuzumab

29. At follow-up in your clinic 1 week after hospital discharge, the patient describes a 4-month history of weight loss and fatigue. He also states that he has had loose, watery stools with a decreased appetite. On exam he appears somewhat flushed, and you appreciate end expiratory wheezes throughout both lung fields. The history and findings are most consistent with which tumor?

    A. Adenocarcinoma
    B. Insulinoma
    C. Lymphoma
    D. Gastrinoma
    E. Carcinoid

30. Which of the following tests is most appropriate in confirming the diagnosis?

    A. Serum gastrin
    B. Serum protein C
    C. Colonoscopy
    D. Urinary 5-hydroxyindoleacetic acid (5-HIAA)
    E. Urinary metanephrine

End of Set

The next two questions (items 31 and 32) correspond to the following vignette.

A 30-year-old male visits your clinic with complaints of drainage around his anus. Perianal pain began 1 week ago and increased until yesterday when it acutely improved, but the patient began noticing drainage from this area. The patient has become constipated due to his reluctance to have a bowel movement. He is otherwise healthy, denies allergies, and is not taking any medication. Examination reveals a slightly erythematous area that appears to have spontaneously drained purulent material and has left an open cavity that is freely draining. It is located just lateral to the anus.

31. What is the best next step in this patient's management?

    A. Pack with wet-to-dry saline-soaked gauze
    B. Rectal irrigations with saline-mixed antibiotics
    C. IV antibiotics
    D. Incision and drainage
    E. Warm sitz baths

32. The dentate line is an important surgical landmark in the anus. Which of the following statements best describes this landmark and its significance?

    A. Below the dentate line the innervation is primarily autonomic.
    B. Stratified squamous epithelium is found above the dentate line, whereas columnar epithelium is found below it.
    C. The blood supply, both above and below the dentate line, is derived from the superior rectal artery.
    D. The dentate line defines the level above which transanal excisions are impossible.
    E. There is embryologic differentiation between endoderm and ectoderm.
    F. Malignant cells from above the dentate line will drain to the inguinal lymph nodes.

End of Set

The next two questions (items 33 and 34) correspond to the following vignette.

A distraught young mother brings her 10-month-old male infant to your clinic. The mother tells you that the child began acting different yesterday afternoon, by not being as playful as usual and not wanting to eat. This behavior was followed by vomiting green fluid. According to the mother, the child has become increasingly lethargic, which prompted her to bring him in. On physical exam, the child appears ill and is lying still, the abdomen is distended and diffusely tender, and no peritoneal signs are present. Abdominal films are obtained and are consistent with an obstructive process.

33. What is the next step in management of this patient?

    A. Upper GI imaging with small bowel follow-through
    B. Esophagogastroduodenoscopy
    C. Barium enema
    D. Emergent exploratory laparotomy
    E. Colonoscopy

34. Imaging is performed, and results are consistent with malrotation and midgut volvulus. What is the most appropriate next step?

    A. Endoscopy
    B. IV resuscitation and observation
    C. Gastrografin enema
    D. Air-contrast enema
    E. Exploratory laparotomy

End of Set

35. A 55-year-old female presents to your outreach clinic complaining of an itchy right breast. The patient tells you that she has noticed a rash for approximately 3 months and the area has now started to "drain." On physical exam, you note an erythematous, oozing, eczematoid rash of the right nipple and areolar complex. There are no palpable breast masses and mammogram is normal. Which of the following treatments is appropriate?

    A. Topical steroids and 2-week follow-up
    B. Biopsy area of rash
    C. Wet-to-dry dressings
    D. Lanolin cream and 1-month follow-up
    E. Dermatology consult

The next two questions (items 36 and 37) correspond to the following vignette.

A 42-year-old female returns to your clinic for her annual breast exam. Three years ago the patient underwent a right breast wide local excision and axillary lymph node dissection for an infiltrating ductal carcinoma diagnosis. All 14 of the lymph nodes were negative, and the patient underwent radiation treatment and was prescribed tamoxifen for 5 years. The patient reports that her health has been excellent, but she is concerned about a new area of fullness in her right breast. On exam you palpate a 2 cm area in her right breast. A mammogram is obtained that is concerning for malignancy. A needle core biopsy demonstrates infiltrating ductal carcinoma. A metastatic work-up is done and all tests are negative.

36. What is the most appropriate treatment option?

    A. Lumpectomy with whole-breast radiation
    B. Modified radical mastectomy
    C. Radiation therapy in combination with chemotherapy
    D. Total mastectomy with postoperative radiation for positive chest wall margins and/or chemotherapy
    E. Chemotherapy alone

37. Which of the following syndromes is associated with an increased risk of breast cancer?

    A. Lynch syndrome
    B. Li-Fraumeni syndrome
    C. Brown-Séquard syndrome
    D. Von Hippel-Lindau syndrome
    E. Crow Fukase syndrome
    F. Beckwith-Wiedemann syndrome

End of Set

The next two questions (items 38 and 39) correspond to the following vignette.

A 35-year-old female is referred to your clinic for a new breast lump. The patient tells you that she has done breast self-exams on a monthly basis for at least the last 3 years, and this past month she noticed a lump in her left breast. The patient also tells you that the mass changes in size and tenderness relative to her menstrual cycle. There has been no nipple discharge, and the patient has not had any recent unexpected weight loss. On physical exam, you note bilateral nodular breasts, and a dominant mass in the upper, outer quadrant of the left breast. There are no palpable axillary, supra, or infraclavicular nodes or breast skin changes. Mammography demonstrates dense breast tissue throughout without findings suggestive of malignancy.

38. The current screening guidelines for breast cancer recommend that all women should begin receiving annual mammograms at what age?

    A. 35
    B. 55
    C. 40
    D. 45
    E. 50

39. The patient is very worried and prefers that you perform an excisional biopsy of the mass. This procedure is completed the following week. The pathology report states that the excised breast tissue is consistent with fibrocystic disease without any evidence of atypia, with lobular carcinoma in situ on the superior, medial margin of the specimen. What further treatment is indicated?

    A. Re-excision of the positive margin
    B. Modified radical mastectomy
    C. Radiation therapy
    D. Close observation
    E. Axillary lymph node staging

End of Set

The next two questions (items 40 and 41) correspond to the following vignette.

A 63-year-old male is seen in your clinic for evaluation of a CT-confirmed mass in the head of the pancreas that was found during a work-up for painless jaundice. You refer the patient for an ERCP, at which time brush biopsies are performed. These biopsies reveal adenocarcinoma. Based on the CT findings, the patient appears to have a resectable tumor and you recommend that he undergo a Whipple procedure.

40. What is the most common complication associated with the standard Whipple procedure that you should discuss with the patient?

    A. Delayed gastric emptying
    B. Pancreatic fistula
    C. Wound infection
    D. Bile leak
    E. Pancreatitis

41. What is the most common location of a pancreatic adenocarcinoma?

    A. Tail
    B. Superior
    C. Head
    D. Body
    E. Anterior

The next three questions (items 42–44) correspond to the following vignette.

A 44-year-old male presents to clinic after finding a small lump on the right side of his neck. The patient first noticed the lump 3 weeks ago and thought it would go away, but it has remained unchanged. The patient states that the lump is not painful. He has no other symptoms, is otherwise healthy, takes no medications, and has had no prior surgeries. On physical exam, you note a well-developed male with a 2 cm nodule on the left lobe of the thyroid gland. No lymphadenopathy is appreciated elsewhere on exam, and the remainder of the physical exam is normal.

42. Which of the following is the most appropriate next step in obtaining a diagnosis?

    A. CT scan of the neck
    B. Fine-needle aspiration
    C. Incisional biopsy
    D. Lobectomy
    E. Total thyroidectomy

43. After the correct procedure is performed, the pathology report reads as follows: cells obtained are suspicious of papillary thyroid cancer. The patient is scheduled for surgery. In the operating room the mass is found to measure approximately 2 cm. What is the most appropriate surgical procedure for this patient?

    A. Enucleation of the mass
    B. Thyroid lobectomy
    C. Thyroid lobectomy with isthmectomy
    D. Subtotal thyroidectomy
    E. Total thyroidectomy

44. Following surgery, the patient undergoes radioiodine ablation and is subsequently started on thyroid hormone replacement therapy. Three years later, at a routine clinic visit with his primary care physician, a 1.5 cm firm cervical mass is noted. What laboratory test is most indicative of recurrent tumor?

    A. Thyroid-stimulating hormone
    B. Free T_4 level
    C. Calcitonin
    D. Thyroglobulin
    E. T_3 reuptake level

End of Set

The next two questions (items 45 and 46) correspond to the following vignette.

A 45-year-old male presents to your clinic complaining of abdominal pain. The patient states this pain has been present for the last 6 months, but it now occurs more frequently. He describes the pain as being dull, mainly localized to the epigastrium, radiating on occasion to the right upper quadrant. The pain occurs during times of stress and fasting, and is usually relieved after eating meals. The patient's father and brother both experience many of the same symptoms and have been treated for *Helicobacter pylori* infection in the past. The patient asks you whether such an infection might also be the source of his problem.

45. Which of the following is most often associated with *H. pylori* infection?

    A. Gastric ulcer
    B. Gastric lymphoma
    C. Esophageal ulcer
    D. Gastric carcinoma
    E. Chronic NSAID use
    F. Gastric Maltoma

46. What is the usual initial therapy for patients with symptomatic *H. pylori* infection?

A. Bismuth subsalicylate and metronidazole
B. Parietal cell vagotomy
C. Proton pump inhibitors
D. H_2 blockers
E. Mucosal barrier drugs

End of Set

47. A 54-year-old African American male presents to your clinic with a 3-month history of increasing difficulty with swallowing. The patient states that the difficulty initially began with only solid foods, but now he is also having trouble with liquids. Past medical history is remarkable for a myocardial infarction 4 years ago, a history of alcohol abuse, and a 1.5-pack-per-day smoking habit. Medications include metoprolol and aspirin. On review of systems the patient complains of a 14-pound weight loss over the last 2 months. Vital signs and physical exam are unremarkable. What is the most appropriate next step in the evaluation of this patient?

A. Upper GI
B. Esophagram
C. Thoracic CT scan
D. Endoscopy
E. Enteroclysis

The next three questions (items 48–50) correspond to the following vignette.

A 45-year-old woman comes to your clinic to discuss cadaveric renal transplantation. The patient has polycystic kidney disease complicated by end-stage renal disease and is currently undergoing hemodialysis three times a week. The transplant team has previously evaluated the patient, and recently she has been placed on the transplant waiting list. You are seeing her for preoperative evaluation. During your discussion of the postoperative course, you explain that despite improved immunosuppressive drugs, rejection may still occur.

48. Which of the following descriptions characterizes acute rejection?

A. Associated with a response to minor histocompatibility antigens
B. Occurs rapidly, usually while in the operating room, and is treated by graft removal
C. Is irreversible despite immunosuppressive therapy
D. Primarily caused by a preexisting humoral response of preformed antibodies
E. Mediated by cellular immunity with graft infiltration of small lymphocytes and mononuclear cells

49. Nine months after your initial clinic visit, the patient undergoes a cadaveric renal transplant and has an uncomplicated postoperative course. She is discharged from the hospital on an immunosuppressive regimen of mycophenolate mofetil (CellCept), tacrolimus (Prograf), and a steroid taper with a creatinine level of 1.2. Four weeks after her surgery, during a routine clinic visit, the patient tells you that she is urinating less, has had some weight gain, and is experiencing right lower extremity edema. Vital signs are as follows: T 37.1°C, HR 75, and BP 135/76. The patient appears nontoxic, with clear breath sounds bilaterally, and the incision is healing nicely without erythema or drainage. On abdominal exam, the graft feels "boggy" and is slightly tender to palpation. Laboratory values are as follows: WBC 9000, HCT 35%, PLT 100,000, Na 140 mmol/L, K 4.3 mmol/L, Cl 109 mmol/L, HCO_3 22 mmol/L, BUN 46 mg/dL, creatinine 2.5 mg/dL, and normal Prograf level. An US is obtained (Figure 5-49). What is the most appropriate next step in the management of this patient?

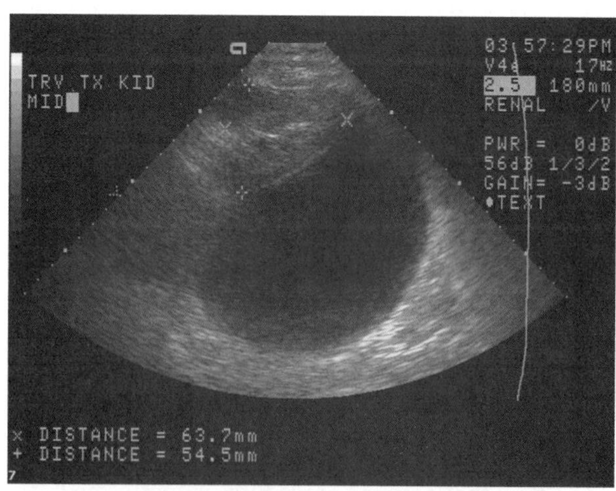

Figure 5-49 • Image Courtesy of the University of Utah School of Medicine, Salt Lake City, Utah.

A. Aspiration of fluid collection for culture and chemistry analysis
B. Reduction of immunosuppressive regimen
C. Percutaneous transplant graft biopsy
D. Prompt increase in immunosuppression to treat acute rejection
E. Reevaluation in 1 week to assess for absorption of fluid collection

50. At the 6-month postoperative clinic visit, the patient complains of pain and pruritis of her back. Vital signs are as follows: T 37.5°C, HR 67, and BP 135/85. On physical exam, you notice an erythematous, papulovesicular rash in a well-defined strip across the right side of the patient's back. Some of the lesions contain scabs. The remainder of the exam is normal. Laboratory values are as follows: WBC 5000, HCT 39%, PLT 120,000, Na 139 mmol/L, K 3.5 mmol/L, Cl 102 mmol/L, HCO_3 24 mmol/L, BUN 12 mg/dL, creatinine 1.0 mg/dL, glucose 99 mg/dL, and Prograf 15 ng/mL. A chest x-ray is normal. What is the most appropriate treatment?

A. Oral acyclovir and follow-up in clinic
B. A reduction in immunosuppressive medications
C. Hospital admission, IV followed by oral acyclovir, and a reduction in the immunosuppressive regimen
D. An increase in the immunosuppressive regimen
E. Close observation

End of Set

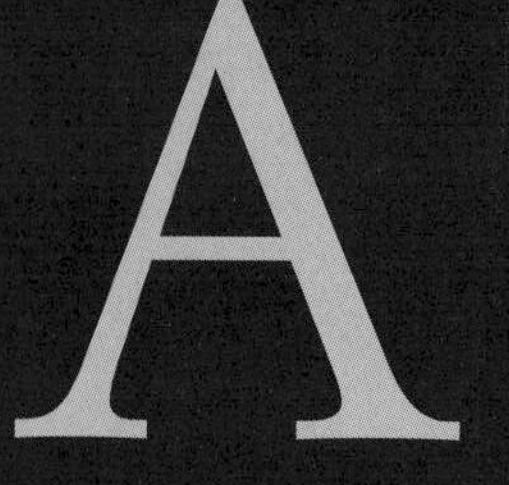

Answers and Explanations

1. D
2. B
3. D
4. C
5. B
6. D
7. B
8. C
9. A
10. C
11. C
12. C
13. C
14. B
15. D
16. E
17. E
18. C
19. D
20. E
21. D
22. B
23. B
24. C
25. A
26. D
27. B
28. A
29. E
30. D
31. A
32. E
33. A
34. E
35. B
36. D
37. B
38. C
39. D
40. A
41. C
42. B
43. E
44. D
45. A
46. A
47. D
48. E
49. A
50. C

1. D. Crohn's disease is a chronic inflammatory disorder of the alimentary tract and can be rapidly progressive or indolent in its course, with a currently unknown etiology. This disease tends to involve transmural inflammation not limited to the mucosa and submucosa like ulcerative colitis. It occurs most commonly between the ages of 15 and 35 years. Most patients present with abdominal pain, weight loss, and diarrhea. Symptoms have usually been present for 2 to 3 years before the diagnosis is confirmed. Intermittent exacerbations are marked by aphthous ulcers, granulomas, and transmural chronic inflammation with fissures and fistulas. Differences between Crohn's disease and ulcerative colitis are demonstrated in Table 5-1.

   A, B, C, E. Sclerosing cholangitis, rectal involvement, treatment via ileoanal pouch procedure, and rectal bleeding are all consistent with ulcerative colitis.

2. B. Medical treatment focuses on immunosuppression with a variety of immunosuppressive medications, such as corticosteroids, sulfasalazine, metronidazole, azathioprine, 6-mercaptopurine, methotrexate, and cyclosporine. Surgical therapy is reserved for complications, including obstruction, bleeding, fistulas, perforation, abscesses, and cancer. The most common cause of obstruction is intraluminal strictures. Small-bowel strictures, like that seen in the abdominal CT (note arrow in Figure 5-2B), are a complication of transmural involvement. Resections of these segments would eventually lead to short bowel syndrome. Strictureplasty is effective at relieving obstructive symptoms without adverse sequelae.

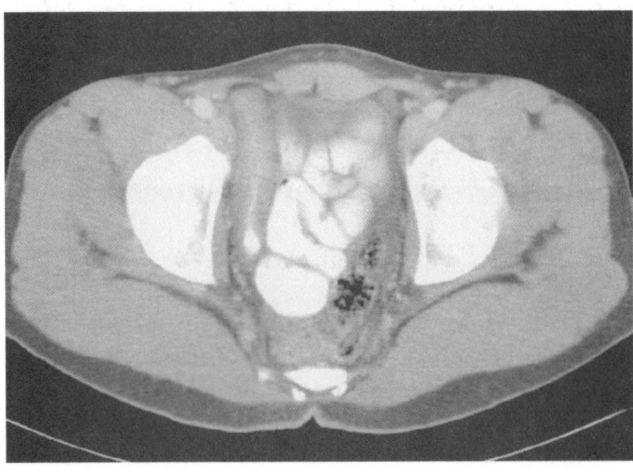

B

Figure 5-2B • Image Courtesy of the University of Utah School of Medicine, Salt Lake City, Utah.

TABLE 5-1 Crohn's Disease versus Ulcerative Colitis

Crohn's Disease	Ulcerative Colitis
Gross Appearance	
Transmural involvement	Mucosal involvement
Segmental disease	Continuous disease beginning in the rectum
Thickened bowel wall	Normal thickness of bowel wall
Creeping fat	Pseudopolyps common
Pseudopolyps rare	Limited to the colon with rare small-bowel involvement
Any section of the alimentary tract may be involved	Perianal disease uncommon
Perianal disease common	
Histological Appearance	
Crypt abscesses uncommon	Crypt abscesses common
Granulomas present	Granulomas absent
Cobblestoning	No cobblestoning
Fistulas	No fistulas
Pseudopolyps absent	Pseudopolyps present
Deep, narrow longitudinal ulcers	Shallow wide ulcers

A. Adhesions would be an extremely rare cause of obstruction because the patient has not had any prior abdominal surgery.
C. Volvulus can be a cause of large-bowel obstruction. It is usually seen in older, debilitated patients. The CT scan obtained demonstrates a small-bowel stricture, not a volvulus.
D. Femoral hernias are more prone to becoming incarcerated, thereby causing obstructive symptoms. The femoral-inguinal area should be thoroughly investigated in anyone with symptoms of bowel obstruction. This patient's clinical picture and CT are most consistent with a Crohn's stricture, however.
E. Intra-abdominal infection may lead to ileus. The CT shows a Crohn's induced stricture, not a pelvic abscess.

3. D. Extra-intestinal manifestations of inflammatory bowel disease (IBD) include aphthous ulcers, pyoderma gangrenosum, iritis, erythema nodosum, sclerosing cholangitis, arthritis, ankylosing spondylitis, and kidney disease. Answers A, B, C, and E are all intestinal manifestations of inflammatory bowel disease.

A. Abdominal pain is more common in Crohn's disease than in ulcerative colitis (UC) but can be seen in both conditions.
B. The risk of carcinoma of the involved bowel is an intestinal manifestation linked to both UC and Crohn's disease.
C, E. Bowel wall thickening is an intestinal manifestation of Crohn's disease, along with creeping fat, segmental involvement, linear ulcers, and lymphoid aggregation.

4. C. This patient has primary sclerosing cholangitis (PSC), which is an idiopathic disorder of the biliary tree. Approximately 50% to 70% of cases are associated with inflammatory bowel disease, most commonly with ulcerative colitis. The risk of PSC remains, even after having a total colectomy. This disease causes multiple intrahepatic and extrahepatic strictures of the bile ducts and is best diagnosed by ERCP. It usually has a characteristic "string of beads" appearance as seen in Figure 5-4 (note arrow).

A. There is no indication for an exploratory laparotomy prior to an appropriate work-up.
B, D. Obtaining either a CT or an MRI of the abdomen is not the preferred way to visualize the biliary tree in this setting.
E. A colonoscopy will not add to the work-up of PSC.

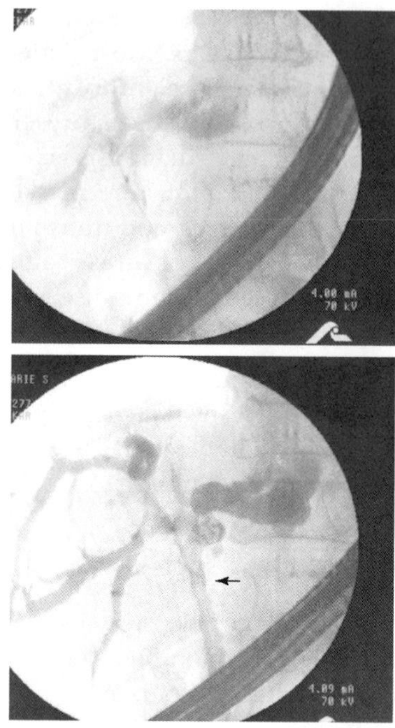

Figure 5-4 • Image Courtesy of the University of Utah School of Medicine, Salt Lake City, Utah.

5. B. PSC is chronic and necessitates a liver transplant in the majority of cases.

A, D. This disease usually involves the entire biliary tree, and removal of only the gallbladder will not address the underlying problem.
C. Although choledochojejunostomy may temporize the complications from extrahepatic involvement, this disease is chronic and progressive. The biliary tree would not be effectively decompressed over the long term by such a procedure.
E. The Whipple procedure is indicated for pathology involving the head of the pancreas, ampulla of Vater, and duodenum. It would not affect the biliary sclerosis seen in this case.

6. D. Hypercalcemia is caused by a variety of disease processes. The most common etiology in an outpatient setting is primary hyperparathyroidism, whereas in hospitalized patients the most common cause is cancer. Other causes

include thiazide diuretics, Paget's disease, vitamins D and A toxicity, sarcoidosis, and milk alkali syndrome. The signs and symptoms of primary hyperparathyroidism are most commonly remembered by the mnemonic "stones, bones, groans, and psychiatric overtones." ECG findings consist of prolonged PR interval with a shortened QT interval. These patients usually present with dehydration, which can be severe in a calcemic crisis as is seen with this patient. The most appropriate initial treatment consists of IV fluid hydration with normal saline.

A, C. A serum PTH level and Sestamibi scan should be used once the patient is stabilized to help identify the source of hypercalcemia.

B, E. Once initial treatment is accomplished, furosemide may be used to reduce the serum calcium level through diuresis. Plicamycin (Mithramycin) may be also used in follow-up treatment for causes of hypercalcemia due to a malignancy.

7. **B. In primary hyperparathyroidism, both calcium and PTH levels are increased, usually due to continued PTH secretion from a parathyroid adenoma. Oversecretion of PTH causes abnormal fluxes of calcium in bone, the kidneys, and the GI tract, resulting in hypercalcemia, hypercalciuria, and increased bone turnover. Serum phosphate level is lowered due to PTH effects on phosphate excretion from the kidney. Although most patients with primary hyperparathyroidism are asymptomatic, as many as 50% will experience subtle neurobehavioral symptoms such as fatigue and weakness ("psychiatric overtones"), 20% will have a history of nephrolithiasis ("stones"), and rarely patients will present with bone pain ("bones" and "groans").**

A. A high PTH level with low or low normal calcium and high serum phosphate levels is most consistent with secondary hyperparathyroidism seen in chronic renal failure. Secondary hyperparathyroidism is caused by low calcium levels, which, in turn, are caused by hypophosphatemia and decreased production of 1,25-dihydroxyvitamin D_2. Severe secondary hyperparathyroidism is an indication for parathyroidectomy if treatment with oral calcium and vitamin D is inadequate.

C. A decreased PTH level is not consistent with primary hyperparathyroidism.

D. Decreased PTH and calcium levels are not consistent with primary hyperparathyroidism, but may be seen with hypoparathyroidism due to damage to all parathyroid glands at surgery, parathyroid agenesis (DiGeorge syndrome), or autoimmune hypoparathyroidism as part of an autoimmune polyendocrinopathy candidiasis ectodermal dystrophy syndrome.

E. Normal levels of serum calcium, phosphate, and PTH are not consistent with the most likely diagnosis of primary hyperparathyroidism.

8. **C. Patients should undergo cystoscopy with directed deep biopsies of suspicious lesions and multiple random biopsies of both the bladder and the prostatic urethra to confirm and stage the disease.**

A. Urine culture is a nonspecific test obtained routinely to evaluate hematuria.

B. Patients suspected of having bladder cancer should eventually undergo an intravenous pyelogram (IVP) to rule out coincident upper urinary tract disease, but an IVP is not specific enough to evaluate a patient for bladder cancer.

D. Bladder washings for cytology would help confirm the diagnosis of bladder cancer, but will not locate or stage the disease.

E. Patients should undergo CT scan of the abdomen and pelvis—not MRI—to rule out metastatic disease and nodal involvement.

9. **A. Transitional tumors account for approximately 90% of all bladder tumors. Approximately 70% of transitional tumors are superficial; the other 30% are invasive or metastatic. Patients in whom the tumor does not invade past the lamina propria do not typically receive adjuvant therapy. Patients with TA and T1 tumors (not invading past the lamina propria) who may be candidates for adjuvant intravesicular chemotherapy include those with high-grade lesions, aneuploid tumors, tumors greater than 5 cm in size, and those with persistently positive cytology. Such patients require close follow-up, because as many as 50% will develop recurrent disease. When recurrence does develop, it is usually at the same stage as the primary tumor.**

B, C, D, E. See the explanation for A.

10. C. **The next step in the work-up of this lung mass is to obtain a tissue biopsy. Definitive diagnosis and staging of the mass are the keys to this patient's management. Because this case involves a centrally located tumor, bronchoscopy with transbronchial biopsy is the most appropriate next step.**

A. Waiting 6 months while looking for advancement of the tumor is not a viable option, because early diagnosis and therapy are key factors in improving survival, particularly with a centrally located mass that may progress to unresectable disease.
B. Because this case involves a centrally located tumor, it would be extremely difficult to biopsy the mass under CT guidance.
D. Mediastinoscopy is indicated for diagnosis if there is CT evidence of lymphadenopathy. With no evidence of a mediastinal mass, mediastinoscopy would be used for staging after diagnosis of a primary lung tumor.
E. Thoracoscopy with biopsy is more easily used in peripherally located masses in the lung.

11. C. **Four types of primary lung tumors exist: adenocarcinoma, squamous cell carcinoma, small cell carcinoma, and large cell carcinoma. Small cell carcinoma (oat cell carcinoma) usually originates in the major bronchus near the hilum. It is known for its rapid growth and early metastasis to both lymphatic and blood vessels. It is therefore considered by many to be metastatic at the time of diagnosis.**

A. Squamous cell carcinoma accounts for 30% of primary malignant lung tumors. It occurs centrally in the segmental, lobar, or mainstem bronchi. Slow growing and late to metastasize, this type of tumor lends itself to resection if diagnosed early enough.
B. Adenocarcinoma accounts for 40% of malignant lung tumors. It is most often peripheral in location. Like squamous cell carcinoma, adenocarcinoma is late to metastasize and may be resectable.
D. Ten percent of malignant lung tumors involve large cell carcinomas, which are also usually located in the periphery. These tumors show rapid growth and early metastasis, but are known to be less aggressive than small cell carcinomas. The majority of large cell carcinomas are poorly differentiated adenocarcinomas.
E. Hodgkin's disease is a lymphoma that usually presents with asymptomatic adenopathy and constitutional symptoms of fever, night sweats, and weight loss. Hodgkin's lymphomas are highly responsive to radiation and chemotherapy.

12. C. **The most likely ectopically produced hormone by squamous cell carcinoma is parathyroid hormone or PTH-like peptide production, leading to hypercalcemia.**

A. SIADH (ADH) is mainly associated with small cell lung cancer.
B. Eaton-Lambert is a neurologic-myopathic syndrome that presents with symptoms similar to myasthenia gravis. This paraneoplastic syndrome is most commonly associated with small cell lung cancer.
D. Cushing's syndrome (ectopic ACTH production) is mainly associated with small cell lung cancer.
E. Ectopic acromegaly is associated with carcinoid tumors of the bronchus, pancreatic islet tumors, and cancers of the lung, breast, colon, and adrenal glands.

13. C. **The Child-Pugh classification of cirrhosis is a method of predicting operative mortality. Patients with cirrhosis are at increased risk for associated morbidity and mortality for any kind of surgery. The operative mortality associated with Child's classes A, B, and C are 2%, 10%, and 50%, respectively. Score A is 5–6, score B is 7–9, and score C is 10 points or higher. See Table 5-13 for the relevant calculation.**

A, B, D, E. Age, history of smoking, ALT and AST levels, and PTT are not used to determine the Child's classification.

TABLE 5-13 Child-Pugh Classification Points

Factor/Points	1	2	3
Serum bilirubin (mg/dL)	<2	2–3	>3
Serum albumin (g/dL)	>3.5	2.8–3.5	<2.8
Ascites	Absent	Mild	Moderate
Hepatic encephalopathy grade	None	1, 2	3, 4
PT (INR)	<1.7	1.7–2.3	>2.3

14. B. A patient with Child's class B cirrhosis and multiple co-morbidities is a poor operative candidate at risk for a significant mortality rate. A transjugular intrahepatic portacaval shunt (TIPSS) is a radiologically guided, percutaneously placed shunt that decompresses the portal venous system to the systemic venous system. It is used in patients who are poor operative candidates, as well as sometimes for sustaining patients who are awaiting a transplant.

A, C, D. The mesocaval shunt, splenorenal shunt, and end-to-side shunt are all portal venous decompressive shunts that require an operative procedure and carry a high mortality rate in a patient with advanced cirrhosis.

E. A patient with Child's class B cirrhosis may eventually be an appropriate candidate for a liver transplant, but in this clinical situation it would not be the best option.

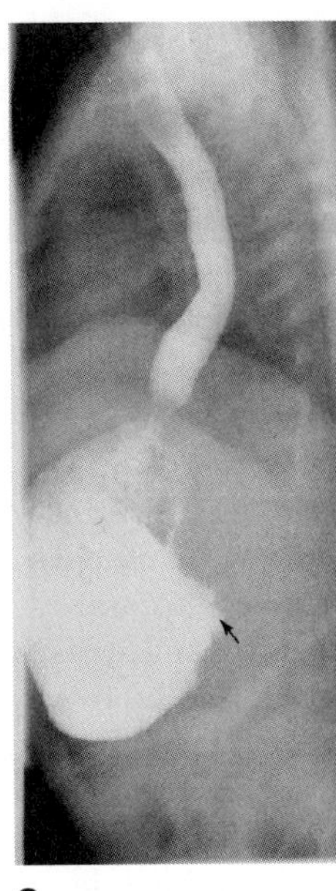

C

Figure 5-15C • Image Courtesy of the University of Utah School of Medicine, Salt Lake City, Utah.

15. D. This is the classic description of hypertrophic pyloric stenosis. Patients present with a history of projectile emesis and often have a palpable, olive-shaped mass in the right upper quadrant. The contrast study images (note the arrows in Figures 5-15C and 5-15D) show the classic gastric outlet obstruction of pyloric stenosis. It is four times more common in male infants and usually presents at 4 to 8 weeks of age. Nonbilious vomiting that increases in volume and frequency is often seen. Dehydration is often seen with a hypokalemic, hypochloremic metabolic alkalosis. All resulting electrolyte abnormalities should be corrected prior to proceeding to the operating room. The Fredet-Ramstedt pyloromyotomy is the classic operation performed. Most patients resume oral intake within 12 hours of surgery.

A. Duodenal atresia presents as bilious emesis in the newborn and is associated with the classic "double bubble" sign on abdominal x-rays.

B. Cholangiocarcinoma is a tumor of the biliary tree; it is not typically seen in children.

C. Hirschsprung's disease presents as a relative colonic obstruction and difficulty passing stool due to an aganglionic segment of the distal colon.

E. Intestinal malrotation is a surgical emergency and must be considered. While infants with malrotation might vomit, they would also have distention and pain, which are not usually found in children with pyloric stenosis.

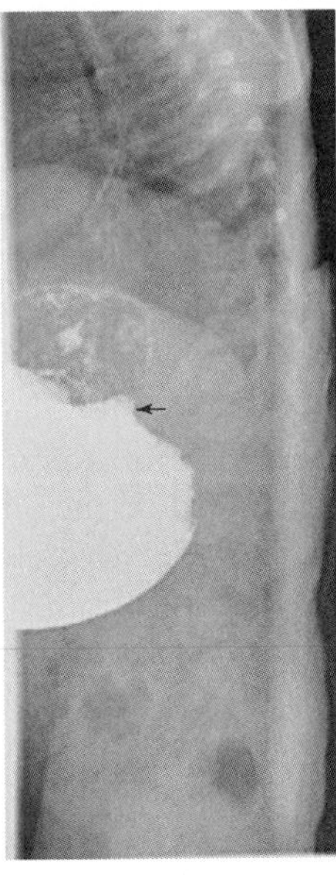

D

Figure 5-15D • Image Courtesy of the University of Utah School of Medicine, Salt Lake City, Utah.

16. E. All incarcerated and strangulated hernias are considered a surgical emergency and should be repaired immediately. Reducible hernias may be repaired on an elective basis. All symptomatic hernias should be repaired with the exception of umbilical hernias in children younger than 4 years of age and adults with severe medical problems such as cirrhosis with ascites.

A. Incarceration of a hernia can lead to ischemia (strangulation) of the contents. Immediate treatment—not reevaluation—is needed. This patient needs to go to the operating room to reduce and repair his hernia and determine whether resection of ischemic bowel is needed.

B, C, D. Nothing found on ultrasound, CT, or upper GI imaging with SBFT would influence the plan for immediate exploration.

17. **E. This patient has a urinary tract infection (UTI) secondary to benign prostatic hyperplasia (BPH). The main symptoms of BPH are categorized as obstructive and irritative voiding symptoms. They are caused by hyperplastic growth of prostatic adenoma in the transition zone of the prostate. BPH is the most common cause of bladder outlet obstruction in men more than 50 years old. Complications include urinary retention, UTIs, bladder stones secondary to stasis, and even renal failure secondary to high-pressure urinary retention. Medical management of BPH includes the use of alpha antagonists (Terazosin) to decrease smooth muscle tone and 5-alpha-reductase blockade (Finasteride) to inhibit the conversion of testosterone to dihydrotestosterone. If medical therapy is unsuccessful, the surgical treatment is transurethral resection of the prostate (TURP). This patient should also be treated with a course of antibiotics for his UTI.**

A. Gonorrhea, a sexually transmitted disease, may cause many of these symptoms and should be included on the differential diagnosis. However, purulent urethral discharge is usually present with this STD.

B. Although a UTI may be present, prostate cancer usually occurs in the peripheral zones of the prostate and does not cause bladder outlet obstruction.

C. Bladder stones, compared to kidney stones, are more likely to cause a UTI. Kidney stones usually result in severe flank pain that radiates into the groin.

D. Although hydronephrosis may be present, it is also a result of bladder obstruction due to BPH.

F. Rectal cancer often presents with rectal bleeding upon bowel movements (hematochezia), alteration in bowel habits, feeling of painful incomplete evacuation (tenesmus), and an intrarectal palpable tumor on rectal exam. Presentation with primarily urinary symptoms would not be the case with rectal cancer.

18. **C. Risk factors that are significant for developing prostate cancer include older age, African ancestry, a positive family history, high dietary fat intake, and cadmium found in cigarette smoke. Unlike most cancers, prostate cancer does not have a peak age of incidence, but its incidence continues to increase with increasing age. Family history is a risk factor, with the age at which the relative was diagnosed being the most significant issue. For example, if the relative was diagnosed at age 70, the patient's relative risk is increased fourfold; this risk increases sevenfold if the relative was diagnosed at age 50. A high fat intake may increase the risk of prostate cancer by almost a factor of 2. Cadmium, found in cigarette smoke, alkaline batteries, and the welding industry, adds to the risk of prostate cancer. Prostate cancer is the most common malignancy affecting men and is the second leading cause of cancer-related death.**

A, D. Prostate cancer is the second leading cause of cancer-related death.

B. African ancestry is a risk factor, with African American patients typically presenting at a later stage of disease as compared to Caucasians.

E. The majority of patients with prostate cancer are asymptomatic. Symptoms suggest the presence of locally advanced or metastatic disease.

19. **D. Cryptorchidism is the failure of normal testicular descent during embryologic development. Its incidence is 1% to 2% in full-term infants and as much as 30% in preterm infants. Placement of the testis into the scrotal sac is indicated after age 1 but prior to age 2. If the testis has not descended into the scrotum by age 1, surgery is indicated to place the testicle in the scrotum. Undescended testes will continue to secrete androgens, but spermatogenic function is progressively impaired. Scrotal placement of the testes should occur prior to age 2 to preserve spermatogenic function. If the testes are not able to be placed successfully into the scrotum, orchiectomy is indicated due to the significantly increased risk of testicular cancer (30 times greater) if the testes are left in an intra-abdominal position.**

A, B. An ultrasound or CT scan would not change the course of management, as described in the explanation for D.

C. After age 2, orchiectomy is indicated due to the increased risk of cancer and spermatogenic failure.

E. Waiting until age 4 would add to the risks of both spermatogenic failure and testicular cancer.

20. **E. A perirectal abscess must be widely opened and drained to heal. Intravenous antibiotics are likewise indicated, but the definitive treatment of the abscess remains surgical drainage. If left undrained, the abscess may progress to a perineal soft tissue infection, especially in immunocompromised patients or in individuals with poorly controlled diabetes. If the abscess recurs after being drained, one should suspect an underlying fistula or ischiorectal abscess.**

A. While admission and IV antibiotics are appropriate therapy, the definitive treatment is surgical drainage.
B. Needle drainage is not adequate management and does not allow for debridement of necrotic tissue.
C. Because the fluctuant mass is easily palpable and the extent will be defined during your exploration of the wound, localization via CT is not needed prior to primary drainage.
D. As in the explanation for C, evaluation using endorectal ultrasound is not needed prior to initial drainage.

21. **D. Approximately 50% of perirectal abscesses will develop a fistula communicating with the anal crypt.**

A, B, C, E. Even in a high-risk diabetic patient, anal incontinence, colovesical fistula, anal stricture, and anal fissure are all much less likely to occur.

22. **B. Ductal carcinoma in situ, also known as intraductal carcinoma, is a premalignant lesion. It is most often found on mammography as microcalcifications. Because it will subsequently develop into infiltrating ductal carcinoma of the breast, surgical treatment is required. Note the arrow and blocked marking of the microcalcifications on Figure 5-22.**

A. DCIS is usually nonpalpable and is primarily found on mammography, rather than on physical exam.
C. The risk of metastasis to lymph nodes is less than 2%, so an axillary dissection is usually not done with the surgical treatment of DCIS.
D. Local treatment of the whole breast is required for DCIS. This is accomplished by lumpectomy and whole-breast radiation, or with a modified radical mastectomy.
E. The chance of lymph node involvement is only 2%, as this condition is usually seen as microinvasion.

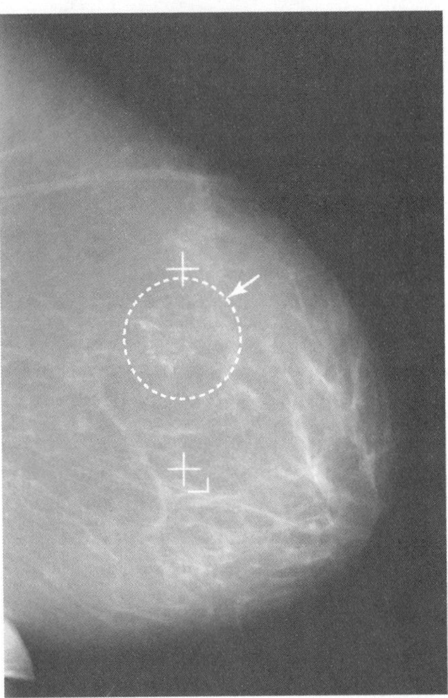

Figure 5-22 • Image Courtesy of the University of Utah School of Medicine, Salt Lake City, Utah.

23. **B. This clinical scenario and CT scan (see the arrow in Figure 5-23B) are characteristic of amebic abscess of the liver, caused by entameba histolytica, which typically occurs in young men who have emigrated from or recently traveled to an endemic area. Symptoms most often include pain in the right upper quadrant, fever, and anorexia. Diagnosis is confirmed with an indirect hemagglutination test with titers greater than 1:512. The CT scan demonstrates the abscess as a single hypodense lesion within the liver.**

A. An elevated alkaline phosphate level (liver function test) is most often present with amebic abscess, but it is nonspecific to this disease.
C. Leukocytosis and anemia are often present with amebic abscess and are nonspecific findings found in a complete blood count test.
D. An indirect Coomb's test is usually obtained to rule out a hemolytic reaction caused by antibodies in the patient's serum.
E. A chemistry panel is a very nonspecific test for an amebic abscess.

[R] [L]

SP:340.0mm
ST: 6.5mm

B

Figure 5-23B • Image Courtesy of the University of Utah School of Medicine, Salt Lake City, Utah.

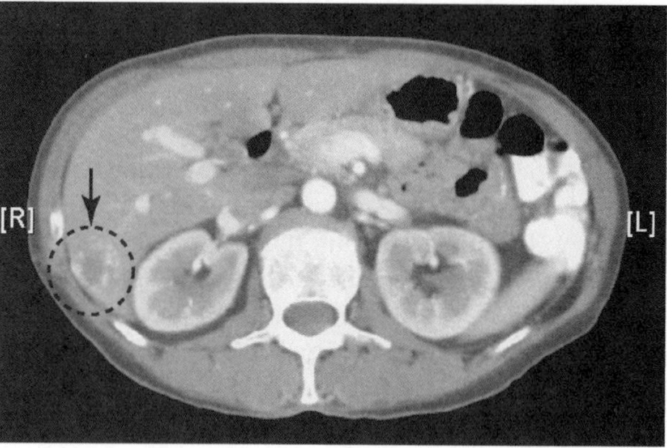

B

Figure 5-25B • Image Courtesy of the University of Utah School of Medicine, Salt Lake City, Utah.

24. **C. Initial treatment of an amebic abscess is oral metronidazole, which cures approximately 75% of patients. Drainage of the abscess is reserved for patients who fail initial therapy.**

    A. Percutaneous drainage is reserved for those who fail an initial trial of oral metronidazole.
    B. Operative drainage would be reserved for patients who do not respond to oral metronidazole and percutaneous drainage.
    D, E. The antibiotic regimen of gentamicin, ampicillin, and metronidazole is more appropriate for a pyogenic abscess of the liver.

25. **A. Hemangiomas are the most common benign masses found in the liver. They are of vascular origin and may be associated with pain in the right upper quadrant, bruits, shock with bleeding, or high-output heart failure. Hepatic hemangiomas are usually found incidentally on CT scan. Biopsy should not generally be performed due to the risk of hemorrhage. Figure 5-25B is a CT scan showing a hepatic hemangioma (note arrow). Notice its hypervascularity compared to the surrounding hepatic parenchyma.**

    B. Although a hamartoma is a possibility, hemangiomas are the most common benign tumors of the liver.
    C. The patient's labs are within normal limits with a negative work-up for hepatic cancer.
    D. A bacterial abscess is unlikely because the patient is afebrile, without any prior intra-abdominal infections.
    E. A hydatid cyst is unlikely because the patient has not traveled to endemic areas.

26. **D. Observation is the treatment of choice for asymptomatic hepatic hemangiomas less than 5 cm in diameter.**

    A. A hepatic wedge resection would be a reasonable choice if the patient was having symptoms, or if the lesion was greater than 5 cm.
    B. Percutaneous drainage is contraindicated due to possible hemorrhage.
    C. Hepatic lobectomy would be an option with multiple symptomatic hemangiomas.
    E. Sclerotherapy is not currently a treatment option for this disease.

27. **B. Although relatively rare, hepatocellular carcinoma (HCC) is one of the most lethal solid tumors in the world. Many different risk factors are associated with it, with the most common cause throughout the world being chronic hepatitis B infection.**

    A. Polyvinyl chloride (PVC), nitrites, and hydrocarbons have all been implicated as hepatic carcinogens.
    C. The hepatitis A virus does not cause chronic hepatitis, so it is not associated with an increased risk of developing HCC.
    D. Alcohol-related cirrhosis is the leading cause of HCC in the United States, Canada, and Western Europe.
    E. Aflatoxins are secondary fungal metabolites that frequently contaminate foods. Exposure to them is associated with development of HCC.

28. **A. Appendiceal carcinoid tumors at the tip of the appendix that are less than 2 cm in size require appendectomy only. For tumors at the base of the appendix or those greater than 2 cm, a right hemicolectomy is advocated. Unfortunately, carcinoid tumors have minimal clinical manifestations until metastases have occurred. Treatment for carcinoid tumors depends on the tumor location and size. Treatment of metastatic disease often consists of palliative care for the symptoms of carcinoid syndrome.**

    B. The role of radiation therapy in the treatment of carcinoid tumors involving metastatic disease, such as in this scenario, is limited to palliation of painful bone metastases. It is not indicated in cases of metastases to the liver.
    C. Surgical resection of hepatic metastases would be considered if they are located in surgically accessible areas of the liver.
    D. Observation alone is an incorrect course of action. The prognosis for malignant carcinoid syndrome is good compared to other malignancies.
    E. Trastuzumab (Herceptin) is a monoclonal antibody used as a chemotherapeutic agent and approved for use in HER-2-positive metastatic breast cancer.

29. **E. Carcinoid syndrome classically presents with flushing (95% of cases), diarrhea (80%), valvular heart disease (40%), and wheezing (20%). Carcinoid tumors secrete serotonin, which is responsible for the symptoms of the syndrome. The systemic effects of the disease do not present until metastatic disease occurs in the liver (Figure 5-29), which filters serotonin. With metastases, some active serotonin passes directly into the central circulation, causing the previously mentioned syndrome. Common sites of tumors include the appendix (most common), ileum, rectum, and bronchi.**

    A. Adenocarcinoma is not associated with the signs and symptoms described here.
    B. Insulinoma symptoms usually present as Whipple's triad: hypoglycemic symptoms produced by fasting, blood glucose less than 50 mg/dL during symptomatic attacks, and relief of symptoms by administration of glucose.
    C. Lymphoma usually presents with constitutional symptoms such as fever, night sweats, and malaise.
    D. Gastrinoma usually presents with symptoms of peptic ulcers, diarrhea, weight loss, and abdominal pain.

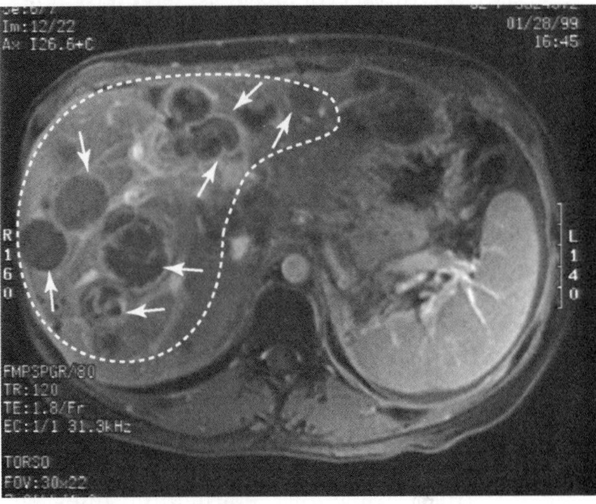

Figure 5-29 • Image Courtesy of the University of Utah School of Medicine, Salt Lake City, Utah.

30. **D. The classic lab test to diagnose carcinoid syndrome is serum serotonin or a 24-hour urinary 5-hydroxyindoleacetic acid (5-HIAA) level.**

    A. Serum gastrin is used to diagnose a gastrinoma.
    B. Serum protein C is a helpful test in diagnosing an insulinoma.
    C. A colonoscopy would help determine whether the lesion in the liver was due to colorectal cancer.
    E. Obtaining urinary metanepherines is important in the diagnosis of pheochromocytomas.

31. **A. This patient has a perianal abscess that appears to have spontaneously drained. Perianal abscesses most often arise from obstruction of an anal gland that becomes infected and overgrown with bacteria. These glands are located between the internal and external anal sphincters. If the infection tracks down this space toward the skin, a perianal abscess occurs. Because this abscess has drained spontaneously and has left an open cavity, it is safe to simply begin wound care with wet-to-dry dressing changes.**

    B. Rectal irrigations are inadequate therapy for an abscess. The abscess needs to be treated with aggressive wound care.
    C. An undrained abscess should be opened surgically. Antibiotics are used if significant cellulitis is present or the patient is immunocompromised, but not as the only treatment.

D. Incision and drainage of a perianal abscess is the proper management. In this case, however, the abscess has already drained spontaneously and no further drainage is required, unless there is evidence of grossly necrotic tissue.
E. Warm sitz baths alone will not adequately treat this type of infection. They can be employed postoperatively to assist with hygiene of the drained area.

32. **E. The upper one-third of the anus originates from endoderm, with the lower two-thirds originating from ectoderm. The dentate line marks this transition point. It is important surgically as the embryologic origin determines the blood supply, innervation, and lymphatic drainage.**

A. The innervation above the dentate line is autonomic; the innervation below it is somatic.
B. Stratified squamous epithelium lines the lumen below the dentate line, whereas columnar epithelium lines the lumen above it.
C. The blood supply above the dentate line originates from the superior rectal artery, a branch of the inferior mesenteric artery that originates from the aorta. The arterial supply below the dentate line originates from the inferior rectal artery, a branch of the internal pudendal artery that originates from the internal iliac artery. The venous system follows the arterial system.
D. A transanal biopsy and excision of benign and malignant tumors are possible well above the dentate line.
F. Lymphatic drainage above the dentate line flows into the lymph nodes along the iliac vessels. These eventually drain into the periaortic lymph nodes. Lymphatic drainage below the line goes to the inguinal lymph nodes.

33. **A. This patient has a proximal bowel obstruction due to the bilious output. It is important to rule out any type of volvulus, which could potentially compromise blood flow to the bowel. The most appropriate study in this setting is upper GI imaging, which would define the location of the obstruction. Such a study will demonstrate distention of the duodenum, abnormal positioning of the duodenojejunal segment (to the right of the midline), and a narrowing (bird's beak) at the point of obstruction.**

B. Upper endoscopy is not indicated in this scenario, as it would not be helpful in ruling out a midgut volvulus.
C. A barium enema is helpful to evaluate distal obstructions, but it is not helpful in case of a proximal obstruction. It may show abnormal positioning of the cecum in the right upper quadrant consistent with malrotation of the intestine.
D. Exploratory laparotomy is indicated in an emergency only in the setting of a midgut volvulus. Because the child has no peritoneal signs, further elucidation of his abdominal pain should be sought prior to emergent surgery.
E. Colonoscopy is not helpful, as it visualizes only the colon and not the proximal small bowel.

34. **E. An intestinal malrotation may result in intestinal obstruction with vascular compromise and is a surgical emergency. Treatment involves exploring the abdomen, untwisting the bowel, and performing lyses of adhesions, also known as the Ladd's procedure.**

A. Endoscopy has no role in the management of intestinal malrotation complicated by volvulus.
B. Although patients with intestinal malrotation require fluid resuscitation, observation is inappropriate because delay in surgical intervention can result in infarction of the bowel.
C. A Gastrografin enema may help relieve the obstruction caused by meconium plug syndrome. Unfortunately, it is not helpful in this clinical scenario.
D. Air-contrast enemas are diagnostic and therapeutic in children with intussusception.

35. **B. All suspicious skin lesions warrant a biopsy. In this case, the patient presents with classic symptoms of Paget's disease of the breast. This disease presents as an eczematous lesion of the nipple-areolar complex associated with itching or burning, as well as possibly erosion and ulceration. A biopsy will demonstrate Paget cells, consisting of invasion of the epidermis by invasive ductal carcinoma. Paget's disease occurs in less than 1% of all breast cancers. Surgical treatment involves a modified radical mastectomy or breast conservation with excision of the nipple areolar complex and breast radiation.**

A. Treatment with topical steroids will merely delay the time until an appropriate biopsy can be obtained.
C. Like steroid use, use of dressings or antibiotic creams will merely delay the diagnosis.

D. Lanolin or other creams that will soothe the area will merely delay the diagnosis.
E. Unfortunately, Paget's carcinoma of the breast is frequently misdiagnosed and initially treated as dermatitis or infection, leading to a delay in its diagnosis. Any suspicious skin lesion of the breast should be biopsied.

36. **D. Women who have undergone previous breast conservation therapy for breast cancer have a 5% to 10% risk of local recurrence at 10 years. These patients should undergo complete restaging of this new diagnosis. Those patients with purely local recurrence should undergo a mastectomy followed by radiation therapy for positive chest wall margins. Chemotherapy is given based on tumor characteristics.**

A. This patient has failed initial breast conservation treatment and must now undergo a mastectomy, not repeat lumpectomy.
B. This patient has previously undergone an axillary node dissection. Most cases will not need a repeat axillary dissection.
C. Given the scenario presented, this patient requires further surgical excision for local control.
E. Isolated local recurrence may be treated without systemic chemotherapy. Mastectomy is the most effective measure for local control.

37. **B. Li-Fraumeni syndrome is an autosomal dominant disorder caused by mutation of the p53 tumor suppressor gene; it is associated with increased incidence of breast cancer. A diagnosis of Li-Fraumeni syndrome is made when all of the following characteristics are present in a family: a sarcoma diagnosis in a person younger than 45 years of age; a first-degree relative with cancer at less than 45 years of age; and a first- or second-degree relative with cancer at age less than 45 years or sarcoma at any age. Approximately 70% of Li-Fraumeni cases are the result of mutations in p53, a gene on chromosome 17. Mutations in p53 confer an increased risk for early-onset breast cancer, childhood sarcoma, osteosarcoma, brain tumors, leukemia, and adrenocortical carcinoma. Individuals with a p53 mutation have a 50% chance of developing one of the associated cancers by age 50. Women with this syndrome have a 60% lifetime risk of developing breast cancer.**

A. Hereditary nonpolyposis colon cancer (HNPCC), also known as Lynch syndrome, is an autosomal dominant disease that is responsible for 1% to 5% of all colon cancers. Patients with this disease have an 85% risk of developing colon cancer at some point in their lifetime. Most cancers are found within the right colon, occur at an earlier age, and are associated with better survival rates. The genetic mutation is found in a DNA mismatch repair gene that prevents replication errors. The affected genes are hMSH2 and hMLH1. No association with breast cancer has been identified with this syndrome, although women with colorectal cancers are at greater risk for developing ovarian or endometrial cancers.
C. Brown-Séquard syndrome is an incomplete spinal cord lesion clinically characterized by hemisection of the spinal cord, often in the cervical cord region. It may result from a penetrating injury to the spine or from other causes such as spinal cord tumors, degenerative disk disease, ischemia, infectious or inflammatory conditions such as meningitis, herpes simplex and zoster, tuberculosis, and syphilis. This syndrome is not associated with an increased risk for developing breast cancer.
D. Von Hippel-Lindau syndrome is an autosomal dominant, inherited, rare genetic disorder characterized by an increased risk of developing tumors. It is characterized by a predisposition to retinal angiomas, central nervous system hemangioblastomas, renal cell carcinomas, adrenal tumors, pheochromocytomas, and islet cell neoplasms of the pancreas. The CNS hemangioblastoma (Lindau tumor) is the most commonly recognized manifestation. Patients often present in the second and third decades of life, and they may present with neurologic symptoms such as headaches, ataxia, and blindness. The deficits depend on the site of the primary lesion. This syndrome is not associated with an increased risk of developing breast cancer.
E. Crow Fukase syndrome is an extremely rare multisystem disorder that is also known as POEMS syndrome (polyneuropathy, organomegaly, endocrinopathy, presence of M-protein, and skin change). It is strongly associated with plasma cell dyscrasia. Common symptoms

include progressive weakness of the nerves in the arms and legs, hepatosplenomegaly, hyperpigmentation, and hypertrichosis. Endocrine abnormalities such as failure of the gonads to function properly and diabetes mellitus type 1 may be present as well. This syndrome is not associated with an increased risk of developing breast cancer.

F. Recently described, Beckwith-Wiedemann syndrome is a rare genetic syndrome for which the cause is unclear. Approximately 80% of children with this syndrome demonstrate genotypic abnormalities of the distal region of chromosome arm 11p. This growth disorder is characterized by macrosomia, macroglossia, hemihypertrophy, visceromegaly, genital tract abnormalities, omphalocele, neonatal hypoglycemia and embryonal tumors such as Wilms tumor, hepatoblastoma, neuroblastoma, rhabdomyosarcoma, adrenal carcinoma and other intra-abdominal neoplasms. This syndrome is not associated with an increased risk of developing breast cancer.

38. C. **Current guidelines for early detection of breast cancer outlined by the American Cancer Society are as follows: All women older than age 20 should perform breast self-examinations. Women 20 to 40 years of age should have a breast exam performed by a health professional every 3 years. After the age of 40, women should have an annual screening mammogram and a breast exam by a trained health professional. The National Cancer Institute guidelines recommend that women in their forties and older should have a mammogram every 1 to 2 years. Issues for obtaining mammograms for women, of all ages, are sometimes confusing and involve insurance as well as financial concerns of which practitioners should be aware. Figure 5-38A is the mediolateral view and Figure 5-38B is the craniocaudal view of normal mammography in a woman with mammographically dense breasts, which can make radiographic diagnosis in younger women difficult.**

A, B, D, E. These are incorrect ages. See the guidelines outlined in the explanation for C.

39. D. **Lobular carcinoma in situ (LCIS) is intraepithelial proliferation of the terminal lobular-ductal unit. It does not present as a palpable mass, has no mammographic findings, and is commonly found incidentally in a breast biopsy**

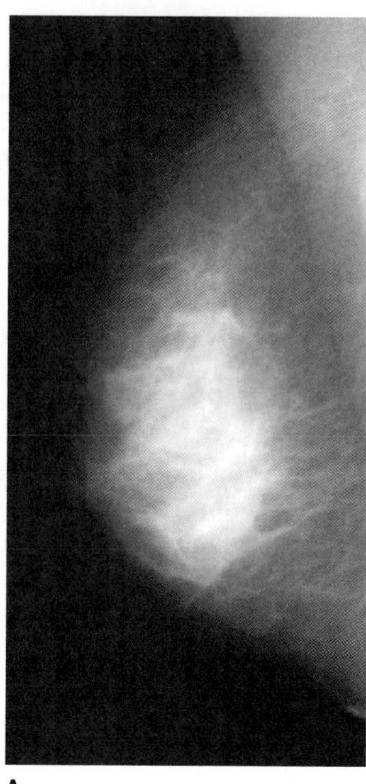

A

Figure 5-38A • Image Courtesy of the University of Utah School of Medicine, Salt Lake City, Utah.

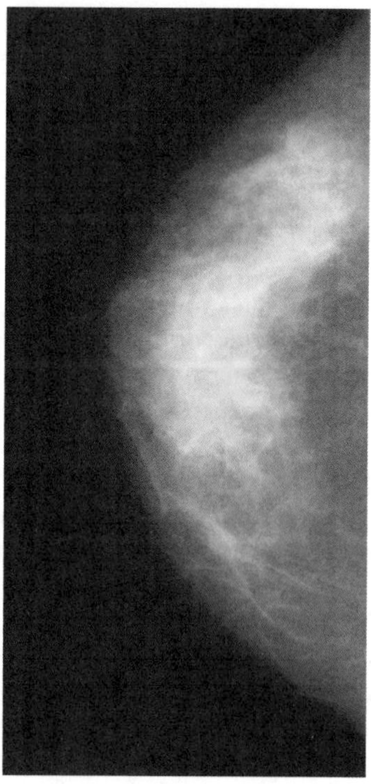

B

Figure 5-38B • Image Courtesy of the University of Utah School of Medicine, Salt Lake City, Utah.

specimen. Although LCIS is not a premalignant lesion, it is considered a marker or predictor for increased risk of breast carcinoma. Future malignancy may occur in the involved breast or in both breasts, usually in the form of infiltrative ductal carcinoma. Treatment consists mainly of close observation, as LCIS places the patient at higher risk for breast cancer. No surgical treatment is indicated at this point, even if the LCIS involves the margins of the specimen.

A, B, C, E. Because LCIS is not considered a premalignant lesion, no further treatment is warranted. The patient should be observed closely because she eventually may develop an invasive ductal or lobular carcinoma.

40. A. A Whipple procedure is more accurately defined as a pancreaticoduodenectomy, often done in a pyloric-preserving fashion. This procedure involves the resection of the pancreas to the level of the superior mesenteric vein, duodenum, gallbladder, and distal common bile duct. The distal stomach and the pylorus may also need to be resected. This technically difficult operation has many potential complications, the most common of which is delayed gastric emptying. This outcome is seen in about one-third of patients.

B. Approximately 20% of patients who undergo a Whipple procedure develop a pancreatic fistula.
C. Approximately 8% of patients who undergo a Whipple procedure develop a wound infection.
D. Approximately 5% of patients who undergo a Whipple procedure develop a bile leak.
E. Approximately 5% of patients who undergo a Whipple procedure develop pancreatitis.

41. C. The most common type (75% to 80% of all cases) of pancreatic cancer is ductal adenocarcinoma. Pancreatic cancers occur most frequently in the head of the pancreas, 70% of the time, followed by the body (20%), and the tail (5% to 10%). Patients typically present with painless jaundice, as well as a history of anorexia and weight loss.

A, D. See the explanation for C.
B, E. These terms are not normally associated with anatomical areas of the pancreas.

42. B. The primary diagnostic maneuver in any patient with a suspicious neck mass is to obtain a fine-needle aspiration (FNA); indeed, this procedure is considered the gold standard for evaluation of a thyroid nodule. The false-negative rate for FNA is less than 5%, and the false-positive rate is less than 2%. The FNA can be performed in an office or clinic setting with minimal discomfort and expense to the patient. If the mass is small or indistinct, ultrasound guidance can be used during the FNA. When positive findings occur, treatment can proceed without further delay. If the FNA result is negative, further diagnostic procedures should be performed.

A. Obtaining a CT of the neck may be an appropriate step, but it should occur following an FNA result.
C. An incisional biopsy is hardly ever performed, especially in a mass of this size, because it may leave involved tissue behind.
D. A lobectomy may eventually be required to obtain a diagnostic result or to treat the mass, but a less invasive means of diagnosis should be attempted initially.
E. Thyroidectomy is not indicated as an initial diagnostic test.

43. E. Papillary thyroid carcinoma is the most common form of thyroid cancer. It is associated with prior exposure to ionizing radiation, has a propensity for local or regional recurrence, and usually spreads via lymphatics. Nearly 50% of patients will have spread to regional lymph nodes at the time of diagnosis. Treatment consists of surgical excision, with the extent of excision being a topic of considerable controversy. Physicians at the M. D. Anderson Cancer Center advocate total thyroidectomy for papillary tumors larger than 1 cm. This procedure is combined with a neck dissection if clinically palpable nodes are present. Total thyroidectomy allows for postoperative radio-iodine ablation, which has been shown to decrease local–regional relapse rates by as much as 50%. Thymoglobulin may also be used as part of monitoring for recurrent disease.

A. Enucleation is inappropriate as it carries the risks of hemorrhage, recurrent laryngeal nerve injury, and incomplete exam of the tumor.
B. A lobectomy is used as a diagnostic measure in thyroid nodules with an unclear diagnosis. In papillary carcinoma, there is no role for lobectomy alone.
C. A lobectomy with isthmectomy is a reasonable treatment for a papillary carcinoma less than 1 cm in size.

D. Subtotal thyroidectomy is reserved for non-cancer thyroid surgery, mainly debulking of a large goiter. Currently, most surgeons would advocate for a complete thyroidectomy with thyroid hormone replacement.

44. **D. Most thyroid carcinomas recur within 5 years of initial treatment. Thyroglobulin values normally drop after thyroidectomy and ablation and, as such, serve as a sensitive indicator of recurrent or persistent disease.**

A, B, E. TSH, free T_4, and T_3 reuptake levels will depend on the adequacy of thyroid replacement. These three levels will not indicate whether recurrent disease is present.

C. Calcitonin is analyzed as part of screening for medullary thyroid cancer, not papillary thyroid cancer.

45. **A. *Helicobacter pylori* infection, one of the most common human bacterial infectious diseases, is causally linked to gastritis, peptic ulcer disease, gastric adenocarcinoma, and gastric B-cell lymphoma. *H. pylori* is a gram-negative spiral organism that is both slow growing and highly motile. Approximately 70% to 90% of patients with duodenal ulcers have concomitant *H. pylori* infections. In the case of gastric ulcers, 50% to 70% will be associated with an *H. pylori* infection. It is believed that such an infection may disrupt the protective mucosal layers, thereby predisposing the patient to ulcer development. Treatment of the *H. pylori* infection will increase healing of the ulcers and decrease the rate of recurrence.**

B. *H. pylori* infection has been implicated in the development of gastric lymphoma, but not to the same degree that it is associated with gastric or duodenal ulcers. It may be linked to as many as 40% of tumors in communities with a low incidence of gastric lymphomas.

C. Esophageal ulcers are most commonly caused by GERD, drug ingestion, and caustic injuries. The relationship between *H. pylori* and GERD is controversial, and involves the prevalence of and protective treatment for *H. pylori* in GERD patients.

D. The incidence of co-morbid gastric carcinoma and *H. pylori* infection is similar to the incidence of co-morbid gastric lymphoma and *H. pylori* infection.

E. Chronic use of NSAIDs increases the risk of ulcer disease but not in association with *H. pylori* infection.

F. Mucosa-associated lymphoid tissue lymphoma (MALToma) is an *H. pylori*–related tumor of B-cell origin. Evidence suggests that a significant proportion of primary gastrointestinal lymphomas are driven by exogenous agents/antigens. In the stomach, *H. pylori* appears to be responsible for most cases of low-grade lymphomas (MALToma).

46. **A. Treatment with bismuth subsalicylate and metronidazole is the least costly initial treatment for *H. pylori* infection.**

B. A parietal cell vagotomy is not indicated unless complications of peptic ulcer disease occur.

C. Proton pump inhibitors are not indicated as treatment for *H. pylori* infection and may obscure test results for the presence of *H. pylori*.

D. H_2 blockers will decrease acid levels but will not treat the infecting organism.

E. Mucosal barrier drugs, such as sucralfate, may protect the mucosa but will not eradicate the *H. pylori* organism.

47. **D. This patient's history is very concerning for an esophageal mass. Symptoms of a mass include unwanted weight loss and dysphagia, which initially is to solids but progresses to liquids. Risk factors include tobacco and alcohol use, male gender, African American ethnicity, nitrosamine ingestion, and history of gastroesophageal reflux disease. Although all of these examination choices may eventually be employed in the total work-up for esophageal carcinoma, endoscopic evaluation provides the most information and allows tissue samples to be obtained for pathology. Endoscopic ultrasound can also be performed, providing information regarding clinical stage.**

A, B. Although a mass in the esophagus may be identified via upper GI imaging or esophagram, an endoscopy will provide even more information because of the access to the mass for biopsy.

C. A thoracic CT will eventually be needed to assist in the staging of an esophageal mass, but it is not the first choice in evaluation.

E. An enteroclysis is a fluoroscopic contrast study of the small bowel. Examination of the small bowel is not part of this study.

48. **E. Acute rejection—a cellular-mediated response—is a result of sensitized lymphocytes and may occur days to weeks following transplantation. The pathology of a kidney biopsy reveals graft infiltration of small lymphocytes and mononuclear cells. High-dose steroids or antilymphocyte medications can usually reverse acute rejection.**

A, C. These options describe chronic transplant rejection. This condition usually occurs months to years following transplantation and is due to both cellular and humoral immune responses. The antigens responsible are usually the minor histocompatibility antigens. Unfortunately, this type of rejection is irreversible.

B, D. These descriptions refer to hyperacute rejection, which occurs when the recipient has preformed antibodies. It begins immediately after revascularization of the graft secondary to neutrophil infiltration and complement-mediated injury to the vascular endothelium. Treatment consists of graft removal.

49. **A. A post-transplant lymphocele occurs in approximately 15% of cadaveric renal transplant cases. It is caused by inadequate ligation of lymphatics transected along the iliac vessels or lymph leakage from the allograft. Diagnosis is made by undertaking needle aspiration of the fluid collection and by obtaining culture and chemistry analyses. Large fluid collections may compromise renal function due to the compression of the kidney, ureter, or bladder. If no improvement is observed in kidney function, or if compression symptoms occur following aspiration, a graft biopsy should be obtained to rule out rejection. Recurrent lymphoceles may be treated by repeated aspiration with a 75% success rate. Multiple aspirations, however, can pose a significant risk of infection. Better long-term solutions include intraperitoneal drainage by removing the lymphocele wall. Omentoplasty is also done to decrease the likelihood of recurrence. This procedure may be performed laparoscopically or via laparotomy, depending on factors such as location and size of the fluid collection, or because of previous abdominal procedures. The US image (see Figure 5-49) shows the large fluid collection adjacent to the kidney, consistent with a lymphocele.**

B. From the information presented, there is no indication of nephrotoxicity from Prograf.

C, D. These choices are appropriate if fluid aspiration of the lymphocele does not lead to improved renal function.

E. Because renal function is already compromised, further observation is not appropriate.

50. **C. This patient has reactivation of herpes zoster, or shingles. This condition affects approximately 30% of transplant patients, usually arising within the first 6 months after transplantation. Treatment initially consists of IV acyclovir followed by an oral course of the same therapy. This treatment helps to prevent systemic dissemination and aids in healing of the skin lesions. Immunosuppression should also be reduced to aid in recovery, an approach that also reduces mortality. In patients with systemic disseminated disease, hyperimmune globulin may be administered as well. Affected patients should undergo a bronchoscopy to rule out superinfection of the lungs.**

A. A more aggressive approach than oral acyclovir should be taken to prevent systemic dissemination, which is associated with a higher mortality rate.

B. A reduction of immunosuppressive medication is only part of the appropriate treatment regimen.

D. Increasing immunosuppressive medications may actually intensify the current infection.

E. Observation alone is not appropriate for this situation.

SETTING 2: OFFICE

Your office is in a primary care generalist group practice located in a physician office suite adjoining a suburban community hospital. Patients are usually seen by appointment. Most of the patients you see are from your own practice and are appearing for regular scheduled return visits, with some new patients as well. As in most group practices, you will often encounter a patient whose primary care is managed by one of your associates; reference may be made to the patient's medical records. You may do some telephone management, and you may have to respond to questions about articles in magazines and on television that will require interpretation. Complete laboratory and radiology services are available.

The next two questions (items 51 and 52) correspond to the following vignette.

A 47-year-old male is seen in your office complaining of left scrotal swelling. The patient states that he first noticed the swelling more than a month ago, while showering. The patient denies dysuria or penile discharge, but over the last 4 months he has inadvertently lost 15 pounds. On examination, you identify the swelling as a varicocele.

51. In this clinical situation, what should you consider as an etiology of this problem?

    A. Testicular cancer
    B. Inguinal hernia
    C. Renal cell carcinoma
    D. Epididymitis
    E. Testicular torsion

52. The left testicular vein most commonly drains into which of the following structures?

    A. Renal vein
    B. Inferior vena cava
    C. Inferior adrenal vein
    D. Internal pudendal vein
    E. Common testicular vein

End of Set

The next three questions (items 53–55) correspond to the following vignette.

A 32-year-old male presents to your office with concerns about a new mole on his right shoulder. The patient's wife was the first to notice it about 2 weeks ago. The patient reports that he has smoked one pack of cigarettes per day for the last 5 years. History also includes work as a lifeguard while in high school, with present employment as a salesman. Family medical history is unremarkable with the exception that his father is treated for hypertension. On exam, you note an irregular, pigmented lesion approximately 7 mm in diameter. There are no palpable lymph nodes. You perform an excision of the lesion in the office and send it to pathology.

53. What risk factor is most significant for disease in the patient's history?

    A. Age
    B. Smoking history
    C. Previous surgery
    D. History of severe sunburn
    E. Fair skin

54. The pathology results are consistent with a 1.2 mm deep melanoma with clear margins. What is the most important prognostic determinant?

    A. Width of the lesion
    B. Patient age
    C. Depth of the lesion
    D. Location of the lesion
    E. Color of the lesion

55. What should the surgical margin of this patient's excised melanoma be?

    A. 0.5 cm
    B. 1 cm
    C. 2 cm
    D. 3 cm
    E. 4 cm

End of Set

The next four questions (items 56–59) correspond to the following vignette.

A 25-year-old male was diagnosed with a pheochromocytoma 6 months ago. The patient underwent a successful adrenalectomy and returns to your office for a follow-up appointment. His physical exam is normal except for a palpable thyroid mass. Lab values obtained reveal a serum calcium level of 11.5 mg/dL.

56. Multiple endocrine neoplasia (MEN) type IIa syndrome is associated with pheochromocytoma, medullary thyroid cancer, and which of the following?

    A. Neurofibromas
    B. Marfanoid habitus
    C. Insulinoma
    D. Pituitary tumor
    E. Parathyroid hyperplasia

57. What is the best way to screen for medullary thyroid cancer?

    A. Serum calcitonin
    B. TSH levels
    C. Serum calcium
    D. Frequent ultrasounds
    E. Random fine-needle aspirations

58. This patient's MEN type II syndrome is associated with which of the following genes?

    A. p53
    B. ras
    C. RET
    D. bcl
    E. n-myc

59. From where are the inferior parathyroid glands derived embryologically?

    A. First pharyngeal pouch
    B. Second pharyngeal pouch
    C. Third pharyngeal pouch
    D. Fourth pharyngeal pouch
    E. Fifth pharyngeal pouch

End of Set

The next two questions (items 60 and 61) correspond to the following vignette.

A 28-year-old female who recently underwent a laparoscopic appendectomy for appendicitis presents to your office for evaluation of a 6 cm liver mass that was incidentally found on a CT scan (Figure 5-60) obtained prior to appendectomy. The patient is otherwise very healthy with no significant medical or surgical history. Medications taken include oral contraceptive pills and acetaminophen for occasional headaches.

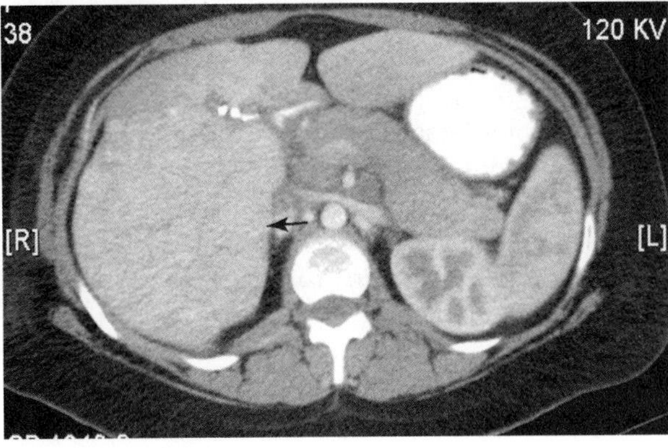

Figure 5-60 • Image Courtesy of the University of Utah School of Medicine, Salt Lake City, Utah.

60. What do you suspect this lesion to most likely be?

    A. Hepatoma
    B. Hepatic adenoma
    C. Focal nodular hyperplasia
    D. Hemangioendothelioma
    E. Hemangioma

61. Which of the following is true regarding this patient's lesion and proper management?

    A. Carries a 60% chance of malignant degeneration
    B. Carries a risk of spontaneous rupture and bleeding
    C. Will regress with cessation of the inciting agent
    D. Caused by chronic use of acetaminophen
    E. Often found to have distant metastases

End of Set

62. A 31-year-old female presents to your office with a history of a pigmented lesion on her shoulder. Recently the lesion has become significantly darker and increasingly irregular in shape. You perform an excisional biopsy, and the pathology comes back as a 0.9 mm deep Clarks II melanoma. What is the most common type of melanoma?

    A. Lentigo maligna melanoma
    B. Superficial spreading melanoma
    C. Acral lentiginous melanoma
    D. Nodular melanoma
    E. Ocular melanoma

The next three questions (items 63–65) correspond to the following vignette:

A 46-year-old female presents to your office and reports a 6-month history of palpitations, diaphoresis, tremulousness, irritability, and weakness. The patient notices the symptoms most frequently after having not eaten for several hours. You suspect she may have an endocrine tumor.

63. Which type of neuroendocrine tumor is most likely associated with this patient's presentation?

    A. Carcinoid
    B. Gastrinoma
    C. Insulinoma
    D. Glucagonoma
    E. Somatostatinoma

64. What is the most appropriate diagnostic step in the work-up of this patient?

    A. CT scan of the abdomen
    B. Ultrasound of the abdomen
    C. Euglycemic C-peptide suppression test
    D. 72-hour fast with measurement of glucose, insulin, and C-peptide levels
    E. Trial course of diazoxide

65. Which triad of symptoms is suggestive of this diagnosis?

    A. Beck's triad
    B. Whipple's triad
    C. Charcot's triad
    D. Virchow's triad
    E. Ostlund's triad

End of Set

The next three questions (items 66–68) correspond to the following vignette.

A mother brings her otherwise healthy 11-month-old male child to your office for evaluation of an abdominal mass the mother first noticed 2 weeks ago while at the swimming pool. The mass has not changed in size and does not seem to bother the child. The child has not experienced any vomiting and his bowel function is unchanged. You suspect the child has a neuroblastoma.

66. What is the most likely location site of childhood neuroblastoma?

    A. Neck
    B. Mediastinum
    C. Adrenal gland
    D. Spleen
    E. Pelvis

67. You take this infant to the operating room and excise the neuroblastoma. The child does well through surgery and recovery, and the tumor is pathologically determined to fit the Stage I classification. Which of the following are factors used to determine stage in childhood neuroblastoma?

    A. Nodal status and tumor crossing the midline
    B. Tumor response to preoperative chemoradiation
    C. Amplification of the c-myc gene
    D. Primary anatomical site
    E. Frequency of constitutional symptoms

68. Amplification of which oncogene is associated with a neuroblastoma?

    A. k-ras
    B. n-myc
    C. c-abl
    D. HER-2/neu
    E. c-myc

End of Set

The next three questions (items 69–71) correspond to the following vignette.

A 52-year-old female presents to your office for evaluation of a 3-day history of abdominal pain. Medical-surgical history includes a total abdominal hysterectomy with bilateral salpingo-oophorectomy 3 years ago, at which time she was found to have an ovarian mass. The mass was a serous cystadenocarcinoma, limited to the ovary. During the last 3 days the patient's pain has worsened and she also complains of feeling bloated. In the last 12 hours she has experienced three episodes of bilious emesis. Her last bowel movement was 2 days ago, and she reports having flatus approximately 2 hours ago. Vital signs are as follows: BP 142/78, HR 98, RR 16, T 38.1°C. All labs are normal. You obtain an abdominal film (Figure 5-69).

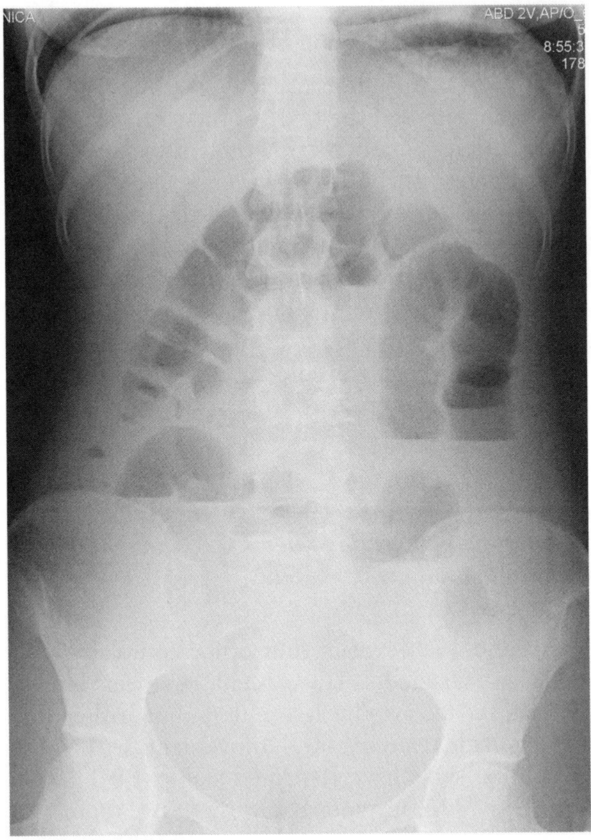

Figure 5-69 • Image courtesy of the University of Utah School of Medicine, Salt Lake City, Utah.

69. What is the most likely cause of this patient's abdominal pain?

   A. Primary small bowel tumor
   B. Metastatic ovarian cancer to the small bowel
   C. Adhesive band
   D. Internal hernia
   E. Ileus

70. Which of the following statements is most appropriate relative to the initial medical management of this patient's disorder?

   A. Bowel rest with immediate use of TPN is recommended.
   B. NGT decompression has no role in modern SBO management.
   C. IV antibiotics should always be given.
   D. Placement of a Foley catheter and fluid resuscitation are standard measures.
   E. Medical management of SBO is never indicated.

71. You decide to admit the patient to the hospital. After starting your initial therapy, she feels somewhat better. Over the next few days there continues to be high output from the NGT. On hospital day 4, the patient's abdomen remains distended and she develops focal tenderness in the right lower quadrant. The CBC shows a WBC count of 15,400 and the patient's temperature is 38.7°C with a heart rate of 113. What is the most appropriate next step in this patient's management?

   A. Three-view image of the abdomen
   B. Enteroclysis
   C. CT scan of the abdomen
   D. Upper endoscopy
   E. Emergent exploratory laparotomy

End of Set

72. A 72-year-old male with a 45-pack-per-year history of smoking comes to your office complaining of blood in his urine. You work up the hematuria and diagnose the patient with a transitional cell carcinoma of the bladder. Based on your preoperative work-up, you believe this to be a T1 tumor. What is the proper management of this tumor?

   A. Local radiation therapy
   B. Chemotherapy
   C. Chemotherapy and radiation therapy
   D. Transurethral resection with chemotherapy
   E. Radical cystectomy with radiation and chemotherapy

The next two questions (items 73 and 74) correspond to the following vignette.

A 35-year-old male who is a known narcotic abuser visits your office complaining of abdominal pain. The patient is unable to sit still and writhes in pain during the examination. He reports that the pain is mainly in the right flank, travels down into the scrotum, began today around 5 P.M., and has progressively worsened. The following labs were obtained: WBC 8000, BUN 15 mg/dL, creatinine 1.0 mg/dL, and UA demonstrated microscopic hematuria. A CT scan is obtained (Figure 5-73A).

73. What is the most appropriate next step in the treatment of this patient?

   A. Emergent ureteroscopy
   B. Narcotics for pain
   C. Exploratory laparotomy
   D. Nonsteroidal anti-inflammatory drugs for pain
   E. No treatment; the patient is seeking narcotics

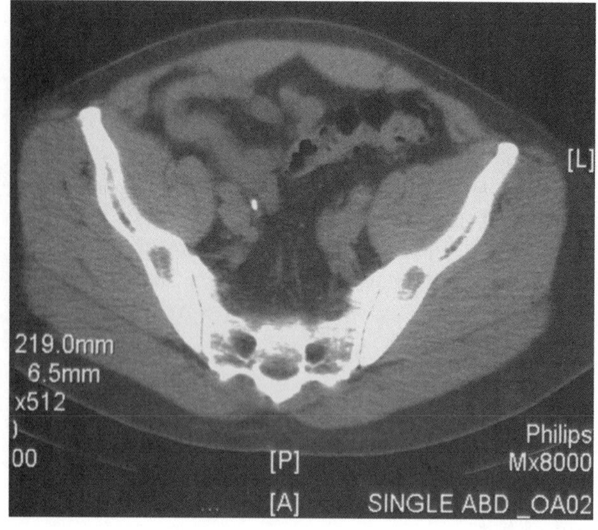

Figure 5-73A • Image courtesy of the University of Utah School of Medicine, Salt Lake City, Utah.

74. What type of renal calculi is most commonly encountered in patients who have undergone small bowel bypass surgery?

    A. Uric acid
    B. Calcium oxalate
    C. Cystine
    D. Struvite
    E. Cysteine

End of Set

The next two questions (items 75 and 76) correspond to the following vignette.

A 51-year-old, previously healthy male presents to your office for evaluation of a gastric carcinoma that was found on an upper endoscopy performed for persistent emesis associated with anemia and a 20-pound weight loss over the last 3 months. The tumor is located in the gastric cardia. CT evaluation shows some enlarged perigastric lymph nodes, but no evidence of distant metastasis.

75. Which of the following factors is associated with an increased risk for developing adenocarcinoma of the stomach?

    A. High-fat diet
    B. Smoked foods
    C. Chewing tobacco
    D. Japanese ancestry
    E. Diet high in fruits and vegetables

76. Which of the following statements best describes the location of gastric tumors?

    A. The distribution is evenly split between the antrum and the body of the stomach.
    B. Tumors rarely occupy the entire stomach.
    C. The distribution is evenly split between the antrum, the body, and the cardia of the stomach.
    D. The distribution is evenly split between the cardia and the body of the stomach.
    E. The distribution is evenly split between the antrum and the corpus.
    F. There is no pattern to gastric tumor location.

End of Set

The next two questions (items 77 and 78) correspond to the following vignette.

A 75-year-old male visits your office complaining of fatigue and dizziness. The patient has been feeling much better during the last 2 days, but earlier this morning had a large bowel movement with gross blood. Vital signs have remained stable: BP 119/82, HR 92, T 37.2°C, and SaO_2 95% on room air. Presently, the patient is alert and the physical exam is unremarkable. Rectal exam shows a moderate amount of gross blood. The following labs are obtained: WBC 7000, HCT 34%, PLT 130,000, Na 141 mmol/L, K 4.1 mmol/L, Cl 108 mmol/L, BUN 35 mg/dL, creatinine 1.0 mg/dL, and glucose 120 mg/dL.

77. What is the most appropriate first step in management of this patient?

    A. Diagnostic laparoscopy
    B. CT scan
    C. Colonoscopy
    D. Angiography
    E. Exploratory laparotomy

78. What is the most likely common cause of this patient's lower GI bleeding?

    A. Ulcerative colitis
    B. Colon cancer
    C. Meckel's diverticulum
    D. Vascular ectasia
    E. Diverticulosis

End of Set

The next three questions (items 79–81) correspond to the following vignette.

An 18-year-old female is referred to your office by a local hematologist. The patient was diagnosed 6 weeks ago with autoimmune hemolytic anemia. Since then she has been treated with glucocorticoids, but continues to require blood transfusions. After discussing the options with the patient's parents, they elect to pursue a splenectomy.

79. To perform the splenectomy, you must know your anatomy. The splenic vein empties into which of the following?
    A. Inferior mesenteric vein
    B. Superior mesenteric vein
    C. Inferior vena cava
    D. Azygous vein
    E. Portal vein

80. When considering splenectomy, this patient will require which of the following?
    A. Vaccinations for encapsulated organisms
    B. Preoperative CT scan to evaluate splenic size
    C. Type and cross for platelet transfusion
    D. An open splenectomy to evaluate for accessory spleens intraoperatively
    E. Routine LUQ drains

81. The patient does well postoperatively and is discharged from the hospital on postoperative day 5. On the return visit to your clinic, you check the patient's CBC and find a stable hematocrit at 36% with a platelet count of 1,400,000. What is the most appropriate next step in her management?
    A. Aspirin
    B. Heparin drip
    C. Coumadin
    D. Lovenox
    E. No treatment needed

End of Set

The next three questions (items 82–84) correspond to the following vignette.

A 68-year-old female visits your office with complaints of constipation for many years, sometimes to the point of self-digitalization. Most recently, the patient experienced the onset of rectal pain along with blood and mucous discharge each time she has a bowel movement. On physical examination, the anus and anoderm are normal but the patient has severe tenesmus.

82. What is the most likely cause of her perirectal pain?
    A. Perirectal abscess with spontaneous drainage
    B. Rectal polyp or cancer
    C. Anal fissure
    D. Solitary rectal ulcer
    E. Anal condylomata

83. What is the best initial therapy for this patient?
    A. Stool softeners, bulking agents, and bowel retraining
    B. Narcotic pain medication with close followup
    C. Surgical closure
    D. Exam under anesthesia
    E. Topical nitroglycerin

84. The patient follows this treatment for several weeks, but returns to your office with complaints of persistent pain and minimal improvement in her condition. What is the next step in management of this patient?
    A. A trial of sucralfate enemas for 6 weeks
    B. Abdominoperineal resection
    C. Internal anal sphincterotomy
    D. Low anterior resection
    E. Diverting colostomy

End of Set

The next three questions (items 85–87) correspond to the following vignette.

A 65-year-old male returns to your office for his annual physical examination. The patient reports that his general state of good health has continued, that he has not been hospitalized recently, and that he has continued to take atorvastatin and aspirin on a daily basis. Laboratory values from a year ago were unremarkable. Physical exam today is unremarkable except for a firm, irregular area felt on his prostate during a digital rectal exam. Laboratory values are as follows: WBC 8000, HCT 42%, PLT 148,000, Na 142 mmol/L, K 3.9 mmol/L, Cl 110 mmol/L, HCO_3 24 mmol/L, BUN 15 mg/dL, creatinine 1.1 mg/dL, glucose 110 mg/dL, Ca 11 mg/dL, alkaline phosphate 112 U/L, PSA 10 ng/mL, total bilirubin 0.8 mg/dL, AST 12 U/L, and ALT 25 U/L.

85. What is the most appropriate initial step in the management of this patient?

A. Cystoscopy with washings
B. Transrectal ultrasound with biopsy
C. Pelvic CT scan
D. Observation
E. Pelvic MRI

86. After further evaluation, the patient is found to have stage B1 prostate cancer (a 1.3 cm nodule in the peripheral zone of the prostate). What is the standard treatment for this patient's stage of prostate cancer?

A. Observation
B. External beam radiation
C. Total prostatectomy with pelvic lymphadenectomy
D. Hormonal therapy alone
E. Repeat pelvic MRI

87. A year later the patient returns to your office for routine follow-up. The patient states that he has been doing relatively well, although he complains of some general malaise as well as body aches. Vital signs are within normal limits, and the physical exam is unrevealing. Laboratory values are as follows: WBC 5000, HCT 40%, PLT 152,000, Na 140 mmol/L, K 3.5 mmol/L, Cl 109 mmol/L, HCO_3 24 mmol/L, BUN 12 mg/dL, creatinine 1.0 mg/dL, glucose 91 mg/dL, Ca 10.5 mg/dL, alkaline phosphate 365 U/L, PSA 8 ng/mL, total bilirubin 0.9 mg/dL, AST 21 U/L, and ALT 22 U/L. Which of the following most likely accounts for these findings?

A. Sarcoidosis
B. Osteoclastic bone metastasis
C. Cholestasis
D. Osteoblastic bone metastasis
E. Vitamin D deficiency

End of Set

The next three questions (items 88–90) correspond to the following vignette.

An 11-year-old male is seen in your office for complaints of left knee pain. Both the patient and his mother tell you that the pain has been present for the last 6 months but has progressively become more severe. The pain is more intense in the evening and usually prevents the patient from sleeping. The child denies any trauma and, according to his mother, is otherwise healthy without any other medical problems. Past history does not include any surgery, and the child is not taking any medications. Currently he attends sixth grade at the local elementary school, where he is an excellent student. Physical exam shows a large, tender mass fixed to the posteromedial distal femur, a knee that is somewhat flexed, and severe pain produced upon passive range of motion.

88. What is the most likely diagnosis?

A. Osteoclastoma
B. Ewing's sarcoma
C. Chondrosarcoma
D. Unicameral bone cyst
E. Osteogenic sarcoma

89. What is a common historical finding in a patient with this disease?

A. Multiple, small skin tumors
B. Premature birth
C. History of loose, bloody stools
D. Prior broken bones
E. A history of retinoblastoma as an infant

90. What is the most appropriate treatment for this patient's mass?

A. Neoadjuvant chemotherapy, limb-sparing surgery, and adjuvant chemotherapy
B. Radiation with delayed amputation
C. Radiation therapy followed by tumor excision
D. Amputation and systemic chemotherapy
E. Limb amputation

End of Set

The next five questions (items 91–95) correspond to the following vignette.

A 48-year-old female member of your staff has been enjoying brownies at the office holiday party when she experiences an acute onset of abdominal pain. The patient states that her pain is primarily in the right upper quadrant, is persistent in nature, and radiates to the subscapular area. The patient has not experienced similar pain in the past. Her abdomen is diffusely tender and rigid on exam. Laboratory values are as follows: WBC 13,000, HCT 39%, PLT 213,000, Na 140 mmol/L, K 3.8 mmol/L, Cl 105 mmol/L, HCO_3

23 mmol/L, BUN 12 mg/dL, creatinine 1.1 mg/dL, glucose 100 mg/dL, amylase 250 U/L, and lipase 35 U/L. A previous right upper quadrant ultrasound, obtained 6 months ago, shows no evidence of stones within the gallbladder or ductal dilatation.

91. What is the next step in this patient's management?

    A. Repeat an abdominal ultrasound
    B. Increase the pain medication
    C. CT scan of the abdomen
    D. Emergent surgery
    E. Fluid bolus

92. The appropriate management is performed, and the patient is found to have a perforated prepyloric gastric ulcer. Which type of gastric ulcer is this?

    A. Type I
    B. Type II
    C. Type III
    D. Type IV
    E. Type V

93. The patient is extremely concerned, and wants to know more about the procedure you recommend. You counsel her that which of the following is the most appropriate surgical procedure for a type I gastric ulcer?

    A. Vagotomy and pyloroplasty
    B. Total gastrectomy
    C. Highly selective vagotomy
    D. Distal gastrectomy, which includes the ulcer with a Billroth II gastrojejunostomy
    E. Vagotomy and gastrojejunostomy
    F. Proximal gastric resection, which includes the ulcer

94. The patient has an uncomplicated hospital stay and is discharged on postoperative day 5. Two weeks later she returns to your office for follow-up. The patient complains of distention and nausea following meals associated with right upper quadrant pain that is relieved by vomiting. This problem consistently occurs with meals. The patient denies fever or chills, and the abdominal exam shows a healing wound. What is the most likely cause of the patient's symptoms?

    A. Recurrent ulcer
    B. Postprandial dumping syndrome
    C. Afferent loop syndrome
    D. Postvagotomy diarrhea
    E. Bile reflux gastritis

95. Which condition following this patient's procedure is associated with abdominal pain and fullness, vomiting, diarrhea, flushing, palpitations, and dizziness?

    A. Recurrent ulcer
    B. Early postprandial dumping syndrome
    C. Afferent loop syndrome
    D. Late postprandial dumping syndrome
    E. Bile reflux gastritis

End of Set

The next two questions (items 96 and 97) correspond to the following vignette.

An 8-year-old female is referred to your office for evaluation of recurrent abdominal pain. The child describes the pain as occurring periodically and not associated with eating. The child's mother notes that her eyes occasionally will appear somewhat yellow. On physical exam, you are able to reproduce some discomfort with deep palpation and you detect a slight fullness in the right upper quadrant. There is no evidence of peritonitis. Past medical history is significant for a similar episode of pain with a slight fever and jaundice approximately 10 months ago, but the patient has otherwise been healthy.

96. You are concerned this patient may have what condition?

    A. Acute cholecystitis
    B. Acute cholangitis
    C. Pancreatic head mass
    D. Choledochal cyst
    E. Choledocholithiasis

97. What is the most appropriate initial diagnostic study in this child?

    A. Right upper quadrant ultrasound
    B. Abdominal CT scan
    C. Hepatobiliary scintigraphy
    D. Endoscopic retrograde cholangiopancreatography (ERCP)
    E. Percutaneous transhepatic cholangiography

End of Set

The next three questions (items 98–100) correspond to the following vignette.

A 67-year-old male with a history of alcoholic cirrhosis is referred to your clinic for evaluation of a liver mass found on a CT scan. The patient has been complaining to his wife of vague, right upper quadrant pain and has lost 20 pounds during the last 4 months. The patient has been previously diagnosed with Child's class A cirrhosis. History includes well-controlled hypertension and a coronary artery bypass graft (CABG) performed 3 years ago. The patient has a 44-pack-per-year history of smoking and quit 3 years ago, after his CABG. Surgical history includes an open appendectomy at age 9 and a laparoscopic cholecystectomy performed 8 years ago.

98. What is the most likely type of mass in this patient's liver?

    A. Hepatocellular carcinoma
    B. Cholangiocarcinoma
    C. Hepatoblastoma
    D. Hemangioma
    E. Adenoma

99. Which tumor marker is most often associated with this type of tumor?

    A. β-hCG
    B. AFP
    C. CA 19-9
    D. Carcinoembryonic antigen (CEA)
    E. CA 125

100. What is the most common site of distant metastasis of this type of tumor?

    A. Brain
    B. Spleen
    C. Small bowel
    D. Pancreas
    E. Lungs

End of Set

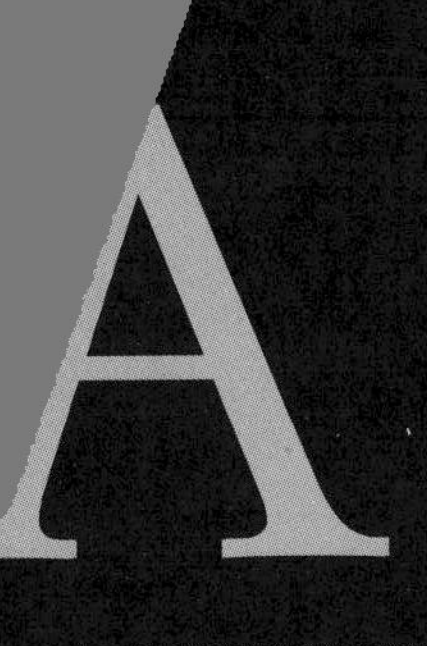

Answers and Explanations

51. C
52. A
53. D
54. C
55. C
56. E
57. A
58. C
59. C
60. B
61. B
62. B
63. C
64. D
65. B
66. C
67. A
68. B
69. C
70. D
71. E
72. D
73. B
74. B
75. B
76. C
77. C
78. E
79. E
80. A
81. A
82. D
83. A
84. A
85. B
86. C
87. D
88. E
89. E
90. A
91. D
92. C
93. D
94. C
95. B
96. D
97. A
98. A
99. B
100. E

51. **C. Renal cell carcinoma (RCC) causes 2% of cancer deaths. It is seen in males twice as often as in females. The classic clinical triad consists of flank pain, hematuria, and a palpable abdominal mass; however, it is seen in only 10% to 15 % of cases. The abdominal CT scan (Figure 5-51) shows a large, left renal mass (note arrows).**

A. Every testicular mass should be investigated with suspicion of testicular cancer and should be included in this patient's differential diagnosis. However, testicular cancer usually presents as a solid, painless testicular mass rather than as a soft venous collection above the testis.

B. An inguinal hernia should be considered, but can usually be ruled out by physical exam.

D. Epididymitis also includes a painful, swollen mass in the scrotum relieved by elevation and antibiotics.

E. Testicular torsion involves a very painful, swollen testis.

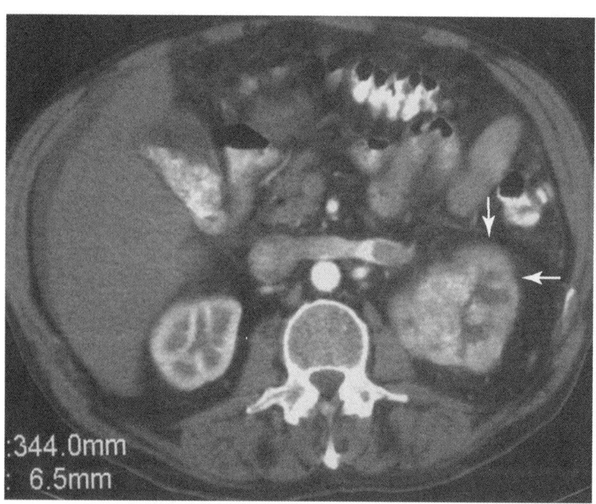

Figure 5-51 • Image Courtesy of the University of Utah School of Medicine, Salt Lake City, Utah.

52. **A. In RCC, the renal vein should be thoroughly investigated, as tumor thrombus may spread into the lumen of the inferior vena cava (IVC). Figure 5-51 demonstrates RCC of the left kidney with probable tumor extension into the left renal vein (note arrows). Because the left testicular vein drains into the left renal vein, IVC involvement may lead to increased pressure within the left testicular vein commonly seen as testicular varicosities, also known as varicoceles.**

B. The right testicular vein will drain into the inferior vena cava.

C. The left inferior adrenal vein usually drains into the left renal vein.

D. The internal iliac vein drains the pelvis but not the testes.

E. There is no common testicular vein.

53. **D. The incidence of melanoma has tripled in the last three decades and currently affects 5 to 25 per 100,000 people. Risk factors include severe sunburn before age 18, giant congenital nevus syndrome, family history of melanoma, multiple dysplastic nevi syndrome, and Caucasian race. Early detection significantly improves the results of treatment. Clinically suspicious lesions include those that change in size or color, itch, ulcerate, or bleed. Work as a lifeguard in high school would suggest significant sun exposure.**

A. Age is a relative risk factor, but not as significant as sun exposure.

B. Smoking history is a relative risk factor, but not as significant as sun exposure.

C. Prior surgery is not a risk factor, unless the procedure was to remove a previous melanoma.

E. Although fair skin is considered a risk factor, it does not correlate with melanoma incidence as much as a history of early severe sun exposure or burns.

54. **C. Tumor depth is the most accurate index of metastatic potential. Breslow's classification of staging is determined by tumor thickness as measured by pathologists: 1.0 mm or less, 1.01 to 2.00 mm, 2.01 to 4.00 mm, and greater than 4.00 mm. The greater the depth involved, the higher the risk of regional and distant metastasis as well as local recurrence.**

A. Although the width of the lesion may make obtaining clear margins difficult, as with facial lesions, it is the depth of the lesion that determines prognosis.

B. Age contributes little to the overall prognosis with melanoma.

D. In terms of location, acral lentiginous melanoma usually occurs on the palms, soles, and under the nails. This type is the most aggressive form of melanoma. Tumor depth still is the most important information for prognosis.

E. The color of the lesion has no effect on prognosis.

55. **C. A full-thickness excisional biopsy is the preferred treatment. The depth of invasion determines the size of the surgical margin. Lesions less than 1 mm thick require 1 cm margins. A surgical margin of 2 cm is adequate for lesions greater than 1 mm thick. There has been much debate in the literature concerning the surgical margin for melanoma. The minimum margin for intermediate-thickness melanoma (1 to 4 mm) is 2 cm. For tumor depths greater than 4 mm, the adequate margin size is 2 to 3 cm.**

A, B, D, E. See the explanation for C.

56. **E. Multiple endocrine neoplasia (MEN) type II syndrome is also known as Sipple's syndrome. It is typically classified as one of two types. Type IIa consists of medullary thyroid carcinoma, pheochromocytoma, and hyperparathyroidism.**

A, B. MEN type IIb is associated with medullary thyroid carcinoma, pheochromocytoma, mucosal neuromas (neurofibromas), and a marfanoid body habitus.

C, D. Pancreatic tumors, such as insulinomas and pituitary tumors, are seen in association with MEN type I.

57. **A. Medullary thyroid cancer (MTC) originates in the parafollicular cells, also known as the "C" cells of the thyroid gland. These cells are responsible for the production and secretion of calcitonin. Patients with pheochromocytomas and hypercalcemia should have a serum calcitonin level drawn to screen for MTC. An elevated level of calcitonin is seen in MTC.**

B. Obtaining TSH levels is an step in evaluating functional thyroid disease, such as hyperthyroidism, but not in the case of thyroid cancers.

C. Serum calcium levels play no role in screening for MTC.

D. Ultrasound is useful in determining the character of the thyroid nodule, but it is not a screening tool for MTC.

E. FNA is used primarily as a safe, cost-effective diagnostic tool in the evaluation of thyroid nodules, when they are found. However, it is not useful for screening for MTC.

58. **C. The RET gene has been implicated in the transmission of MEN type II syndromes.**

A, B, D, E. MEN type II syndrome is not associated with these genes.

59. **C. The parathyroid glands are derived embryologically from the third and fourth pharyngeal pouches. The inferior parathyroid glands arise from the dorsal portion of the third pouch and migrate inferiorly into the neck along with the thymus.**

A. The first pharyngeal pouch will become the eustachian tube and middle ear.

B. The second pharyngeal pouch contributes to the development of the palatine tonsils.

D. The superior glands arise from the fourth pharyngeal pouch, and their migration is limited.

E. The fifth pharyngeal pouch is a rudimentary structure that becomes part of the fourth pouch.

60. **B. Hepatic adenomas are benign lesions of the liver, most often found in women in their thirties and forties. Oral contraceptives are a risk factor for developing a hepatic adenoma. The lesions are usually solitary but can occur in multiples; they most often arise in the right lobe of the liver. Such lesions are often found incidentally on CT scan. Patients may present with abdominal pain and a palpable mass. The diagnosis can be made radiographically. A large adenoma of the right hepatic lobe is seen on the CT (see Figure 5-60; note arrow).**

A. A hepatoma is a malignant tumor of the liver. It would be very uncommon in a young female with no history of cirrhosis of the liver.

C. Focal nodular hyperplasia is a benign liver tumor often seen in young women. It is associated with tissue ischemia and regeneration. Such a tumor appears as a central stellate scar on CT scan.

D. A hemangioendothelioma is a rare, benign lesion that usually appears in the first 2 years of life.

E. A hemangioma is the most frequently seen benign liver tumor. Most are small and asymptomatic. When they become larger, however, they can cause significant pain. Delayed-phase CT scan reveals pooling of contrast in the lesion, thus distinguishing it from other benign tumors.

61. **B. Hepatic adenomas larger than 5 cm should be resected because one-third of patients present with bleeding or rupture of the adenoma.**

A. Hepatic adenomas have a 10% risk of malignant degeneration.
C. A number of smaller adenomas may regress with cessation of the inciting agent—in this case, oral estrogens. Such cases may be followed rather than proceeding directly to surgery.
D. Acetaminophen is not a cause of hepatic adenomas, but can be related to liver damage as a result of overdosage.
E. Hepatic adenomas are not malignant and do not metastasize.

62. B. Superficial spreading is the most common type of melanoma, accounting for approximately 70% of melanomas. This lesion typically grows radially for months to years, having little surface elevation, but may eventually enter a vertical growth phase in which it develops a nodular component.

A. Lentigo maligna are cutaneous melanomas that are usually confined to chronically sun-damaged sites, such as the hands and neck. They are usually found in older adults and account for less than 10% of all melanomas.
C. Acral lentiginous are cutaneous melanomas that are usually found on the palms, soles of the feet, nail beds, and mucous membranes. They account for less than 10% of all melanomas.
D. Nodular melanomas do not grow radially, and usually present as deep, invasive lesions. They are dark brown-black or blue-black in color. They account for 15% to 30% of all melanomas.
E. Ocular melanomas are rare and often are not diagnosed until they become quite large. The most common site for them to develop is along the uveal tract. They account for 2% to 5% of all melanomas.

63. C. An insulinoma is a functional islet cell tumor that presents with symptoms of hypoglycemia (such as those described in this patient), often brought on by fasting or exercise. Other symptoms include *palpitations, diaphoresis, tremulousness, irritability, weakness,* vision changes, and neurologic changes. Carcinoid, gastrinoma, glucagonoma, somatostatinoma, and insulinoma are all forms of amine precursor uptake and decarboxylation (APUD) cell tumors.

A. Carcinoid tumor presentation symptoms can include diarrhea and flushing.
B. Gastrinoma tumor presentation symptoms can include abdominal pain and symptoms caused by gastric acid hypersecretion.
D. Glucagonoma tumor presentation symptoms can include dermatitis, glucose intolerance or diabetes, and weight loss.
E. Somatostatinoma tumor presentation symptoms can include diabetes mellitus, gallbladder disease, diarrhea, and steatorrhea.

64. D. An insulinoma is diagnosed using a 72-hour fast followed by measurement of glucose, insulin, and C-peptide levels. An insulin/glucose ratio greater than 0.30 or an insulin level greater than 6 μU during a fast is diagnostic for an insulinoma.

A, B. CT scan and ultrasound of the abdomen are useful imaging tests, but because of the small size of insulinomas, they are successful only 50% of the time in localizing the lesion. Angiography with subtraction techniques or intraoperative ultrasound are the two most accurate tests.
C. A euglycemic C-peptide suppression test may be useful, but it is rarely used.
E. Diazoxide (Hyperstat) is used to inhibit insulin release and to decrease peripheral glucose utilization. Secondary to its multiple side effects, it is used for a short period to help briefly control symptoms and is inappropriate until the diagnosis of insulinoma has been made.

65. B. Whipple's triad consists of hypoglycemic symptoms with fasting, blood glucose less than 50 mg/dL, and relief of symptoms with administration of glucose. It is associated with an insulinoma diagnosis.

A. Beck's triad (shock, distant heart sounds, and distended neck veins) is associated with pericardial tamponade.
C. Charcot's triad (jaundice, fever, and upper quadrant pain) is associated with cholangitis.
D. Virchow's triad (abnormal vessel wall, circulating blood abnormalities, and stasis) is associated with venous thrombosis.
E. There is no such thing as Ostlund's triad.

66. C. A neuroblastoma is the most common childhood tumor. The majority of patients present with an asymptomatic abdominal mass. These tumors most often arise in the adrenal gland, originating from neural crest cells of the adrenal medulla or sympathetic chain.

A. The neck is the least common location for a neuroblastoma.
B. The mediastinum is the second most common location for a neuroblastoma.
D. Neuroblastomas are not found in the spleen.
E. The third most common location for a neuroblastoma is in the pelvis.

67. A. The stage of the tumor is determined by the size, such as a tumor crossing the midline, nodal status, and distant metastases. Patients with a Stage I neuroblastoma have a 100% survival rate with therapy. Radiotherapy is used only when incomplete excision has been performed. Preoperative chemoradiation is used when the tumor appears unresectable on imaging studies. Staging and survival rates are listed in Table 5-67.

B, C, D, E. These factors are unrelated to staging the tumor.

TABLE 67 Neuroblastoma Staging

	Stage	Survival Rate with Therapy
I:	Confined to the origin	100%
IIa:	Completely excised unilateral tumor, (−) nodes	80%
IIb:	Completely excised unilateral tumor, (+) nodes	70%
III:	Tumor across midline or contralateral (+) nodes	40%
IV:	Distant metastasis	15%

68. B. Amplification of the n-myc gene correlates with poor outcomes in neuroblastomas.

A. The k-ras gene is associated with colorectal, lung, and prostate cancer.
C. The c-abl gene is associated with the Philadelphia chromosome in CML.
D. The protein HER-2/neu is overexpressed in approximately 30% of breast cancers.
E. The c-myc gene is associated with Burkitt's lymphoma.

69. C. This patient presents with a partial small bowel obstruction (SBO). In the setting of previous abdominal surgery, the most likely cause of the obstruction is an adhesive band. The leading cause of SBO in developed countries is postoperative adhesions, which account for approximately 50% to 70% of all cases. Surgeries most commonly related to SBO are appendectomy and upper gastrointestinal, colorectal, and gynecologic procedures. Small bowel obstructions can be partial or complete, simple or strangulated.

A. Primary small bowel tumors are an extremely rare cause of partial bowel obstruction. Neoplasms account for approximately 10% of cases.
B. Metastatic ovarian cancer to the bowel is a cause of partial bowel obstruction. Given that adhesive bands are the cause of 50% to 70% of all SBOs in patients with previous abdominal surgery, metastatic cancer is less likely in this case.
D. Hernias are the second most common cause of partial obstructions, accounting for approximately 25% of all cases. They are the most common cause in patients who have not undergone prior abdominal surgery.
E. An ileus is a mechanical or functional intestinal obstruction resulting in dysfunctional motility of the bowel. It is most commonly seen immediately following abdominal surgery, in patients with metabolic abnormalities, or with infectious processes. The x-ray findings in this case are not consistent with an ileus.

70. D. Initial nonoperative management of a partial SBO includes strict bowel rest, nasogastric tube (NGT) decompression, IV fluids, and placement of a Foley catheter to monitor urine output closely.

A. Total parenteral nutrition is not part of the initial management of SBO.
B. NGT placement is indicated in all except mild cases of SBO. It will decompress the stomach, eliminate vomiting, minimize discomfort of reflux of intestinal contents, and assist in monitoring intestinal output.
C. Antibiotics do not have a role in the initial management of SBO. They will, however, have a role if the patient requires surgery.
E. Medical management or nonoperative management for SBO is prudent and appropriate. Most episodes of obstructions from adhesions resolve without surgical intervention.

71. E. The four cardinal signs indicating the need for prompt operative intervention are persistent focal tenderness, fever, leukocytosis, and tachycardia. Given this patient's current findings, she should go directly to the operating room for exploratory laparotomy.

A, B, C, D. These are all inappropriate choices in this scenario because this patient has failed conservative management of a bowel obstruction and has now deteriorated as indicated by the leukocytosis, tachycardia, fever, and persistent focal tenderness.

72. D. Ninety percent of bladder cancers are transitional cell tumors, with the remainder being either squamous cell or adenocarcinoma. Men are more prone to developing bladder cancer than are women. The risk of developing bladder cancer is increased by smoking and exposure to β-naphthylamine and/or paraminodiphenyl. Treatment of T0 and T1 tumors includes transurethral resection of the bladder tumor with or without chemotherapy.

A. The use of *postoperative* radiation therapy is controversial; it is considered only in T2 and T3 stage disease.
B. Chemotherapy alone is not sufficient; resection of the tumor is required.
C. Chemotherapy and radiation therapy alone are not sufficient; resection of the tumor is required.
E. Radical cystectomy is indicated in T2 and T3 tumors.

73. B. Patients with kidney stone disease usually present with acute onset of pain in the flank that radiates to the groin. The patient is often unable to find a comfortable position, and vomiting is common. Dysuria, frequency, and hematuria may be present. Evaluation of the urine will reveal hematuria unless the affected ureter is totally obstructed. An abdominal x-ray may be helpful because 90% of stones are radio-opaque. Most commonly, a CT scan without contrast is used to evaluate for stones. Pain is usually severe. Although this patient is a known narcotic abuser, narcotic pain medication should not be withheld with objective proof that the patient is actually suffering from nephrolithiasis. Figure 5-73B shows the CT scan typically ordered to rule out kidney stones; note the arrow, which points to a nephrolith.

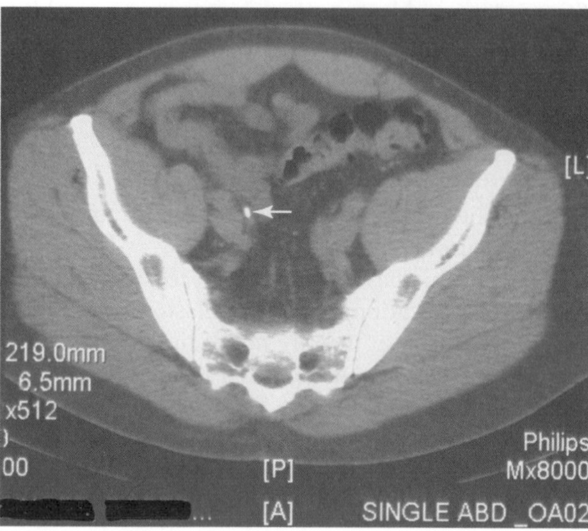

B

Figure 5-73B • Image Courtesy of the University of Utah School of Medicine, Salt Lake City, Utah.

A. An emergent ureteroscopy may be needed if the patient is unable to pass the stones due to their size. The initial therapy, however, is IV fluid hydration and pain control.
C. There is no indication at this time for an exploratory laparotomy.
D. NSAIDs are a reasonable choice, but the pain relief they offer would most likely be insufficient.
E This patient has clinical and radiographic signs of kidney stone disease and should be treated appropriately, regardless of the history of narcotic abuse.

74. B. Kidney stones are most commonly calcium phosphate and calcium oxalate (80%), followed by struvite (15%), uric acid (5%), and cystine (1%). Calcium and struvite stones are more common in women. Uric acid stones are twice as common in men, and cystine stones occur in both men and women with the same frequency. Absorptive hyperoxaluria occurs in approximately 10% of people who have undergone surgical removal of a portion of the bowel. It causes unabsorbed fatty acids to combine with calcium. This results in excess oxalate absorption by the gut, resulting in formation of calcium oxalate stones.

A. Uric acid stones are found in approximately 5% of cases. These radiolucent stones are associated with gout, Lesch-Nyhan syndrome, and a low urine pH.

C. Cystine stones are rare, being found in fewer than 1% of cases. Affected individuals have a genetic predisposition for developing such stones.

D. Struvite stones are composed of magnesium, ammonia, and phosphate. They occur in approximately 15% of cases and are associated with UTIs with urea-splitting bacteria, such as *Proteus* and *Pseudomonas.* Infection with these organisms may cause staghorn calculi that fill the entire renal pelvis.

E. Cysteine is not a component of kidney stones.

75. **B. Gastric adenocarcinoma encompasses 90% to 95% of all gastric tumors. It is the eighth most common cause of cancer mortality in the United States. This type of cancer is seen more frequently in males than in females (2:1 ratio), and 70% of patients are more than 50 years old. The incidence of gastric cancer is highest in Asia, with the incidence in Japan being 80 times higher than the incidence in the United States. Risk factors include diet (smoked foods), exposure to nitrosamine compounds, low consumption of fruits and vegetables, occupational exposures (heavy metals, rubber, and asbestos), cigarette smoking, alcohol use, and low socioeconomic status.**

A, C. Chewing tobacco and high-fat diets are not associated with an increased risk for developing gastric cancer.

D. While the Japanese do have a much higher incidence, it is believed to be due to their diet and is not a genetic-related risk.

E. See the explanation for B.

76. **C. Tumors can be located anywhere in the stomach, although there is a general pattern to their distribution. Thirty percent are located in the pyloric canal or antrum, 20% to 30% in the body, 37% in the cardia, and 12% in the entire stomach (Linitis plastica). Many remember the distribution as approximately one-third in the antrum, one-third in the body, and one-third in the cardia. The corpus is another name for the body of the stomach.**

A, B, D, E. These distribution patterns are incorrect. See the explanation for C.

77. **C. Continuous bleeding from the rectum with or without hemodynamic instability is known as an acute lower GI hemorrhage. This patient appears stable, as evidenced by the stable vital signs and unchanged hematocrit. Nevertheless, the patient should be closely observed. A nasogastric tube should be placed to rule out the possibility of rapid upper GI bleeding. Once this diagnosis is ruled out, the patient should have a colonoscopy to help determine the cause of lower GI bleeding. According to the results of clinical trials, colonoscopy is successful in localizing the bleeding sites 50% to 90% of the time. Therapy consisting of cauterization can also be employed if the site of active bleeding is identified.**

A. Diagnostic laparoscopy would not be helpful in this situation, as the source of the bleeding usually cannot be identified by simply looking into the abdomen with a laparoscope. A localizing study, such as a colonoscopy, should be performed first.

B. A CT scan would not be helpful in diagnosing the source of ongoing bleeding within the colon.

D. Angiography may be used to localize the bleeding vessel and treat it by embolization. Identification in this manner typically requires a fairly rapid rate of bleeding to localize the source of bleeding. This procedure is more invasive than colonoscopy and would not be the first choice. It is an option, however, if the bleeding cannot be controlled at the time of colonoscopy.

E. Exploratory laparotomy may be required in an unstable patient after unsuccessful endoscopy. If the source of bleeding is not localized, a total colectomy may be the only option.

78. **E. There are multiple causes of lower GI bleeding, with the most common etiology in the United States being diverticulosis. Approximately 80% to 90% of lower GI bleeds stop spontaneously, with a 25% rate of rebleeding. It is imperative to attempt to localize and treat the underlying disorder to prevent any future bleeding.**

A. Inflammatory bowel disease is the fourth most common cause of lower GI bleeding.
B. Neoplasms are the fifth most common cause of lower GI bleeding.
C. Meckel's diverticulum is the sixth most common cause of lower GI bleeding.
D. Vascular ectasia are the second most common cause of lower GI bleeding.

79. **E. The splenic vein empties directly into the portal vein.**

A. The inferior mesenteric vein empties into the splenic vein.
B. The superior mesenteric vein empties into the portal vein.
C. Blood returns to the vena cava after going through the liver and out the hepatic veins to the vena cava.
D. The azygous vein empties into the superior vena cava in the chest.

80. **A. Immunologic function of the spleen is needed to prevent overwhelming infections from encapsulated bacteria such as *Streptococcus pneumoniae, Haemophilus influenzae,* and *Meningococcus.* When considering splenectomy, patients should receive vaccinations protecting against all of these organisms. This measure helps to prevent the condition known as overwhelming post-splenectomy infection (OPSI), which can be fatal. Children are more susceptible to this complication and are often kept on prophylactic antibiotics.**

B. A preoperative CT scan is not needed, either to evaluate splenic size, which is usually near normal in AHA, or to look for other problems.
C. Platelet count and function are not affected in AHA, and transfusion of platelets should not be necessary.
D. Today, most normal-sized spleens would be removed laparoscopically. There is no advantage to open surgery in the evaluation for accessory spleens.
E. Unless pancreatic injury or other unusual complications occurs, the routine use of left upper quadrant (LUQ) drains is not needed.

81. **A. A patient who is post-splenectomy and who presents with an increased number of platelets should be started on aspirin to prevent spontaneous clotting. Aspirin does not destroy platelets, but rather makes them dysfunctional and thus decreases the risk of thrombus formation.**

B, C, D. Systemic anticoagulation is not necessary, nor are preventive doses of Coumadin or Lovenox, as long as the patient can continue to take aspirin.
E. The increased risk of spontaneous thrombus formation requires treatment.

82. **D. A solitary rectal ulcer is a *much less common* cause of acute rectal pain and is thought to be due to excessive straining during which the anterior rectal mucosa is forced into the anal canal, causing congestion, edema, and ulceration.**

A. A perirectal abscess typically causes severe anal pain, worsened by defecation. Diagnosis is made by rectal exam and palpation of an indurated perirectal mass.
B. Rectal neoplasms tend to be occult in terms of symptoms; they do not cause sudden acute pain.
C. An anal fissure occurs after forceful dilatation of the anal canal. It usually occurs after constipation with forceful defecation. An anal fissure most frequently occurs in the posterior midline, leading to increasing pain with defecation and reluctance to have further bowel movements. This results in further constipation, which in turn worsens the problem. The diagnosis is made by simply separating the buttocks, revealing a tear in the anoderm of the posterior midline.
E. Anal condylomata are caused by infection with human papillomavirus (HPV) types 6 and 11. Affected individuals complain of a perianal growth that appears as a cauliflower-like lesion on physical exam. Minimal disease may be treated in the office with bichloracetic acid or podophyllum; larger lesions may require surgical excision.

83. **A. The goals of treatment for a solitary rectal ulcer (SRU) include patient reassurance that the lesion is benign and cessation or minimization of symptoms, which can be achieved with conservative therapy consisting of dietary fiber, stool softeners, bowel retraining, and bulking agents.**

B. Narcotic pain medication is often needed, and it should be used in conjunction with stool softeners. Narcotics should be used conservatively, as they may increase the patient's constipation.
C. Surgical treatment is an option, and it is typically indicated for those patients who fail conservative management.
D. An exam under anesthesia is not required to obtain a diagnosis in this case.
E. Nitroglycerin topical ointment has been reported to be an effective treatment for anal fissures but not for SRU. Its use is limited because of the high incidence of side effects, which include headaches and tachyphylaxis.

84. **A. For patients who fail dietary measures, a trial of sucralfate enemas is the next therapeutic step. A rectopexy or other surgical procedure should be reserved for failures of all other measures.**

B. Abdominoperineal resection is used to treat rectal tumors less than 5 cm from the anal verge.
C. Lateral internal anal sphincterotomy is the procedure of choice after failure of medical management for anal fissures, not SRU. In this procedure the internal anal sphincter is divided, relieving the spasm that causes pain and limits healing. Fecal continence is maintained by the external anal sphincter. This procedure has a success rate exceeding 90%.
D. A low anterior resection is used to treat rectal cancer that is more than 5 cm from the anal verge.
E. While a diverting colostomy might allow the SRU to heal, it is a morbid operation and requires a second operation.

85. **B. Prostate cancer is the most common neoplasm, after skin cancer, in men and the second most common cause of cancer-related death. Prostate cancer occurs more commonly in African American men and in men older than age 50. Ninety-five percent of prostate tumors involve adenocarcinoma, and they occur primarily in the peripheral zone. A transrectal ultrasound is used to evaluate tumor volume, and with the acquisition of biopsies.**

A. A cystoscopy with washings is not required except in cases of large lesions with suspected bladder involvement.
C. A pelvic CT scan will most likely eventually be required to assist in the staging of this disease, but it would not be the initial step in this patient's management.
D. Because the patient's history and physical exam are very concerning for prostate cancer, further diagnostic evaluation is warranted, not observation.
E. A pelvic MRI has no role in the initial workup of prostate cancer.

86. **C. Patients with nonpalpable tumors and more than 5% prostate involvement (stage A2), or with localized nodules of 1 to 1.5 cm in diameter in one lobe (stage B1), or with a tumor greater than 1.5 cm in diameter in one or more lobes (stage B2) are candidates for total prostatectomy.**

A. Observation is usually reserved for stage A1 disease, which includes nonpalpable tumors with an incidental finding of low-grade cancer seen in less than 5% of the prostate.
B. Radiation therapy is used in stage C disease, which includes periprostatic extension of tumor.
D. Hormonal therapy alone should be used in men with stage D cancer, which consists of distant metastases.
E. Pelvic MRI has no role in the initial work-up for, or treatment of, prostate cancer.

87. **D. Any patient with a history of prostate cancer and elevated alkaline phosphatase should be evaluated for metastatic disease to the bones. Prostate metastases cause osteoblastic lesions. Treatment is usually palliative and consists of hormonal therapy and irradiation of symptomatic lesions.**

A. Sarcoidosis is a disease of unknown etiology characterized by noncaseating granulomas in multiple tissues. Hypercalcemia results from excessive secretion of $1,25(OH)_2$ D and occurs in 20% of patients.
B. Metastatic prostate cancer results in hypercalcemia due to osteoblastic—not osteoclastic—bone metastases.
C. Cholestasis refers to delay or obstruction of bile secretion. It does not cause elevated calcium levels.
E Vitamin D deficiency results in hypocalcemia. Dietary rickets is uncommon today in the United States, especially since vitamin D has been added to milk products.

88 **E. The most common—albeit rare—primary malignant bone tumor is osteogenic sarcoma. Males between 10 and 20 years of age are most often affected. The lesion occurs on the metaphysic of the distal femur or proximal tibia. The presenting symptoms are usually pain, tenderness, and swelling near a joint. Limitation of motion may also be present. Serum alkaline phosphatase is usually elevated, and plain films reveal a destructive lesion in the metaphysic with periosteal elevation known as Codman's triangle.**

A. An osteoclastoma is a benign tumor that contains highly vascular cellular stroma and occurs on the ends of long bones. Radiographically they appear as clear cystic tumors. Treatment is via surgical excision, and the local recurrence rate is as high as 50%.

B. Ewing's sarcoma is a small, round, blue cell malignancy that occurs at the diaphysis of long bones. Affected individuals are usually younger than 20 years of age. The radiographic characteristic of "onion-skinning" is caused by the tumor extending from the medulla with new bone formation parallel to the shaft. This tumor is extremely malignant, with early metastases being observed.

C. Chondrosarcomas arise from chondroblasts and usually occur in older age groups. They are found most commonly in the pelvis, ribs, sternum, or femur. Plain films demonstrate destruction of the involved bone with an expanding soft tissue mass containing irregular calcifications.

D. Unicameral bone cysts are common benign bone cysts of uncertain etiology, which most often arise during childhood. The lesions are often asymptomatic and discovered incidentally, although some may present as pathologic fractures. The most frequent site for their development is the proximal humeral metaphysis. Radiographically one observes a well-defined metaphyseal lucency that may expand the bone. Small cysts may be treated with steroid injections; larger cysts may require surgical curettage and bone grafting.

89. **E. Patients born with familial retinoblastoma inherit a defective copy of the retinoblastoma (Rb) tumor suppressor gene located on chromosome 13q14. Mutation of the normal Rb gene early in development leads to the emergence of retinoblastoma at an early age. Treatment is surgical excision. These children are at an increased risk for developing an osteogenic sarcoma and other soft tissue sarcomas.**

A. Neurofibromatosis, also known as Von Recklinghausen's disease, is associated with multiple neurofibromas of the skin. Affected individuals also have café au lait spots. This disease is associated with pheochromocytomas and osteitis fibrosa cystica. There is no association with osteosarcoma.

B, C, D. Premature birth, history of loose, bloody stools, and prior broken bones are all nonspecific findings.

90. **A. The natural history of an osteogenic sarcoma is relentless growth, early metastasis to the lungs, and death if not appropriately and aggressively treated. Current therapy combines limb salvage surgery with preoperative and postoperative chemotherapy consisting of multiple cytotoxic drugs. The 5-year survival rate is greater than 70% with this therapy.**

B. At one point, radiation with delayed amputation was the standard treatment for osteosarcoma, with a 5-year survival rate of less than 20%.

C. Osteosarcomas are radiation resistant. For that reason, radiation therapy is now limited to large, unresectable tumors.

D, E. Limb-sparing surgery is the current standard of care in the treatment of this tumor.

91. **D. While this patient initially presented with what appeared to be acute cholecystitis, this condition has progressed to an acute abdomen. The patient needs to be emergently taken to the operating room for exploratory abdominal surgery.**

A, C. Regardless of any new radiographic study finding, based on the clinical signs of an acute abdomen, the patient needs to be emergently taken to the operating room.

B. Increasing pain medication will make the patient comfortable, but it will not solve the underlying problem. If the patient has been given too much medication, it may affect the ability to truly evaluate her clinical abdominal exam.

E. Fluid boluses may be required as a result of the global inflammatory response seen with an acute abdomen, in which the fluid requirements increase. The patient should be closely followed, with frequent monitoring of her vital signs and urine output.

92. C. This case involves a type III ulcer, which is located in the prepyloric region of the stomach. An antrectomy and vagotomy, with incorporation of the ulcer into the specimen, is an appropriate procedure for treating a type III ulcer.

A. A type I ulcer is located along the lesser curvature of the stomach.
B. A type II ulcer is a combination of an ulcer in the body of the stomach and a duodenal ulcer.
D. A type IV ulcer is an ulcer at the gastroesophageal junction.
E. There is no type V ulcer category.

93 D. Because type III ulcers are less likely to be associated with hyperacidity and can carry a risk of being malignant, removal of the ulcer via a distal gastrectomy without vagotomy is the best choice. Ninety-five percent of gastric ulcers occur on the lesser curvature of the stomach, making them type I ulcers.

A. A vagotomy and pyloroplasty is a procedure used for management of peptic ulcer disease. This approach would not remove the ulcer for pathologic evaluation.
B. While a total gastrectomy would obviously remove the ulcer, this procedure involves significant morbidity not justified in this scenario.
C. A highly selective vagotomy is a procedure used to lower acidity in peptic ulcer disease. It would not be indicated in treatment of type I ulcers and would not allow pathologic evaluation of the ulcer.
E. Vagotomy and gastrojejunostomy is a procedure that was used and then discarded as an acid-reducing strategy. It would not be appropriate in this case and would not remove the ulcer for pathologic examination.
F. Proximal gastric resection is not a standard gastric procedure and therefore is inappropriate in this case.

94. C. Afferent loop syndrome presents with postprandial distention, nausea, and RUQ pain, all of which are relieved by emesis, typically bilious in nature. The acute form may be due to edema at the gastrojejunostomy, thus obstructing the afferent loop. If symptoms persist, conversion to a Roux-en-Y gastrojejunostomy may be required.

A. Recurrent ulcers are more common with duodenal ulcers and occur at the anastomotic site. They usually present with pain and postprandial vomiting.
B. Postprandial dumping syndrome is the most common complication of gastrectomy. Symptoms include pain, vomiting, diarrhea, palpitations, and flushing usually within 30 minutes of a meal.
D. Postvagotomy diarrhea occurs episodically and may be associated with nausea and vomiting. Typical treatment consists of dietary adjustments and antidiarrheals.
E. Bile reflux gastritis presents with epigastric pain associated with nausea and vomiting. Initial therapy consists of H_2 blockers.

95. B. Early postprandial dumping syndrome is the most common postgastrectomy complication. Rapid emptying of hyperosmolar chyme causes intravascular fluid shifts, resulting in symptoms that include pain, vomiting, diarrhea, palpitations, and flushing usually within 30 minutes of a meal. Frequent consumption of high–protein, low-carbohydrate meals is recommended to decrease the incidence and severity of this syndrome.

A. Recurrent ulcers are more common with duodenal ulcers and occur at the anastomotic site. They usually present with pain and postprandial vomiting.
C. Afferent loop syndrome presents with postprandial distention, nausea, and RUQ pain, which are relieved by emesis, typically bilious in nature.
D. Late postprandial dumping syndrome is also known as reactive hypoglycemia. Ingestion of large amounts of carbohydrates stimulates insulin release, causing hypoglycemia several hours after eating.
E. Bile reflux gastritis presents with epigastric pain associated with nausea and vomiting. Initial therapy consists of H_2 blockers.

96. D. This patient's history and physical exam are concerning for a possible choledochal cyst. A choledochal cyst is a congenital malformation of the bile ducts that results in cystic dilations. Five types of choledochal cysts exist:

- **I: Dilation of the common bile duct**
- **II: Diverticulum of the common bile duct**

- **III: Choledochocele**
- **IV: Multiple intrahepatic and extrahepatic choledochocysts**
- **V: Single or multiple intrahepatic cysts (Caroli disease)**

Patients present with a triad of symptoms: recurrent abdominal pain, mild episodic jaundice, and a right upper quadrant mass. Choledochal cysts are frequently seen in older children. Excision of the cyst is the treatment of choice.

A. Acute cholecystitis is an unlikely choice, based on the child's age, history, and physical exam.
B. Acute cholangitis in a child without a fever is unlikely.
C. A mass in the head of the pancreas would be an unlikely choice, for the same reason of age, as well as the episodic jaundice. A mass of the pancreas would be more likely to present with persistent jaundice.
E. Choledocholithiasis is a possibility, but the history is not consistent with biliary colic and this condition would be less likely at this age. Obtaining an ultrasound of the right upper quadrant would be the study of choice, and would help eliminate this possibility.

97. **A. The initial study of choice is a right upper quadrant ultrasound. Diagnosis can often be made from an ultrasound alone. Other studies, such as an abdominal CT scan, hepatobiliary scintigraphy, ERCP, or cholangiography, may be obtained later as needed to formulate a treatment plan.**

B. An abdominal CT scan would not be considered the initial diagnostic study in this case. Compared to an US, its higher cost is an important factor.
C. Hepatobiliary scintigraphy is useful in detecting associated intrahepatic cystic disease or obstruction, but in this scenario it is not the initial study of choice.
D. An ERCP would be useful later to define the location of the cyst and to aid in placement of a stent if necessary.
E. Cholangiography is used to define the anatomy and location of the cyst. It would be performed secondary to an initial ultrasound of the right upper quadrant.

98. **A. The most common primary malignant tumor of the liver is hepatocellular carcinoma (HCC). It is also one of the most common solid cancers in the world, with an annual incidence estimated at 1 million new patients per year. Patients with cirrhosis, hepatitis B, history of alcohol abuse, hemochromatosis, schistosomiasis, aflatoxin, and α-1-antitrypsin disease all have an increased risk of developing HCC. Patients typically present with dull RUQ pain, weight loss, hepatomegaly, and an abdominal mass. Treatment consists of surgical resection if possible. Unfortunately, only 5% to 15% of newly diagnosed patients with HCC undergo a potentially curative resection. Figure 5-98 shows an obvious tumor in the right lobe of the liver.**

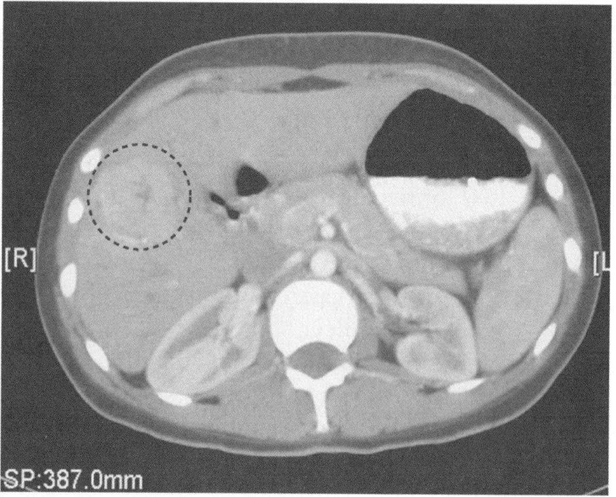

Figure 5-98 • Image Courtesy of the University of Utah School of Medicine, Salt Lake City, Utah.

B. While cholangiocarcinoma is included in the differential diagnosis, it accounts for only 7% of all primary hepatic tumors. Cholangiocarcinoma is associated with chronic cholestasis, congenital cystic disease of the liver, and infection with the liver fluke, *Clonorchis sinensis.* Given this patient's history of cirrhosis and alcohol abuse, HCC is a more likely diagnosis.
C. A hepatoblastoma is a tumor seen in infants and children.
D. A hemangioma is a benign liver tumor, which rarely causes symptoms such as presented in this case.
E. An adenoma is a benign lesion that occurs primarily in young females taking oral contraceptives.

99. **B. Alpha fetoprotein (AFP) is associated with hepatocellular carcinoma. More than 70% of patients with a HCC larger than 3 cm will have an elevated AFP level.**

A. β-hCG is associated with intrauterine pregnancy, as well as testicular and trophoblastic tumors.

C. CA 19-9 is associated with pancreatic cancer; it may also be elevated in colorectal and gastric cancers.

D. CEA is associated with colorectal cancer; it may also be elevated in HCC, pancreatic, breast, and testicular cancers.

E. CA 125 is associated with ovarian tumors.

100. **E. The most common site of distant metastasis for a hepatocellular carcinoma is to the lungs. Local invasion into the diaphragm is also common.**

A, B, C, D. The brain, spleen, small bowel, and pancreas are unlikely locations for metastasis of HCC.

SETTING 3: INPATIENT FACILITIES

You have general admitting privileges to the hospital. You may see patients in the critical care unit, the pediatrics unit, the maternity unit, or recovery room. You may also be called to see patients in the psychiatric unit. A short-stay unit serves patients who are undergoing same-day operations or who are being held for observation. There are adjacent nursing home/extended-care facilities and a detoxification unit where you may see patients.

101. A 3-day-old male infant is transferred to the newborn intensive care unit from an outside facility with abdominal distention, bilious emesis, and failure to pass meconium. You evaluate the infant and, after obtaining a contrast enema (Figure 5-101A), determine that he has meconium ileus. Which other condition is this child at risk for having?

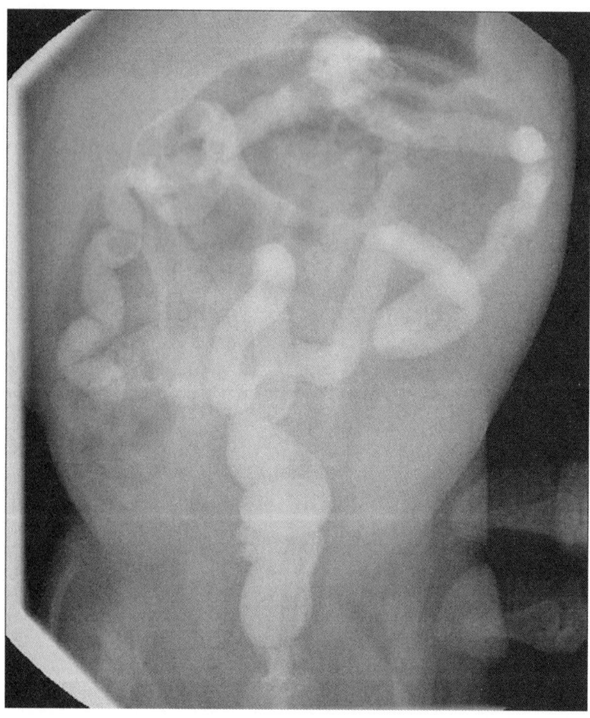

A

Figure 5-101A • Image Courtesy of the University of Utah School of Medicine, Salt Lake City, Utah.

A. Budd-Chiari syndrome
B. Down syndrome
C. Von Hippel-Lindau syndrome
D. Eaton-Lambert syndrome
E. Cystic fibrosis

102. You are called to the newborn intensive care unit to evaluate a 36-hour-old infant whose abdomen has become distended, associated with bilious emesis. After performing your history and physical exam, you obtain an abdominal x-ray (Figure 5-102A). What is the most likely diagnosis in this case?

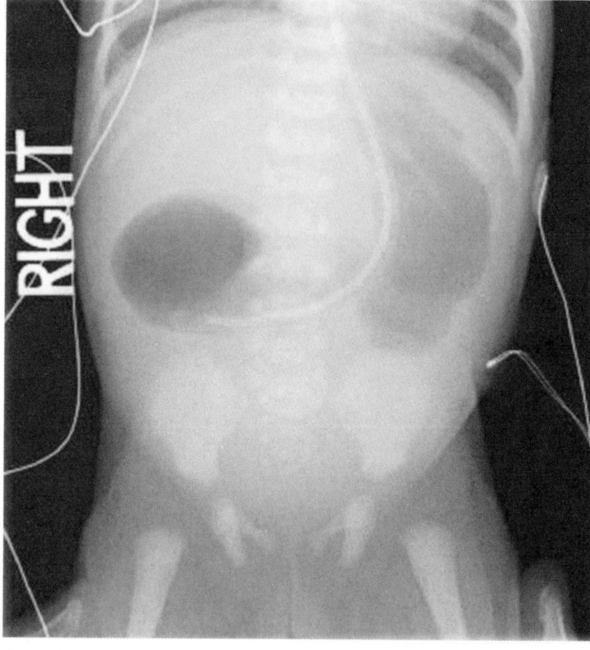

A

Figure 5-102A • Image Courtesy of the University of Utah School of Medicine, Salt Lake City, Utah.

A. Midgut volvulus
B. Hypertrophic pyloric stenosis
C. Duodenal atresia
D. Meconiumileus
E. Hirschsprung's disease

The next three questions (items 103–105) correspond to the following vignette.

A 50-year-old female patient scheduled to be discharged from the hospital the next day is suffering from a unrelated 2-week history of extreme pain upon defecation. The patient denies any associated abdominal pain, nausea, vomiting, fever, or chills. She reports a long history of constipation, which has been severe lately. She has also noticed slight spotting of blood on tissue paper, but denies any anal drainage, bright red blood per rectum, or melena.

103. On examination, what is the most likely physical finding in this patient?

A. Disruption of anoderm in the posterior midline.
B. Protrusion of an internal hemorrhoid
C. Fistula in ano
D. Perirectal abscess
E. Anal condyloma

104. What is the best initial therapy for this patient?

A. Surgical treatment
B. 0.2% nitroglycerin topical ointment
C. Stool softeners, bulking agents, and sitz baths
D. Botulinum toxin
E. No treatment is necessary

105. The patient returns to your outpatient office with the same complaints and physical findings 6 weeks after completing initial management. What is the next best step in the management of this patient's problem?

A. Diverting colostomy
B. Lateral internal anal sphincterotomy
C. Low anterior resection
D. Incision and drainage
E. Hemorrhoidectomy

End of Set

106. You are called to evaluate a 33-year-old female on the cardiology service who recently delivered a healthy baby girl. During the course of her pregnancy, the patient developed dilated cardiomyopathy that progressed to complete heart failure. The patient has remained in the cardiac intensive care unit on multiple inotropes, which the cardiologists have been unable to wean. The patient recently had a balloon pump placed. The transplant cardiology service is likewise seeing this young woman to evaluate for a heart transplant. What is the next best option you could offer this patient prior to receiving a transplant?

A. Aortic valve replacement
B. Placement of a biventricular assist device
C. Coronary artery bypass grafting
D. Extracorporeal membrane oxygenation (ECMO)
E. Vigorous diuresis and physical therapy

107. A 66-year-old male is undergoing coronary artery bypass grafting to the left anterior descending, circumflex, and right coronary arteries. Despite maximizing volume status and optimizing inotropic agents, the patient is unable to be weaned from the cardiopulmonary bypass machine, at which time an intra-aortic balloon pump is placed. Which of the following statements is true regarding intra-aortic balloon pumps?

A. They decrease afterload by inflating during systole.
B. They augment coronary artery flow during diastole.
C. They assist in afterload reduction in aortic regurgitation.
D. They increase mesenteric flow by inflating during systole.
E. Immediate postoperative use is contraindicated secondary to bleeding risks.

The next three questions (items 108–110) correspond to the following vignette.

The orthopedic surgery service asks you to evaluate a 78-year-old female who underwent total hip replacement 8 days ago. The patient was initially tolerating her diet, but over the last 3 days she has become distended and has begun having nausea and vomiting. On exam, the patient's abdomen is distended and nontender.

108. Based on the abdominal film shown (Figure 5-108), what is the most likely diagnosis?

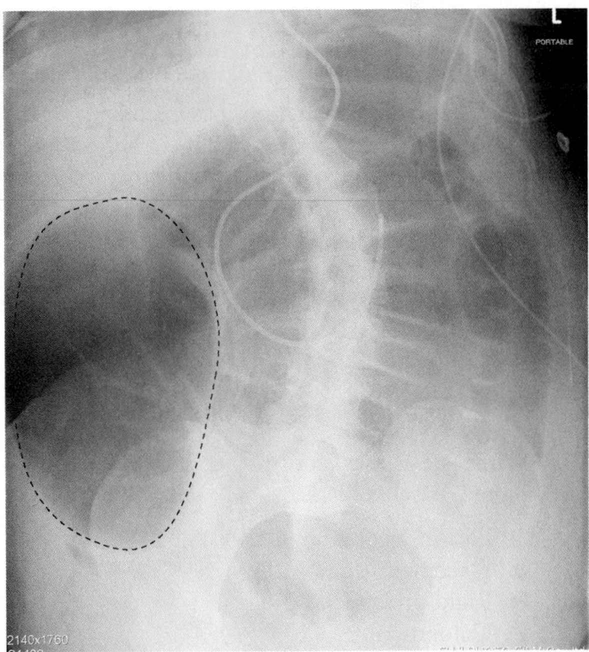

Figure 5-108 • Image Courtesy of the University of Utah School of Medicine, Salt Lake City, Utah

A. Ogilvie syndrome
B. Acute SBO
C. Toxic megacolon
D. *C. difficile* colitis
E. Mesenteric ischemia

109. What is the best initial approach to this patient's problem?

A. Immediate exploratory laparotomy
B. IV antibiotics and proton pump inhibitors
C. Total parenteral nutrition
D. Institution of nasojejunal feedings
E. Neostigmine

110. Prior to treatment, the patient should have correction of serum electrolytes and which of the following procedures?

A. Chest x-ray
B. ECG
C. Continuous pulse oximetry
D. Continuous cardiac monitoring
E. Baseline arterial blood gas

End of Set

The next two questions (items 111 and 112) correspond to the following vignette.

You are called to see 73-year-old male in the medical ICU for evaluation of a GI bleed. The medicine service intern reports that bright red blood was first noticed in the patient's stool this morning. Throughout the day, the patient has become progressively more tachycardic despite a 250 cc bolus of normal saline (NS). The patient has a history of colon cancer, which was resected via a left hemicolectomy 8 years ago. The vital signs are as follows: BP 110/72, HR 116, and RR 14. You examine the patient, and see that he has difficulty talking due to the CPAP mask he is wearing. The rectal exam is unremarkable except for gross blood. To ensure a good IV, you place a central line.

111. What is the first step in this patient's management?

A. Barium enema
B. Placement of a NGT
C. Rigid proctoscopy
D. Colonoscopy
E. Urgently operative procedure

112. You choose to send the patient to angiography for embolization of the bleeding vessel. What is the main limiting factor of angiography?

A. Difficult to visualize if the bleed is in the proximal duodenum
B. Difficult to visualize if it is a small bowel bleed
C. Difficult to visualize if the bleed is less than 1 cc/min
D. Difficult to visualize if cauterization was attempted during colonoscopy
E. Difficult to localize recurrent tumor by angiography

End of Set

113. During an elective repair of a right inguinal hernia in a 6-year-old male, an undescended testicle is encountered in the inguinal canal. In addition to a high ligation repair of the indirect hernia sac, an orchiopexy is performed. Which of the following statements is true regarding testicular tumors?

A. Germ cell tumors are the least common type of testicular cancer.
B. An elevated serum human chorionic gonadotropin (HCG) level is almost always found in association with seminoma.
C. Orchiopexy does not reduce the likelihood that this patient will develop testicular cancer.
D. A biopsy of suspected testicular cancer may be safely performed under local anesthesia via a scrotal incision.
E. Seminomas are insensitive to radiation therapy.

The next three questions (items 114–116) correspond to the following vignette.

An 81-year-old male undergoes an elective abdominal aortic aneurysm repair. The surgery is uncomplicated, and the patient is transported to the SICU in guarded condition. When the patient is examined on postoperative day 1, he is unable to move his legs. There is decreased sensation to both the posterior and anterior aspects of his legs, and rectal sphincter tone is absent.

114. What is the most appropriate next step in the work-up of this patient?

A. Electromyography of the lower extremities
B. Lumbar puncture
C. MRI of the spinal cord
D. CT scan of the head
E. Lumbar myelogram

115. The artery that had become occluded resulting in this complication is found most commonly between which vertebral levels?

A. T1 to T5
B. T5 to T10
C. T10 to L2
D. L4 to S2
E. S2 to S4

116. Which of the following neurological findings is commonly associated with this syndrome?

A. Loss of proprioception
B. Loss of pain and temperature sensation
C. Quadriplegia
D. Constipation
E. Loss of vibration sensation

End of Set

117. During your morning rounds, a 45-year-old male patient you admitted the night before with a small subdural hematoma is found to have new mental status changes. Although a painful sternal rub is applied, the patient fails to open his eyes, proceeds to extend his legs while flexing his upper extremities, and makes a low-pitched moan as his only verbal response. What is this patient's Glasgow Coma Score (GCS)?

A. 3
B. 4
C. 5
D. 6
E. 7

The next two questions (items 118 and 119) correspond to the following vignette.

A 48-year-old male is admitted to the ICU after being found unconscious in a neighborhood park. The patient was intubated while in the emergency department, and he remains on a ventilator with maintenance IV fluids running. You are called emergently to the bedside because the patient has become progressively hypotensive over the last 45 minutes, with a present blood pressure of 78/40 and a heart rate of 130, which is down from 116/64 an hour ago. In addition to giving the patient a fluid bolus, you place a pulmonary artery catheter. The cardiac index is 6.1 L/min/M^2, CVP is 4 mm Hg, PCWP is 10 mm Hg, and SVR is 400 dynes/s/cm^5.

118. What type of shock is this patient experiencing?

A. Septic shock
B. Obstructive shock
C. Hypovolemic shock
D. Neurogenic shock
E. Cardiogenic shock

119. What is the most appropriate next step in the management of this patient?

A. Vasopressin
B. IV fluids
C. Fresh frozen plasma transfusion
D. Dobutamine drip
E. Norepinephrine drip

End of Set

The next two questions (items 120 and 121) correspond to the following vignette.

You admit a trauma patient involved in a motorcycle accident who was brought to the emergency department by helicopter in critical condition. The patient has multiple injuries identified on physical exam and with CT scans of his head, chest, abdomen, and pelvis. His injuries include a subdural bleed, two right rib fractures without evidence of a pneumothorax, a traumatic bowel perforation that required a bowel resection, and a tibial fracture. Following your exploratory laparotomy, the patient was taken to the surgical intensive care unit. You are called 5 hours later by the SICU nurse, who is concerned because the patient has a blood pressure of 82/58 and a heart rate of 116. The nurse gives you the following pulmonary artery numbers: CI of 3.1 L/min/M^2, CVP of 2 mm Hg, PCWP of 9 mm Hg, and SVR of 1600 dynes/s/cm^5.

120. What type of shock is this patient experiencing?

A. Hypovolemic shock
B. Cardiogenic shock
C. Septic shock
D. Neurogenic shock
E. Obstructive shock

121. On admission to the hospital, this patient's hematocrit was 42%. You tell the nurse to check this level, and when you arrive to the SICU you find it to be 22%. The patient remains intubated and continues to follow commands. Where is the patient most likely bleeding to cause a 20% decline in hematocrit?

A. Pleural cavity
B. Abdominal cavity
C. Retroperitoneal space
D. Intracranial
E. Leg
F. Unidentified injury

End of Set

The next two questions (items 122 and 123) correspond to the following vignette.

You are called to the ICU bedside of a 53-year-old female who has been on a ventilator for the last 2 days after undergoing a sigmoid colectomy with diverting colostomy for perforated diverticulitis. The patient remains on IV antibiotics but has been showing signs of sepsis; however, she has not required any vasopressors. Vital signs are BP 102/76, HR 98, RR 20, and T 37.6°C. The ventilator is set on pressure support ventilation, FiO_2 0.50, PIP 14, PEEP 5, and ventilator set rate of 14. The most recent arterial blood gas shows a pH of 7.28, PCO_2 53, PO_2 88, HCO_3 23, and BE –2.

122. What is the proper interpretation of this blood gas reading?

A. Metabolic acidosis
B. Metabolic alkalosis
C. Respiratory acidosis
D. Respiratory alkalosis
E. Combined metabolic and respiratory acidosis

123. How can you best correct this abnormality?

A. Give 2 amps of $NaHCO_3$
B. Increase the FiO_2
C. Increase the respiratory rate
D. Change the IV fluids to 0.9% NS
E. Increase the PIP

End of Set

The next two questions (items 124 and 125) correspond to the following vignette.

You are called to evaluate a 3-week-old premature female infant born with a Tetralogy of Fallot. The child has recently become distended and is having bilious emesis. The patient's vital signs are stable, and an abdominal film is obtained (Figure 5-124A).

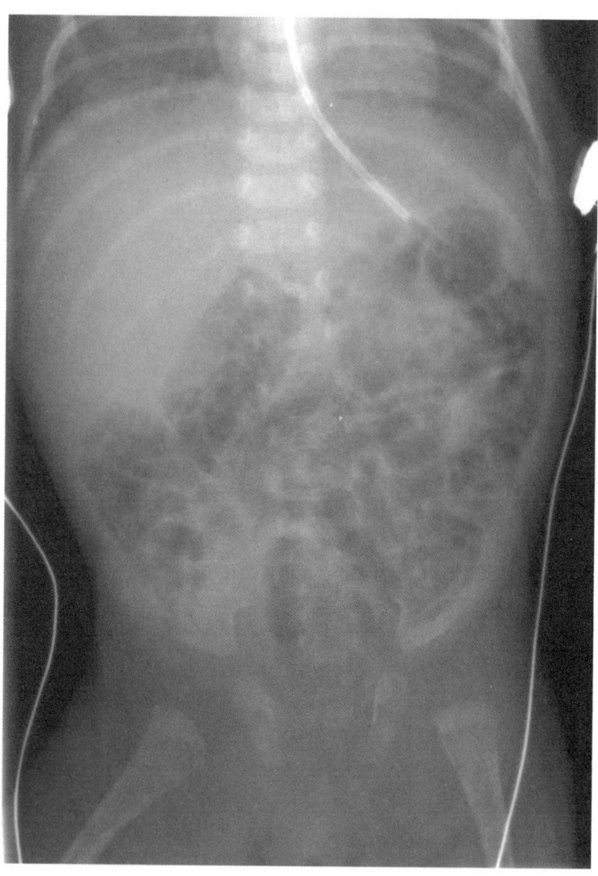

A

Figure 5-124A • Image Courtesy of the University of Utah School of Medicine, Salt Lake City, Utah.

124. What diagnosis concerns you most at this point?

A. Malrotation
B. Necrotizing enterocolitis
C. Jejunal atresia
D. Meconium ileus
E. Meconium plug syndrome

125. Which of the following is part of the initial management of this condition?

A. Nasogastric decompression
B. Anaerobic antibiotic coverage
C. Placement of a feeding tube
D. Emergent laparotomy
E. Diagnostic laparoscopy

End of Set

The next four questions (items 126–129) correspond to the following vignette.

A 37-year-old male is involved in an industrial accident in which he sustains total body surface area burns consisting of 56% of partial- and full-thickness burns. The patient is transferred to your facility, where he undergoes proper resuscitation with ringer's lactate and albumin. After having a feeding tube placed, you need to calculate his daily caloric requirements.

126. What will be his estimated resting energy expenditure?
    A. 10 to 20 kcal/kg/day
    B. 20 to 30 kcal/kg/day
    C. 30 to 40 kcal/kg/day
    D. 40 to 50 kcal/kg/day
    E. 50 to 60 kcal/kg/day

127. After 2 weeks of enteral feeding, you want to check your patient's nitrogen balance to ensure that he is receiving adequate nutrition. A 24-hour urine nitrogen sample is collected. How do you convert the grams of urinary nitrogen collected to grams of protein?
    A. [urinary nitrogen (g) per 24 hours] × 6.25
    B. [urinary nitrogen (g) per 24 hours + 4] × 6.25
    C. [urinary nitrogen (g) per 24 hours + 8] × 6.25
    D. [urinary nitrogen (g) per 24 hours + 4] × 13.5
    E. [urinary nitrogen (g) per 24 hours + 8] × 13.5

128. Which of the following complications of overfeeding can be corrected by increasing fat calories as a percentage of nonprotein calories?
    A. Increased CO_2 production
    B. Hepatic failure
    C. Slower recovery
    D. Impaired immune system
    E. Catheter sepsis

129. In which of the following situations is enteral feeding potentially possible?
    A. Severe pancreatitis
    B. Short gut syndrome
    C. High-output enterocutaneous fistula
    D. Prolonged ileus
    E. Prolonged intubation

End of Set

The next three questions (items 130–132) correspond to the following vignette.

A 23-year-old obese male is brought to the hospital today by ambulance after being involved in a motor vehicle accident the day before. Initially the patient was evaluated and found to have no injuries, and he had been wearing a seat belt. The morning after the accident, the patient's abdomen became acutely tender after eating, at which time he called for an ambulance. Upon arrival to the hospital, the patient is hemodynamically stable but has an acute abdomen. He is taken to the operating room, where you perform an exploratory laparotomy and find an area of small bowel ischemia without significant spillage. The small area of injured bowel is resected and the abdomen is irrigated prior to closing. Nevertheless, you remained concerned about this patient developing a wound infection.

130. How would this patient's level of contamination be classified?
    A. Clean
    B. Sterile
    C. Clean contaminated
    D. Contaminated
    E. Dirty

131. On postoperative day 2, this patient develops a fever of 38.9°C. You are called by the nursing staff to evaluate the patient, who has otherwise been doing well. What is the most likely cause of fever at this point in his hospital course?
    A. Urinary tract infection
    B. Atelectasis
    C. Intra-abdominal abscess
    D. Line infection
    E. Medications

132. The patient is slow to progress and remains in the hospital on postoperative day 7. He is febrile and the incision is erythematous. Upon removal of some of the skin staples to check for a suspected wound infection, you note bilious fluid draining from the wound. A diagnosis of enterocutaneous fistula is made. What is the initial step in the treatment of this complication?
    A. Percutaneous drainage of abdominal abscess
    B. Control of fistula output
    C. Initiation of enteral nutrition
    D. Exploratory laparotomy
    E. IV fluids and electrolyte repletion

End of Set

The next two questions (items 133 and 134) correspond to the following vignette.

A 34-year-old male is transported to the ED by firefighters after he sustained minor burns to both lower extremities upon falling near a bonfire. The patient is admitted to the hospital as a trauma/burn case. Initial evaluation shows the patient to be coherent and talking, with the following vital signs: BP 188/82, HR 119, RR 18, and SaO_2 of 100% on 2 liters oxygen. The burns are approximately 14% of total body surface area in size, involving both lower extremities, with the right lower extremity having circumferential full-thickness burns below the knee.

133. Which potential acute injury concerns you most in this patient?
    A. Fluid losses from burn wounds
    B. Infection of burns
    C. Rhabdomyolysis
    D. Compartment syndrome
    E. Inhalation injury

134. How do you best evaluate the severity of this patient's injury?
    A. Central venous pressure monitoring
    B. Urine myoglobin
    C. Sputum gram stain and cultures
    D. Blood cultures
    E. Check compartment pressures

End of Set

The next two questions (items 135 and 136) correspond to the following vignette.

A 28-year-old male is seen in the clinic with a 3-day history of crampy abdominal pain accompanied by nausea and vomiting. The patient denies any bowel movements for 3 days and has not passed any gas in 2 days. At age 8, the patient underwent surgical resection of a Wilm's tumor through a midline laparotomy. On exam, his abdomen is grossly distended and tender with high-pitched bowel sounds. There is a well-healed midline scar and no evidence of any inguinal or incisional hernia. The patient is afebrile, with a HR of 108 and a BP of 114/88. This morning's WBC count is 10,800.

135. What is the next step in this patient's management?
    A. Surgical exploration
    B. NGT decompression, IV fluid resuscitation, and reevaluation in 24 to 48 hours
    C. Abdominal CT scan
    D. Colonoscopy
    E. Enteroclysis

136. What is the most likely cause of this clinical entity in this patient?
    A. Recurrent cancer
    B. Intussusception
    C. Hernia
    D. Adhesions
    E. Midgut volvulus

End of Set

137. A 46-year-old female is in the hospital on postoperative day 3 after undergoing an exploratory laparotomy for a small bowel obstruction. An ischemic bowel was found during the procedure, and a resection with primary anastomosis was performed. The patient continues to have an ileus and over the last 24 hours there has been 625 cc of drainage from the nasogastric tube. The nurse calls you because the patient has spiked a fever of 38.9°C.The physical exam is essentially normal. At this point in this patient's hospital course, you should be suspicious for what process?
    A. Wound infection
    B. Intra-abdominal abscess
    C. Urinary tract infection
    D. Deep venous thrombosis
    E. Pneumonia

The next two questions (items 138 and 139) correspond to the following vignette.

A 58-year-old female returns to the emergency department 10 days after undergoing a sigmoid colectomy for chronic diverticulitis. The patient's vital signs are as follows: T 102.3°F, HR 123, BP 83/42, RR 28, and SaO_2 of 88% on RA. On physical exam, the abdomen is distended, diffusely tender in the lower quadrants, with no peritoneal signs present. A CBC reveals a WBC count of 23,000. The patient is admitted to the ICU and receives 4 liters of ringer's lactate, but remains hypotensive at 96/47. A central venous catheter is placed and the initial CVP is 5 mm Hg.

138. What is the most likely cause of this patient's hypotension?

A. Myocardial infarction
B. Hypovolemia
C. Pulmonary embolism
D. Spinal shock
E. Sepsis

139. What is the most appropriate treatment once the patient is clinically stable?

A. IV antibiotics and observation
B. Barium enema
C. Surgical exploration
D. CT scan of abdomen and pelvis
E. Oral antibiotics

End of Set

140. A 62-year-old Native American female patient with a 10-year history of GERD is found to have a 1.4 cm adenocarcinoma limited to the submucosa of the distal esophagus upon routine endoscopy. There is no evidence of lymph node involvement or distant metastasis. The patient undergoes a transhiatal esophagectomy. On postoperative day 7, the patient has a temperature of 39.4°C, but is otherwise stable. Laboratory values reveal a mild leukocytosis. On physical exam, the abdomen is soft, nondistended, and nontender. Breath sounds are decreased in both bases, with some crackles in the left base. The neck incision is erythematous, tender, and indurated, with some cloudy drainage noted. What is the most likely cause of this patient's fever?

A. Superficial wound infection
B. Wound hematoma
C. Pneumonia
D. Anastomotic leak
E. Intra-abdominal abscess

The next two questions (items 141 and 142) correspond to the following vignette.

A 25-year-old female involved in a motor vehicle accident was admitted to your service 4 days ago. The injuries that this patient sustained included facial lacerations and a severely broken left radius and ulna, requiring external fixation by the orthopedic surgery service. Pain control has been difficult for this patient, and she has been slow to ambulate. You are called by the nursing staff to assess the patient due to an abrupt increase in oxygen requirements and complaints of chest pain. Initial impression reveals a patient in mild distress, complaining of chest pain and a feeling of suffocation, which began 30 minutes ago when she returned to bed after ambulating. The patient is presently receiving 4 L of O_2 by nasal cannula with saturations in the low 90s. Your exam reveals the following: Cognition is intact, without focal neurological deficits, tachycardia, and few crackles in the right lung base. The left arm is dressed, and other extremities are warm, without edema. An ECG demonstrates sinus tachycardia, at a rate of 130. The recorded heart rate an hour earlier was 75. Other vital signs are T 37.6°C and BP 124/76. A CXR obtained is unchanged from 2 days ago, which was normal.

141. What test should be ordered next for this patient?

A. CT scan of the thorax
B. Ventilation perfusion lung scan
C. Duplex scanning of lower extremities
D. Pulmonary angiography
E. Transthoracic echocardiogram

142. The test ordered confirms your suspected diagnosis. What treatment should be immediately initiated?

A. β-Blocker, aspirin, and nitroglycerin
B. Lorazepam taper
C. IV fluid bolus
D. Systemic anticoagulation
E. Thoracentesis

End of Set

143. After surgically repairing your patient's ruptured abdominal aneurysm, the intubated patient is transferred to the ICU, where massive fluid resuscitation continues. Despite a stable hematocrit, 24 hours postoperatively the patient becomes progressively more oliguric, with elevated peak airway pressures, and tense distention of his abdomen on physical exam. The patient's BP is 110/80 with a HR of 120. What is the best option for this patient at this point?

A. Emergent angiogram to evaluate for possible renal artery damage during AAA repair
B. Abdominal decompression
C. Increase positive end expiratory pressure and give diuretics
D. Transesophageal echo and Swan Ganz placement
E. Increasing IV fluid rate with an epinephrine drip infusion

The next two questions (items 144 and 145) correspond to the following vignette.

The medical ICU service consults you about a patient with pancreatitis. The patient has no history of alcohol abuse, and a recent ultrasound shows no evidence of gallstones or acute cholecystitis. The patient has been experiencing severe nausea and vomiting and is beginning to have mental status changes. Labs are reviewed: WBC 18,000, hematocrit 32%, amylase 466 U/L, lipase 1176 U/L, serum creatinine 1.2 mg/dL, and calcium 14 mg/dL.

144. What is the proper management of this patient at this time?
    A. Start imipenem
    B. Start parenteral nutrition
    C. Transfuse 2 units packed red blood cells
    D. Increase IV fluids to maintain urine output of 80 to 100 cc/h
    E. Perform laparoscopic cholecystectomy

145. What medication may be indicated to assist in the emergent management of this condition?
    A. Ondansetron
    B. Furosemide
    C. Ticarcillin/clavulanate
    D. Promethazine
    E. Phosphate

End of Set

The next three questions (items 146–148) correspond to the following vignette.

A 36-year-old female is referred to you for evaluation of periodic abdominal pain that occurs 30 to 40 minutes after eating. The pain and vomiting are most common after she consumes a fatty meal, and the patient reports having symptoms for the last 3 to 4 weeks. A right upper quadrant ultrasound reveals cholelithiasis. You take her to the operating room, where you perform an uncomplicated laparoscopic cholecystectomy. After removing the gallbladder, you open it and find multiple brown stones.

146. Development of brown gallstones is frequently associated with which of the following conditions?
    A. Infection
    B. Hyperbilirubinemia
    C. Cholangiocarcinoma
    D. Complete cystic duct obstruction
    E. Hypercholesterolemia

147. Which of the following ethnic groups has an increased incidence of brown pigment stone formation?
    A. African Americans
    B. Caucasians
    C. Asians
    D. Scandinavians
    E. Hispanics

148. Which of the following bacteria most commonly produce the enzyme, bacterial β-d-glucuronidase, that is involved in the formation of brown pigment stones?
    A. *Staphylococcus aureus* and *Enterococcus*
    B. *Staphylococcus aureus* and *Streptococcus*
    C. *Pseudomonas* and *E. coli*
    D. *E. coli* and *Bacteroides fragilis*
    E. *E. coli* and *Klebsiella*

End of Set

The next two questions (items 149 and 150) correspond to the following vignette.

A 32-year-old male presents to your clinic for evaluation of gallstones. The patient describes multiple episodes of biliary colic to you and brings a report of an ultrasound that confirmed the presence of multiple gallstones. You recommend that he undergo a laparoscopic cholecystectomy with an intraoperative cholangiogram. The evening following the cholecystectomy, the patient develops a fever of 40°C. The morning WBC count is elevated to 21,000 and all of the liver function tests are slightly elevated. You start the patient on antibiotics to treat the cholangitis.

149. Which bacteria are most commonly associated with cholangitis?
    A. *Enterobacter*
    B. *E. coli*
    C. *Enterococcus*
    D. *Klebsiella*
    E. *Proteus*

150. The triad of right upper quadrant pain, fever, and jaundice—commonly known as Charcot's triad—is associated with cholangitis or an active infection in the biliary system. This combination of symptoms can be associated with which two additional symptoms of severe cholangitis?

A. Nausea and elevated WBC
B. Hypertension and chills
C. Mental status changes and hypotension
D. Diarrhea and elevated alkaline phosphatase
E. Oliguria and vomiting

End of Set

A Answers and Explanations

101. E
102. C
103. A
104. C
105. B
106. B
107. B
108. A
109. E
110. D
111. B
112. C
113. C
114. C
115. C
116. B
117. D
118. A
119. B
120. A
121. A
122. C
123. E
124. B
125. A
126. D
127. B
128. A
129. E
130. C
131. B
132. E
133. D
134. E
135. A
136. D
137. C
138. E
139. D
140. D
141. B
142. D
143. B
144. D
145. B
146. A
147. C
148. E
149. B
150. C

101. E. Meconium ileus is an obstruction of the distal ileum from inspissated meconium and is often associated with cystic fibrosis. Approximately 10% to 15% of infants with meconium ileus have cystic fibrosis. Meconium ileus presents with failure to pass meconium within 48 hours of birth in conjunction with progressive abdominal distention and bilious emesis. Abdominal films show the classic "soap bubble" appearance in the proximal colon, and a contrast enema shows a microcolon with small plugs of meconium (note the arrows in Figure 5-101B).

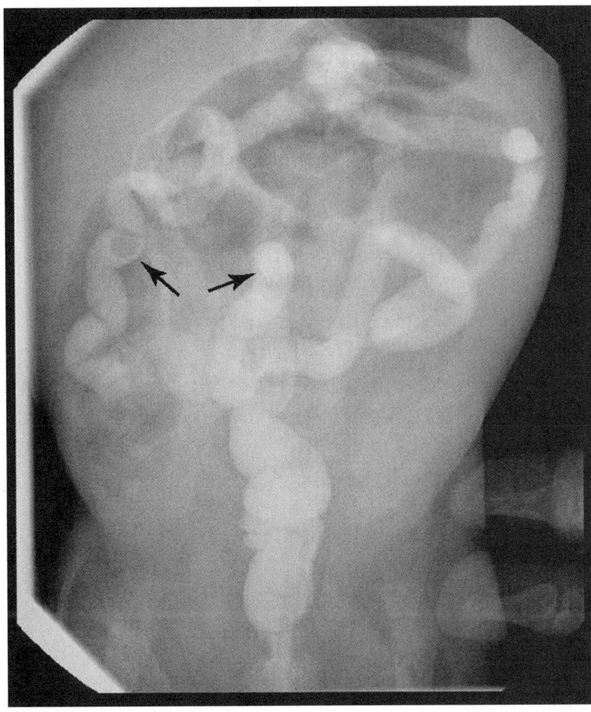

B

Figure 5-101B • Image Courtesy of the University of Utah School of Medicine, Salt Lake City, Utah.

A. Budd-Chiari syndrome is hepatic veno-occlusive disease, mostly seen in adults and not associated with meconium ileus.
B. Down syndrome (trisomy 21) is most often associated with cardiac and renal abnormalities. Associated abdominal abnormalities include imperforate anus, duodenal or jejunal atresia, duodenal or jejunal stenosis, and Hirschsprung's disease.
C. Von Hippel-Lindau syndrome is associated with pancreatic, central nervous system, and renal tumors in adults.
D. Eaton-Lambert syndrome is a paraneoplastic neurologic-myopathic syndrome that presents with symptoms similar to myasthenia gravis.

102. C. Bilious emesis in a newborn should be evaluated immediately to rule out malrotation and midgut volvulus. The "double bubble" sign seen in Figure 5-102B (note the arrows) is associated with duodenal atresia. Duodenal atresia is frequently associated with other anomalies such as anal atresia, tracheoesophageal fistula with esophageal atresia, and vertebral defects. Obstruction can be due to a duodenal web, duodenal atresia, duodenal stenosis, or annular pancreas.

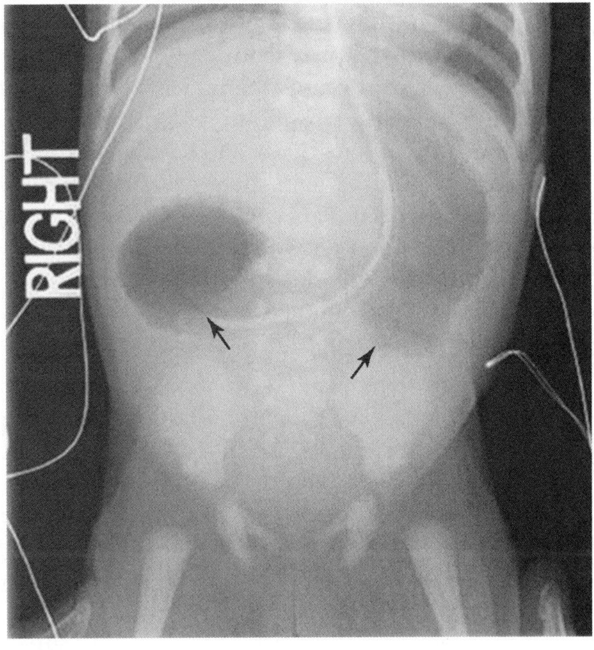

B

Figure 5-102B • Image Courtesy of the University of Utah School of Medicine, Salt Lake City, Utah.

A. A midgut volvulus is a surgical emergency due to compromised blood supply to the bowel and increases the risk for developing ischemic bowel. It is part of the differential diagnosis for newborns with bilious emesis, but a "double bubble" sign is virtually pathognomonic for duodenal atresia.
B. Pyloric stenosis presents as rapid, nonbilious projectile vomiting of feeding in infants approximately 6 to 8 weeks of age. It is more common in males than in females (4:1 ratio), and is most common in first-born males.

D. Meconium ileus is a distal ileal obstruction caused by thick, inspissated meconium. It is frequently associated with cystic fibrosis. X-ray findings include dilated loops of bowel and a ground-glass appearance of meconium mixed with air in the right lower quadrant (soap bubble sign).

E. Hirschsprung's disease involves an aganglionic colonic segment with secondary colonic obstruction. It is not associated with bilious emesis.

103. **A. An anal fissure is a disruption of the anoderm. It most commonly occurs in the posterior midline as a result of forceful dilatation of the anal canal, most often during defecation. Initially it is felt as a tearing pain upon defecation. This pain causes the patient to ignore the urge to defecate, resulting in constipation and further disruption to the anoderm upon defecation. A cycle of pain, poor sphincteric relaxation, and reinjury occurs. The patient presents with pain upon defecation and minimal bleeding on tissue of stool. Physical exam by simply separating the buttocks will reveal a tear in the anoderm in the posterior midline.**

B. Protrusion of an internal hemorrhoid usually results in anal fullness and discomfort along with bright red blood per rectum. Occasionally, an internal hemorrhoid can prolapse through the anus and incarcerate, requiring surgical intervention. Hemorrhoids can usually be distinguished from a fissure on physical exam.

C. A fistula in ano presents as a draining site on the buttock skin, usually as a complication of an anorectal abscess. It presents with drainage, not extreme pain.

D. Perirectal and anorectal abscesses most often arise from obstruction of an anal gland that subsequently becomes infected and overgrown with bacteria. These glands are located between the internal and external anal sphincters. If the infection tracks down this space toward the skin, an anorectal abscess occurs.

E. Anal condylomas are caused by infection with human papillomavirus (HPV) types 6 and 11. Patients complain of a perianal growth that appears as a cauliflower-like lesion on physical exam. Minimal disease may be treated in the office with bichloracetic acid or podophyllum. Larger lesions may require surgical excision.

104. **C. Initial treatment with stool softeners, bulking agents, and sitz baths will heal 90% of all anal fissures. A second episode may be treated in the same manner with a 70% success rate.**

A. Surgical treatment is reserved for patients who fail conservative management.

B. A 0.2% nitroglycerin topical ointment is an effective treatment, although some studies call its use into question. Side effects may include headaches and tachyphylaxis.

D. Botulinum toxin has been found to be an effective treatment in the healing of anal fissures. However, due to its expense and concerns about paralysis of the anal sphincter, it has not been widely accepted as a therapy for this indication.

E. Patients with this disorder are very uncomfortable and require treatment.

105. **B. Lateral internal anal sphincterotomy is the procedure of choice after failure to respond to medical management. Patients with ulcers of the anus persisting for longer than 1 month, as well as patients with chronic, recurring ulcers should be considered candidates for surgery. In this procedure, the internal anal sphincter is divided, relieving the spasm that causes the pain and limits the healing. Fecal continence is maintained by the external anal sphincter. This procedure has a success rate exceeding 90%.**

A. Although a diverting colostomy would allow the anal ulcer to heal, it is a drastic measure and not appropriate in this patient.

C. A low anterior resection is used to treat rectal tumors that are located more than 5 cm from the anal verge.

D. Incision and drainage is more appropriate in the treatment of a perianal abscess.

E. Hemorrhoidectomy would be appropriate for the treatment of hemorrhoids.

106. **B. This patient has developed severe heart failure and will likely need a transplant to survive. Assist devices are intended as a bridge to transplant. A left ventricular assist device (LVAD) is used for left heart failure, and a right ventricular assist device (RVAD) is used for right heart failure. A biventricular assist device is the best choice in this scenario because the patient has developed bilateral heart failure.**

A. The patient's aortic valve is unlikely to be contributing to her condition, and its replacement would not help the situation. The patient is suffering from a severe dilated cardiomyopathy, which will likely be definitively cured only with a heart transplant.
C. A coronary artery bypass graft is performed for ischemic myocardium, which is not the case here.
D. ECMO is used most commonly in children as a means of delivering oxygen to the circulation and removing carbon dioxide in pulmonary or cardiopulmonary failure.
E. This patient's medical management has already been maximized.

107. **B. An intra-aortic balloon pump decreases afterload by deflating during systole, and by decreasing both the pressure against which the left ventricle must pump, and the work of the heart during systole. The balloon inflates during diastole, increasing aortic pressure, which augments coronary and visceral perfusion.**

A. A balloon pump deflates during systole.
C. A balloon pump is contraindicated in aortic regurgitation.
D. Use of a balloon pump increases mesenteric flow by inflating during diastole.
E. Although bleeding is always a concern when placing an intra-aortic balloon pump, this alone would not prevent its use.

108. **A. This patient has pseudo-obstruction (Ogilvie syndrome), which is a paralytic ileus of the large intestine. Painless distention is a common presenting finding. Risk factors include severe blunt trauma, orthopedic trauma or procedures, cardiac disease, acute neurologic disease, and acute metabolic derangements. This condition is dangerous, because the cecum can expand by as much as 10 to 12 cm and possibly become perforated.**

B, C, D, E. Acute SBO, toxic megacolon, C. *difficile* colitis, and mesenteric ischemia are all possibilities, but are inconsistent with this patient's clinical presentation.

109. **E. The best initial management of this problem is the correction of metabolic derangements and minimization of narcotic use. When the cecum becomes extremely distended, however, decompression is needed to prevent perforation. Decompression can be accomplished by using neostigmine or by performing a colonoscopy.**

A. Exploratory laparotomy is not indicated unless colonic perforation is suspected by clinical exam.
B. Neither antibiotics nor proton pump inhibitors have a role in this situation.
C. It is too early to consider TPN, and its use would not influence the bowel distention.
D. The patient should remain on strict bowel rest until the ileus resolves and should not be started on nasojejunal feedings.

110. **D. Neostigmine therapy works by preventing destruction of acetylcholine by acetylcholinesterase, and by overcoming the parasympathetic paralytic ileus present. However, neostigmine use carries a risk of life-threatening AV node block, so this patient must be on continuous cardiac monitoring. α-blocking agents are contraindicated during neostigmine administration. Atropine should be available at the bedside.**

A, B, C, E. Chest x-ray, ECG, continuous pulse oximetry, and a baseline ABG are all unnecessary prior to administration of neostigmine. Due to the risks of sudden heart block associated with the administration of neostigmine, continuous cardiac monitoring is the only required treatment.

111. **B. The most common cause of hemodynamically significant lower GI bleeding is angiodysplasia or an arteriovenous malformation (AVM) within the colon. Overall, the most common source of lower GI bleeding (bright red blood per rectum) is upper GI bleeding with rapid intestinal transit. This condition is often seen in the ICU setting. The quickest and easiest way to diagnose upper GI bleeding is to place a nasogastric tube (NGT).**

A. A barium enema is not an indicated test in an emergent situation.
C. Rigid proctoscopy limits visualization to the rectum, which does not allow you to define any colonic sources of bleeding.
D. Colonoscopy is, in most centers, the first diagnostic option after an upper GI bleeding source has been ruled out. It allows the operator to definitively treat a bleeding source once it is located and to mark the area for surgery by using ink injections if needed.

E. Proceeding to the operating room is not indicated until the source of the bleeding has been located. It is difficult to locate an intraluminal source of bleeding in the operating room.

112. **C. Angiography offers an opportunity for definitive treatment with embolization of the bleeding arteries, but there is the potential for bowel ischemia and infarction after the procedure. The bleeding must be fairly rapid, at least 1 cc/min, to be detected by angiography. For elderly patients with multiple co-morbidities, this is a valuable option due to the increased risk of surgery associated with multiple co-morbidities.**

A, B. Bleeding of a small bowel source can be identified with angiography.

D. Cauterization does not affect your ability to visualize the anatomy during angiography.

E. Angiography is a tool used to locate bleeding vessels and define anatomy of the vasculature, but not to diagnose intestinal tumors.

113. **C. Testicular cancer is the most common solid tumor found in young adult men. Cryptorchidism is the failure of the testicle to descend into the scrotum; it significantly increases the affected individual's risk of testicular cancer. Although cryptorchid testicles should be placed back in the scrotum (orchiopexy), this step does not alter their malignant potential; however, it does facilitate examination and tumor detection.**

A. Ninety-five percent of testicular tumors arise from germ cells. These tumors include seminomas, non-seminomas, embryonal cell carcinomas, choriocarcinomas, and teratomas.

B. Human chorionic gonadotropin (HCG) is found in almost 100% of choriocarcinomas, but not seminomas.

D. Seeding of malignant cells can occur along the biopsy tract site. Therefore, orchiectomies should be approached through an inguinal incision.

E. Seminomas are highly sensitive—not insensitive—to radiation therapy.

114. **C. This patient suffers from anterior cord syndrome, which occurs as a result of ischemia of the spinal cord either from cross-clamping of the aorta or from a low flow state. It is a rare complication of repair of a thoracolumbar aortic aneurysm, or ruptured abdominal aortic aneurysm. When this syndrome is suspected, the most sensitive and specific exam is an MRI of the spinal cord to confirm the diagnosis and delineate the extent of the injury. Figures 5-114A and 5-114B are T2 weighted MRI images of the spinal cord. The arrows identify the area damaged by an ischemic event leading to anterior cord syndrome.**

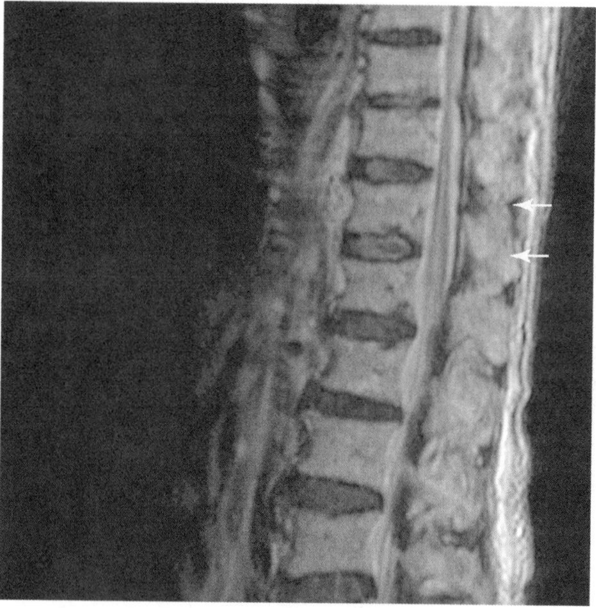

A

Figure 5-114A • Image Courtesy of the University of Utah School of Medicine, Salt Lake City, Utah.

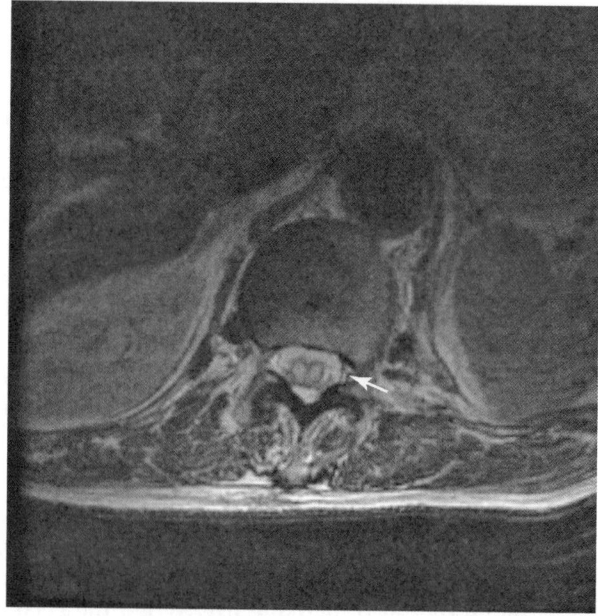

B

Figure 5-114B • Image Courtesy of the University of Utah School of Medicine, Salt Lake City, Utah.

A. Electromyography of the lower extremities would be more helpful in determining a progressive neurological loss to the lower extremities, not an acute event.
B. A lumbar puncture should be used in cases of suspected meningitis which is not the case here.
D. The patient has clinical signs that localize the neurological injury to the spinal cord, not the head.
E. Lumbar myelogram would be helpful in visualizing a mass lesion causing these symptoms, but would be of little use in identifying an injury to the parenchyma of the spinal cord.

115. **C. The great anterior radicular artery (artery of Adamkiewicz) is usually found in the inferior thoracic (T10 to T12) or superior lumbar (L1 to L2) region. It is larger than the other radicular arteries and is of clinical importance because it supplies the major arterial contribution to the anterior spinal artery. This artery provides the main blood supply to the inferior two-thirds of the spinal cord. It is most likely to be damaged or occluded during a thoracolumbar aortic aneurysm repair.**

A, B, D, E. These levels do not usually correspond to the origin of the great anterior radicular artery.

116. **B. The anterior spinal artery supplies the anterior two-thirds of the spinal cord with blood via the sulcal artery. An occlusion of the great anterior radicular artery (artery of Adamkiewicz) causes an infarction of the anterior two-thirds of the spinal cord, sparing the posterior one-third that is supplied by the posterior spinal artery. Loss of pain and temperature sensation occurs because of infarction of the lateral spinothalamic tracts, which carry pain and temperature sensation to the thalamus.**

A. The dorsal columns, which carry sensory fibers for proprioception, remain intact.
C. Infarction of the lateral and ventral corticospinal tracts causes paralysis below the affected level, usually resulting in paraplegia, not quadriplegia.
D. Damage associated with the conus medullaris or inferior-most portion of the spinal cord will cause loss of bowel and bladder control, not constipation.
E. Vibration is sensed via fibers in the dorsal columns, which remain intact.

117. **D. The Glasgow Coma Scale is a scoring tool used to quantify level of consciousness; it is used to initially assess prognosis in patients with a head injury. The grading system evaluates verbal, motor, and ocular responses (Table 5-117). A coma is usually seen with a score less than 8. This patient's scores as follows: eye opening—does not open eyes (1); motor response—decorticate posture (3); and verbal response—incomprehensible sounds (2).**

A, B, C, E. These options all give incorrect calculations for the GCS.

TABLE 5-117 Glasgow Coma Grading System

Assessment	Score
Eye opening	4: Opens spontaneously 3: Opens to voice (command) 2: Opens to painful stimulus 1: Does not open eyes
Motor response	6: Obeys commands 5: Localizes painful stimulus 4: Withdraws from pain 3: Decorticate posture 2: Decerebrate posture 1: No movement
Verbal response	5: Appropriate and oriented 4: Confused 3: Inappropriate words 2: Incomprehensible sounds 1: No sounds

118. **A. This patient is demonstrating symptoms of septic shock. The low systemic vascular resistance combined with an elevated cardiac index is indicative of septic shock. Septic shock is characterized by microvascular permeability mediated by the cytokines TNF-α and IL-1, reactive oxygen radicals, vasoactive peptides, complement, and platelet-activating factor. This cascade of events leads to decreased intravascular volume and third-space fluid losses. Treatment of septic shock is directed at adequate fluid resuscitation followed by vasopressors as needed.**

B. Obstructive shock is seen in conditions such as tension pneumothorax and cardiac tamponade. In this type of shock, the PCWP, CVP, and SVR values would he higher.

C. Hypovolemic shock is caused by significant intravascular volume loss, such as with blood loss during trauma or surgery. In this scenario, the CVP and PCWP values would be low and the SVR value would be high.

D. Neurogenic shock is seen with spinal cord injury or anesthetic blocks. Diagnosis is made based on history and physical exam, which shows decreased blood pressure with a paradoxically low pulse rate.

E. Cardiogenic shock is seen with cardiac events that cause depressed cardiac function, such as in a myocardial infarction or with tamponade. In this type of shock, there would be a low CI value, and high CVP and PCWP values.

119. **B. Prior to starting any type of vasoactive agent, it is vital to ensure that the patient is intravascularly fluid resuscitated. With a CVP of 4 mm Hg and a PCWP of 10 mm Hg, it is appropriate to give this patient more fluid or volume to increase the CVP.**

A. Vasopressin increases the cAMP level, which subsequently increases water permeability at the renal tubules. Its use is becoming more common in the management of sepsis. This patient needs adequate fluid resuscitation before starting a vasoactive agent.

C. A fresh frozen plasma transfusion is not indicated in this case, as the patient is not coagulopathic. While he does need volume, it is safest to start with crystalloid fluids.

D. Dobutamine is a vasoactive agent that is primarily a β-agonist. As such, it increases myocardial contractility but does not produce peripheral vasoconstriction.

E. Norepinephrine is the drug of choice in septic shock, but only after the patient is fluid resuscitated. Its potent α-agonist activity provides peripheral vasoconstriction to counteract the global inflammatory response associated with septic shock.

120. **A. In this scenario, the patient's cardiac index is normal and the systemic vascular resistance is compensating for his being intravascularly volume depleted or hypovolemic. The CVP and PCWP values are both low, so the patient needs volume, starting with crystalloid and following with blood products as needed.**

A, B, D, E. See the explanation for question 118 for more detail.

121. **A. This patient is exhibiting hypovolemic shock and had a 20% drop in his hematocrit. There are multiple areas in which a trauma patient may bleed, including the pleural space (rib fractures, great vessel injuries), abdomen (solid organ or great vessel injuries), retroperitoneal space (kidneys, pelvis), legs (femur fractures, not lower leg fractures), or bleeding out exteriorly. The pleural cavity is the most likely place in which this patient would be bleeding, as a result of his rib fractures and likely associated intercostal vessel injuries.**

B. Abdominal cavity bleeding is likely from the liver, spleen, or other vessel injuries. There were no solid organ injuries by CT, and a bowel perforation would be less likely to cause this type of hematocrit drop.

C. The retroperitoneal space is a possible source of bleeding, as with pelvis fractures or renal injuries. However, this patient did not have any identified retroperitoneal injuries.

D. It is very unlikely that an individual could bleed enough into his or her head that the hematocrit level would change by 20%. This patient is alert and following commands, which would also argue against a head bleed.

E. While a patient with a femur fracture can bleed a large amount into the thigh, this does not happen with below-the-knee fractures.

F. Unidentified injuries are always possible and should not be forgotten or discounted.

122. **C. This patient has a respiratory acidosis due to underventilation. The elevated PCO_2 of 53 properly accounts for the acidemia. For every unit increase of PCO_2 that occurs, the pH will fall by 0.8. Thus, when you correct the pH for a PCO_2 of 53 to a the pH for a PCO_2 of 40, the pH would reflectively show an increase to 7.38, which is normal. From this result, you can conclude that the acidosis is due to underventilation.**

A, E. With a base excess of –2 and a HCO_3 of 23, it is safe to say that this patient does not have metabolic acidosis.

B, D. With a pH less than 7.4, the patient is acidotic, not alkalotic.

123. E. When a patient is experiencing retained CO_2, ventilation needs to be improved. This is accomplished by increasing the minute ventilation, which entails increasing the respiratory rate or increasing the tidal volume. This patient is already over-breathing to a rate of 20 the ventilator set rate of 14, so increasing the rate would not be helpful. The tidal volume can be increased by raising the peak inspiratory pressure (PIP) to improve ventilation status.

A. Giving sodium bicarbonate ($NaHCO_3$) is helpful in a metabolic acidosis situation to increase the pH. It is not indicated in respiratory acidosis.
B. Increasing the FiO_2 would help to increase the oxygenation, but it would not improve the minute ventilation.
C. The patient is over-breathing the set ventilator rate, and a further increase in the rate would not change her minute ventilation. Increasing the PIP, in this case, would increase the minute ventilation.
D. Changing the IV fluids to normal saline (NS) would not change the overall situation.

124. B. Bilious emesis in a newborn is considered a surgical emergency and needs to be evaluated immediately. The x-ray in Figure 5-124B (see the arrow) shows extensive pneumatosis intestinalis in the descending colon. This finding is concerning for necrotizing enterocolitis (NEC). The etiology of NEC is unknown, but is believed to be associated with ischemic intestine damage and bacterial colonization.

A. Three-fourths of patients with malrotation present with obstruction in infancy due to Ladd's bands (adhesions) or volvulus around the superior mesenteric vessels. Newborns with pneumatosis intestinalis are more likely to have NEC.
C. Jejunal atresia presents with bilious vomiting, but not pneumatosis intestinalis as seen on the abdominal film for this patient.
D. Meconium ileus occurs in 10% to 20% of infants with cystic fibrosis. By history, those babies fail to pass meconium and abdominal films show a "soap bubble" sign in the right lower quadrant. Nonoperative treatment is successful in 60% to 70% of cases.
E. Neonatal small left colon syndrome (meconium plug syndrome) is due to a narrow left colon with proximal dilation of the transverse and right colons on plain abdominal films.

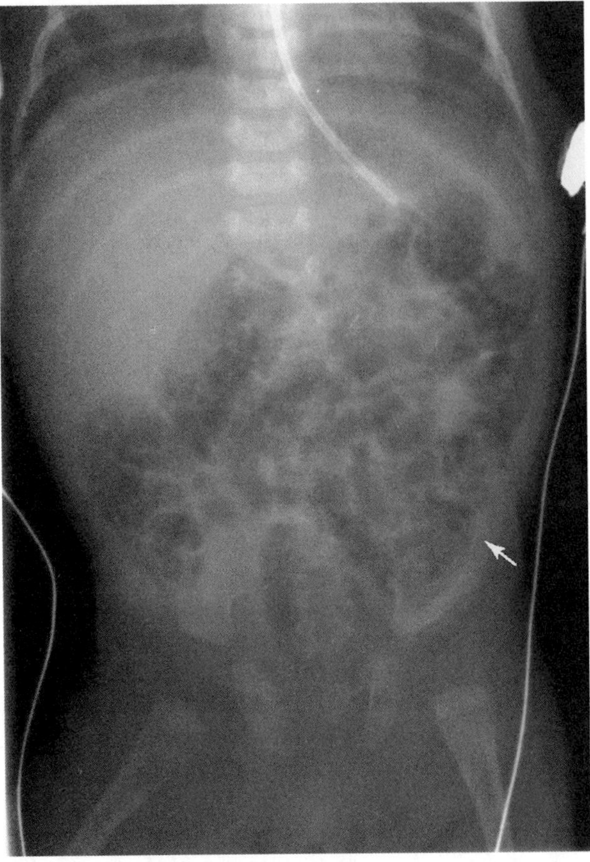

B

Figure 5-124B • Image Courtesy of the University of Utah School of Medicine, Salt Lake City, Utah.

125. A. The pathophysiology of necrotizing enterocolitis (NEC) has been somewhat controversial. Some authors suggest it is related to hypoxic stress during delivery, while more recent studies relate it to infectious causes in a compromised host with immature immune and gut barrier defenses. Proper initial management of NEC includes nasogastric decompression, broad-spectrum antibiotics, bowel rest with TPN, and IV hydration. Once a perforation has occurred and free air is seen on an x-ray, the patient needs an exploratory laparotomy.

B. While anaerobic antibiotic coverage is necessary, broad-spectrum coverage is the most appropriate choice (gram-positive, gram-negative and anaerobic coverage).
C. Strict bowel rest is necessary for management of NEC. TPN is appropriate for nutritional support.

D. Emergent laparotomy is necessary if the infant has a perforated bowel. Otherwise, it is not part of the initial management.
E. Laparoscopy has no role in the management of NEC.

126. **D. The caloric requirements of an injured person increase substantially, depending on the severity of the injury. An average individual requires an REE of 30 to 40 kcal/kg/day. Severely stressed individuals, as in this scenario, require 40 to 50 kcal/kg/day.**

A, B. Even for a healthy individual, 10 to 30 kcal/kg/day is not adequate.
C. The requirement for maintenance of weight in a nonstressed individual is 30-40 kcal/kg/day.
E. Even for a severely stressed individual, 50 to 60 kcal/kg/day is too many calories.

127. **B. By measuring the nitrogen balance, nitrogen synthesis and breakdown can be evaluated. Nitrogen intake is the amount of protein taken in, and the output is the total of all excretions and secretions. The urinary urea nitrogen is converted to grams of protein by the following equation: [urinary nitrogen (g) per 24 hours + 4] × 6.25. A correction factor of 4 is added to account for the losses in stool.**

A, C, D, E. These are all incorrect formulas.

128. **A. Increased CO_2 production is a direct result of overfeeding and can be reduced by increasing the percentage of fat calories consumed relative to total calories.**

B. Hepatic failure is usually part of the picture for multiple organ dysfunctions due to sepsis.
C, D. Overfeeding can cause prolonged recovery and impaired immune response, but these problems will not necessarily be corrected with consumption of an increased percentage of fat calories.
E. Central line sepsis is not directly related to the percentage of fat calories consumed.

129. **E. Whenever a patient is able to feed using the GI tract, this approach is the method of choice. Nasojejunal tube feedings should be started for patients without conditions that would preclude use of enteral feeding, such as patients with prolonged intubation.**

A, B, C, D. Sometimes parenteral nutrition is required, including in the following situations: severe pancreatitis, where strict bowel rest is necessary; short gut syndrome, due to inadequate bowel length for enteral feeding absorption; a enterocutaneous fistula, to decrease secretions and output, thereby allowing the fistula to close; and a prolonged ileus, which precludes enteral feeding until the source of the problem is treated.

130. **C. A small bowel resection with minimal, contained spillage is considered to be a clean contaminated operative case. Wound infection rates are associated with the level of contamination seen during the surgical case. In a clean contaminated case (GI or respiratory tract entered without significant spillage), a 5% to 8% wound infection rate is seen.**

A. A clean case, such as a breast biopsy, has a 1% to 3% rate of wound infection.
B. There is no such classification as a sterile case.
D. A contaminated case, such as a colon injury with bowel spillage, has a 10% to 15% rate of wound infection.
E. A 15% to 40% wound infection rate is seen in a dirty or infected case, such as an intra-abdominal abscess from a colonic anastomosis leak.

131. **B. Many conditions may cause a postoperative fever. A commonly used mnemonic is the 5 W's: wind, water, wound, walking, and weird drugs. On postoperative day 2, it is less likely that a patient would have pneumonia, a wound infection, or a urinary tract infection. The most common cause of an "early" postoperative fever is atelectasis.**

A. Indwelling Foley catheters are foreign bodies and predispose patients to develop urinary tract infections. Postoperative day 2 would be early for a UTI to emerge, but this possibility is easily checked by obtaining a urinalysis.
C. A central line is a foreign body that can easily cause an infection, but a line placed under sterile conditions is unlikely to be the cause of infection so early in the postoperative course.

D. Some medications may induce a fever and should be taken into consideration when making the diagnosis. The vast majority of fevers (approximately 90%) that occur within the first 48 hours, however, are secondary to atelectasis.
E. An intra-abdominal abscess is always a consideration in a surgical case that is considered a contaminated case, but usually the presentation is closer to postoperative day 5.

132. **E. The initial priority in patients with an enterocutaneous fistula (ECF) is fluid resuscitation and repletion of electrolytes. The difficulty of this task depends on the location of the fistula and the amount of output present. Proximal fistulas usually have a higher output with more electrolyte irregularities. It is imperative to aggressively treat these patients, as their electrolyte levels can rapidly become depleted.**

A. The abdomen should be studied by CT scan, looking for the presence of abscesses. If present, they should be drained percutaneously. Ongoing infections limit spontaneous closure of the fistula and increase the risk of death.
B. Control of the fistula entails protecting the skin from enteric contents and assisting in fluid replacement by accurate measurement of output.
C. It is important to begin nutritional support early in the treatment of ECF. Preventing malnutrition decreases the septic mortality and increases the likelihood of spontaneous closure.
D. The decision to perform an exploratory laparotomy is a difficult one in treating patients with an ECF. After resuscitation, this procedure should be performed in patients who continue to have sepsis and a worsening course despite maximal support. In stable patients without ongoing signs of sepsis, it should be done after the patient is nutritionally stable and free from infection.

133. **D. Whenever a patient sustains burns that are circumferential in nature on an extremity, you must be concerned about compartment syndrome. It is important to check baseline compartment pressures and follow them serially. Escharotomies should be performed as needed for increasing compartment pressures above 30 mm Hg. This procedure releases the pressure within the compartment and reestablishes blood flow distal to the injury.**

A. With every burn injury, concern arises regarding significant fluid losses. Fluid resuscitation is based on standard burn fluid calculations, which should address fluid issues.
B. Infection of burns is a significant complication, but would not occur in the acute injury situation.
C. Rhabdomyolysis occurs in severe crush injuries or anytime muscle is severely damaged. It is unlikely in a 14% TBSA burn.
E. Inhalation injuries occur most often in closed-space fires (indoors) and with patients who are symptomatic in terms of respiratory distress. Signs and symptoms can include carbonaceous sputum; burns near the nose, mouth, and face; raspy voice; and hoarseness.

134. **E. The best way to evaluate for compartment syndrome in an involved area is to evaluate the pressures in the compartment. Elevated compartment pressures in the presence of hypoperfusion are diagnostic for compartment syndrome.**

A. CVP measurement is used to evaluate a patient's fluid status.
B. Urine myoglobin measurement is used to evaluate for rhabdomyolysis.
C. Sputum cultures are used to evaluate for pneumonia.
D. Blood cultures are unlikely to be helpful in the acute injury setting.

135. **A. This patient has a complete small bowel obstruction. The most common presentation includes abdominal distention, diffuse pain, persistent nausea and vomiting, and decreased flatus or bowel movements. It is important to differentiate between a complete versus partial obstruction. Complete obstruction is accompanied by obstipation, or the failure to pass gas or stool within the last 12 hours. Abdominal films usually demonstrate a paucity of gas within the colon and rectum. Complete obstruction is an absolute indication for surgery. This patient complains of obstipation for 2 days. Exploratory laparotomy is warranted to correct the underlying cause of obstruction.**

B. Partial obstruction can be accompanied by flatus or diarrhea as well as colonic or rectal gas on abdominal plain films. In both cases, plain abdominal films will demonstrate multiple air-fluid levels and dilated loops of small bowel. Partial small bowel obstructions are usually seen in patients with previous abdominal surgery, which results in adhesion formation. Non-operative management consists of NPO status, NGT decompression, IV hydration, electrolyte repletion, and close observation. Failure to resolve the obstruction within 48 hours or any change in stability or increased tenderness noted on abdominal exam warrants surgical intervention.

C. An abdominal CT scan may demonstrate a transition point, but it would not change the immediate treatment plan in this case.

D. A colonoscopy would not allow you to visualize the small bowel and would not be helpful.

E. An enteroclysis is the study of choice to localize the obstructed area, but it would not change the initial management of this patient.

136. **D. The most common causes of small bowel obstruction in the United States are adhesions, hernias, and small bowel tumors (in that order). An incarceration of a hernia (femoral, inguinal, or ventral) is the second most common cause of SBO. Tumors may result in occlusion of the bowel lumen or intussusception if the tumor is intrinsic, and twisting or entrapment of the small bowel by extrinsic tumors. Intussusception is a possibility, especially in children, but is infrequent in adults.**

A, B, C, E. These options are all causes of small bowel obstructions, with adhesions being by far the most common cause in a patient with previous abdominal surgery.

137. **C. Urinary tract infections typically occur after postoperative day number 3 and are usually accompanied by dysuria and low-grade fever. Diagnosis is made with urinalysis and confirmed by cultures. Discontinuation of the Foley catheter and antibiotic therapy are usually sufficient treatment.**

A. A wound infection is easily diagnosed by erythema, warmth, and tenderness on physical exam, as well as fever. Treatment would consist of opening the wound and packing it with moist gauze until the wound heals.

B. Intra-abdominal abscesses generally occur 7 to 10 days after surgery. Patients will have complaints of fever, abdominal pain, and abdominal distention with food intolerance. A leukocytosis is usually present. Abdominal and pelvis CT scan is used to diagnose abscesses. If an abscess is identified by CT, it can often be drained percutaneously.

D. Surgery significantly increases the risk for developing a deep vein thrombosis (DVT), due to prolonged stasis of blood during surgery and shortly thereafter. Patients with DVT will often present with fevers early in their course; for that reason, it is important to be aware of the possibility of thrombus formation. Calf, thigh tenderness, and hypoxia with chest pain should also be evaluated for pulmonary embolus from a DVT.

E. Pneumonia often presents with productive cough, fever, tachypnea, decreased breath sounds on auscultation, and dullness to percussion. Management includes antibiotics and aggressive pulmonary toilet. The overall mortality rate from postoperative pneumonia is 20% to 40%.

138. **E. This patient presents with clinical evidence of shock. Given her recent history, it is very likely that she has an intra-abdominal abscess leading to septic shock. Sepsis results in the release of circulating cytokines during the inflammatory response, causing fever, leukocytosis, and loss of systemic vascular resistance. Ultimately, the patient develops hypotension refractory to fluid resuscitation.**

A, C. Cardiogenic shock results from depressed cardiac function. It may occur secondary to myocardial infarction, pulmonary embolus, arrhythmias, cardiac tamponade, pneumothorax, and toxic doses of medication. This type of shock and its potential causes need to be kept in mind with elderly patients, but this scenario is more consistent with septic shock symptoms.

B. While septic shock patients experience a relative hypovolemia due to all the third-space fluid and decreased vascular tone, the underlying process is a global inflammatory response that causes microvascular leaking of intravascular fluid into the interstitium. Fluid resuscitation alone will not always correct the hypotension due to the loss of systemic vascular tone; consequently, vasopressors may be needed.

D. Damage to the cervical spinal cord may result in loss of autonomic innervation, causing depressed myocardial function as well as loss of vascular tone. This type of shock occurs with a history of trauma and would be unlikely in this scenario. It is usually treated with fluid resuscitation and dopamine.

139. **D. Most septic patients need management in an intensive care setting including central venous access and invasive hemodynamic monitoring. Once the patient has been adequately stabilized with fluids and vasoactive agents, if necessary, the underlying cause of the sepsis needs to be identified and treated. With this patient's recent clinical history, it is likely that she has an intra-abdominal abscess. This problem can best be diagnosed by a CT scan of the abdomen and pelvis.**

A. While IV antibiotics are necessary to treat sepsis, an intra-abdominal abscess will not respond to administration of antibiotics alone. Instead, it will require drainage as well, which can be done either percutaneously or surgically.

B. A barium enema helps define the intraluminal anatomy of the bowel; it will not give a picture of an intra-abdominal process.

C. Surgical exploration is necessary if the abscess cannot be adequately drained percutaneously, or if the patient has ongoing contamination from an anastomotic leak that fails to close.

E. Oral antibiotics alone are an inadequate treatment. Drainage of the abscess and IV antibiotics are needed.

140. **D. A transhiatal esophagectomy consists of an abdominal incision with mobilization of the stomach and dissection of the esophagus up to the level of the neck. A left cervical incision is made, and the remainder of the esophagus is mobilized. The esophagus is then removed and an esophagogastric anastomosis is created in the neck. An anastomotic leak occurs in approximately 10% of all patients who undergo esophagectomy with esophagogastrectomy. The risk of a leak is higher with a cervical anastomosis than with an intrathoracic anastomosis. However, the mortality from a cervical anastomotic leak is significantly lower than that associated with an intrathoracic leak. Symptoms of a leak usually appear 5 to 10 days postoperatively and consist of fever, leukocytosis, subcutaneous crepitus, erythema, and wound drainage. If this problem is suspected, the cervical wound should be opened widely and drained. The wound is then packed with dry gauze. Almost all cervical leaks heal with conservative management. One-third of these complications subsequently develop strictures, requiring repeat dilatation.**

A. Although this scenario describes a classic wound infection, in patients undergoing a cervical esophagogastric anastomosis, the description would represent an anastomotic leak until proven otherwise.

B. Hematoma, while included in the differential diagnosis, should not be considered first in this scenario.

C, E. Although both of these complications are important in the differential diagnosis of postoperative fever, this presentation with cervical wound changes is most consistent with an anastomotic leak.

141. **B. Polytrauma patients are at an increased risk of deep vein thrombosis (DVT), and a pulmonary embolus (PE) is the most severe complication of a DVT. Because of this risk, aggressive DVT prophylaxis along with early ambulation should be started in all high-risk patients. The most common symptoms of a PE include dyspnea, chest pain, and a cough. Increased oxygen requirements, tachypnea, and tachycardia are often present when examining a suspected patient with a PE. Given that these signs and symptoms are associated with other cardiopulmonary disorders, it is imperative that you obtain further tests. The ventilation-perfusion lung scan is the pivotal study in hemodynamically stable patients suspected of having a PE. It is safe, noninvasive, and widely available. A normal perfusion scan excludes the diagnosis of PE, whereas a scan with perfusion defects and normal ventilation is highly suggestive of a PE. An indeterminate scan should be followed by a more specific test such as a CT angiogram.**

A. CT angiograms of the thorax are becoming increasingly more popular in the diagnosis of a pulmonary embolus. Figure 5-141 shows a large clot in the right pulmonary artery (note the arrows). A simple chest CT scan would not be of any diagnostic value in this case.

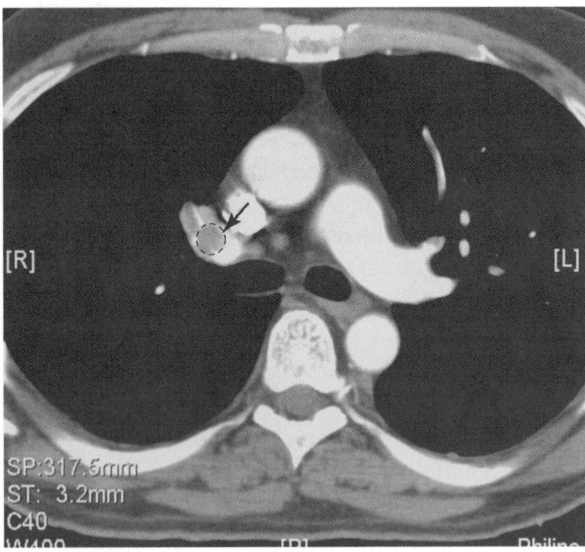

Figure 5-141 • Image Courtesy of the University of Utah School of Medicine, Salt Lake City, Utah.

C. Duplex scanning of the lower extremities is used to evaluate for DVT, but it cannot diagnose a pulmonary embolism. It may be an appropriate study in patients with signs of a PE and simultaneous signs of a DVT. In this case, the patient does not demonstrate symptoms of a DVT.

D. Pulmonary angiography is the most sensitive and specific test in diagnosing a pulmonary embolus, but it is invasive and expensive.

E. A transthoracic echocardiogram may be obtained in a critically ill or hemodynamically unstable patient. Right heart dysfunction is usually identified by right ventricular dilation, demonstrating aberrant motion of the interventricular septum. Transesophageal studies can visualize thrombi within the pulmonary trunk.

142. D. This patient should be started on systemic heparinization immediately. Once a therapeutic range is obtained and the patient can tolerate oral medications, she should be switched over to warfarin, with the heparin being continued until the PT/INR is therapeutic. Oral anticoagulation is then continued for 3 to 6 months.

A. This choice is the appropriate initial treatment for a patient you suspect of having a myocardial infarction.

B. A lorazepam (Ativan) taper should be initiated in patients suspected of suffering from acute alcohol withdrawal.

C. An IV fluid bolus would be appropriate in the treatment of a patient with hypovolemic shock.

E. A thoracentesis would be indicated in a patient with respiratory embarrassment secondary to a significant pleural effusion.

143. B. This case is a classic presentation of abdominal compartment syndrome (ACS) after a repair of a ruptured AAA. ACS may be seen after massive fluid resuscitation as encountered in conjunction with emergent repairs of a ruptured AAA, abdominal trauma, pancreatitis, severe intra-abdominal infections, and severe burns. Increased intra-abdominal pressure results in renal venous compression and increased pressure in the renal parenchyma, which produce oliguria. Alteration in microvascular permeability leads to a progressive increase in intra-abdominal pressure and subsequently decreased cardiac output due to decreased venous return and increased systemic vascular resistance. The transmission of the intra-abdominal hypertension to the chest reduces compliance and necessitates increased airway pressures to maintain adequate ventilation. The diagnosis of ACS is based on recognition of the clinical syndrome of tense abdominal distention, signs of decreased cardiac output, elevated airway pressures, and oliguria. Intra-abdominal pressure (IAP) is measured indirectly and easily by measuring the bladder pressure using a Foley catheter and pressure transducer system, with pressures greater than 15 mm Hg being consistent with ACS.

A. The majority of abdominal aortic aneurysms have a "neck" of normal aorta between the renal artery ostia and the beginning of the aneurysm, allowing for their repair without renal vascular injury. While oliguria may be related to either renal vascular injury or prolonged hypotension leading to acute tubular necrosis (ATN), in this case oliguria and increased ventilatory pressures are the most overt clinical ramifications of ACS.

C. Increased positive end expiratory pressure (PEEP) may be needed to temporarily support ventilation, but it will not treat—and may actually exacerbate—the increased intra-abdominal pressure found in ACS. Diuretics should not be given to a patient who is relatively hypotensive with classic signs of ACS.

D. Transesophageal echo (TEE) and Swan Ganz (SG) pressure measurements would show decreased cardiac output due to decreased venous return and artificially elevated left and right heart pressures secondary to increased intrathoracic pressures. In ACS, the TEE and SG catheter measurements would show the effects of increased intra-abdominal pressure rather than primary cardiac dysfunction. The patient would still require abdominal decompression, given the information derived from the TEE and SG placement.

E. Increasing the amount of intravenous fluids may potentiate the ACS rather than relieve the problem. Added vasoactive support may transiently improve the hemodynamic status but it will not improve renal perfusion or urine output in the clinical condition of ACS described.

144. D. The two most common causes of pancreatitis are alcohol and gallstones. This patient does not show any evidence of gallstones on the ultrasound and has no history of alcohol abuse. Among the other causes of pancreatitis is hypercalcemia. In this case, the patient's calcium level is 14 mg/dL. With the onset of mental status changes, aggressive therapy must be started. Aggressive fluid resuscitation should be instituted and monitored by following the patient's urine output.

A. There is no indication for antibiotic therapy at this time.

B. While total parenteral nutrition (TPN) may be needed if the pancreatitis does not resolve, it is not indicated at this time.

C. There is no need for blood transfusion with a hematocrit of 32% and no evidence of bleeding.

E. A cholecystectomy is not indicated in a patient with a negative US for gallstones and acute cholecystitis.

145. B. Once the patient is adequately hydrated, administration of a loop diuretic such as furosemide (Lasix) promotes calcium excretion. Other medications that may be used include steroids, mithramycin, and calcitonin. Renal dialysis may be required if medication proves ineffective or if the situation is critical.

A, D. Antiemetics do not have a role in the management of hypercalcemia.

C. Antibiotics do not have a role in calcium reduction.

E. Phosphate does not have a role in the management of hypercalcemia.

146. A. Gallstones are composed of bile salts, cholesterol, and lecithin. They are typically classified as either cholesterol or pigmented stones (black or brown). The cholesterol stones account for 75% of all gallstones, while the black and brown pigmented stones account for 20% and 5%, respectively. Brown stones are frequently associated with infection and are typically found in Asian patients. Primary common duct stones are frequently brown gallstones.

B. Hyperbilirubinemia associated with gallstones occurs when the hepatic duct or common duct becomes obstructed. Brown stones are not directly related to increased levels of bilirubin.

C. There is no increase in the incidence of cholangiocarcinoma with brown gallstones.

D. Cystic duct obstruction occurs with any type of gallstone, resulting in pain and nausea following consumption of a fatty meal. There is no increase in the incidence of cystic duct obstruction with brown stones.

E. Brown gallstones are not associated with hypercholesterolemia.

147. C. Asians have a higher incidence of developing brown gallstones than non-Asian individuals. The reasons for this propensity are not clearly understood.

A, B, D, E. These ethnic groups are not associated with an increased incidence of brown gallstones.

148. E. The enzyme β-d-glucuronidase drives the hydrolysis of bilirubin glucuronide into free bilirubin and glucuronic acid. The free unconjugated bilirubin can then combine with the calcium in bile to form pigmented stones. This enzyme is produced by *E. coli* and *Klebsiella*, both enteric bacteria commonly found in bile.

A. *Enterococcus* is an enteric bacterium that is found in bile and does not produce the enzyme β-d-glucuronidase. *Staphylococcus aureus* is common skin flora; it is not usually found in bile.

B. *Staphylococcus* and *Streptococcus* are not usually found in bile and do not produce the enzyme β-d-glucuronidase.

C, D. *E. coli* is commonly found in bile and produces the enzyme β-d-glucuronidase. *Pseudomonas* and *Bacteroides fragilis* do not produce the enzyme and are not commonly found in bile.

149. **B. Numerous bacteria are associated with cholangitis. Not surprisingly, they are most commonly related to normal gut flora. *E. coli* is the most common bacteria associated with cholangitis at 35%, followed by *Enterococcus* (16%), *Klebsiella* (14%), *Proteus* (12%), *Pseudomonas* (9%), and *Enterobacter* (5%).**

A, C, D, E. See the explanation for B.

150. **C. Mental status changes and hypotension are grave signs of biliary sepsis and demand urgent treatment to decompress the biliary tree. This grouping is termed Reynolds' pentad.**

A. Nausea and an increased WBC count may occur in severe cholangitis, but not as a part of Reynolds' pentad.

B. Hypotension—not hypertension—is a sign of biliary sepsis and severe cholangitis.

D. Diarrhea and elevated alkaline phosphatase may be seen, but they do not complete the pentad of symptoms.

E. Oliguria and vomiting may be seen, but they do not complete the pentad of symptoms.

SETTING 4: EMERGENCY DEPARTMENT

Generally, patients encountered here are seeking urgent care; most are not known to you. A full range of social services is available, including rape crisis intervention, family support, child protective services, domestic violence support, psychiatric services, and security assistance backed up by local police. Complete laboratory and radiology services are available.

The next three questions (items 151–153) correspond to the following vignette.

A 66-year-old male presents to the emergency room with acute onset of right leg pain. The patient states that the pain started 2 hours ago and is unrelenting, and he claims that the leg is "tingling." On your examination, it looks pale and feels cold to touch, and there are no Doppler-able pedal signals.

151. What is the most appropriate next step in the management of this patient?

 A. CT scan
 B. IV heparin drip
 C. Ankle-brachial index
 D. Bedrest with lower extremity elevation
 E. Venous duplex

152. What is the most common cause of the condition shown in this patient's angiogram (Figure 5-152A)?

 A. Deep vein thrombosis
 B. Abdominal aortic aneurysm
 C. Blue toe syndrome
 D. Fat embolism
 E. Atrial fibrillation

153. What is the most appropriate treatment for this patient?

 A. Systemic anticoagulation
 B. Stent placed angiographically
 C. Femoral artery to tibial artery bypass
 D. Embolectomy
 E. Medical management

End of Set

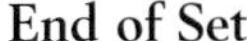

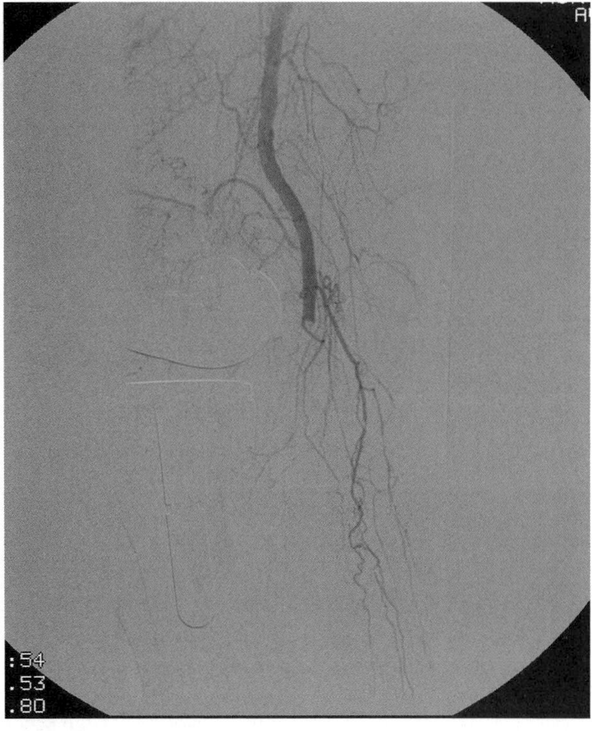

A

Figure 5-152A • Image Courtesy of the University of Utah School of Medicine, Salt Lake City, Utah.

154. You are the general surgery intern on call at a busy university hospital. You are called by the ER physician to see a 57-year-old female complaining of abdominal pain. Six months ago the patient was diagnosed with metastatic breast cancer and she has been receiving chemotherapy, with her last dose being 6 days ago. The patient states that the abdominal pain started this morning and has become progressively worse, with multiple bouts of emesis. The patient's abdomen is very tender to the touch and demonstrates rebound tenderness throughout. The patient also denies flatus or a bowel movement. A CBC reveals WBC 0.15K, HCT 20%, and PLT 65,000. A chest x-ray is obtained (Figure 5-154A). What is the most appropriate next step in this patient's management?

 A. CT scan of the abdomen
 B. Fluid resuscitation and pain control
 C. Exploratory laparotomy
 D. Colonoscopy
 E. Plan for discharge with narcotics

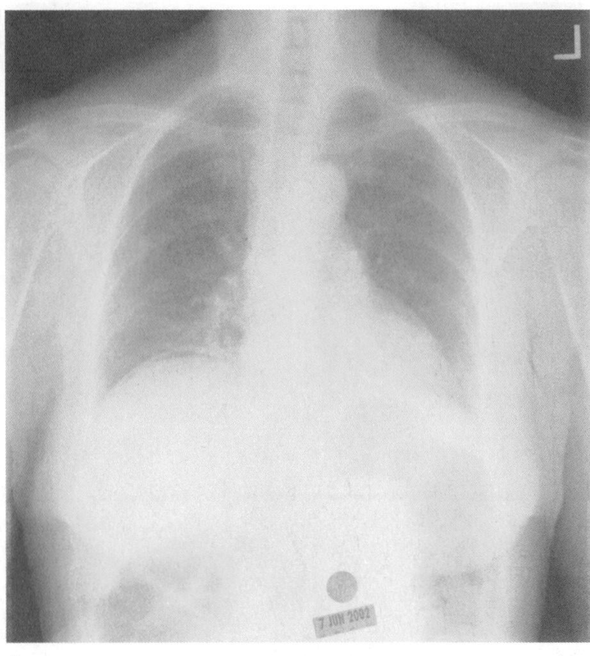

A

Figure 5-154A • Image Courtesy of the University of Utah School of Medicine, Salt Lake City, Utah.

155. A 12-year-old male is seen in the ED after being hit by a car. His only injury is a left closed tibia/fibula fracture. The orthopedic surgeon on call takes the patient to the operating room and performs an open reduction with internal fixation. Later that night the patient complains of increasing left leg pain, unrelieved with morphine. After the dressings are removed, a tight left lower leg is noted. The dorsal pedal pulse is palpable, but the patient is unable to move his toes and cries out in pain upon passive dorsal flexion. What is the most appropriate next step?

   A. Four-compartment fasciotomies
   B. A different narcotic
   C. Surgical embolectomy
   D. Duplex Doppler scan
   E. Nothing, as long as you can feel pulses

156. An 18-year-old motorcycle rider is admitted to the ER after suffering a closed head injury with loss of consciousness. The patient's vital signs are as follows: BP 128/74, HR 85, RR 18, T 38°C, and GCS 10. The patient is also confused and combative. The trauma evaluation shows no associated injuries other than a scalp laceration. After appropriate treatment you suspect post–head injury diabetes insipidus. Which of the following findings is most consistent with this diagnosis?

   A. High urine specific gravity
   B. Low urine output
   C. Polydipsia
   D. Low serum sodium
   E. Fluid restriction

The next two questions (items 157 and 158) correspond to the following vignette.

A 75-year-old male is transferred from a nearby skilled nursing facility to the emergency department because of increasing abdominal pain. The patient has a history of dementia and has been a resident of this facility for approximately 5 years. A nurse who accompanies him to the hospital tells you that the patient has not eaten anything for 2 days and has been vomiting. On exam, the patient is in mild distress and has a palpable right upper quadrant mass, with a distended, tender abdomen, without peritoneal signs. Vital signs are as follows: T 36.5°C, BP 115/65, HR 95, RR 12, and SaO_2 95% on room air. Labs results are as follows: Na 145 mmol/L, K 3.5 mmol/L, Cl 103 mmol/L, HCO_3 30 mmol/L, BUN 25 mg/dL, creatinine 1.1 mg/dL, glucose 115 mg/dL, WBC 10,000, HCT 45%, PLT 450,000, and lipase 33 U/L. An abdominal film is obtained (Figure 5-157A).

157. What is this patient's most likely diagnosis?

   A. Perforated duodenal ulcer
   B. Diverticulitis
   C. Pancreatitis
   D. Appendicitis
   E. Sigmoid volvulus

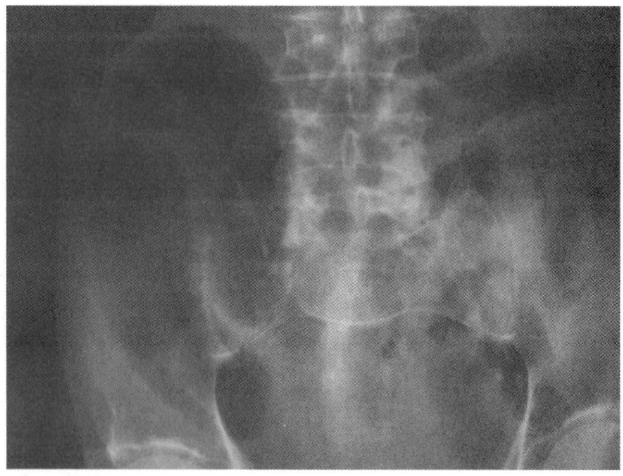

A

Figure 5-157A • Image Courtesy of the University of Utah School of Medicine, Salt Lake City, Utah.

158. What is the most appropriate next step in his management?

A. Abdominal ultrasound
B. Endoscopic reduction
C. CT scan of the abdomen
D. Exploratory laparotomy
E. Observation

End of Set

159. A 55-year-old obese female with a history of longstanding renal failure requiring dialysis is admitted to the ER with a clotted AV fistula. The patient has missed her regular dialysis and complains of fatigue, nausea, and feeling puffy. The patient's BP is 178/101, HR is 101, and RR is 22. Labs are drawn and show K 6.8 mmol/L. The patient's EKG tracing shows peaked T waves with a prolonged PR interval and widening of the QRS complex. What is the initial step in the emergency treatment of hyperkalemia?

A. Calcium gluconate
B. Metoprolol
C. Insulin and glucose
D. Dialysis
E. Albuterol

160. A 33-year-old female comes to the emergency room to be evaluated for frequent spontaneous nose bleeds. The CBC obtained reveals a WBC 9500, HCT 37%, and PLT 19,000. The patient is eventually diagnosed with ITP and given oral steroids for treatment, with follow-up appointments scheduled in oncology. Lacking a health care insurance provider, she returns to the emergency room 2 weeks after her discharge for increasing frequency and duration of nose bleeds. The patient has a platelet count of 500. What is the most appropriate next step in management of this patient?

A. Outpatient follow-up only
B. Prednisone, 1 mg/kg/day for 6 months
C. Splenectomy
D. Technetium 99-m colloid liver spleen scan
E. Platelet transfusion until the count is normal

The next three questions (items 161–163) correspond to the following vignette.

A 64-year-old male presents to the emergency room with a 12-hour history of acute-onset abdominal pain. The patient states that the pain is located primarily around his umbilicus and is unremitting and intense in nature. The physical exam is concerning for pain out of proportion to his exam. Past medical history is significant for diabetes mellitus and atrial fibrillation, for which the patient takes insulin and aspirin, respectively.

161. What is the most likely diagnosis?

A. Gastritis
B. Ruptured abdominal aortic aneurysm
C. Mesenteric ischemia
D. Ulcerative colitis
E. Gastric tumor

162. You order a panel of labs, including a CBC, metabolic panel, hepatic panel, and an arterial blood gas. Which of the following abnormalities consistent with your diagnosis would you expect in this patient?

A. Decreased hematocrit
B. Metabolic acidosis
C. Metabolic alkalosis
D. Hyponatremia
E. Decreased albumin

163. Of the following, which is the most appropriate study to obtain to confirm your diagnosis?

A. Right upper quadrant ultrasound
B. Colonoscopy
C. Enteroclysis
D. Angiogram
E. Upper endoscopy

End of Set

The next two questions (items 164 and 165) correspond to the following vignette.

A 33-year-old female who is 5 weeks postpartum comes to the emergency department with a 3-day history of nausea and vomiting. The patient reports normal bowel function and states that the nausea usually occurs about 1 hour after eating. On exam, the patient's abdomen is soft and nondistended, with right upper quadrant tenderness. Vital signs are as follows: BP 118/72, HR 97, and T 38.8°C. Labs are as follows: WBC 13,000, total bilirubin 1.3 mg/dL, AST 70 U/L, ALT 62 U/L, amylase 81 U/L, and lipase 110 U/L. An ultrasound of the gallbladder (Figure 5-164) shows gallbladder wall thickening with a small amount of pericholecystic fluid and evidence of multiple gallstones. There is no intrahepatic ductal dilation.

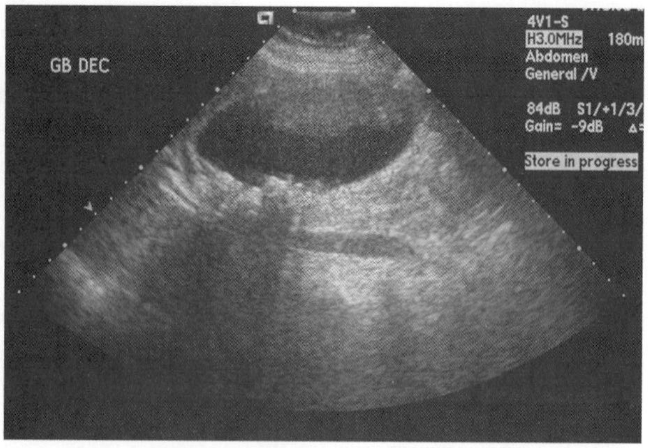

Figure 5-164 • Image courtesy of the University of Utah School of Medicine, Salt Lake City, Utah.

164. What is this patient's diagnosis?

A. Symptomatic cholelithiasis
B. Acute acalculous cholecystitis
C. Acute calculus cholecystitis
D. Ascending cholangitis
E. Biliary dyskinesia

165. Had the ultrasound of this patient's gallbladder been normal, what study would be the next best choice to evaluate the gallbladder?

A. Abdominal CT scan
B. HIDA scan
C. Oral cholecystogram
D. Percutaneous transhepatic cholangiography
E. ERCP

End of Set

The next three questions (items 166–168) correspond to the following vignette.

A 33-year-old male construction worker comes to the emergency room with the acute onset of right groin pain after vomiting 1 hour prior to his arrival at the ER. The patient reports the pain to be constant and denies any radiation of the pain. Vital signs are as follows: BP 168/88, HR 122, and T 36.6°C. The patient's abdomen is soft and nondistended, but he has a tender, palpable mass on the right side of the right scrotum. The right testicle is nontender. The patient's WBC count is 7500.

166. What is this patient's most likely diagnosis?

A. Direct inguinal hernia
B. Incarcerated inguinal hernia
C. Strangulated inguinal hernia
D. Testicular torsion
E. Hiatal hernia

167. Upon taking this patient to the operating room, what is the procedure of choice?

A. Reduction of the hernia via a groin incision
B. Exploratory laparotomy via a midline incision
C. Orchiopexy
D. Reduction in the OR under anesthesia if possible
E. Exploration and hernia repair via the groin

168. At the time of surgical repair of the hernia, you diagnose the patient with an indirect inguinal hernia based on what finding?

A. Hernia sac located anterior to the epigastric vessels
B. Hernia sac located posterior to the epigastric vessels
C. Hernia sac located medial to the inferior epigastric vessels
D. Hernia sac located lateral to the inferior epigastric vessels
E. Hernia sac protruding through Hesselbach's triangle

End of Set

The next two questions (items 160 and 170) correspond to the following vignette.

A 70-year-old female comes to the emergency department 3 weeks after being discharged from the hospital for acute, uncomplicated diverticulitis that required IV antibiotic administration. Currently she complains of pain that has increased over the last 5 days. The pain is mainly in the right upper quadrant and is associated with fever, chills, and decreased appetite. Vitals signs are as follows: T 38.6 °C, HR 65, BP 123/63, RR 15, and SaO_2 93% on room air. On physical exam, the patient is a slightly obese female, who has tenderness in the right upper quadrant without rebound or rigidity. A CT scan is obtained (Figure 5-169).

169. Which of the following conditions is the most likely cause of this patient's problem?

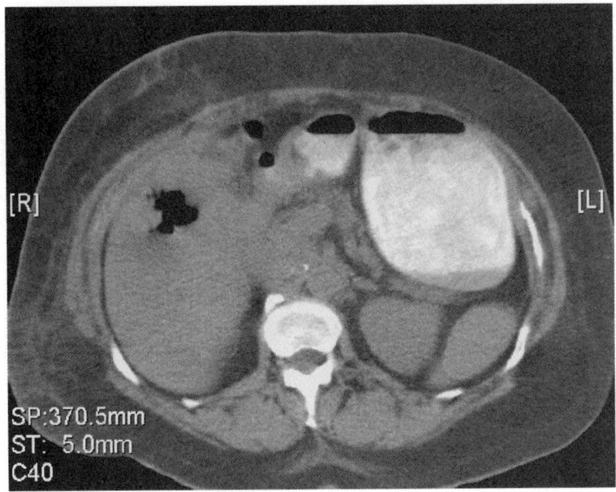

Figure 5-169 • Image Courtesy of the University of Utah School of Medicine, Salt Lake City, Utah.

A. Pelvic inflammatory disease
B. Sigmoid volvulus
C. Irritable bowel syndrome
D. Appendicitis
E. Urosepsis

170. What is the most appropriate initial therapy for this patient?

A. Broad-spectrum IV antibiotics
B. Exploratory laparotomy and hepatic resection
C. Broad-spectrum IV antibiotics with drainage via surgical laparotomy
D. Broad-spectrum IV antibiotics and percutaneous drainage
E. Oral antibiotics with follow-up in the clinic

End of Set

The next two questions (items 171 and 172) correspond to the following vignette.

A 66-year-old male comes to the emergency department with the acute onset of abdominal pain that began 3 hours ago. The pain is constant and radiates to his back. Past medical history is significant for hypertension, type 2 diabetes, a significant drinking history, and a 40-pack-per-year history of smoking. The patient is anxious and diaphoretic with the following vital signs: BP 88/48, HR 122, RR 34, and T 36.2°C. You palpate his abdomen and feel a pulsatile mass.

171. What is the next step in this patient's management?

A. Ultrasound of the abdomen
B. CT scan of the abdomen
C. Placement of 2 large-bore peripheral IVs
D. Intubation
E. Placement of a central line for central IV access

172. If the same patient were to present with an asymptomatic abdominal aortic aneurysm, which was found during a routine physical exam by his primary care provider, what would be the indication to repair it electively?

A. Extension of the aneurysm above the renal arteries
B. Extension of the aneurysm into at least one of the iliac arteries
C. Diameter greater than 5 cm
D. Growth in diameter greater than 3 mm annually
E. Should never be electively repaired due to high operative risk

End of Set

The next three questions (items 173–175) correspond to the following vignette.

A 27-year-old male is the unrestrained passenger in a car when it is broadsided at high speed. The patient is transported by air to the hospital. On arrival to the ER, he is difficult to rouse. Vitals are as follows: HR 125, BP 84/62, RR 30, and T 36.5°C. On exam, the patient has facial abrasions, decreased breath sounds on the left, a distended abdomen, and external rotation of the right femur.

173. What is the most appropriate first step in this patient's management?

A. Exploratory laparotomy
B. Endotracheal intubation
C. Chest x-ray
D. Infusion of crystalloid
E. Tube thoracostomy

174. On further assessment, the patient continues to have hypotension with systolic pressures in the 80s. He is also difficult to ventilate. The chest x-ray obtained in the trauma bay is shown in Figure 5-174A. What action is critical in helping to stabilize this patient?

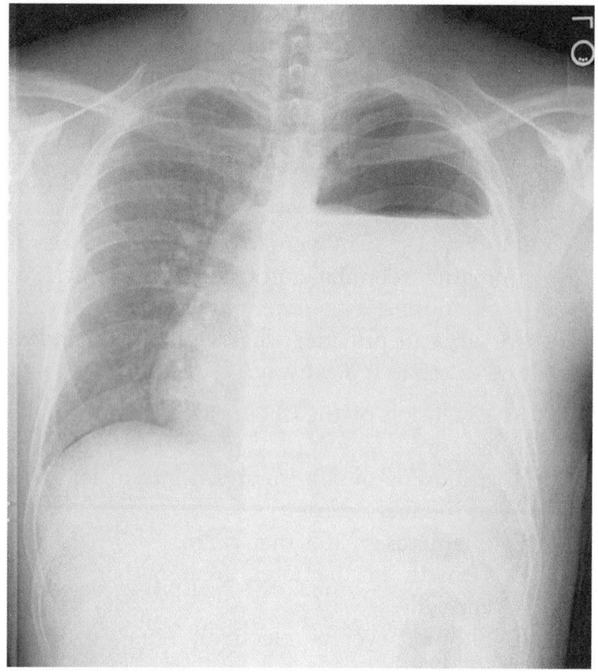

Figure 5-174A • Image Courtesy of the University of Utah School of Medicine, Salt Lake City, Utah.

A. Exploratory laparotomy
B. Endotracheal intubation
C. Chemical paralysis
D. Infusion of crystalloid
E. Tube thoracostomy

175. Despite attempts to correct this patient's hemodynamic instability, the hypotension continues. The patient has received 4 units of O-negative, packed red blood cells in addition to 4 liters of crystalloid. The blood pressure remains 82/41, with a heart rate of 123. What is the most appropriate next step in the management of this case?

A. Exploratory laparotomy
B. Endotracheal intubation
C. CT scan of the chest
D. Infusion of crystalloid
E. Tube thoracostomy

End of Set

176. A 28-year-old, obviously intoxicated and possibly chemically impaired, unrestrained male driver is admitted to the ER after rolling his car while attempting to evade the police. Vital signs are BP 116/62, HR 116, and RR 32. Intravenous lines were placed at the scene, and a NGT is in place. The patient is uncooperative, as well as physically and verbally abusive to the staff. Full four-point restraints are in place. The patient complains of abdominal pain, is short of breath, and randomly screams for intravenous pain medication. Which portion of this patient's management is best delayed until the secondary survey?

A Exposure
B. Abdomen
C. Circulation
D. Disability
E. Airway

177. A 16-year-old female restrained driver is involved in a head-on collision with oncoming traffic. The patient arrives intubated to the trauma bay. After your primary assessment, the vital signs are T 36.9°C, HR 135, and BP 100/60. You obtain the chest x-ray shown in Figure 5-177A. Assuming the patient remains in stable condition, what study will be required to further assess for intrathoracic injury?

A. PA and lateral chest x-ray
B. CT of the chest
C. Thoracic arch aortogram
D. Mediastinoscopy
E. Video-assisted thoracoscopic surgery

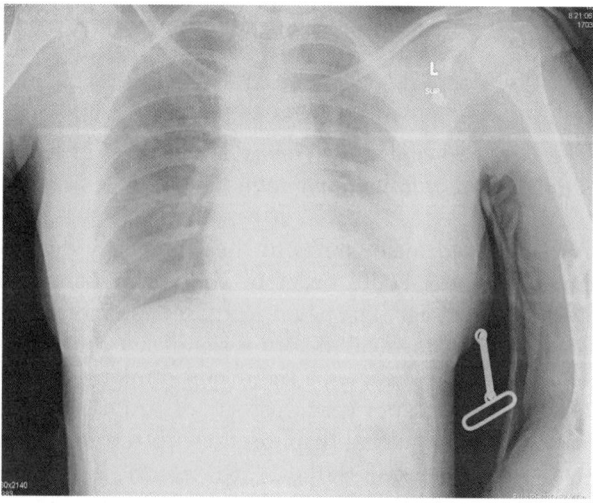

Figure 5-177A • Image Courtesy of the University of Utah School of Medicine, Salt Lake City, Utah.

The next two questions (items 178 and 179) correspond to the following vignette.

A 40-year-old male involved in an auto-versus-pedestrian accident arrives in the ER. The patient's vital signs are T 36.5°C, HR 140, and BP 85/40. The GCS is 15. Your exam reveals the following findings: left-sided hemotympanum with some clear discharge, multiple abrasions to the right face, the pelvis unstable to rock, and blood in the urethral meatus. On rectal exam, the tone is normal, although the prostate is difficult to palpate and gross blood is found. There is an obvious deformity to the left femur and an open fracture to the right tibia.

178. Which of the following statements is true regarding this scenario?

    A. Foley catheter placement is critical in this patient to help drain the traumatized bladder.
    B. Immediate head CT takes precedence over other treatments.
    C. Colonoscopy should be performed to diagnose the site of bleeding.
    D. The extraperitoneal urethral injury will require emergent surgery to repair it.
    E. External fixation of pelvic fracture may help maintain hemodynamic stability by reducing retroperitoneal bleeding.

179. After stabilizing the patient, your further work-up reveals a transverse process fracture of the fifth cervical vertebrae. What artery must be further examined to rule out an associated injury?

    A. Deep cervical artery
    B. Vertebral artery
    C. Ascending cervical artery
    D. Common carotid artery
    E. Internal carotid artery

End of Set

180. A 77-year-old obese male with a known AAA is brought to the ER with sudden, severe abdominal pain, which radiates to his back. The patient is on diuretics for hypertension and oral medication for adult-onset diabetes. Vital signs are HR 125 and BP 88/57. The patient's abdomen is distended and mildly tender. What is the best initial management for this patient?

    A. Vigorous fluid resuscitation, ICU admission for stabilization prior to operative repair
    B. Paracentesis to evaluate for possible ruptured AAA
    C. Emergent surgical exploration
    D. Abdomen/pelvic CT scan to evaluate the AAA prior to repair
    E. Emergency angiogram to confirm a ruptured AAA diagnosis

The next three questions (items 181–183) correspond to the following vignette.

A 6-year-old male is brought into the emergency room as a trauma patient after being struck by an automobile while playing in his front yard. The patient is hypotensive and has bilateral open femur fractures, from which he is hemorrhaging severely. The child is crying but his SaO_2 level is 99% on room air. You are very concerned that he will exsanguinate from his femur fractures.

181. What is the first step in the management of this patient?

    A. Apply direct pressure to the bleeding vessels
    B. Apply a tourniquet
    C. Transfuse type O-negative RBCs
    D. Obtain control of the airway
    E. Transfuse 2 units FFP

182. After the patient is stabilized in the trauma bay, a CT scan is obtained (Figure 5-182A). What injury are you concerned about after seeing this scan?

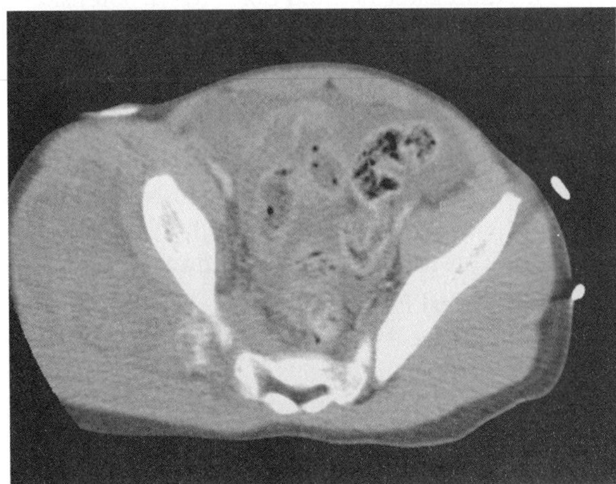

A

Figure 5-182A • Image Courtesy of the University of Utah School of Medicine, Salt Lake City, Utah.

A. Traumatic bowel perforation
B. Splenic laceration
C Intraperitoneal bladder rupture
D. Extraperitoneal bladder rupture
E. Internal iliac artery injury

183. Based on your presumed diagnosis, what is the best management of this patient's condition?

A. Small bowel resection
B. Splenectomy
C. Arterial embolization
D. Suprapubic catheter placement
E. Observation

End of Set

The next three questions (items 184–186) correspond to the following vignette.

A 28-year-old female is ejected from her car after it is struck from the side by a car traveling approximately 50 mph. At the accident scene, her initial GCS is 10. The patient was intubated by the paramedic for respiratory distress and is brought to the emergency department in critical condition. The paramedic reports that the patient's blood pressure has been slowly falling during transport. The last pressure was 64/40 with a heart rate of 133 and an oxygen saturation rate of 62%. You notice obvious deformities of multiple ribs of the left chest.

184. What is the first step in managing this seriously injured patient?

A. Administer IV fluid bolus for hypotension
B. Stabilize her chest injury
C. Obtain a chest x-ray
D. Reevaluate the airway
E. Place a central line

185. If this patient remained hypotensive and had a trachea that deviated to the right, you would be most concerned about which injury?

A. Tracheal injury
B. Esophageal injury
C. Open pneumothorax
D. Tension pneumothorax
E. Flail chest

186. You determine that the patient needs a left thoracostomy tube. After placement, the chest x-ray shown in Figure 5-186A is obtained. What injury does this patient have?

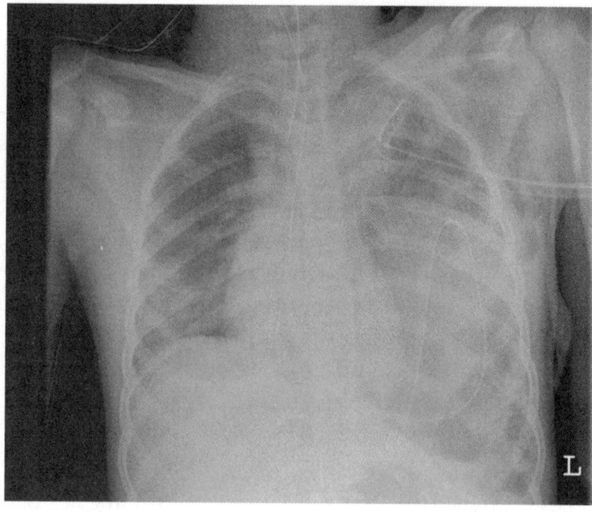

A

Figure 5-186A • Image Courtesy of the University of Utah School of Medicine, Salt Lake City, Utah.

A. Pulmonary laceration
B. Aortic dissection
C. Ruptured diaphragm
D. Gastric perforation
E. Cardiac contusion

End of Set

187. A 32-year-old female who rolled her jeep down a highway embankment is brought to the trauma bay. The patient is awake and answers questions appropriately. Primary examination shows her ABCs to be intact. The patient claims that she is unable to feel or move anything below the nipple line. Vital signs are as follows: T 37.8°C, HR 98, and BP 82/48. Fluid resuscitation is initiated. Secondary survey reveals thoracic spine tenderness and midline deformities, and a large, deep abrasion to the left thigh, which is contaminated with dirt and grass. The abdomen is soft, nondistended, and nontender. An abdominal ultrasound shows no free peritoneal fluid, and laboratory values are unremarkable. One liter of crystalloid is infused without improvement in blood pressure. What is the most important medication for this patient to receive at this point?

A. Cefazolin
B. Methylprednisolone
C. Norepinephrine
D. Phenylephrine
E. Morphine sulfate

End of Set

The next three questions (items 188–190) correspond to the following vignette.

An 18-year-old female is seen in the ED with a 1-day history of abdominal pain. The patient states that the pain began periumbilically as a dull ache, but it has since migrated to the right lower quadrant. It is now sharp and constant in nature. This morning, the patient began vomiting and had one episode of diarrhea. She is sexually active and her last menstrual period ended 7 days ago. On exam, she is ill appearing and tachycardic. There is involuntary guarding in both quadrants of the lower abdomen. A pelvic exam reveals tenderness noted upon movement of the cervix and during rectal exam. A CBC demonstrates a leukocytosis of 13,000, and β-hCG is negative.

188. What is the most appropriate next step in the management of this patient?

A. Surgical exploration
B. Abdominal ultrasound
C. CT scan of the abdomen
D. IV hydration and observation
E. Oral antibiotics and follow-up in 2 days

189. In order of decreasing frequency, what are the potential causes of appendicitis in this patient?

A. Foreign body, tumor, fecalith
B. Tumor, fecalith, lymphoid hyperplasia
C. Fecalith, lymphoid hyperplasia, tumor
D. Lymphoid hyperplasia, fecalith, tumor
E. Fecalith, tumor, lymphoid hyperplasia

190. Further radiographic imaging demonstrates acute appendicitis. The patient is taken to the operating room for surgical exploration. Two days later, the pathology report reveals a 1 cm carcinoid tumor at the tip of the appendix. What further treatment should be implemented?

A. CT scan of the abdomen and pelvis for metastatic staging
B. No further treatment
C. Radiation therapy
D. Right hemicolectomy
E. Chemotherapy

End of Set

The next two questions (items 191 and 192) correspond to the following vignette.

A 15-year-old female presents to the emergency department with a 2-day history of lower abdominal pain. The patient states that the pain began in the right lower quadrant, but has progressively worsened over the last 24 hours, becoming quite intense. She denies having a fever but complains of nausea, vomiting, and a poor appetite. Her last menstrual period was 6 weeks ago, and she reports being sexually active only twice. Currently she takes no medications and denies allergies. On physical exam, she appears acutely ill and has diffuse tenderness in the lower abdomen, with the right side being worse than the left, with no peritoneal signs. Rectal and pelvic exams are normal. A serum β-hCG level is 5500 mIU/mL.

191. What initial test is most appropriate in the work-up of this patient?

A. CT scan of abdomen and pelvis
B. Pelvic ultrasound
C. Abdominal series
D. Culdocentesis
E. Diagnostic laparoscopy

192. What is the most likely diagnosis?

A. Acute appendicitis
B. Acute diverticulitis
C. Ruptured ovarian cyst
D. Tubo-ovarian abscess
E. Ectopic pregnancy

End of Set

The next two questions (items 193 and 194) correspond to the following vignette.

A 45-year-old male skier is brought to the emergency room by helicopter after being struck by an out-of-control snowboarder. Initially the patient was dazed and confused but these symptoms quickly resolved and he continued to ski to the lodge. The patient's wife noticed that he was acting strangely, so she took him to the clinic at the resort. From there, he was transported to the hospital. On exam, the patient has a GCS of 14, and he demonstrates some confusion, perseveration, and a slightly dilated right pupil. The patient is taken for a CT scan (Figure 5-193A).

193. What is the etiology of this patient's current condition?

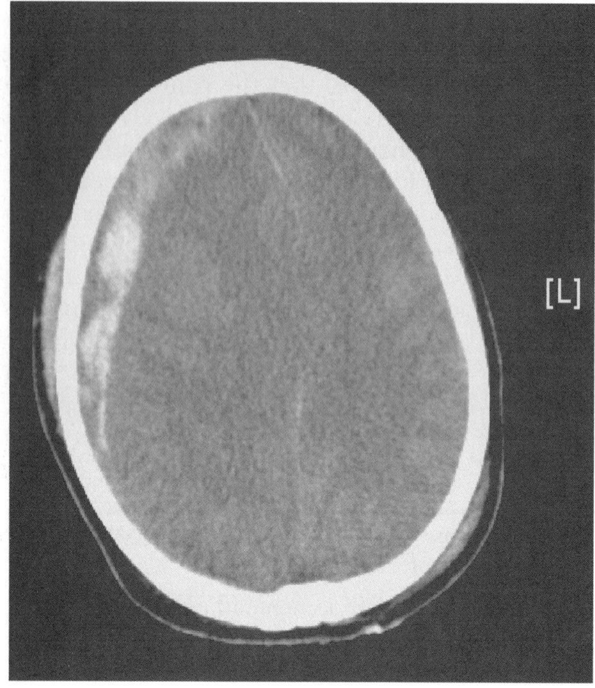

A

Figure 5-193A • Image Courtesy of the University of Utah School of Medicine, Salt Lake City, Utah.

A. Subdural hematoma
B. Epidural hematoma
C. Subarachnoid hemorrhage
D. Intraparenchymal hemorrhage
E. Axonal shear injury

194. What is the most appropriate management option?

A. Evacuation of the hematoma
B. Angiographic embolization
C. Ventriculostomy
D. Mannitol and hyperventilation
E. Serial neurological exams

End of Set

The next two questions (items 195 and 196) correspond to the following vignette.

You evaluate a 42-year-old male driver in the emergency room who has previously been involved in a high-speed, head-on, motor vehicle accident. His GCS is 15. After the initial ABCs of trauma care are completed, you note that the only significant injury appears to involve the patient's abdomen. The abdominal exam shows diffuse tenderness, peritoneal signs, and seat belt imprint on the lower chest and abdomen. The patient is taken to the OR; during the ensuing surgical exploration, you repair a small bowel mesentery laceration and find a large, right retroperitoneal hematoma surrounding the right kidney.

195. In what zone is this retroperitoneal hematoma found?

A. Zone I
B. Zone II
C. Zone III
D. Zone IV
E. Zone V

196. What is the most appropriate management of this hematoma at this time?

A. Close the abdomen and obtain a CT
B. Obtain an intraoperative angiogram
C. Explore the hematoma if it is expanding
D. Remove the involved kidney
E. Open the hematoma

End of Set

The next two questions (items 197 and 198) correspond to the following vignette.

While on call in the ED, you are contacted by the medical team to see a patient with bright red blood per rectum. The patient is a 67-year-old male who was admitted 3 days ago for pneumonia. Approximately 3 hours prior to your being contacted, the patient complained of abdominal pain that was followed by passage of a large amount of stool containing gross blood. Vital signs are as follows: T 37.5°C, BP 115/76, HR 95, and SaO_2 92% on 2 L by nasal cannula. Your exam reveals an alert and responsive patient in no apparent distress. Cardiopulmonary exam reveals a regular heart rate and rhythm, skin warm and pink throughout, decreased breath sounds, and dullness to percussion in the right lower lung field. The abdominal exam is unremarkable.

197. What is the most appropriate first step in management of this patient?

A. Exploratory laparotomy
B. Endoscopy
C. Tagged RBC scan
D. CT scan
E. Angiography

198. Your initial work-up does not reveal any obvious source of bleeding but there is clearly evidence of blood in the descending colon. The patient's hematocrit remains stable and his vital signs are unchanged over the course of the next 2 days, despite ongoing bright red blood in his stool. What is the next step in this patient's management?

A. Left hemicolectomy with primary anastomosis
B. Left hemicolectomy with diverting colostomy
C. Total abdominal colectomy with ileoanal anastomosis
D. Repeat colonoscopy
E. Close observation

End of Set

The next two questions (items 199 and 200) correspond to the following vignette.

A 53-year-old male presents to the emergency department after falling and striking his right lower chest. The film in Figure 5-199A is obtained.

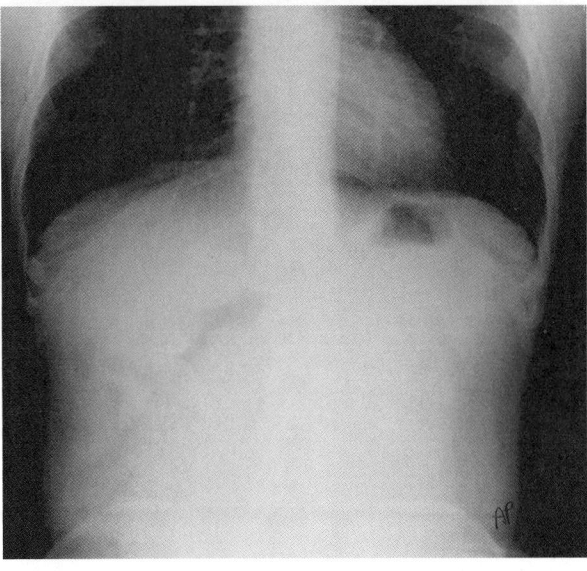

A

Figure 5-199A • Image Courtesy of the University of Utah School of Medicine, Salt Lake City, Utah.

199. What is the abnormal incidental finding on the x-ray?

A. Free intraperitoneal air
B. Dilated small bowel
C. A calcified gallbladder
D. Dilated large bowel
E. Kidney stone

200. What is the most appropriate step in this patient's management?

A. Percutaneous transhepatic cholangiography (PTC)
B. Elective cholecystectomy
C. Endoscopic retrograde cholangiopancreatography (ERCP)
D. Emergent cholecystectomy
E. Observation

End of Set

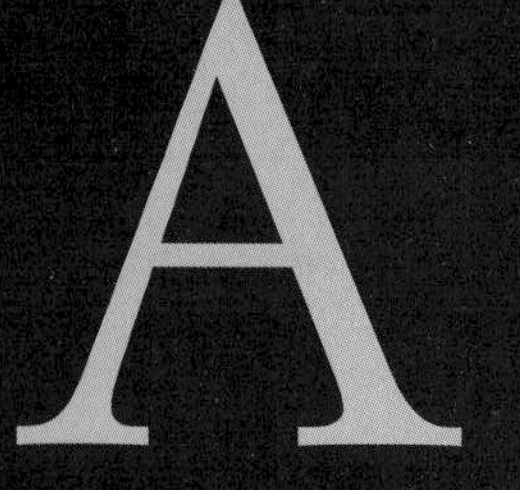

Answers and Explanations

151. B
152. E
153. D
154. C
155. A
156. C
157. E
158. B
159. A
160. C
161. C
162. B
163. D
164. C
165. B
166. B
167. E
168. D
169. D
170. D
171. D
172. C
173. B
174. E
175. A
176. B
177. C
178. E
179. B
180. C
181. D
182. E
183. C
184. D
185. D
186. C
187. B
188. C
189. D
190. B
191. B
192. E
193. A
194. A
195. B
196. C
197. B
198. E
199. C
200. B

151. **B. Acute arterial occlusion is an acute event typically caused by embolization. It can also be seen in thrombosis of an atheromatous plaque or in vascular trauma. Rapid intervention is required to avoid permanent sequelae. The diagnosis is made by physical exam and is characterized by the "six P's": pain, paralysis, pallor, paresthesia, poikilothermy, and pulselessness. The most appropriate immediate treatment consists of anticoagulation with IV heparin.**

A. A CT scan is an inappropriate choice for imaging because it does not evaluate peripheral arterial disease.
C. An ankle brachial index (ABI) is used to evaluate arterial insufficiency. In this patient with no Doppler-able pedal signals, it will not assist in the diagnosis.
D, E. A venous duplex and bedrest with lower extremity elevation would be more appropriate in patients with venous stasis, not in patients with arterial disease.

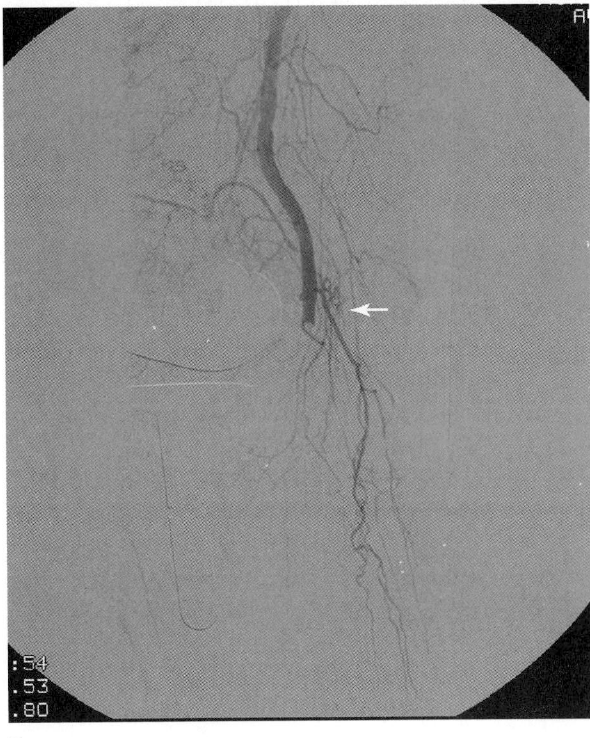

B

Figure 5-152B • Image Courtesy of the University of Utah School of Medicine, Salt Lake City, Utah.

152. **E. An arteriogram is important to define the anatomy and demonstrate the location of vessel occlusion. The superficial femoral artery is the most common site of occlusion, as shown in the angiogram in Figure 5-152B (note the arrow). The cause of a sudden occlusion should be determined. The most common source involves the heart; atrial fibrillation is seen in approximately 85% of all such cases. Other sources include aneurysms and atheromatous plaques proximal to the site of occlusion.**

A. Deep vein thromboses are caused by venous stasis, not seen by angiography.
B. Although an abdominal aortic aneurysm can be the source of an embolism to the lower extremities, it is less likely than the most common cause, which is from the heart.
C. Blue toe syndrome occurs when atheromatous plaques are showered from the artery into the periphery. It is usually seen after cardiac catheterization.
D. A fat embolism can be seen in cases of long bone fractures. It usually occurs in the pulmonary vasculature.

153. **D. Surgical management consists of an embolectomy, which involves cutdown of the occluded artery proximal to the occlusion with insertion of a catheter. The catheter is threaded distally until it passes the thrombus. The balloon is inflated and the catheter is withdrawn, bringing the clot along with it.**

A. Anticoagulation with heparin and/or Coumadin is used as an adjunct to surgery to prevent extension or recurrence of clot formation.
B, C. Stent placement and bypass surgery are reserved for areas of atherosclerotic stenosis, not acute occlusion due to an embolism.
E. This disease is a surgical emergency, not a medically treated condition.

154. **C. In the evaluation of an acute abdomen, the observance of pneumoperitoneum(i.e., "free air") on the chest x-ray (note the arrow in Figure 5-154B) or physical exam findings of peritonitis, including rebound tenderness,**

warrant an exploratory laparotomy. This is a surgical emergency; therefore, the other choices are inappropriate. No further radiologic evaluation is needed when a patient demonstrates peritoneal signs on physical exam and free air under the diaphragm on chest x-ray.

A. Obtaining a CT scan will delay surgical treatment and will merely show the free air already noted on the chest x-ray.
B. IV resuscitation and pain control are very appropriate, but not without an urgent laparotomy.
D. Colonoscopy would delay treatment and possibly exacerbate the problem.
E. Discharge is obviously not appropriate for a patient with an acute abdomen and free air.

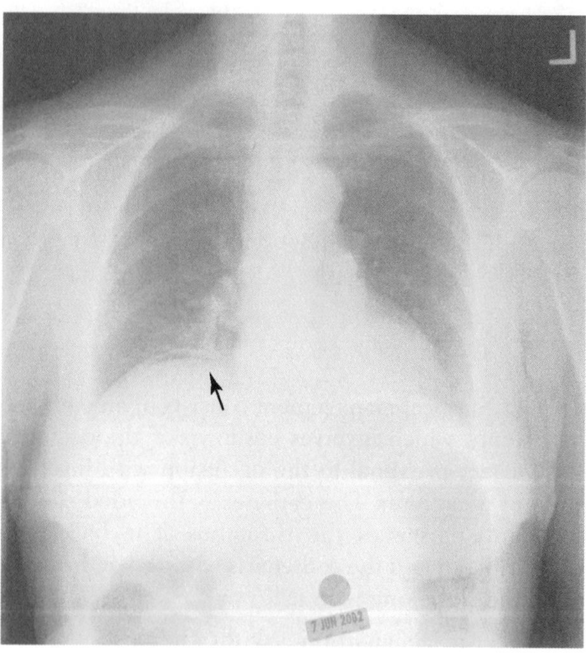

B

Figure 5-154B • Image Courtesy of the University of Utah School of Medicine, Salt Lake City, Utah.

155. **A. This case is a classic example of lower extremity compartment syndrome. Patients are at risk when reperfusion follows an extended period of ischemia. Early signs of compartment syndrome include pain out of proportion to exam, decreased sensation in the first web space, and increased pain with passive dorsiflexion of the foot. The diagnosis can be confirmed by measurement of compartment pressures; any value higher than 30 mm Hg is considered diagnostic. Patients with compartment syndrome may not lose peripheral pulses, as the pressures would have to be elevated above systolic arterial pressure to compromise arterial perfusion. Emergent four-compartment fasciotomies is the appropriate treatment.**

B. Inadequate pain control is not the issue in this patient. The pain associated with compartment syndrome is significant, and trying a different narcotic will not resolve the problem.
C. There is no evidence of thrombosis formation in this case.
D. A duplex Doppler scan would show evidence of arterial flow but would miss the problem of decreased tissue perfusion.
E. Pulses may be palpable despite the presence of compartment syndrome.

156. **C. Diabetes insipidus results from a deficiency (central DI) or unresponsiveness (nephrogenic DI) of antidiuretic hormone (ADH). Because of insensible water loss, patients experience extreme thirst.**

A, B. Voluminous urine output—not low urine output—with a low specific gravity—not high specific gravity—are symptoms seen with DI.
D. Hypernatremia—not hyponatremia—is seen with DI.
E. Vasopressin and intravenous fluid replacement—not fluid restriction—are the usual means of treatment.

157. **E. Colonic volvulus occurs when the colon twists around its mesentery, resulting in obstruction and vascular compromise. If prolonged, this condition can result in necrosis and eventually perforation. It may occur in the sigmoid colon or cecum. Sigmoid volvulus is most common, occurring in approximately 80% of cases. It is usually seen in elderly institutionalized patients with chronic constipation and history of prior abdominal surgery or distal colonic obstruction. It is characterized by acute abdominal pain, abdominal distention, and obstipation. On plain film, the "omega" sign—a loop of colon aiming toward the right upper quadrant—is commonly seen (note the arrows in Figure 5-157B).**

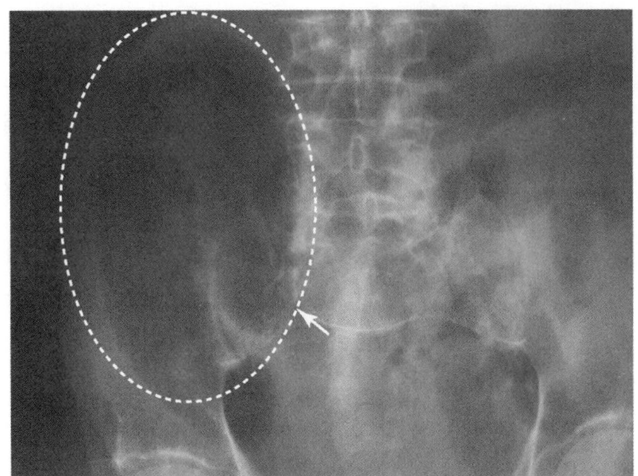

B

Figure 5-157B • Image Courtesy of the University of Utah School of Medicine, Salt Lake City, Utah.

A, B, C, D. Although all of these options should be part of the differential diagnosis, the history, laboratory values, and radiographic imaging help one come to the proper diagnosis.

158. **B. Sigmoidoscopy is both diagnostic and therapeutic for sigmoid volvulus and is successful in treatment of 80% of cases. Indications for surgery include free air or pneumatosis on abdominal films, peritoneal sign on exam, or unsuccessful endoscopic reduction. Most patients should undergo an elective sigmoid colectomy after reduction, as the recurrence rate for this condition approaches 40%.**

A, C. Abdominal ultrasound and CT scan will help confirm the diagnosis, but they are not therapeutic.

D. The patient will require an exploratory laparotomy if the sigmoidoscopy is unsuccessful.

E. Observation is inappropriate, as continuation of this disease process will lead to bowel necrosis and perforation.

159. **A. Hyperkalemia is seen in cases involving renal failure, crush injuries, burns, blood transfusions, and iatrogenic potassium containing infusions, and secondary to some medication use. Potassium is critical to the electric physiology of the heart, and hyperkalemia can result in ventricular fibrillation and cardiac arrest. EKG findings include peaked T waves, prolongation of the PR interval, and widening of the QRS complex. Levels exceeding 6.5 mmol/L are considered critical and should be immediately addressed. Immediate treatment includes cardiac stabilization by administration of IV calcium gluconate.**

B. Metoprolol is a β-antagonist and causes potassium to leave the cells and enter circulation, thereby causing hyperkalemia.

C, E. Following administration of IV calcium gluconate, you must take action to reduce the serum concentration of potassium. These steps include shifting potassium into the cells with infusion of insulin and glucose or administration of an albuterol nebulizer, diuresis of potassium with furosemide, and binding of potassium in the intestinal tract with sodium polystyrene (Kayexalate), resulting in excretion.

D. Dialysis can be used if the measures described in the explanation for C and E are ineffective or contraindicated.

160. **C. Idiopathic thrombocytopenic purpura (ITP) is an immune condition involving antiplatelet antibodies that is most commonly seen in children younger than the age of 6 years and in women in their thirties. In children, ITP is typically self-limiting, and strict bedrest with avoidance of contact sports is recommended. The spleen is the source of the IgG specific for platelets and the site of the phagocytosis of the coated platelets. Signs and symptoms of ITP include bleeding following minor trauma, easy bruising, mucosal bleeding, and petechiae. In adults, the initial treatment includes prednisone 1 mg/kg/day, but only 25% of patients sustain their platelet levels after steroid treatment alone. In those who do not achieve a sustained response to steroid therapy, IVIG is also given. When a patient fails to respond to these medical therapies, a splenectomy is indicated. Splenectomy is successful in 85% of cases. If ITP recurs after splenectomy, it may be due to the presence of an accessory spleen. Using a technetium-99 colloid scan or infusion of indium-111–labeled platelets, accessory spleens can be localized.**

A. Outpatient follow-up for a patient with severe thrombocytopenia is inappropriate and risks life-threatening complications such as spontaneous intracranial bleeding.
B. Prednisone therapy is an option but 6 months of unmonitored therapy is not indicated.
D. A radiolabeled study is used to localize remaining splenic tissue (accessory spleens) following splenectomy. It is not indicated prior to splenectomy.
E. The spleen will continue to make antibodies to platelets, and the transfused platelets will eventually be destroyed.

161. **C. Pain out of proportion to findings on physical exam is always concerning for mesenteric ischemia. Acute mesenteric ischemia can be caused by arterial thrombosis or embolus, venous occlusion, or "low flow" nonocclusive mesenteric ischemia. This patient is at higher risk for embolic disease due to his history of atrial fibrillation without adequate anticoagulation.**

A. Gastritis may be painless or may be associated with less severe pain, which is typically localized in the epigastric—not periumbilical—area.
B. A patient with a ruptured abdominal aortic aneurysm is likely to be in hemorrhagic shock and have severe abdominal pain radiating to the back or groin and possibly a pulsatile abdominal mass.
D. Ulcerative colitis typically presents with crampy abdominal pain and bloody stools with a past history of the same, as well as diarrhea.
E. A gastric tumor typically presents with prolonged history of weight loss and vague upper abdominal discomfort.

162. **B. In addition to the classic findings on a physical exam, patients with mesenteric ischemia often present with leukocytosis and metabolic acidosis (lactic acidosis). This acute condition is associated with a high mortality rate, and prompt diagnosis and treatment are imperative.**

A. As a later sign of ischemic bowel, patients may develop gastrointestinal bleeding with a decrease in hematocrit, but only as a late finding, not as a presenting symptom.
C. Metabolic alkalosis may be due to overaggressive diuresis, persistent emesis, exogenous bicarbonate loading, or a so-called contraction alkalosis. None of these findings would be expected with ischemic bowel.
D. The sodium level is not usually directly affected by ischemic bowel.
E. Decreased albumin is seen in states of chronic malnutrition, not acutely in ischemic bowel.

163. **D. Visceral angiography is used to definitively confirm the diagnosis. Papaverine may be injected at the time of angiography to promote vasodilation.**

A. Ultrasound of the right upper quadrant is used to evaluate biliary tract disease, not bowel ischemia.
B. Colonoscopy may show areas of ischemia but it is not indicated in the acute setting of bowel ischemia.
C. Enteroclysis would likely be abnormal but the test is too nonspecific and time-consuming to be helpful.
E. Upper endoscopy would likely be normal and therefore unhelpful in this acute setting.

164. **C. This patient's condition is consistent with acute calculus cholecystitis. Cholecystitis is characterized by fever, leukocytosis, right upper quadrant tenderness, and pain. The multiple risk factors for developing gallstones include female gender, obesity, age 30 to 40 years old, and multiparity.**

A. Symptomatic cholelithiasis presents with right upper quadrant pain, usually postprandially, which may be associated with nausea and vomiting. This presentation differs from that of cholecystitis, as there is typically no fever or elevated WBC count—both indicators of inflammation.
B. Acalculous cholecystitis is not associated with gallstones. This condition is commonly seen in ICU patients or in cases where patients are NPO for acute illness.
D. Ascending cholangitis is a serious infectious process of the entire biliary tree in which bacteria (*E. coli, Klebsiella, Pseudomonas, and Enterococcus*) enter the bloodstream secondary to biliary obstruction. The condition is marked by fever, jaundice, and right upper

quadrant pain (Charcot's triad). The addition of hypotension and mental status changes in the later stages is known as Reynolds' pentad.

E. Biliary dyskinesia is the inability of the gallbladder to empty in a normal fashion due to uncoordinated contraction of the gallbladder wall. It is not associated with a fever and elevated WBC count.

165. **B. The test of choice to document acute cholecystitis is a HIDA scan. In the presence of a stone obstructing the cystic duct, the labeled, intravenously administered iminodiacetic acid cannot pass into the gallbladder. The usual work-up begins with an ultrasound to document stones. When stones are not seen, a HIDA scan is the next test of choice. A normal HIDA scan shows the gallbladder as having prompt drainage into the duodenum.**

A. An abdominal CT scan is not helpful in documenting gallbladder function.
C. The oral cholecystogram is a test of historical interest, often unavailable today.
D. A PTHC is an invasive test to evaluate possible biliary obstruction.
E. An ERCP is an invasive procedure used to evaluate the common bile duct.

166. **B. This patient has an incarcerated inguinal hernia. When a hernia is not able to be reduced into the abdomen, it is considered incarcerated. When blood flow is compromised, it is considered strangulated.**

A. A direct inguinal hernia passes medial to the inferior epigastric vessels and through Hesselbach's triangle. This patient could have a direct hernia or indirect inguinal hernia, both of which could become incarcerated.
C. This scenario is unlikely to involve a strangulated inguinal hernia, because these patients usually present with a fever or elevated WBC count and diffuse abdominal pain. A strangulated hernia cannot be completely excluded from the list of possibilities, however, due to the short time frame of incarceration and the lack of systemic symptoms.
D. A torsed testicle is very painful, but this patient is not experiencing such discomfort.
E. A hiatal hernia occurs through the hiatus of the diaphragm, and is not seen in the groin.

167. **E. The operation of choice is exploration with reduction and repair of the hernia. Operative options include the Marcy, Bassini, Shouldice, and McVay repairs, as well as tension-free mesh repairs such as the Lichtenstein repair. Complications to surgical repair include recurrence, hematomas, hydroceles, paresthesias, chronic pain, seromas, and testicular ischemia.**

A. Reducing the hernia is part of the procedure, but repairing the defect is important to prevent recurrence.
B. A midline incision is inappropriate for a groin hernia unless compromised or dead bowel is suspected.
C. Orchiopexy is the wrong procedure, because the testicle is not involved in this case.
D. Reducing the hernia is part of the procedure, but the defect still needs to be repaired and the hernia contents inspected to ensure viability.

168. **D. Hesselbach's triangle is formed by the inguinal ligament inferiorly, the rectus sheath medially, and the inferior epigastric vessels laterally and superiorly. A direct hernia protrudes through the triangle, medial to the epigastric vessels. An indirect hernia protrudes through the internal ring and lateral to the epigastric vessels following the path of the cord.**

A, B. These are incorrect locations.
C, E. These are incorrect locations, as this case involves a direct inguinal hernia.

169. **D. In an older woman with a recent history of diverticulitis, the most likely etiology of such a lesion is a pyogenic (bacterial) hepatic abscess. These abscesses typically arise secondary to (1) portal vein bacteremia from diverticulitis or appendicitis, (2) biliary obstruction and cholangitis, (3) hepatic artery bacteremia from endocarditis, (4) direct extension from gangrenous cholecystitis of subhepatic abscess, (5) superinfection from a necrosing malignancy, or (6) necrosis after hepatic trauma and secondary to seeding of the hematoma.**

A, E. While PID and urologic infections may present with similar symptoms, they are not associated with bacterial hepatic abscesses.
B, C. Sigmoid volvulus and irritable bowel syndrome are not associated with bacterial hepatic abscess.

170. D. Left untreated, a pyogenic liver abscess is uniformly fatal. Initial therapy consists of broad-spectrum IV antibiotics and CT-guided percutaneous drainage. This approach is successful approximately 80% of the time.

A. Broad-spectrum IV antibiotics alone have been used successfully in some patients, but results vary widely, and this is not the standard of care. Antibiotics alone might be used for a patient with multiple, widely distributed, small abscesses.
B. Drainage of the hepatic abscess—not hepatic resection—is needed.
C. Indications for surgical drainage would include the necessity for laparotomy for the underlying disorder, such as diverticular abscess, as well as failure to drain the abscess percutaneously.
E. Oral antibiotics with follow-up would be inadequate treatment for this seriously ill patient.

171. D. This patient has a pulsatile abdominal mass and is hemodynamically unstable. He should be considered as having a ruptured aneurysm until proven otherwise. In this emergency situation, the first step is to obtain a secure airway, then address breathing issues, and finally monitor circulation. This patient should be intubated immediately.

A. An abdominal ultrasound is a good method to follow the size of an aneurysm, but it should not be used in the emergent management of an unstable patient.
B. A CT scan of the abdomen would be helpful to confirm the diagnosis of an abdominal aortic aneurysm, but obtaining it before stabilizing the patient is not appropriate.
C, E. Ideally, while you are intubating the patient, someone else is achieving IV access, either with large-bore peripheral IVs or a large central line, such as a cordis. Establishing a secure airway is the first priority.

172. C. Indications for elective repair of an abdominal aortic aneurysm include a diameter greater than 5 to 5.5 cm or growth in diameter of greater than 5 mm over a 1-year period.

A. While it makes the repair more difficult, extension above the renal arteries alone is not an indication to repair the aneurysm.
B. Extension into the iliac arteries is not an indication for surgery. This problem is commonly encountered and is fixed at the time of repair, but by itself it is not an indication to operate.
D. The aneurysm must grow more than 5 mm in a 1-year period to warrant elective repair.
E. This is a false statement in this scenario.

173. B. In all traumas, the ABCs (airway, breathing, and circulation) are the medical practitioner's first priority. In an alert patient, the airway can be assessed by asking the patient to speak and obtaining an appropriate response. In patients who are difficult to rouse, control of the airway is mandatory.

A. Although an exploratory laparotomy may eventually be necessary, the most important initial treatment is to address control of this patient's airway.
C. A chest x-ray will be required, but not before addressing the ABCs of resuscitation and trauma.
D. Infusion of crystalloid should be addressed as soon as possible, but not before a secure and patent airway is obtained.
E. A tube thoracostomy may be indicated on the right side, but securing the airway is the priority.

174. E. A large hemo-pneumothorax should be suspected due to the patient's continuing unstable vital signs and decreased breath sounds. This condition is easily treated in the emergency department by tube thoracostomy. An initial output of 1500 mL or 200 mL per hour for 4 hours of sanguinous fluid demands an emergent thoracotomy. The initial chest x-ray (see Figure 5-174A) shows a large hemo-pneumothorax with air fluid levels. Figure 5-174B shows resolution after proper placement of a tube thoracostomy.

A. Currently, the most important problem this patient faces is the inability to ventilate. Taking the patient to the OR for a laparotomy is not yet indicated in this scenario.
B. The patient should already have been intubated.
C. The patient should be treated based on the physical signs. Treating the hemo-pneumothorax should improve ventilation. Chemical paralysis may merely mask an underlying

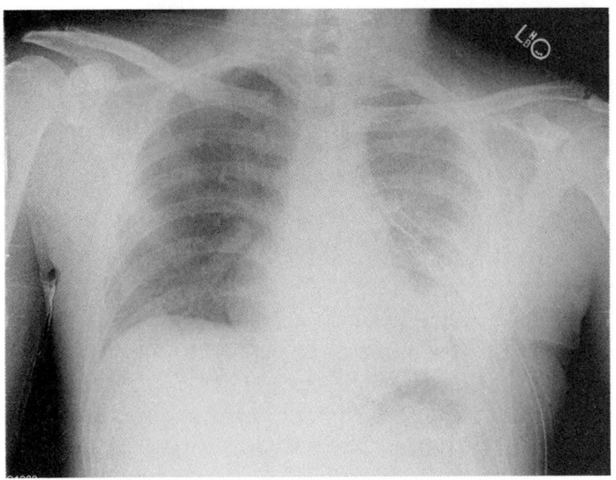

B

Figure 5-174B • Image Courtesy of the University of Utah School of Medicine, Salt Lake City, Utah.

situation and should be used after completing the primary and secondary trauma surveys.

D. Crystalloid infusion is a reasonable choice, but it will not correct the hemo-pneumothorax.

175. **A. Because the airway and breathing are controlled and the patient remains in shock, the hypotension is likely due to intra-abdominal hemorrhage. The patient has not responded to an adequate trial of crystalloid infusion and blood products. To treat the patient's ongoing shock, it is imperative to take the patient to the operating room for an exploratory laparotomy.**

B. The patient in this scenario should already be intubated.

C. The patient is hemodynamically unstable and should go to the operating room rather than to radiology. In situations where abdominal injury is suspected in a trauma victim with very stable vital signs, this might be the correct answer.

D. The patient has already failed infusion of 4 liters of crystalloid as well as 4 units of blood products, without improvement of vital signs.

E. A chest tube should have already been placed for the hemo-pneumothorax.

176. **B. Abdominal evaluation for injury—in particular, for blunt injury—is part of the secondary trauma survey. The secondary survey follows the primary survey and resuscitation and involves a head-to-toe systemic assessment of the patient. It may include blood and radiologic testing as well as reassessment of the primary survey.**

A. Exposure is part of the primary survey and includes completely removing all clothing and jewelry, as well as keeping the patient warm with blankets.

C. Ensuring adequate tissue circulation can be assessed through the palpation of pulses and is part of the primary survey. Once blood pressure and heart rate are assessed, resuscitation can proceed if indicated.

D. Disability is a component of the primary survey and is assessed by determining mental status, looking at the equality and reactiveness of the pupils, and performing a gross motor and sensory exam.

E. Airway is the first component of the primary survey, termed the ABCs (airway, breathing, circulation) in trauma management.

177. **C. The chest x-ray demonstrated several nonspecific findings suggestive of an aortic injury, including widened mediastinum, apical pleural capping, loss of aortic knob, and depression of left main stem bronchus (note the arrows in Figure 5-177B). Traumatic aortic disruption is a highly morbid injury, with more than 85% of patients dying at the scene of the accident. In addition, there is a 50% in-hospital mortality rate for every 24 hours this injury goes undiagnosed. For these reasons, it is absolutely critical to have a high index of suspicion in trauma patients. The gold standard for diagnosing aortic injury remains angiography. The injury usually occurs just proximal to the left subclavian take-off. Treatment consists of surgical placement of an aortic interposition graft. (Note the arrows in Figures 5-177C and 5-177D.) Transesophageal echocardiogram (TEE) is rapidly becoming a useful adjunct in the rapid diagnosis of this type of injury. Because it is relatively noninvasive, it should be considered in blunt chest trauma cases. Intensive care practitioners, anesthesiologists, and cardiologists are the most likely disciplines to be trained in the use of this diagnostic method.**

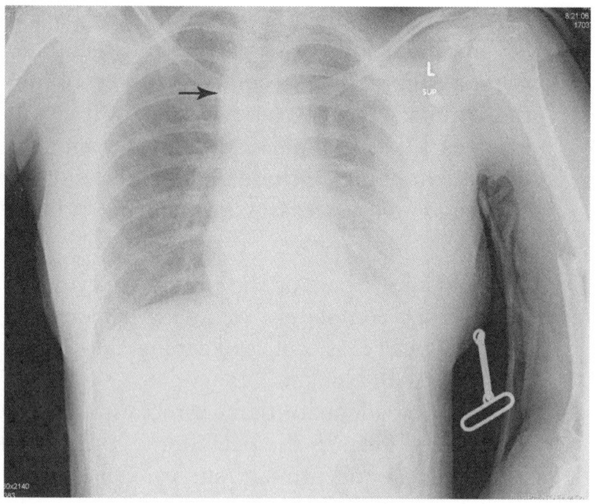

B

Figure 5-177B • Image Courtesy of the University of Utah School of Medicine, Salt Lake City, Utah.

A. A plain film would give only the nonspecific findings mentioned in the explanation for C.
B. A routine chest CT scan is not specific enough to define this injury, although the CT angiogram is gaining acceptance for screening this injury (note the arrow in Figure 5-177E).

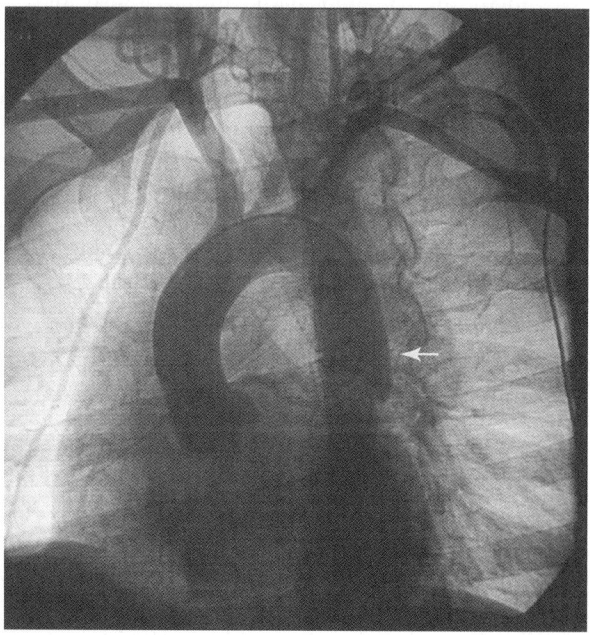

C

Figure 5-177C • Image Courtesy of the University of Utah School of Medicine, Salt Lake City, Utah.

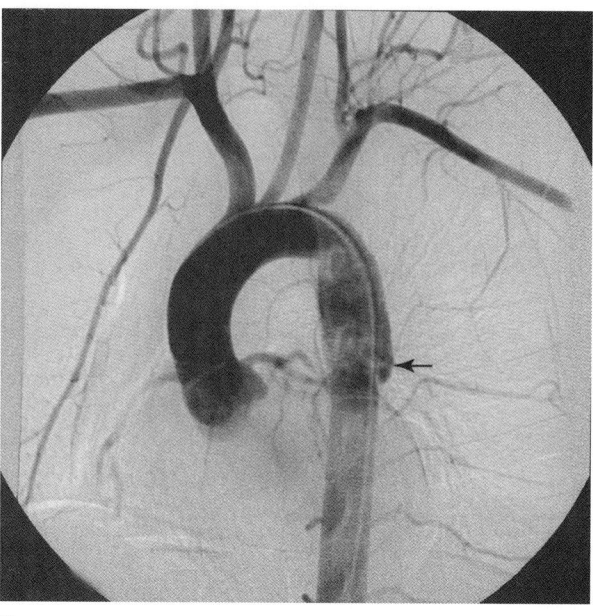

D

Figure 5-177D • Image Courtesy of the University of Utah School of Medicine, Salt Lake City, Utah.

Nevertheless, the aortogram remains the gold standard for diagnosis.

D. A mediastinoscopy is not indicated for assessing an intrathoracic injury, even in a stable trauma patient.
E. Video-assisted thoracoscopic surgery is not indicated in a trauma patient to evaluate a possible aortic disruption.

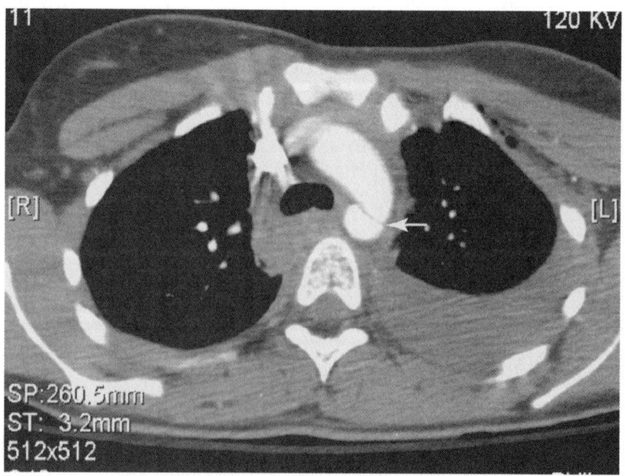

E

Figure 5-177E • Image Courtesy of the University of Utah School of Medicine, Salt Lake City, Utah..

178. E. An open book fracture of the pelvis is common in trauma and is associated with disruption of the vertebral venous plexus along the sacrum. This type of fracture can lead to a large amount of retroperitoneal bleeding, requiring blood transfusions and aggressive resuscitation. In this orthopedic emergency, the patient should be stabilized as soon as possible to prevent massive blood loss and third spacing. An easy way to accomplish this goal is application of mast trousers until arrival at the trauma center. Once the patient is at the hospital, an external fixation device should be placed to reduce the fracture and help minimize retroperitoneal bleeding.

A. This patient has blood found at the external meatus, which is an indication of urethral injury. A retrograde urethrogram should be obtained prior to placement of a Foley catheter.

B. Following the ABCs of trauma is of utmost priority, and this care should be delivered first before obtaining any imaging modality.

C. Rectal injuries can occur with traumatic pelvic fractures. Proctoscopy or flexible sigmoidoscopy can be used to help diagnose the location of the lesion, although this is not the most appropriate treatment option at this time.

D. Extraperitoneal injuries to the bladder are associated with pelvic fractures, especially when the superior and inferior pubic rami are involved. This type of injury is treated nonsurgically with placement of a Foley catheter for a prolonged period of time.

179. B. The vertebral artery courses through the transverse foramina of the second through sixth cervical vertebrae. Any fracture through the transverse foramen at this level may cause a disruption or dissection of the vertebral artery. This type of fracture warrants a CT angiogram or invasive angiogram of the vertebral artery to verify patency.

A, C, D, E. The deep cervical, ascending cervical, common carotid, and internal carotid arteries do not flow through the cervical transverse foramina.

180. C. Survival after ruptured AAA is dependent on rapid diagnosis and immediate surgical exploration for repair. A ruptured AAA carries a 90% overall mortality rate, which can be reduced to 50% for patients who reach a hospital that is capable of providing appropriate care via immediate exploration and repair. Figure 5-180 is an abdominal CT showing a rim of calcium at the borders of the AAA and surrounding retroperitoneal hematoma from rupture (note the arrow).

A. While fluid resuscitation for hypovolemic shock is needed, once the diagnosis of AAA rupture is made, surgical exploration and repair should not be delayed for attempts at stabilization.

B. An acute AAA rupture, as described in this case, usually consists of a rupture with the surrounding hematoma contained within the retroperitoneum. Paracentesis in an effort to find evidence of rupture would therefore be fruitless and needlessly delay the proper surgical treatment.

D. The CT scan is an excellent diagnostic tool for evaluating patients suspected of having an AAA. However, in the setting of suspected ruptured AAA, obtaining a CT scan would merely delay the move to immediate surgical care.

E. While abdominal angiography is a test for work-up of some aortic aneurysms, it should not be used to confirm a ruptured AAA. Time wasted in obtaining the study could potentially be lethal due to delay in definitive surgical care.

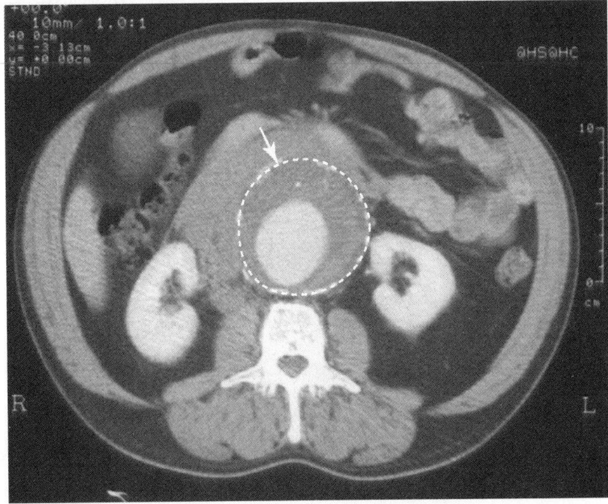

Figure 5-180 • Image Courtesy of the University of Utah School of Medicine, Salt Lake Ci0ty, Utah.

181. **D. This critically ill young boy may be bleeding to death from his numerous injuries. Despite the severity of his injuries and the fact that he appears to be oxygenating well, the first step is to establish a secure airway. In a trauma situation, airway, breathing, and circulation take priority, and should be addressed in that order. Controlling the bleeding and giving red blood cells (RBCs) and fresh frozen plasma (FFP) are secondary to obtaining a secure airway.**

A, C, E. These steps are all important measures and need to be performed expediently, but only after the airway is secure.

B. A tourniquet is not used in the trauma situation. Direct pressure to the bleeding vessels is required.

182. **E. Figure 5-182B is a single image of the pelvis that shows a thickened bowel wall, consistent with prolonged hypotension, as well as a large gluteal hematoma (note the arrows). Adjacent to the hematoma is a blush indicating ongoing bleeding, which would be consistent with an arterial injury.**

A. There is no evidence of free air indicating bowel perforation. Often in a trauma situation, bowel perforations are late findings that present 12 to 24 hours after the injury.

B. The spleen is not seen, and a diagnosis of splenic laceration cannot be made based on this scan.

C, D. There is no evidence of either intraperitoneal or extraperitoneal bladder rupture on this film.

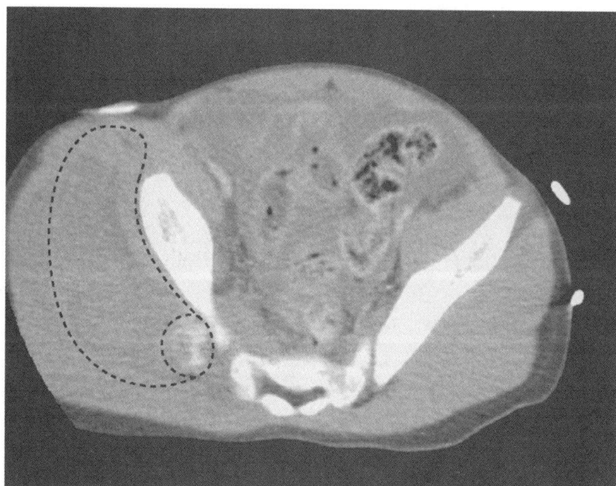

B

Figure 5-182B • Image Courtesy of the University of Utah School of Medicine, Salt Lake City, Utah.

183. **C. With ongoing bleeding from an arterial source in a patient who is hypotensive, arterial embolization is indicated. Pelvic bleeding is difficult to control operatively; thus angiography is a valuable option. Patients may bleed from fractures, the sacral venous plexus, the major venous vessels, or arterial sources. Venous bleeding can often be controlled with external fixation, while embolization is a better option with arterial bleeds.**

A. A bowel resection would not be indicated as this patient has not suffered a bowel injury.

B. A splenectomy is not indicated, as no splenic injury is seen (see Figure 182B).

D. Suprapubic catheter placement is not an option, as no bladder injury or rupture is noted.

E. Observation of a hemodynamically unstable patient is never a correct answer.

184. **D. This critically ill patient is in shock and has obvious serious injuries. In any trauma situation, one always begins with the basics: airway, breathing, and circulation. Because this patient is critically injured, it is vital to secure the airway. Despite the fact that she is already intubated, it is important to confirm the placement of the endotracheal tube, which is evident by the poor oxygen saturation level. Often it is easier to reintubate the patient to guarantee that the endotracheal tube is in the correct position. This measure should be taken before moving to the next step.**

A. While this patient's hypotension is very concerning and needs to be promptly addressed, you still start by securing the airway before addressing the other issues. Often, these tasks are being accomplished simultaneously; if not, always follow the ABCs.

B. If tension pneumothorax is suspected, a needle thoracostomy may be indicated. The first step, however, is always to make sure the airway is secure.

C. A chest x-ray is important to evaluate for chest injuries but securing the airway takes precedence.

E. Placing a central line falls under circulation, which is secondary to establishing an airway.

185. D. In a patient who is hypotensive, is hypoxic, and has tracheal deviation, tension pneumothorax is the diagnosis until proven otherwise. This life-threatening condition must be addressed immediately. If a tube thoracostomy is not immediately available, you might start by needling the chest to relieve the tension pneumothorax, followed by placement of a chest tube.

A, B. Tracheal and esophageal injuries are much less common in the acute, blunt trauma setting. Nevertheless, they should be kept in mind during the trauma work-up.

C. An open pneumothorax is a life-threatening injury but it does not cause tracheal deviation.

E. Flail chest occurs when a segment of chest wall does not have continuity with the rest of the thoracic cage, due to multiple rib fractures. A free-floating segment of ribs moves inward on inspiration, while the rest of the chest moves outward, referred to as paradoxical respiration. Tracheal deviation is not a usual sign of this type of injury.

186. C. The chest x-ray (see Figure 5-186A) clearly demonstrates a nasogastric tube that is in the stomach and located above the normal level of the diaphragm. This finding is consistent with a diaphragmatic rupture. Figure 5-186B is a CT scan that shows the stomach in the left chest, which is also consistent with a diaphragmatic rupture. Diaphragmatic rupture is a severe injury, and one that is seen most often with blunt trauma. The diagnosis is usually and easily made with a chest x-ray, with the bowel seen within the chest. The left hemidiaphragm is injured more often, as the liver is thought to offer some protection to the right hemidiaphragm.

A. Pulmonary laceration is difficult to diagnose via chest x-ray alone. It would present with lung density due to parenchymal bleeding.

B. Aortic dissection would show a widened mediastinum on chest x-ray in a hemodynamically labile patient.

D. A gastric perforation should show free air on chest x-ray.

E. A cardiac contusion would not be seen on chest x-ray.

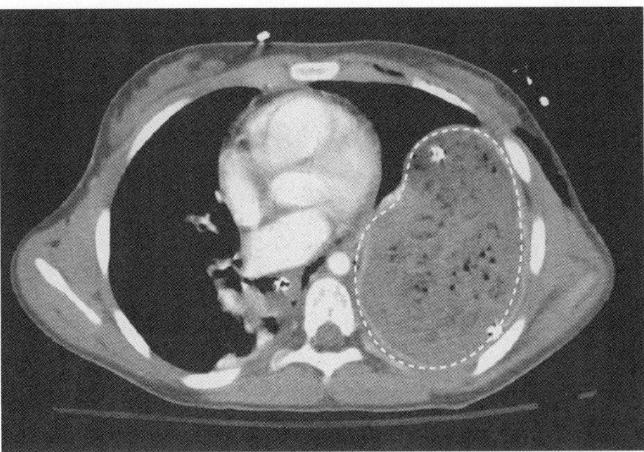

B

Figure 5-186B • Image Courtesy of the University of Utah School of Medicine, Salt Lake City, Utah.

187. B. Injury or disruption of the spinal cord at the cervical or high thoracic level can result in the loss of autonomic innervation. The severity of complications from spinal cord injury can be significantly decreased by limiting the swelling around the cord. Steroids are known to improve the outcome if they are given within 8 hours of injury. There is no proven benefit to giving steroids after that time frame.

A. Cefazolin is a first-generation cephalosporin that provides good antibiotic coverage for skin flora. Although the patient should receive an appropriate antibiotic, it is not the most important medication at this time.

C, D. This patient is hypotensive due to decreased vascular tone from the spinal cord injury. Initially, the patient needs fluids to help maintain blood pressure. Vasoactive agents are not needed at this time.

E. Morphine sulfate is a narcotic that is commonly prescribed for trauma patients. This patient is not having any sensation due to the spinal cord injury and is not in need of pain medication. She is also hypotensive, and narcotics typically decrease blood pressure, which at this point may further complicate the picture.

188. C. The CT scan is becoming an important tool in diagnosing acute appendicitis, especially in young females and in patients with atypical symptoms. This patient is a good candidate for CT scan because the management of her case would likely change depending on the

radiographic findings. An appendix with a diameter greater than 6 mm, with thickened walls and periappendiceal fat stranding, is diagnostic for appendicitis.

A. This patient has a history and exam that are consistent with acute appendicitis. However, women of reproductive age pose a diagnostic dilemma when it comes to lower abdominal pain. Ectopic pregnancy, ovarian torsion, pelvic inflammatory disease, tubo-ovarian abscess, and ruptured ovarian cysts should all be included in the differential diagnosis. A CT scan of the abdomen would be the next step in this scenario rather than surgical exploration.

B. Abdominal ultrasound is especially helpful to diagnose lower abdominal pain in women of reproductive age, looking for ovarian pathology. Ultrasound is user dependent and not as reliable as a CT scan, however.

D. Although IV hydration is required, the appendicitis will not get better with fluids alone. Instead, this condition requires an operation before perforation of the appendix occurs. Observation is not an appropriate choice in this scenario.

E. Acute appendicitis is a surgical emergency, for which giving oral antibiotics with a 2-day follow-up is entirely inappropriate.

189. **D. All of the choices listed are causes of appendiceal lumen obstruction that cause appendicitis, with the proper order of incidence being lymphoid hyperplasia, fecalith, and tumor. Sixty percent of cases are caused by lymphoid hyperplasia, with peak incidence occurring in the teenage years. The hyperplasia leads to venous obstruction, followed by arterial insufficiency and ischemic necrosis of the appendix, which causes the pain to become localized to the right lower quadrant. Fecaliths are identified in 20% to 30% of appendicitis cases and are more commonly seen in adults. They can sometimes be identified in the right lower quadrant on abdominal plain films or on CT scans, and they need to be removed with the appendix at the time of surgery. The most common appendiceal tumor is a carcinoid. These uncommon tumors are usually located in the tip of the appendix and are unlikely to cause acute appendicitis.**

A. Foreign bodies, such as seeds, can result in luminal obstruction leading to appendicitis. This is rare, however.

B, C, E. These options are all causes of appendiceal lumen obstruction, but are not arranged in the correct order of frequency.

190. **B. The most common tumor of the appendix is a carcinoid tumor. Benign tumors, including carcinoids, are found in fewer than 5% of appendix specimens examined microscopically. They are most commonly found incidentally at the time of an appendectomy being performed for acute appendicitis. Tumors smaller than 2 cm in the tip of the appendix are unlikely to metastasize. Most authors recommend appendectomy for tumors less than 2 cm. Appendectomy alone is adequate treatment unless lymph nodes are visibly involved, the tumor is larger than 2 cm in diameter, mucinous elements are present in the tumor (adenocarcinoid), or the mesoappendix or base of the cecum is invaded.**

A. No staging is required due to the low probability of metastatic disease.

C, E. Radiation therapy and chemotherapy have no role in the treatment of localized carcinoid tumors.

D. For tumors larger than 2 cm or with more aggressive lesions, the patient should undergo a right hemicolectomy.

191. **B. A pelvic ultrasound is a safe, accurate, and useful technique in pregnant patients suspected of having an ectopic pregnancy. This procedure can identify an intrauterine pregnancy with considerable accuracy, effectively ruling out ectopic pregnancy. It should be the first imaging study performed.**

A. Although a CT scan may ultimately be needed, it is not the test of choice in a female with an early pregnancy because of the risks associated with radiation exposure.

C. An abdominal series is a nonspecific test that would not be helpful in ruling out an ectopic pregnancy and would expose an early pregnancy to unnecessary radiation.

D. Culdocentesis is a diagnostic procedure that was more commonly used prior to the advent of ultrasonography. It entails placing an 18-gauge needle in the cul-de-sac of Douglas and aspirating the contents. A negative culdocentesis cannot definitively confirm or rule out an ectopic pregnancy.

E. A diagnostic laparoscopy is a reasonable option, but only in cases in which other non-invasive modalities are unable to confirm a diagnosis.

192. **E. Ectopic pregnancy should be high on the differential diagnosis of a woman of reproductive age with abdominal pain. Its incidence has increased over the past few years secondary to an increase in the incidence of pelvic inflammatory disease (PID). An ectopic pregnancy usually occurs after implantation of the embryo in the fallopian tube; this tube is not suited to accommodating the conceptus. The growing conceptus will eventually erode into blood vessels or cause the fallopian tube to rupture. Delay in diagnosis can lead to catastrophic bleeding and maternal death. Patients usually present with abdominal pain, amenorrhea, and vaginal bleeding. The diagnosis is made by obtaining a β-hCG level and a pelvic ultrasound. Traditional treatment has consisted of surgical removal, although some ectopic gestations may be treated with methotrexate.**

A. Acute appendicitis should always be on the differential diagnosis list at this point. The clinical presentation in this case and the positive pregnancy test warrant investigation of an ectopic pregnancy, however. Pelvic ultrasound usually reveals a noncompressible, fluid-filled tubular structure in the right lower quadrant with a diameter greater than 6 mm.

B. Acute diverticulitis is more common in older patients. It would be extremely unlikely in such a young female.

C. A ruptured ovarian cyst should be high on the differential diagnosis list in a woman of reproductive age. A CT scan can be helpful for distinguishing the etiology of the pain. A ruptured cyst would most likely demonstrate free pelvic fluid without an adnexal mass.

D. Tubo-ovarian abscesses develop in approximately 15% of women with PID and can often mimic appendicitis. Risk factors for developing PID include multiple sexual partners, previous PID, and use of an intrauterine device for birth control. Treatment of an abscess would include surgical drainage and IV antibiotics. Complications of infertility may occur from severe scarring caused by PID, and affected women have an increased risk for ectopic pregnancy.

193. **A. Transection of the cerebral veins as they enter the superior sagittal sinus is the most common cause of a traumatic subdural hematoma. Blood collects below the dura and above the subarachnoid membranes. Initially, the bleeding is not enough to cause noticeable symptoms. As the hematoma increases in size, however, the underlying brain becomes compressed, causing symptoms of increased intracranial pressure. The CT in Figure 5-193B (note marked area) shows a concave-shaped hematoma on the right, which is displacing the brain to the left.**

B. Epidural hematomas are usually the result of blunt trauma to the head leading to arterial bleeding from the middle meningeal artery. They are often associated with a temporal skull fractures. The patient typically experiences a brief loss of consciousness, which is followed by several hours of lucid behavior, and then by a rapid decline in consciousness.

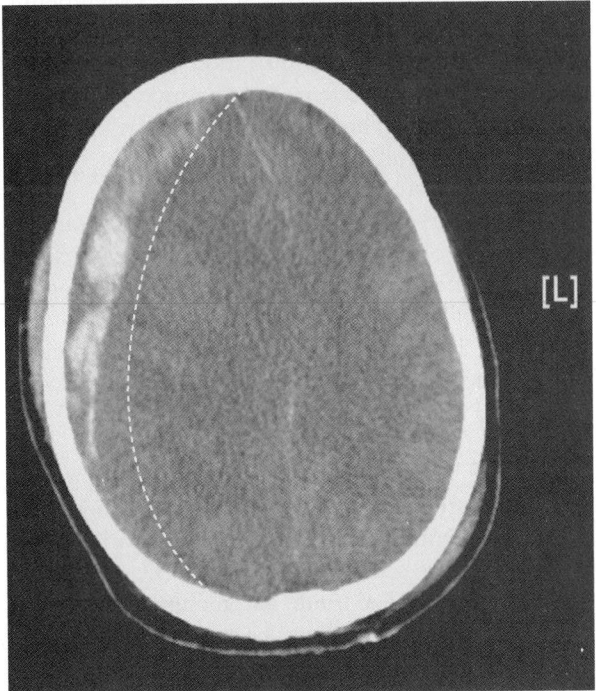

Figure 5-193B • Image Courtesy of the University of Utah School of Medicine, Salt Lake City, Utah.

Diagnosis is made by CT scan of the head, demonstrating a convex-shaped hematoma with or without mass effect.

C. A subarachnoid hemorrhage usually occurs due to rupture of a cerebral aneurysm.

D. Intraparenchymal hemorrhage presents with blood within the brain parenchyma. The CT scan shown here is not consistent with an intraparenchymal bleed.

E. Axonal shear injury occurs with angular acceleration–deceleration injuries. Shearing of deep white matter tracts leaves the patient with a very low GCS and poor prognostic outcome. An MRI is the most useful radiographic modality to delineate areas of shear injury.

194. **A. Although the majority of patients with a small subdural hematoma can be observed, any alteration in consciousness or the neurological function of the patient requires emergent surgical evacuation of the hematoma.**

B. Angiographic embolization will not fix the mass effect of the hematoma, and embolizing the cerebral vessels is very unlikely.

C. Ventriculostomy is performed to monitor intracranial pressures. It is not a therapeutic maneuver.

D. IV mannitol administration and hyperventilation are used to help reduce intracranial pressure. These measures can be initiated, but definitive treatment consists of evacuation of the hematoma.

E. Observation, with serial neurologic exams, is appropriate in individuals with small hematomas and minimal neurological deficits. These patients should be observed in a critical care setting with frequent neurological examinations and immediate access to drainage if required.

195. **B. In evaluation of abdominal trauma, the retroperitoneum is divided into three zones. Zone I (the central zone) contains the majority of the vasculature within the abdomen (i.e., the aorta, vena cava, celiac trunk, and mesenteric arteries). This zone should always be explored in both penetrating and blunt trauma. Zone II (the lateral zone) lies on either side of Zone I. The kidneys and their vasculature are found within this area. Exploration should be undertaken in penetrating trauma, or in blunt trauma with a pulsatile expanding hematoma. Zone III consists of the pelvic retroperitoneum; the iliac vessels and the hypogastric plexus are found here. This is a difficult area to explore, and obtaining hemostatic control is challenging. Mandatory exploration should occur in penetrating trauma cases. In cases involving blunt trauma, exploration should be undertaken if the hematoma is expanding or is pulsatile. Otherwise, no exploration is the best management choice.**

A, C. See the explanation for B.

D, E. There are only three zones of the retroperitoneum.

196. **C. Exploration of the hematoma—but only if it is expanding or is very large—is the correct choice. Although most lateral retroperitoneal hematomas are small and nonexpanding and, therefore, do not require exploration, large, expanding, or pulsatile hematomas around the kidney require this step to control bleeding.**

A. To close the abdomen and obtain a CT scan is a reasonable option if the hematoma is small and not expanding.

B. It would be technically difficult, if not impossible, to obtain an intraoperative angiogram that accesses the renal blood flow and offers the detail needed to evaluate a renal vascular injury.

D. Removing the involved kidney may be needed for major vascular injuries. In the majority of cases, blunt renal trauma is contained by Gerota's fascia. When this condition is conservatively treated with observation, patients have a reasonable rate of healing with normal renal function.

E. Opening the hematoma regardless of size or position is incorrect. Lateral retroperitoneal injuries (Zone II) and pelvic hematomas (Zone III) do not routinely require exploration, unlike upper central retroperitoneal hematomas (Zone I), which should be explored because of the high rate of associated vascular and pancreatic injuries.

197. **B. Acute lower gastrointestinal (GI) hemorrhage is defined as continuous bleeding from the rectum, with or without hemodynamic instability. Aggressive fluid resuscitation should be initiated in an ICU setting during work-up of the etiology. A nasogastric tube should be**

inserted and aspirated to eliminate the possibility of a massive upper GI bleed. Endoscopy, including colonoscopy and esophagogastroduodenoscopy, is a critical step in the management of a lower GI bleed. Cauterization can be therapeutic if the site of active bleeding is identified. Colonoscopy is successful in localizing the bleeding site(s) in 50% to 90% of cases, according to clinical trials.

A. Exploratory laparotomy may be required in an unstable patient or after unsuccessful endoscopy. If the source of bleeding is not localized, a total colectomy may be the only option.

C. Tagged RBC scans may be obtained to localize the bleeding following a negative endoscopy in a stable patient. Unfortunately, localization with this procedure is not entirely dependable. If the scan is positive, the patient should proceed to angiography for further delineation and treatment.

D. A CT scan would yield little information in an acute intestinal bleeding scenario.

E. Angiography may be used to localize the bleeding vessel and treat it with embolization. This technique is best employed following localization with a tagged RBC scan.

198. **E. Given that the patient is not currently experiencing any hemodynamic compromise and does not require transfusions for his hematocrit, there is no urgency for surgery. Approximately 80% to 90% of lower GI bleeds will stop spontaneously, making close observation the appropriate next step.**

A, B, C. Given that the patient is hemodynamically stable and does not require transfusions, there is no need for urgent surgery.

D. Repeating the colonoscopy at this time is not necessary, as the patient is clinically doing well. If the bleeding became more brisk and intervention became necessary, repeating the colonoscopy would be the next logical step.

199. **C. Figure 5-199B shows a calcified gallbladder (see the arrows). Also known as a porcelain gallbladder, it is usually discovered incidentally radiographically, on physical exam, or during surgery for another condition. It is thought to develop secondary to recurrent inflammation from gallstones, although most patients remain asymptomatic.**

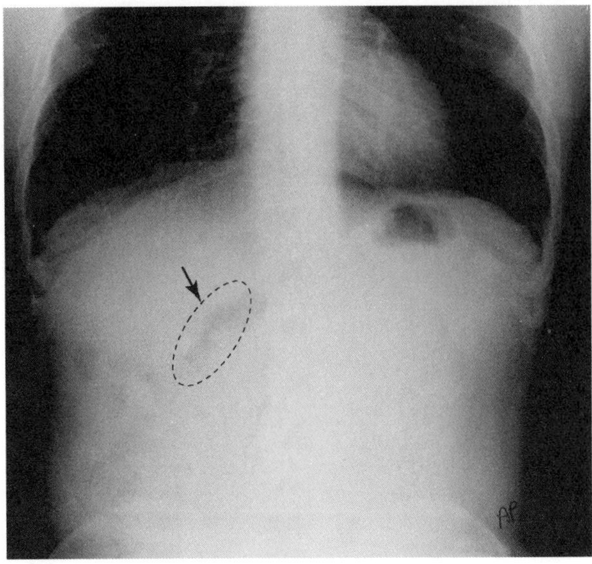

B

Figure 5-199B • Image Courtesy of the University of Utah School of Medicine, Salt Lake City, Utah.

A. Free intraperitoneal air below the diaphragm would be evident on an upright film. In patients who are unable to be upright, a left lateral decubitus can be obtained, where free air will be seen overlying the liver. This patient does not have any free air on this film.

B, D. The bowel gas patterns are normal on this film.

E. Approximately 80% of all renal stones are visible on abdominal plain films, but they are not seen here.

200. **B. Elective cholecystectomy is the treatment of choice, as there may be an increased incidence of gallbladder carcinoma in patients with a porcelain gallbladder.**

A. A PTC would be used to evaluate or drain the biliary tree, but it is not indicated here.

C. An ERCP would be used to evaluate the biliary and pancreatic ductal systems, but it is not indicated here.

D. Although cholecystectomy is strongly recommended, it can be done as an elective procedure as there is no indication for emergency surgery.

E. Observation is not recommended due to the risk of gallbladder cancer.

Index

Index note: Page numbers with an f indicate figures; those with a t indicate tables on designated page; page references in bold indicate discussion of the subject in the Answers and Explanations sections